Textbook of
Forensic Medicine, Medical Jurisprudence and Toxicology
Including Forensic Psychiatry

Textbook of
Forensic Medicine, Medical Jurisprudence and Toxicology
Including Forensic Psychiatry

GK Sharma MBBS, MD

Former
Director-Professor and Head
Department of Forensic Medicine and Toxicology and
Director
Lady Hardinge Medical College and Associated Hospitals
New Delhi

Additional Director General of Health Services
Ministry of Health and Family Welfare

Dean, Faculty of Medical Sciences, University of Delhi

Member, Ethics Committee, Medical Council of India

Member, Delhi Medical Council

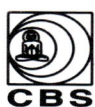

CBS

CBS Publishers & Distributors Pvt Ltd

New Delhi • Bengaluru • Chennai • Kochi • Kolkata • Mumbai
Hyderabad • Jharkhand • Nagpur • Patna • Pune • Uttarakhand

Textbok of
Forensic Medicine, Medical Jurisprudence and Toxicology
Including Forensic Psychiatry

ISBN: 978-93-86478-33-7

Copyright © Author and Publisher

First Edition: 2017

Published by Satish Kumar Jain and Produced by Varun Jain for

CBS Publishers & Distributors Pvt Ltd
4819/XI Prahlad Street, 24 Ansari Road, Daryaganj, New Delhi 110 002, India.
Ph: 23289259, 23266861, 23266867   Fax: 011-23243014   Website: www.cbspd.com
e-mail: delhi@cbspd.com; cbspubs@airtelmail.in.

Corporate Office: 204 FIE, Industrial Area, Patparganj, Delhi 110 092
Ph: 4934 4934   Fax: 4934 4935   e-mail: publishing@cbspd.com; publicity@cbspd.com

Branches

- **Bengaluru:** Seema House 2975, 17th Cross, K.R. Road,
  Banasankari 2nd Stage, Bengaluru 560 070, Karnataka
  Ph: +91-80-26771678/79   Fax: +91-80-26771680   e-mail: bangalore@cbspd.com
- **Chennai:** 7, Subbaraya Street, Shenoy Nagar, Chennai 600 030, Tamil Nadu
  Ph: +91-44-26680620, 26681266   Fax: +91-44-42032115   e-mail: chennai@cbspd.com
- **Kochi:** Ashana House, No. 39/1904, AM Thomas Road, Valanjambalam,
  Ernakulam 682 016, Kochi, Kerala
  Ph: +91-484-4059061-65   Fax: +91-484-4059065   e-mail: kochi@cbspd.com
- **Kolkata:** 6/B, Ground Floor, Rameswar Shaw Road, Kolkata-700 014, West Bengal
  Ph: +91-33-22891126, 22891127, 22891128   e-mail: kolkata@cbspd.com
- **Mumbai:** 83-C, Dr E Moses Road, Worli, Mumbai-400018, Maharashtra
  Ph: +91-22-24902340/41   Fax: +91-22-24902342   e-mail: mumbai@cbspd.com

Representatives

- **Hyderabad** 0-9885175004   • **Jharkhand** 0-9811541605   • **Nagpur** 0-9021734563
- **Patna** 0-9334159340   • **Pune** 0-9623451994   • **Uttarakhand** 0-9716462459

Printed at: Shree Maitrey Printech Pvt. Ltd., Noida, UP, India

Contributors

Dr Mukta Rani MD
Professor, Department of Forensic Medicine
Lady Hardinge Medical College and Associated Hospitals
New Delhi
(Infanticide, Sexual Offences)

Dr Arvind Kumar MD
Associate Professor, Department of Forensic Medicine
Lady Hardinge Medical College and Associated Hospitals New
Delhi
(Forensic Toxicology)

Dr SK Naik MD
Professor, Department of Forensic Medicine
Lady Hardinge Medical College and Associated Hospitals New
Delhi
(History of Forensic Medicine)

Dr Sukhdeep Singh MD
Associate Professor, Department of Forensic Medicine
Lady Hardinge Medical College and Associated Hospitals New
Delhi
(Medical Jurisprudence)

Foreword

I t is indeed a great pleasure and honour to write a Foreword for the book *Textbook of Forensic Medicine, Medical Jurisprudence and Toxicology including Forensic Psychiatry*, written by my senior colleague Prof Dr GK Sharma, who has more than four decades of rich experience in the field of forensic medicine.

The book has been written in a lucid style, is up-to-date, and covers almost every topic in forensic medicine and toxicology. I hope that it will be immensely useful for both the undergraduate and postgraduate medical students.

I wish Prof GK Sharma all the success in his endeavour.

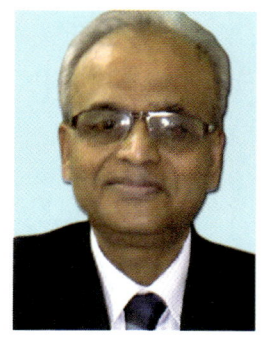

Dr Atul Murari
Director-Professor
Department of Forensic Medicine
and
Former Director
Lady Hardinge Medical College
New Delhi 110 001.

Foreword

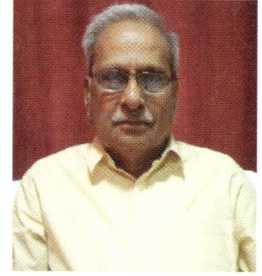

This book from my long-time friend and colleague Dr GK Sharma comes as no surprise for I have always known him to be academically inclined and respected professionally, by all his peers. He has had a wide practical and teaching experience and his participation in conferences and seminars has been appreciated and well received.

The book by him covers the undergraduate syllabus on the subject as prescribed by the Medical Council of India and followed in institutes beyond purview of the Medical Council. His clarity on the principles of the subject translates into simple and easy material for the undergraduate. I have no doubt that this book will be popular with the students and teachers alike for being technically correct, covering all the required areas with appropriate explanations and yet being crisp.

I congratulate Dr GK Sharma on this endeavour and hope the book becomes available to the undergraduate students all over the country.

Dr BP Dubey
Former Dean and Professor and Head
Department of Forensic Medicine,
Gandhi Medical College, Bhopal

Preface

It is an endeavor to provide a textbook on forensic medicine in a simplified and student friendly manner so that undergraduate medical students are able to understand the subject both for clinical and examination purposes. Postgraduate students may also refer this book as a basic guide to buildup proper understanding of the subject.

The book covers the prescribed undergraduate MCI curriculum and the format helps the students to remember and reproduce the subject during examinations. There are various upshots of this subject, especially in osteology, dentistry, crime scene visit, forensic pathology, firearm investigations and transport accident investigations, to name a few. Even though these topics have been discussed in the book but for postgraduate students, references from other books may be required to advance their knowledge.

Concerned portions of the Indian law has been incorporated in various chapters to make them more relevant in their application in providing evidence in the courts. Advance scientific techniques and histopathology may help the practitioners of forensic medicine to interpret changes seen during crime investigations.

At the end of the book Multiple Choice Questions are given for revision of the topics as well as for postgraduate entrance examinations.

I am indebted to Dr KS Rai, Professor of Forensic Medicine, Govt Medical College, Patiala, for initiating me in this subject; Dr Bishnu Kumar, Professor of Forensic Medicine, and Dr BN Reddy, Associate Professor, Maulana Azad Medical College, New Delhi, for making me understand the intricacies of practical aspects of forensic medicine, and all my friends and colleagues for helping me in compiling this textbook.

I am thankful to CBS Publishers & Distributors. I would like to put on record the sincere efforts of Mr YN Arjuna and his team, comprising Mrs Ritu Chawla, Mr Sanjay Chauhan (Sanju), Mr Parmod Kumar and Mr Mukund Kumar, for bringing out the book in the present form.

I welcome comments, suggestions and corrections from the readers.

GK Sharma

Contents

SECTION 2 MEDICAL JURISPRUDENCE

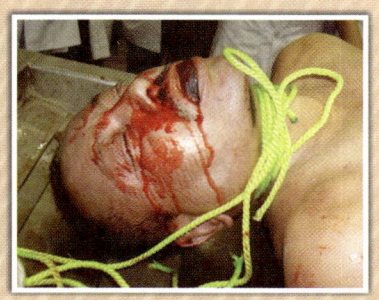

Section 1

Forensic Medicine

1 | Introduction

Medicine and Law has been related to each other from ancient times. Forensic medicine acts as a bridge between medicine and law. Medicolegal relationship has three aspects:

1. Forensic medicine
2. Medical jurisprudence
3. Toxicology

Even though forensic medicine and medical jurisprudence are not synonymous but sometimes they are used to denote this medicolegal relationship.

Forensic medicine (forensic = court of law)
It deals with application of medical knowledge for the better administration of the Justice. In short it is the medical aspects of law. It is also known as legal medicine. Therefore, it deals with examination of injured or dead person, observe various findings, interpretation of those findings and finally giving evidence in the court of law.

Medical jurisprudence (juris = law, prudence = knowledge): It deals with legal aspects of the practice of medicine, like responsibilities of a *medical professional,* medical negligence, ethics, duties, etiquette and law governing medical practice, etc.

Medical toxicology: Toxicology deals with source, properties, action, diagnosis, management and medicolegal aspects of various poisonous substances.

HISTORY OF LEGAL MEDICINE

History of legal-medicine can be divided in to four periods.

Ancient Period

During the ancient period there was no separate entity of forensic medicine. The primitive people united medicine with law through superstition, religion and magic. The priest used to function as jurist and medical man. Diseases during this period were attributed to supernatural powers or magic, hence the treatment consisted of prayers to appease the supernatural powers and used religious rites, talismans, amulets, etc. to counter evil magic. Medical knowledge as per mythology confined to gods and the priests were the intermediary between god and the masses.

According to Indian mythology lord *Brahma* (The creator of earth as per hindu mythology) was first to make compilation of the Ayurveda into eight parts. *Ashwani kumars (sons of sun god)* imparted this science to lord *Indra*. Medicine and surgery were gifts from the god *Indra* to sages *Bharadwaja*, the patron saint of medicine, and *Dhanvantari*, the patron saint of surgery.

Early Period

Hammurabi, the king of babylon dated about 2200 BC enacted the oldest known law code on the practice of medicine. Medical malpractice was discussed in detail along with the punishments which included cutting of hands to monetary compensation.

Manu Smriti by sage *Manu* scripted around the same period was the first to provide laws related to medical practice, criminal acts like sexual offences, adultery, seduction and persons who were not permitted to give evidence in the courts.

Atreya samhita is one of the oldest medical books in the world. Sage *Atreya* headed the medical school in taxila. His treatise on medicine is contained in 46,500 verses. This was considered to be the origin of Medical ethics in India. The treatise, *Susruta Samhita*, on surgery, indicates that he was probably the first surgeon to perform a rhinoplasty and ear lobe reconstruction. Both sages *Atreya* and *Susruta* practiced around 600 BC.

Hippocrates around 400 BC made major contributions towards medial ethics. Modified hippocratic oath is still being taken by the medical graduate before they practice medicine.

In 44 BC Julius Caesar was assassinated by his close trusty Brutus. On his body, autopsy was conducted by physician *Antistius*, to find out which of the twenty-three wounds was fatal.

Intermediate Period or Medieval Period

The *Justinian* code, which made its appearance in rome between 529 and 564 AD, a number of provisions were made to treat medicolegal cases. Within its provisions it was clearly indicated that physicians are not ordinary witnesses but having special position of expert witnesses to act as impartial arbitrator.

There was also the recognition of medico-legal problems in the Far East. In China, in approximately 1236 AD, a volume entitled the *Hsi Yuan Lu* (*Washing Away of Wrongs*) was compiled that outlined procedures to be followed in investigating suspicious deaths. The book urged the medical examiner to make a thorough and systematic examination of every corpse, however unpleasant its condition. Chapters were devoted to wounds caused by blows from fists or from kicking and to deaths caused by strangulation or drowning. It also discussed procedure for distinguishing between the bodies of drowned persons and those thrown into the water after death, and for distinctions between antemortem and postmortem burns.

During 12th to 16th century, Italy and France made good progress in the field of Legal-medicine. Surgeons were required to compile reports on the basis of external examination of the body for presence of any injuries. However, no detailed autopsies were done. Detailed medicolegal autopsy was conducted by *Bartoloneo DE Varignana* in Bologna (Italy) in 1302 AD. However, the right to conduct autopsy was given to the faculty of montpellier by the pope in 1374.

In 1507 the George Prince Bishop of Bamberg in Germany, a systematized code of penal law was drawn which required presence of physicians in all cases of violent deaths. The *Costitutio Criminalis Carolona* was instituted in 1532. As penalties were made proportion to the injuries or its effects, the evidence of a physician to evaluate them was of great importance.

Progressive Period

Meanwhile, in Italy, a physician named *Fortunato Fedele* in 1602, published a fairly comprehensive volume on forensic medicine entitled, *De Relationes Medicorum*. Another Italian, Paola Zacchia, a papal physician, published the huge *Questions Medicina Legales*, which quickly overshadowed Fedele's work. Zacchia's book discussed in detail questions of age, legitimacy, pregnancy, death during delivery, resemblance of children to their parents, dementia, poisoning, impotence, feigned diseases, miracles, rape, mutilation, and the matters concerning public health. The work has deficiencies that can easily be explained by the era in which it was written; for instance, the knowledge of anatomy and physiology was sketchy and erroneous. The book also contains sections on the different methods of torture then in existence, and it has a section that deals with miracles. Despite these shortcomings, it was a worthwhile and influential volume. *Valantini* published *Corpus Juris Medico-legale* in 1722 which challenged the work of zacchis.

Legal medicine was not treated as being just a theoretical pursuit; it was eventually brought into the courtroom. For example, in 1667 *Schwammerdamm,* in Germany, claimed that the lungs of a newborn baby would float in water if the baby had actually breathed, that is, if it was not stillborn and had lived and subsequently died, either by natural causes or by homicide. In 1681, the German physician *Schreger* used this test forensically, and secured the acquittal of a girl who had been accused of murdering her illegitimate child.

MP Orfila professor of Chemistry and legal-medicine at Paris published his work in 1815 and was considered as the founder of modern toxicology.

The first book on legal medicine written in english was authored by *Samuel Farr* in 1788 and was entitled *Elements of Medical Jurisprudence*. Number of books were published but prominent amongst them was "Principle and practice of medical jurisprudence" by *Alfred Swaine Taylor*, which is still a standard book on the specialty.

Advent of modern medical science happened with the British coming to India. In 1824 a Native medical institute was established in Kolkata. Which was converted into medical college in 1835. This was followed by opening of medical colleges in Madras (Chennai) and Bombay (Mumbai). By the year 1857 there were 27 Medical colleges in India. Majority of medical colleges in independent India came in the private sector. As per medical council of India, in September 2016 there were 426 medical colleges in India.

In 1916 Indian medical Degree act was promulgated to regulate and recognize medical degrees and to penalize fake medical degrees/certificates. In 1933 Indian medical council act was passed to maintain uniformity in medical education which was modified and replaced by MCI act of 1956.

Indian courts are following criminal procedure code (CrPC), 1973; Indian penal code (IPC), 1860 and Indian evidence act (IEA), 1872 to conduct and try various offences.

2   Legal Procedures

Legal procedures which are followed in India are based on the constitution of India and various codes or acts enforced for the same. However, this chapter primarily deals with the procedures followed in cases of sudden, unnatural or suspicious deaths.

INQUEST

An inquest is a legal enquiry or investigation to find out cause and manner of death in sudden or suspicious death. There are different types of inquests held all over the world:

1. Police inquest
2. Magistrate's inquest
3. Coroner's inquest
4. Medical examiners system
5. Procurator fiscal system

Police Inquest: (174 Cr PC)

All over India police officer incharge of a police station or designated police officer conducts the inquest. On receipt of information of unnatural or accidental death, he informs the area magistrate and proceeds to the site. In presence of two witnesses (panchas) he prepares a report of the apparent cause of death. This inquest report (panchnama) is signed by the witnesses and the police officer. If no foul play is suspected the dead body is ordered for disposal. In case, there is any doubt of foul play, the body is sent for postmortem examination. In order to complete investigations police officer can summon a witness under section 175 Cr PC.

Magistrate's Inquest: (176 Cr PC)

This type of inquest or investigation is conducted by the district, subdivisional or first class magistrate (or a magistrate empowered by the State Govt.) in following cases:

a. Death in prison
b. Death in police custody
c. Death in police firing.
d. Dowry deaths.
e. Exhumation
f. In addition to police inquest in certain cases.

The magistrate shall inform the relatives, wherever practicable, record the evidence and order postmortem examination of the dead body. Differences between police and magistrate's inquest are mentioned in Table 2.1.

Coroner's Inquest

Coroner's system prevails in England, wales and some states of USA. Coroner used to be a representative of the crown but gradually all other powers were taken away and only investigation into sudden and suspicious deaths remained with him. There are approximately one hundred and fifty coroners in England and wales. Most of the coroner's are solicitors by profession and hold the post of coroner as a part-time office. Each coroner

Table 2.1: Differences between Police and magistrate's inquest		
Feature	*Police inquest*	*Magistrate's inquest*
Conducting officer	Police officer	District Magistrate/SDM, assisted by police
Under section	174 CrPC	176 CrPC
Informing when visiting scene of crime	Must inform area magistrate	Need not inform
Types of cases	All cases of unnatural and suspected deaths except deaths in custody, jail, police firing and dowry deaths.	As specified under 176 CrPC
Warrant or arrest	Cannot issue but can arrest in cognizable offences	Can issue
Impose fine	Cannot impose fine	Can impose fine
Exhumation	Cannot order	Can order
Importance of inquest	Less important	More important

presides over a certain geographical area. In large cities the coroners are generally appointed on a full-time basis and many have both legal and medical qualifications. The office of coroner is an independent one and only the high court can issue instructions to coroners.

Any sudden, unexpected, unattended death; death due to vehicular accident; death from injuries; overdose of drugs or homicidal deaths when reported to the coroner's office through police, medical practioners or general public. Coroner's office investigates circumstances of death with the help of the police. If required, a postmortem is conducted to find out the medical cause of death. In case of natural death, a certificate to that effect is issued for disposal of the dead. Otherwise, in cases of unnatural or deaths in custody hearing is held in open court with or without injury. If any person is named for the crime, he issues a warrant for the arrest of the accused and commits him to stand trial in the court. When accused is not traceable, coroner returns an *"open verdict"*. Such a case is kept in abeyance and the matter can be reopened when further information is available regarding cause and manner of death.

In India under coroner's act (1871) a coroner used to conduct inquest in all cases of sudden, un-natural and suspected deaths in the cities of Mumbai and Kolkata. Initially it was abolished from Mumbai and then finally from 1999 onwards it was discontinued from Kolkata also. Differences between coroner's inquest and magistrate's inquest are mentioned in Table 2.2.

Table 2.2: Differentiation between coroner's inquest and magistrate's inquest		
Feature	*Coroner's inquest/court*	*Magistrate's inquest/court*
Status in India	Not prevalent in India	Conducted all over India
Type of court	Only court of enquiry	Court of trial
Presence of accused	Not required	Required during trial
Punishment	Cannot award any punishment	Can impose punishment
Contempt of court	Punish if committed within precinct of his court	Can punish whether committed within or without the precinct of his court

Medical Examiner's System

Medical examiner's system is prevalent in most of the states in USA. A medical practitioner is appointed to conduct inquest in sudden and unexpected deaths. On being informed about any such death he visits the site and if required, conducts postmortem examination to find out the cause and manner of death.

Procurator Fiscal System

Criminal law in Scotland is administered by a public procurator. The procurator fiscal is appointed by the lord advocate and is always a lawyer. One procurator fiscal is appointed for each sheriff court district. The procurator fiscal has wide powers in the investigation of criminal matters. Amongst his roles is the investigation of sudden, unexplained or suspicious deaths. His main interest is in excluding criminality. He requests either an external examination or autopsy to be performed by a forensic pathologist.

COURTS OF LAW

There are two types of courts:
1. Civil courts: They try only civil cases.
2. Criminal courts: They try criminal cases along with civil cases.
   a. Supreme court
   b. High courts
   c. Session Courts
   d. Magistrate's courts

Supreme Court

It is the highest court in India. The law passed by it is binding on all lower courts. It is located in New Delhi and can pass any sentence under Indian law. Normally it considers appeals from lower courts.

High Courts

They are the highest court of a state and are located mostly in the state capital. They can also award any punishment under Indian laws. There are 24 high courts at the state and union territory levels in India.

Session courts

This is highest court in a district of a state. A Session judge or Addl. Session judge can award any punishment prescribed by the Indian law. However the death sentence has to be confirmed by the high court. Assistant Session judge can pass any penalty authorized by law except death sentence and imprisonment for more than 10 years.

Magistrate's Courts

a. *Chief judicial magistrate:* The court of chief judicial magistrate can award imprisonment up to 7 years and any amount of fine.
b. *First class magistrate:* They can award Imprisonment up to 3 years and fine up to ₹ 5000.
c. *Second class magistrate:* Imprisonment up to 1 year and fine up to ₹ 1000 can be awarded by these courts.

SUMMONS/SUBPOENA: (Sub = under, Poena = penalty)

It is a document compelling the attendance of a witness in a court of law under penalty on a particular day and time for giving evidence.
a. Subpoena duces tacum: For giving documentary evidence.
b. Subpoena ad testificandum: For giving oral evidence.

Summon is issued in duplicate to a witness. When summon is served to a witness, he should return one copy after signing it and should retain other copy. The attendance can be excused only on urgent and valid reasons. Failure to attend the court can lead to fine or damages in civil court and fine or imprisonment in a criminal court.

When a witness is summoned by two courts on the same day, higher court has priority over lower court and criminal courts have priority over civil courts. In case the summons are from two similar courts then the witness should attend the court from which summon was received first and the other court must be informed about the reason for non-attendance.

CONDUCT MONEY

It is the fee offered to a witness in civil cases at the time of serving summons. In civil cases the witness can ignore summons when no conduct money is offered or bring it to the notice of the presiding officer of the court. In case he feels that offered conduct money is less, he can also bring it to the notice of the judge before giving evidence. Judge will decide the amount to be paid to the witness.

In criminal cases no fee is paid. However, conveyance and daily allowance is paid as per court rules or a certificate is issued to a witness in government service, so that he can claim the same from his office.

RECORDING OF EVIDENCE

a. *Oath:* Before deposition a witness is required to take oath in the name of the god by placing his hand on the religious book e.g. Geeta, Quran or Bible, etc. that he shall tell the truth, whole truth and nothing but the truth or can solemnly affirm in case the witness is atheist.

b. *Examination in chief:* This is conducted by the party who has called that witness. In this examination *leading questions* (questions which suggest their answers) are not allowed.

c. *Cross examination:* Conducted by the opposite party. During this examination leading questions are allowed. There is no time limit for this; however the presiding officer of the court may not permit irrelevant questions.

d. *Re-examination and re-cross examination:* In case some fresh leads are brought forward in cross examination.

e. *Questions by the judge:* Under section 311 CrPC the presiding judge can ask certain questions to clarify doubts at any stage of Trial.

PERJURY

Telling a lie under oath is perjury and is punishable under section 193 IPC.

MEDICAL EVIDENCE

Medical evidences which are produced before the courts are of two types:
a. Documentary
b. Oral

A. Documentary Evidences

1. Medical certificates
2. Medicolegal reports
3. Dying declaration

Medical Certificates

They generally refer to ill health, unsoundness of mind or death, etc. These certificates are only accepted in the court if issued by a registered medical practitioner (RMP).

Certificate of ill health must be issued after properly examining the person and his signature or thumb impression taken at the bottom of the certificate.

Death certificate must mention proper cause of death as per ICD-10 requirements. Brodrick's committee recommended that a doctor should not issue a death certificate unless he has attended the deceased at least once during the seven days preceding the death. No fee can be collected for issuing a death certificate. If a doctor is not sure about the cause of death, in such a case he must decline to issue the death certificate. Death certificate is of great importance in organ transplantation; hence the certificate in such cases should be issued as per the organ transplantation Act.

Medicolegal Reports

A doctor is required to make various types of reports, e.g. injury report or age report. This report basically consists of three parts:
a. *Preliminary information:* In which personal data of that individual is collected, along with his consent.
b. *Observations:* All the findings are recorded in a systematic manner
c. *Inference* or *opinion:* Based on the findings or observations opinion is expressed at the end under signatures of the doctor.

Dying Declaration

A statement made oral or written by a person since deceased, relating to the cause of his/her death or any circumstances of the transaction resulting in death.

In case time permits, a doctor must call the area magistrate to record the dying declaration otherwise he should record himself in presence of independent witnesses. A doctor must record the answers given by the person in the same words without inferring the meaning of those words.

Under Indian Evidence Act this is admissible in courts, whether the person who made it was or was not under expectation of death, but must be of sound mind. A mute person can also make a dying declaration.

Dying deposition: This is evidence taken by Magistrate on oath in presence of accused or his lawyer who can cross examine. Presence of a doctor is required to certify the mental condition of the patient (*compos mentis*) and may also act as a witness. Differences between dying declaration and dying deposition are mentioned in Table 2.3.

B. Oral Evidence

Under section 60 IEA direct oral evidence is required. This is considered more important than documentary evidence because it is recorded under oath and cross examination is permitted.

Exceptions are as follows:

a. Dying declaration (section 32 IEA)
b. Expert opinion expressed in treatise (section 60 IEA)
c. Evidence in lower court (section 291 Cr PC)
d. Report of certain Govt. scientific experts (section 293 Cr PC)
e. Hospital and police records
f. Evidence in previous judicial proceedings.

Witnesses

Witnesses appearing in the court are of following types:

1. *Common witness:* Any person who has actually seen or observed any fact and inform the same to the court (first-hand knowledge).
2. *Expert witness:* They help the court by inferring any observation by their expert knowledge in their field of expertise. All doctors are considered by law as expert witnesses. They act both as common witness (when they inform their observations in a case) and expert witness (when they express their opinion on observed facts).
3. *Hostile witness:* It is an individual who has some interest in concealing the truth. In case a witness is declared hostile the party who has called him can ask leading questions in examination in chief.

Table 2.3: Differences between dying declaration and dying deposition		
Feature	*Dying declaration*	*Dying deposition*
Person recording	Any person	Magistrate only
Procedure	It is recording of a statement	It is recorded as if in a court
Presence of lawyer or accused	Not required	Accused or lawyer representing accused must be present
Administration of oath	Not required	Oath is administered
Cross examination	Not required	Allowed by accused or his lawyer
Witnesses	required	Not required to verify statement
Leading questions	Recorded as verbatim	Allowed in cross examination
Value	Less	More
If person survives	Loses its importance	Retains its value
Presence of doctor	Can record statement when magistrate is not available	Certify mental status and act as a witness

3 | Identification

Identity or identification means establishment of individuality of a person. In medicolegal practice identification is of great importance both in living as well as in dead.

In living person identification is required of a person accused of any crime such as murder, rape or assault and also in cases of inheritance or absconding soldiers, etc. Whereas identification is of importance and should be undertaken with extreme care in a dead person where there is decomposition, mutilated or fragmentary remains are recovered, air crash, fire or railway accidents. When the identity of a person is fully established it is known as **complete identification**, however where some features of identity are known but the identity is not fully established, it is called **partial identity** or **incomplete identity**.

Corpus delicti (body of offence): The corpus delicti refers to the body of a victim and other facts which prove death from foul play. The main features of the corpus delicti are establishment of the identification of the dead body recovered and commission of crime resulting in the death of that individual.

Identification of a person could be established by other individual like a friend or a relative and is known as *third party identification*. When identification is done by noting certain physical characteristics like colour of the hair, height, weight, shape of the nose or colour of the iris this is *subjective identification*. Circumstances of death may also assist in identification of a person like location of the body, presence of certain documents or objects on the body, even presence of clothing with laundry marks are known as *circumstantial identity*.

However in forensic practice reliable identification is done by noting morphological features which can be analyzed and documented, known as *objective identification*. Following features are useful in identification of an individual:

1. Race and religion
2. Sex
3. Age
4. Complexion and features
5. Hair
6. Anthropometry (Bertillon's system)
7. Dactylography (Galton's system) including Poroscopy (Locard's system)
8. Footprints
9. Teeth
10. Scars
11. Deformities
12. Birth marks
13. Tattoo marks
14. Occupational marks
15. Handwriting
16. Gait
17. Manner and habits

18. Mental power and memory
19. Height and weight
20. Clothes and personal effects
21. Superimposition technique
22. DNA fingerprinting
23. Miscellaneous methods like facial reconstruction, lip prints, palato prints, etc.

RACE AND RELIGION

Race

The race depends upon geographical location and climatic conditions. It is of importance when individuals of various races are involved in a mass disaster like plane crash or railway accident.

Primarily there are three races:
a. Caucasians
b. Negroid
c. Mongoloid.

Indians are a mixture of caucasian and negroid characteristics.

Race can be differentiated by following means:

1. *Complexion:* Skin colour is fair in europeans, black in negroes and brown in Indians. however it may be of limited use as after decomposition or burning the skin colour may change.
2. *Eyes:* Europeans have blue or grey eyes whereas other races have dark brown iris.
3. *Hair:* Negroes have wooly and curly hair with bean shaped cross-section. Medulla is also not fragmented. Mongols have coarse and dark hair with round cross-section. Caucasians have light brown or reddish hair and oval cross-section. People in the Indian subcontinent have long, black and straight hair.
4. *Skull:* Skull gives reliable information about the race.
   i. Race can be determined by cephalic index.
      "**Cephalic index** = maximum transverse breadth/maximum anteroposterior length × 100"
      Based on the cephalic index the skulls can be classified into following types:

a. *Dolichocephalic:* They are also called long headed with the cephalic index from 70 to 74.9 and mostly seen in Negroid or Aryan race.
b. *Mesaticephalic:* They are medium headed with cephalic index between 75 and 79.9 and are present in europeans.
c. *Brachycephalic:* They are short headed with cephalic index varying from 80 to 84.9. Indians are mostly covered under this category.
   ii. Zygomatic arch which determines the width of the face is more prominent and may exceed head width in mongoloid race.
   iii. Nasal opening width is more in negroid in comparison with caucasian race.
5. *Long bones:* Femur is slightly straighter in Negroid race. Some indices of long bones like *brachial index* (length of radius/length of humerus × 100) or *crural index* (length of tibia/length of femur × 100) may be of some help but are not reliable.
6. *Teeth:* Shovel shaped upper medial incisors are seen in mongoloid race. Negroid race have bigger teeth with thicker enamel in comparison with caucasoid race; however, largest teeth are seen in Australians.

Religion

Two main religions in the Indian subcontinent, i.e. Hindus and Muslims can be differentiated in the following manner:

Hindu males: They are not circumcised, wear sacred thread, may have cast mark on the forehead, tuft of hair on the back of head and piercing of ear lobes are present in few cases.

Muslim males: They are circumcised, have religious marks or corns on the forehead and lateral aspects of knees due to posture adopted during prayers.

Hindu females: They may have vermilion on the head, nose ring aperture on the left nostril and tattoo marks.

Muslim females: Nose ring aperture in the septum, several ear rings apertures along the helix and no tattoo marks may be observed.

SEX

Sex determination is of importance in medico-legal cases like for identification of living or dead, for purposes of marriage, divorce, impotency, legitimacy, paternity, rape, eligibility for army service or for participation in competitive sports.

Presumptive evidence of sex: This is primarily based on the physical appearance of an individual like features, distribution of hair over the face and body, voice, clothes, habits and manners.

Highly probable signs: This is based on external sexual structures like in females' presence of developed breasts, distribution of subcutaneous fat and presence of female external genitalia, whereas in males it is the muscularity and male external genitalia.

Confirmatory evidence of sex: In males the presence of testis with emission of semen and in females presence of ovaries, uterus and periodic menstrual discharge.

Sex of a person is determined on medical examination by:

1. *Secondary sex characters:* These characters develop after a person has attained puberty and include built of a person, development of breasts, voice changes, beard, pubic hair distribution and fat distribution over the body.

2. *External genitalia:* Presence of penis and scrotum in males and vagina in females.

3. *Internal sex organs:* Presence of functioning testes in males and ovaries and uterus in females.

4. *Hormonal sex determination:* Presence of male hormones like androgen in males and estrogen and progesterone in females.

5. *Nuclear sex:*
   a. *Barr bodies:* Presence of barr bodies, representing inactive X-chromosome, condensed on the nuclear membrane of the cell (Fig. 3.1) and is detected in more than 20% of cells indicating female sex (chromatin positive), whereas in males

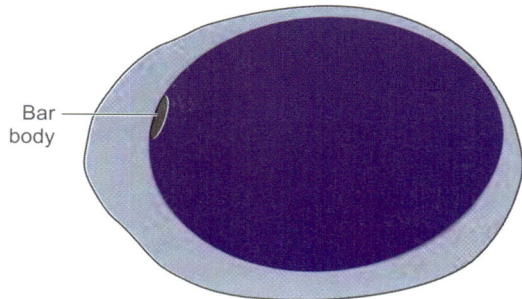

Fig. 3.1: Sex chromatin in cells

these may be detected but not in more than 4–5% cells. Buccal smears are commonly used to look for barr bodies. However, in a putrefied dead body scalp hair roots sections are used.

   b. *Davidson's body:* Neutrophils in females have a drum stick like attachment to the nucleus known as davidson's body which is helpful in sex determination (Fig. 3.2).

   c. Staining of Y-chromosome: Y-chromosome in male cells can be stained by quinacrine dihydrochloride and is seen as a fluorescent body in the nucleus of the cell.

   d. Staining of X-chromosome: X-chromosomes can also be stained with fluorescent Feulgen method which stains the X-chromosome as bright yellow spot. This is seen in much abundance in females.

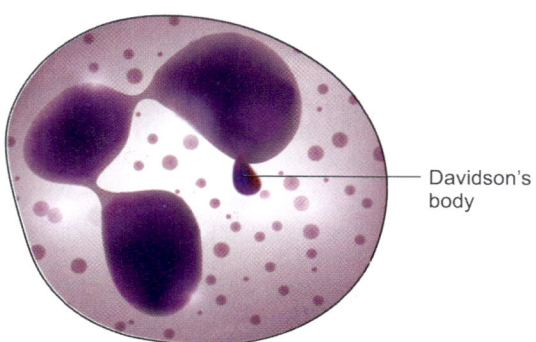

Fig. 3.2: Sex chromatin in polymorphs

6. *Gonadal biopsy:* This can be done to know the functioning status of the gonads in a person and to determine the sex of that individual.

7. *Psychological sex:* It is the mental makeup and behaviour of a person regarding his assigned sex. In rare cases, a person behaves opposite to the actual sex, and may wear the clothing of the opposite sex. Such transsexual person experience a gender identity inconsistent or not culturally associated with their assigned sex, i.e. in which a person's assigned sex at birth conflicts with their psychological gender.

Intersex

This is a general term used for a variety of conditions in which a person is born with a reproductive or sexual anatomy that does not seem to fit the typical definitions of female or male. This can be divided into four groups:

1. *Gonadal agenesis:* In such a condition sexual organs like testis or ovaries have not developed. Nuclear sexing is negative.

2. *Gonadal dysgenesis:* The external genitalia are present but at puberty the testes or ovaries fail to develop and function. There are two syndromes bases on the nonfunctioning testes or ovaries:

   a. *Klinefelter's syndrome:* In external appearance they are males but testes fail to develop, however they are chromatin positive. Testes are small, firm to feel, aspermic and hyalinised, mostly associated with gynecomastia, signs of eunuchoidism like tall stature but proportionately having long extremities, mental deficiency, scanty pubic hair and no beard. Their chromatin pattern is XXY. Serum testosterone is usually low. This condition can be diagnosed during pregnancy by karyotyping of aminocytes or chorionic villi.

   b. *Turner's syndrome:* They look like females, but have non-developed ovaries. They are chromatin negative with chromatin pattern of XO is diagnostic. They are of short stature, webbed neck, with congenital abnormalities like coarctation of aorta, bicuspid aortic valve, aortic stenosis or hydronephrosis, amenorrhea hence sterile, lack of breast tissues and scanty pubic hair.

3. *True-hermaphroditism:* In such cases both testes and ovaries are present, and such persons are chromatin positive.

4. *Pseudohermaphroditism:* They are classified as males or females depending on the presence of ovaries or testes independent of external genitalia, which may be of the opposite sex. Sex in such cases is determined by nuclear sexing. Hence in male pseudohermaphroditism the nuclear sex is of male and the anatomical sex is of female (testicular feminization), and in female pseudohermaphroditism the nuclear sex is of female and the anatomical sex is of male (adrenal hyperplasia).

AGE

Along with identification of a person, age determination is of vital importance in following conditions:

1. *Identification:* Age is one of the criteria used for identification of an individual.

2. *Criminal responsibility:* According to section 82 IPC a child under 7 years of age is not capable of committing an offence. When proved by the defence, that the child is above 7 years but below 12 years has not attained sufficient maturity of understanding, to judge the nature and consequences of his act, is not held responsible for the crime (section 83 IPC).

3. *Marriage:* Age for marriage in India is 18 years for girls and 21 years for boys. However for a person under legal guardianship under direction of a court, the marriage age is 21 years.

4. *Consent:* A person below 12 years of age cannot give legally valid consent for any procedure. In such cases consent has to be obtained from the legal guardian. A person

above 18 years of age can give consent to suffer any harm for an act not intended and not known to cause death or grievous hurt (section 87 IPC).

5. *Kidnapping or abduction:* Whoever takes or entices any minor, less than 16 years of age if a male or 18 years if a female from the legal guardianship commits the offence of kidnapping (section 361 IPC). However kidnapping or abducting a child with intention to steal from his person the age of such a child should be under 10 years. If a female is abducted with intention of marrying against her will or forced to illicit sexual intercourse the age of the female being 18 years the person abducting such female is punished under section 366 of IPC. To import a girl for prostitution is punishable under section 366B IPC provided the age of the girl is below 21 years.

6. *Sexual offences:* Sexual act with or without consent with a girl who is under 18 years of age is rape. Sexual act with a wife provided she is below 15 years of age is also rape.

7. *Attainment of majority:* A person attains majority at the age of 18 years except when such an individual is under the legal guardianship, under direction of a court; in such a case the age of majority is 21 years.

8. *Employment:* Age limit for government service is 25 years. A person above 14 years but below 15 years can work on non-hazardous jobs in a factory with conditions that he will not work for more than 8 hours and will not be posted on night shift. A person below 17 years cannot work in an underground coal mine.

9. *Judicial punishment (juvenile justice act):* According to Juvenile act any person below 18 years is tried in a juvenile court. No capital punishment or imprisonment can be awarded to a juvenile. They are kept in Juvenile homes. Bill was passed by the upper house of parliament in december, 2015 to replace the juvenile justice (care and protection of children) act, 2000. It addresses children in conflict with law and children in need of care and protection. The Bill shall permit juveniles between the ages of 16–18 years to be tried as adults for heinous offences on the recommendations of juvenile justice board. Current age of criminal responsibility in England and Wales is 10 years, in france it is 13 years, Italy it is 14 years, and 16 years in Spain to understand what they are doing and that it is wrong.

10. *Infanticide:* Infanticide is unlawful destruction of a newly born viable infant up to the age of one year and is punishable under section 302 IPC.

11. *Criminal abortion:* A woman who is not in the child bearing age cannot be punished for criminal abortion.

12. *Will Making:* A person who has attained the majority can make his will, however a person under guardian appointed by a court can make a valid will only after 21 years of age.

13. *Impotency:* A boy before puberty is sterile but not impotent. A woman becomes sterile after attaining menopause.

14. *Eligibility for certain posts:* Age eligibility for some of the constitutional posts is variable, e.g. to become a member of the lok sabha or Prime Minister of India an Indian citizen must be above 25 years of age and for the president of India a person must be above 35 years of age.

Determination of Age

Age of an individual can be determined from features mentioned below.

General Physical Characters

a. *Height and weight:* A person attains maximum height with full development and growth of the bones. Height and weight can be of some help to roughly assess the age of an individual. An infant triple their weight from birth weight, by the end of one year. Average height and weight charts are available for a given population in relation to the age.

b. *Secondary sex characters:* In males at puberty there is increase in the size of the testes at about 12 to 14 years with growth of pubic hair which becomes moderately thick by 15 years, fully grown with male distribution by 16 years. Facial hair and hoarse voice are seen by 16 years and facial hair gets well developed by 20 years. Use of certain drugs like cimetidine, spironolactone or nifedipine may lead to enlargement of breasts in males.

In females there is development of breasts along with appearance of pubic hair which starts about 2 years before menarche. The development of breast happens in five stages. Stage one small breast bud is formed (11–12 yrs.). In stage two breast and nipple show some enlargement (13 yrs.). In the stage three there is general enlargement with darkening of areola (14 yrs.). Stage four is indicated by formation of a secondary swelling under the areola which is seen in early teens (15 yrs.). In stage five the breast is fully developed (> 15 yrs.). Pubic hair are well developed by 14 to 15 years, axillary hair also appear at this time. In **McCune-Albright syndrome** secondary sex characters may appear early.

c. *Age related degenerative changes:* Graying of hair and baldness in males usually starts by 50 years; however this is variable and may occur early in a genetically predisposed or due to debilitating diseases.

Arcus senilis an opaque ring at the periphery of the cornea may be noticed after 50 years of age.

Age from Dentition

a. *Dental eruption:*
   i. Alveolar cavities are formed around 3rd and 4th intrauterine month.
   ii. Rudiments of all temporary teeth and 1st permanent molars are present in the jaw at birth.
   iii. Temporary teeth are 20 in number, start erupting by 7th or 8th month and are completely erupted by 30th month Table 3.1.
   iv. Eruption of teeth depends upon nutritional status, heredity, and endocrinal factors. In syphilis teeth may be present at birth or erupt early. Differences between temporary and permanent teeth are mentioned in Table 3.2.
   v. Permanent teeth are 32 in number and start erupting from 6th year onwards and 3rd permanent molar erupts between 17 and 25th years of age Table 3.3.

b. *Gustafson's method:* Gustafson devised a method for age estimation from teeth depending on the age related changes taking place in the teeth after 21 years of age (Fig. 3.3). Anterior teeth are primarily used to observe various changes. Main disadvantage of this method is that it can be used only in dead as teeth are required

S.No.	Teeth	Age of eruption of temporary teeth	Calcification of root completed	Reabsorption of root begins at
1.	Central incisors			
	a. lower	6–8 months	2 years	4 years
	b. Upper	7–9 months	2 years	5 years
2.	Lateral incisors			
	a. Upper	7–9 months	2 years	5 years
	b. lower	10–12 months	2 years	5 years
3.	First molar	12–14 months	$2\frac{1}{2}$ years	6 years
4.	Canine	17–18 months	3 years	8 years
5.	Second molar	20–30 months	3 years	7 years

Table 3.1: Age of eruption of temporary teeth

Table 3.2: Differences between temporary and permanent teeth

Feature	Permanent teeth	Temporary teeth
Total number	32 replaces temporary teeth	28
Size	Bigger	Smaller
Weight	Heavy	Lighter
Colour	Ivory white	China white
Position of incisors	Vertical	Forward inclined
Neck	Less constricted	More prominent
Ridge between neck and body	Absent	Present
Roots of molars	Less divergent	Divergent
Replaced by different type tooth	Premolars replaces temporary molars	Do not replace any teeth
Number of molars	3 in each quadrant	2 in each quadrant

Table 3.3: Age of eruption of permanent teeth

S.No.	Teeth	Beginning of calcification	Eruption	Completion of calcification
1.	Central incisors	3–4 months	6–8 years	10 years
2.	Lateral incisors	1 year	7–9 years	11 years
3.	Canines	4–5 months	11–12 years	12–13 years
4.	First premolars	1–2 years	9–11 years	12–13 years
5.	Second premolars	2 years	10–12 years	12–14 years
6.	First molars	At birth	6–7 years	9–10 years
7.	Second molars	3 years	12–14 years	14–16 years
8.	Third molars	8–10 years	17–25 years	18–25 years

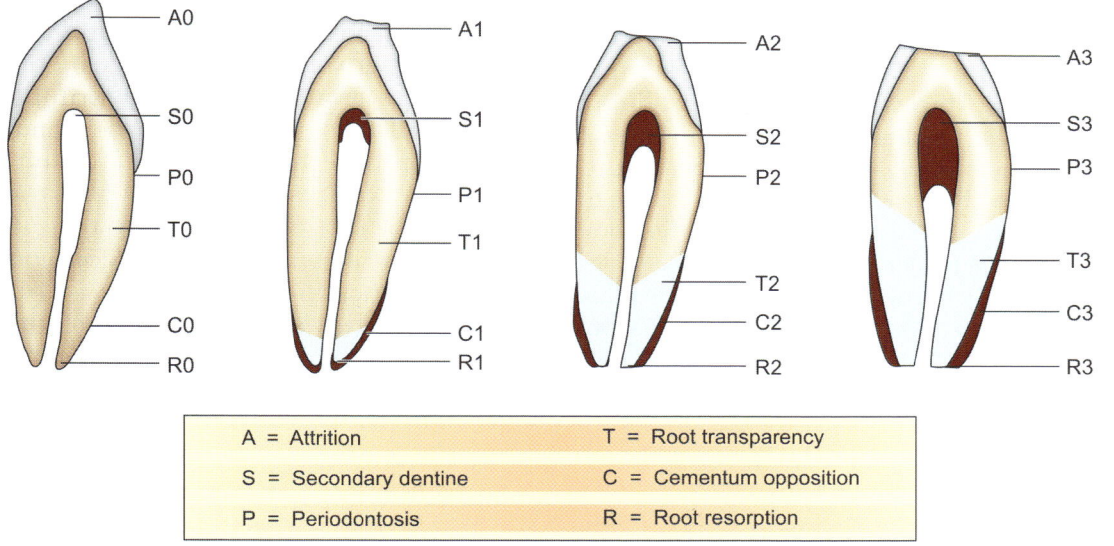

A = Attrition	T = Root transparency
S = Secondary dentine	C = Cementum opposition
P = Periodontosis	R = Root resorption

Fig. 3.3: Age related changes in teeth (Gustafson's method)

to be extracted. Before the teeth are extracted the periodontosis changes are noted. The extracted tooth is then grinded from lateral sides up to 1 mm thickness to note the transparency of the root. After which the tooth is further grinded on a glass slab up to 0.25 mm thickness to note the remaining changes. All the six changes are graded in four stages from 0 to 3. Individual grading are then added and compared with a plotted regression equation to find out the age of a person. The error is up to ± 5 years in age calculations with this method.

i. Attrition: It is the loss of the masticating surface of the tooth due to friction.

ii. Periodontosis: There is regression of gums and exposure of the root.

iii. Secondary dentine: There is deposition of secondary dentine tissue in the pulp cavity with age. The size of the cavity goes on diminishing.

iv. Root reabsorption: Apex of the root start eroding with age, which gradually extends upwards.

v. Cementum apposition: Layer of cementum on the root surface gets on becoming thicker with age.

vi. Root transparency: Root start to become transparent with age as the canals in the dentine are gradually filled with minerals. The area is calculated by measuring the graph paper squares visible through the transparent area or transparency is observed by reading through the transparent area. This is the most reliable method out of the above criteria (Miles, 1963).

Initially narrowing of root canal was also considered as one of the criteria, but was discarded and is not being used these days.

c. *Incremental lines and apatite crystal size:* Age can also be determined within few months after birth from daily increments of growth known as incremental lines in the enamel. Age of the individual is calculated by counting number of lines from neonatal line onwards (**Boyd's method**). The crystallinity of the dental hydroxyl-apatite decreases with the age.

d. *Chemical changes:* The a-lattice constant that is associated with the carbonate content in carbonate apatite decreases with age in a systematic way, whereas the c-lattice constant does not change significantly. Thermogravimetric measurements demonstrate an increase of the carbonate content with the age.

e. *Stack's method:* This method uses the height and weight of the erupting teeth during infancy and early childhood to determine age of the child.

Age from Bones

a. *Size of the bones:* With age the bones of the body goes on growing till the growth stops. Out of the long bones femur length has been examined against the crown-rump length during intrauterine period and stature during childhood.

b. *Appearance of ossification centers:* Even though adult person has 206 bones but these bones develop from multiple ossification centers. First ossification centers are seen in the clavicle bone between 4 and 5 weeks of intrauterine period. Most of the long bone shafts have ossification centers by 8th week of intrauterine period which are known as primary centers. At birth there are about 450 ossification centers. Secondary ossification centers appear after birth. Appearance of ossification centers is a very good indicator of age of a person.

c. *Epiphyseal union:* Most of the long bone shafts are ossified before birth however ends of the bones, i.e. epiphyses ossify after birth. These centers join with the diaphysis at different time intervals by which the age of an individual can be determined.

d. *Suture closure:* Posterior fontanel closes at birth to 6 months and anterior fontanel closes between 1½ years to 2 years. Metopic suture closes by 2 to 4 years, however may persist in 5 to 10% cases (Fig. 3.4). The

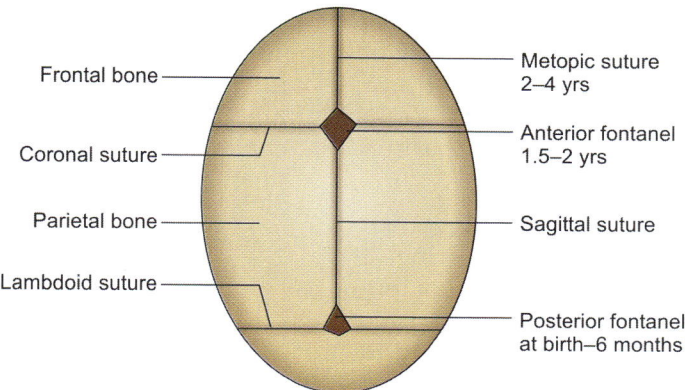

Fig. 3.4: Skull fontanel

sutures start closing from inside first. Last to close is the temporal suture, which closes by 70 to 80 years (Fig. 3.5).

e. *Joint lipping:* With advancing age the joint cavities start showing lipping of the margins.

f. *Changes at pubic symphysis:* Pubic symphysis also show various changes related to the age of a person.

g. *Scapular changes:* Scapular changes have also been studied in relation to the age of a person.

h. *Sternum and hyoid bone:* Four segments of sterna body fuses from below upwards between 14 and 25 years and xiphoid process joins at 40 years with the body. Greater cornua of hyoid bone joins with body at about 40 to 60 years.

(Findings in detail are mentioned in the chapter on forensic osteology).

COMPLEXION AND FEATURES

Complexion and detailed features are of help in visual identification of a person. Friends and relatives identify a person for medico-legal purposes from detailed features only. Even during criminal identification parade a witness identifies a criminal from the complexion and features. These features may change with time, mental stress or disease. In **Bhowal Sanyasi** case complexion and features were taken into account in deciding by the court that he was actually Kumar Ramendra Narayan Roy of Bhowal estate in Dhaka.

HAIR

Hair and fibers are helpful in crime detection. They resist decomposition for a considerable time after death. Hair consists of hair bulb and shaft. Hair bulb is formed in the follicle of skin and is the growing end. A hair follicle has period of growth during which the hair increases in length. During resting phase the follicle shrinks and the hair may readily shed.

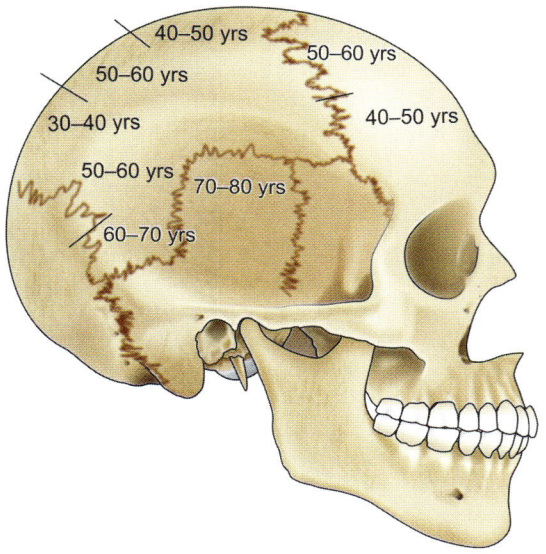

Fig. 3.5: Closure of skull sutures

In certain poisoning like thallium or during chemotherapy, there is extensive shedding of hair. Hair follicles are not formed in a scar tissue. Scalp hair normally grows at 0.3 mm per day. Beard growth is faster in comparison to other body hair.

Hair shaft is the portion which grows out of the skin. The shaft has outer covering of scales known as cuticle. It is composed of thin microscopic, non-pigmented scales of variable size and shape, attached at the lower end to the cortex. Outer portion of hair is cortex, made of keratinized mass. It is made of longitudinally placed elongated cells without nuclei. Pigmented granules are present in the fibrils inside these cells giving colour to the hair. In human hair the pigmented cells are present near the periphery of the cortex. Central portion of the hair is known as medulla. Human has thin medulla which may be interrupted at places. Medulla in animal hair is thick and may even show different patterns. Hair terminates into a pointed non-modulated portion known as tip. Tip may be split with repeated damage to the cuticle.

Medicolegal Questions

i. *Hair or some other fibers:* Hair can be identified from other fibres. Whereas the fibers could be natural fibers or artificial fibers. Natural fibers like cotton fiber are flattened and twisted with long tubular cells with blunt pointed ends. Silk fibers are long clear threads without any cells. Jute fibers are smooth without transverse lines. Wool is an animal hair and show characteristics of animal hair. Manmade fibers produced from synthetic polymers or mixtures of various polymers are commonly used for various applications. Scientific identification of fibers is based on microscopic examination, staining tests, solubility tests, fiber density, identification of chemical composition, chromatographic analysis and infrared spectroscopy.

ii. *Human hair or animal hair:* Human hair can be differentiated from animal hair by noting the physical characteristics under a microscope. Human hair are fine and thin, more over the cortex is thick; more than 3 times the medulla, cuticular scales are short broad and thin in comparison to animal hair. Detailed differences are mentioned in Table 3.4.

iii. *Race:* Negroid scalp hair has close spirals, black or very dark brown, thick, woolly and transverse shape is of flattened eclipse. Mongoloid hairs are long cylindrical brown or light yellow. Caucasian have features between Negroid and mongoloid hair and are normally of light brown, reddish or yellowish in colour.

iv. *Derived from which part of the body:* physical appearance indicate the origin of that hair. Scalp hairs are long, soft and circular in

S.No.	Feature	Human hair	Animal hair
		TAble 3.4: Differences between human and animal hair	
1.	Texture	Fine and thin (50–150μ)	Thick and course
2.	Colour	Black, gray, reddish or brown	Any colour even banded
3.	Cuticle	Scales are short, broad, annular and thin	Large having step like wavy projections.
4.	Cortex	Thick; more than 3 times medulla	Thin; less than two times medulla
5.	Pigment	Distributed peripherally in cortex	No fixed pattern. Mostly near medulla.
6.	Medulla	Thin and interrupted or fragmented	Wider and continuous
7.	Root	Bulb shaped	Brush shaped
8.	Medullary index	<0.25	>0.4
9.	Precipitin test	Specific for human	Specific for animal

cross-section. Beard and moustache hair are thick and triangular in cross-section. Axillary and pubic hair are curly and oval on cross-section. Body hair are soft and thin.

v. *Sex:* Male hair is thick and dark as compared to female hair. Beard and moustache hair are specific to males. Detection of Barr bodies in more than 20% of hair bulb cells indicates female sex.

vi. *Age:* Hair can be of limited use in age determination. In newborn lanugo hair are fine, soft, and non-pigmented. There is graying of hair in old age. Loss of scalp hair may be seen after third decade of life.

vii. *Has it been altered by dyeing:* Colour of the hair can be changed by dyeing or bleaching. Some persons use Henna or artificial dyes to colour their hair. Growing portion of the hair will show the actual colour of the hair. Such hair become lusterless rough and dry on dyeing. Individuals working in some metallurgic factories may get some colouration to their hair like persons working in copper factories has greenish tinge to their hair or in cobalt factories have bluish colouration.

viii. *Matching with victim or assailant:* Hair bulb cells are used to detect ABO blood group for cross matching, but is not reliable. DNA profiling can also be done from the hair bulb cells. Mitochondrial DNA from shaft cells can be used to match the hair with victim or assailant. Hair present on the weapon of offence or on the vehicle involved in an accident or on the body of the victim of the assailant provides valuable evidence. In bestiality presence of animal hair around the genitalia of the accused is commonly seen.

ix. *Did it fall naturally or forcibly removed:* The naturally fallen hair has atrophied hair bulb and the hair sheath is absent. In case the hair is forcibly pulled out the hair sheath is ruptured and the bulb is swollen.

x. *What was the cause of injury or death:* Injury caused by a sharp cutting weapon also causes clean cut of the shaft, whereas in blunt force the hair show splitting with ragged margins. In burn injuries or near range firearm injuries the hair show singeing with swelling of the singed end which show enlarged and vacuolated appearance of cells on microscopy. Few poisons especially heavy metals can be detected from hair.

ANTHROPOMETRY (BERTILLON'S SYSTEM)

Alphonse Bertillon was a French criminologist who first developed this anthropometric system of physical measurements of body parts, especially components of the head and face. His method was based on the fact that body measurements do not normally change after a person reaches 21 years of age. This system, invented in 1879, became known as the Bertillon system, or *bertillonage*, and quickly gained wide acceptance as a reliable, scientific method of criminal investigation. In 1884 alone, French police used Bertillon's system to help capture 241 repeat offenders, which helped establish the system's effectiveness. Law enforcement agencies began to create archives of records of known criminals, which contained fourteen identical anthropometric measurements, as well as full-face and profile photographs of the perpetrator (now commonly known as "mug shots," which are still in use).

Bertillon's system was based on body measurements which included; head length; head breadth; span of outstretched arms; length and breadth of right ear; length of the middle finger; length of left little finger; the length of the left foot; the length of the "cubit" (the forearm from the elbow to the extremity of the middle finger) apart from colour of the hair and eyes; shape of the nose and eyes; tattoo marks; scars or birthmarks.

It was eventually displaced by fingerprint analysis, although bertillon measurements were commonly used in conjunction with fingerprinting into the early decades of the 20th century. The reliability of bertillon system was questioned as the measurements required expert technicians, leading to errors and photographs were not always reliable. These days fingerprint analysis is used by law enforcement agencies all over the world to track down criminals and conclusively identify them.

DACTYLOGRAPHY (GALTON'S SYSTEM) INCLUDING POROSCOPY (LOCARD'S SYSTEM)

A fingerprint is an impression of the friction ridges of all or any part of the finger. A friction ridge is a raised portion of the epidermis on the palmar (palm and fingers) or plantar (sole and toes) skin, consisting of one or more connected ridge units of friction ridge skin. Some other animals, including gorillas and koalas have their own unique prints. In fact, koala fingerprints are remarkably similar to human fingerprints. Gorillas have fingerprints while chimpanzees do not, even though the latter are more closely related to humans.

Fingerprint identification (dactylography) or palm-print identification is the process of comparing questioned and known friction skin ridge impressions from fingers or palms to determine if the impressions are from the same finger or palm; this system is known as **Henry Galton's** system of identification. These ridges on the palmar surface develop by fourth month of intrauterine period and remain unchanged throughout life.

Fingerprint identification is based on the fact that each individual has permanent, characteristic pattern and even in uniovular twins the fingerprints are different even though the DNA profiling is same.

History of Fingerprinting for Identification

In ancient babylon fingerprints were used on clay tablets for business transactions around 1500 BC. In ancient China thumbprints were found on clay seals, around 1000 BC. In 14th century Persia government officials would use their fingerprint in much the same way we use signatures today.

In 1823, Jan Evangelista Purkyne, a professor of anatomy at the university of Breslau, in his thesis discussed 9 fingerprint patterns, but he did not mention the use of fingerprints to identify persons.

In 1880, Dr. Henry Faulds published his first paper on the subject in the scientific journal nature. Returning to the UK in 1886, he offered the concept to the metropolitan police in London but it was dismissed.

In 1892, Sir Francis Galton published a detailed statistical model of fingerprint analysis and identification and encouraged its use in forensic science in his book on fingerprints.

Juan Vucetich in 1892, an argentine police officer who had been studying Galton pattern types for a year, made the first criminal fingerprint identification. He successfully proved Rojas guilty of murder after showing that the bloody fingerprint found at the crime scene was hers, and could only be hers.

The world's first fingerprint bureau was opened in Kolkata, India in 1897, after the council of the Governor general approved a committee report that fingerprints should be used for classification of criminal records. Azizul Haque and Hem Chandra Bose were the Indian fingerprint experts credited with primary development of the fingerprint classification system, expanding Galton's system, eventually named after their supervisor, Sir Edward Richard Henry.

The first united kingdom fingerprint bureau was founded in scotland yard in the year 1901. The henry classification system, devised by Sir Edward Richard Henry with the help of Haque and Bose was accepted in England and Wales.

In 1902, Dr. Henry P. De Forrest used fingerprinting in the New York civil service.

New York City Police Department Deputy Commissioner Joseph A. Faurot introduced fingerprinting of criminals to the United States in 1906.

Fingerprint Classification Systems

Before computerization replaced manual filing systems in large fingerprint operations, manual fingerprint classification systems were used to categorize fingerprints based on general ridge formations, for filing and retrieval of paper records. The most popular classification systems include the roscher system, the vucetich system, and the henry classification system. The roscher system was developed in Germany and implemented in both Germany and Japan, the vucetich system was developed in Argentina and implemented throughout South America and the henry system was developed in India and implemented in most english-speaking countries.

Basic fingerprint patterns: On the basis of patterns present on the terminal phalanx of fingers, they are divided into following types:

a. *Loops:* Ridges are arranged in a loop formation; starting from one side and ending on the same side. In case they start from medial side; are known as ulnar loop and if starting from lateral side are known as radial loop. They are quite common and seen in about 60–70% of fingers (Fig. 3.6b).

b. *Whorls:* This pattern has ridges arranged in circular or oval formation and are seen in about 30–35% of cases (Fig. 3.6c).

c. *Arches:* In this pattern the ridges start from one side and after making an arch ends on the other side of the finger. These are seen in about 5–10% of cases. They can be sub-grouped into plain or tented arches (Fig. 3.6a).

d. *Composite:* There is combination of two or more patterns and are seen in 1–2% of cases (Fig. 3.6d).

Types of fingerprints available at scene of crime:

a. ***Latent prints:*** Latent prints mean any chance or accidental impression left by friction ridge skin on a surface, invisible at the time of deposition. Electronic, chemical and physical processing techniques permit visualization of invisible latent print residue from natural secretions of the eccrine glands present on friction ridge skin (made of palmar sweat, electrolytes, sebum and various kinds of lipids).

Latent fingerprints are normally processed for identification either by using contrast powders or by chemicals reacting with the substances which are present in the fingerprints.

i. *Powders:* Mostly dark powders like black or dark grey powders are used. However, in cases where the background is dark other light coloured powders like aluminum powder can be used. Magnetic or fluorescent powders are also used by the forensic scientists. Once the fingerprint is made visible by dusting with above powders and using light brushing, they are lifted with transparent cellulose tape of 4–5 cm width and preserved by fixing them on a contrast coloured paper. They can also be lifted with rubber lifter.

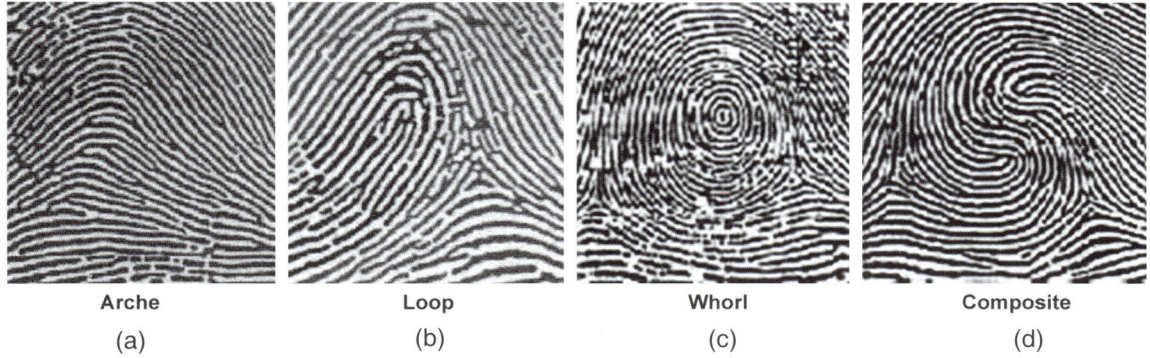

Arche	Loop	Whorl	Composite
(a)	(b)	(c)	(d)

Figs 3.6a to d: Types of fingerprints

ii. *Chemicals:* Most of the chemicals used react with fatty acids present in the fingerprints. Some of the chemicals used are iodine fumes, ninhydrin, silver nitrate, cyanoacrylate, osmic acid or tannic acid, etc. Once the print becomes visible it is photographed immediately as the colour may fade or disappear with time.

iii. *Autoelectronography:* Lead dust on the fingerprints is irradiated with high energy beam of X-rays. The X-ray beam is first passed through copper plate to get a homogenous beam. The beam results in emission of electrons which is captured on a radiographic film, for visualization of the latent fingerprints even from the skin surface.

b. *Patent (visible) prints:* These are friction ridge impressions obvious to the human eye and are caused by a transfer of foreign material on the finger such as motor oil, blood or ink, onto a surface. Because they are already visible they need no enhancement, and are generally photographed instead of being lifted in the manner as is done for latent prints.

c. *Plastic prints:* These are the prints made in some soft pliable material which can retain the print impression. Commonly encountered examples are melted candle wax; putty removed from the perimeter of window panes and thick grease deposits on car parts. Such prints are already visible and also need no enhancement. After photographically recording such prints, attempts should be made to develop other nonplastic impressions deposited.

Fingerprints from decomposed bodies: In cases of advanced putrefaction especially in drowning the skin of the hands may get separated in the form of a glove. This is preserved in formalin and once the skin hardens the fingerprint impressions can be obtained. Ridges are also present in the dermis up to a depth of 0.6 mm; hence impressions can be obtained from histological sections. In case the fingers are shriveled up they are immersed in 20% acetic acid for a day.

Taking samples of fingerprints for record or comparison:

a. *Manual:* Fingerprint sample for comparing are normally taken on a paper with printers ink applied on the terminal portion of the fingers. They can be taken as:
   i. plain prints
   ii. rolled prints

b. *Live-scan prints:* There are different types of fingerprint readers in the market, but the basic idea behind each capture approach is to measure in some way the physical difference between ridges and valleys. All the proposed methods can be grouped into solid-state fingerprint readers and optical fingerprint readers. The procedure for capturing a fingerprint using a sensor consists of rolling or touching with the finger onto a sensing area, which according to the physical principle in use (capacitive, optical, thermal, etc.) captures the difference between valleys and ridges.

Comparison of fingerprints

Friction ridges do not run evenly and unbroken across our fingers, hands, toes and feet. Rather, they display a number of characteristics known as minutiae (Fig. 3.7). The principle categories of minutiae are as follows:

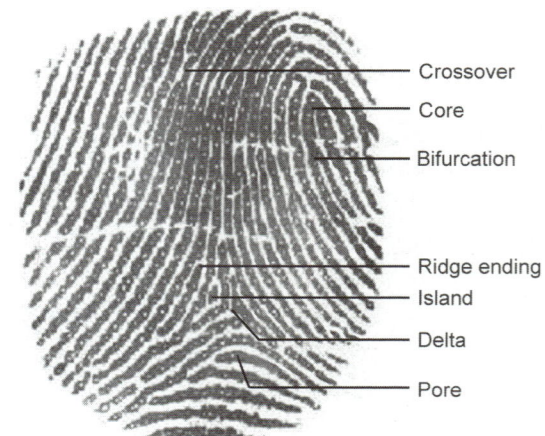

Fig. 3.7: Various minutiae for comparison

a. *Ridge ending:* A ridge that ends abruptly.

b. *Bifurcation:* A single ridge that divides into two ridges.

c. *Lake or enclosure:* A single ridge that bifurcates and reunites shortly afterwards to continue as a single ridge.

d. *Short ridge, island or independent ridge:* A ridge that commences travels a short distance and then ends.

e. *Dot:* An independent ridge with approximately equal length and width.

f. *Spur:* A bifurcation with a short ridge branching off a longer ridge.

g. *Crossover or bridge:* A short ridge that runs between two parallel ridges.

Fingerprints can be compared to each other by examining the minutiae to determine whether: (i) the same minutiae are present (e.g. a bifurcation); (ii) the minutiae flow in the same direction (e.g. the bifurcation is on a ridge running horizontally and the two divided ridges are to the right of the bifurcation); and (iii) the minutiae occupy the same relative positions to each other (e.g. the bifurcation is separated from an enclosure below it by six intervening ridges).

Where minutiae on two different fingerprint impressions meet these criteria, they are referred to as points of similarity. As soon as a fingerprint examiner identifies a single unexplainable point of dissimilarity between two fingerprint impressions, then he or she assumes there is not a match between the two fingerprints. However, there is no international standard for the number of points of identification required for a match between two fingerprints. (Some countries have set minimum numbers of points of identification for a match from 8 to 16). Central fingerprint bureau at Kolkata has set the minimum matching point at 9 for fingerprint identification.

Poroscopy

This technique to match fingerprints is used when only a fragment of the fingerprint is available. Microscopic pores of the sweat gland opening are present on the ridges of the hand. These pores vary in size, shape, position and numbers over a given length of the ridge which can be compared for matching. This technique is known as Poroscopy and was developed by **Edmond Locard** in 1912. (In crime reconstruction he also advocated **Locard's exchange principle**, which states that when two objects or person comes in contact there is cross transfer of physical evidence.)

Footprints

Friction ridge skin present on the soles of the feet and toes (plantar surfaces) is as unique as ridge detail on the fingers and palms. When recovered at crime scenes or on items of evidence, sole and toe impressions are used in the same manner as finger and palm prints to effect identifications.

Footprints of infants, along with thumb or index fingerprints of mothers, are still commonly recorded in hospitals to assist in verifying the identity of infants.

It is not uncommon for military records of flight personnel to include bare foot inked impressions. Friction ridge skin protected inside flight boots tends to survive the trauma of a plane crash (and accompanying fire) better than fingers.

TEETH (Odontology)

Dental evidence for determination of identification has been used on many occasions. Apart from determination of age, sex and race (discussed earlier), teeth can be helpful in identification from physical features. Morphology of a tooth is shown in Figs 3.8 and 3.9. Teeth are important as they resist putrefaction, moreover, bite marks left at the scene of crime may leave certain characteristic features for the identification of the criminal.

Identification from Teeth

Dental characteristics of each individual is unique, hence detailed examination of teeth are undertaken. The dental charting include; (a) number of teeth present; (b) decayed teeth if any; (c) permanent or temporary teeth

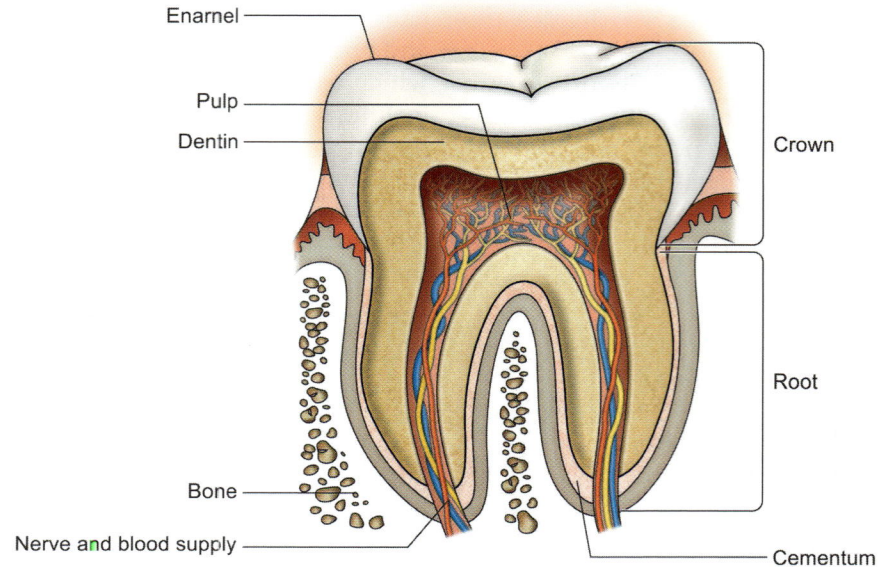

Fig. 3.8: Morphology of tooth

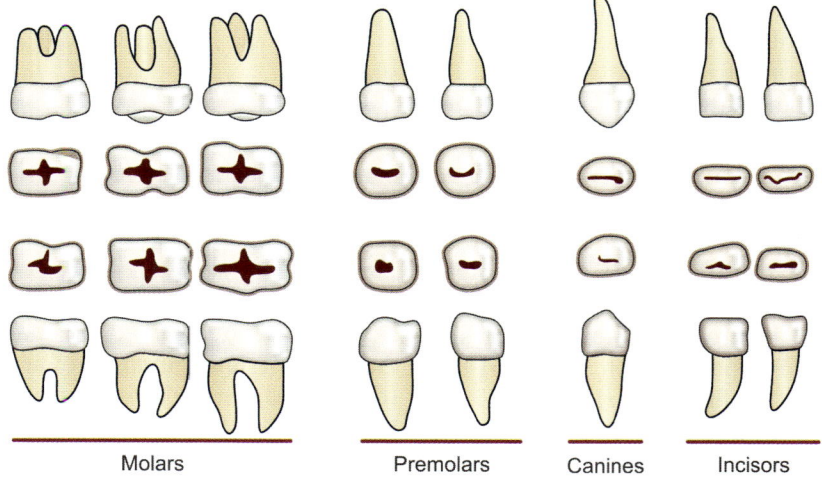

Fig. 3.9: Shape of permanent teeth in adult person

present in mouth; (d) any extractions; (e) fillings present and the filling material used; (f) any irregularities in teeth; (g) special treatment carried out like root canal or apicectomies; (h) any stain present on the teeth like nicotine or pan stains and (i) dentures present: type of denture, material used, technician's mark, etc.

Detailed records are made in the form of "Dental charting" so that the data can be compared easily. Most commonly used charting methods are mentioned below:

a. *Palmer's notation:* This notation is commonly practiced by orthodontists. Permanent teeth in each quadrant are represented by numerical from 1 to 8 and temporary teeth by alphabets from A to E (Fig. 3.10). This system has been replaced by FDI system.

b. *Universal system:* Permanent teeth are numbered from 1 to 32 and starting from right to left side and from 17 to 32 from left to right side for the mandibular teeth (Fig. 3.11).

c. *Haderup method:* Teeth are similarly numbered as in Palmer's notation, however the upper jaw teeth are donated with + mark and mandibular teeth with–mark (Fig. 3.12).

d. *FDI notation:* The general assembly of Federation Dentaire Internationale adopted two digit numbering system for each tooth both for permanent set and temporary set. The first number represents the tooth's quadrant and second number represents the tooth placement (Fig. 3.13). This system has advantage of easy transmission and easy recovery from computerized records. This system is also known as ISO system of WHO.

e. *Modified FDI notation:* FDI system has been modified to change the numerical representing each quadrant of the jaw.

f. *Zsigmondy notation:* Roman numerology was used for temporary teeth and 1 to 8 for permanent teeth in this system. Roman numbers were replaced by A to E by Palmer in his system. However, presently this system is not in common use.

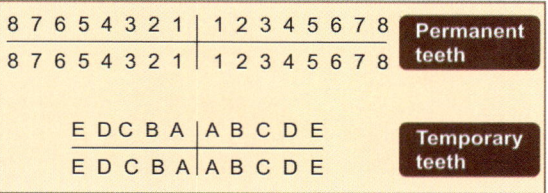

Fig. 3.10: Palmer's notation

Fig. 3.11: Universal system

Bite Marks

On numerous occasions bite marks are seen on a person or foodstuff at the scene of crime. Bite marks are made from the incisal surface and cusps of the anterior teeth. Females may defend themselves by inflicting bite marks on the body of an accused especially in sexual assault. These may vary from indentation and

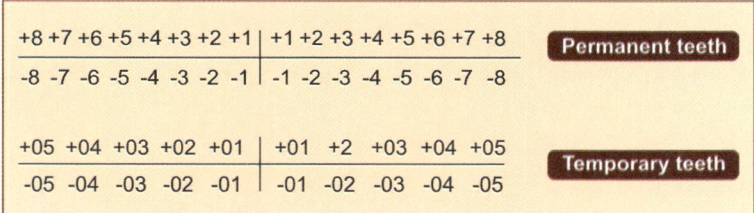

Fig. 3.12: Haderup method

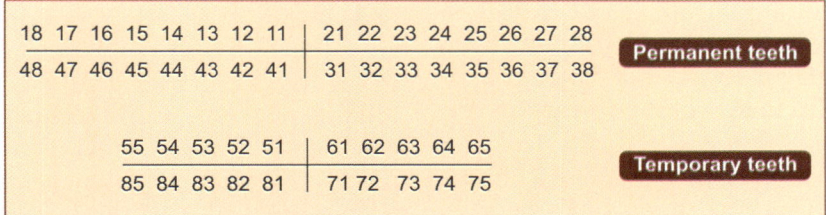

Fig. 3.13: FDI notation

bruising to lacerations of the tissues. Bite marks on foodstuffs may show dimensional variation depending on the manner in which the bite was made and also due to shrinkage of the foodstuff from drying.

Presence of saliva at the bite location is used to confirm the bite, moreover, detection of ABO blood group from the saliva in secretors also help in identification.

Details of the bite marks are recorded by means of measurements, photographs and making cast models. In some cases ultraviolet lamps may be used to highlight the faint bite marks. Inked impression on a wet paper or a photograph is taken from inked cast made from the person suspected to have produced that bite. A positive transparency is the prepared and placed on the bite mark or real size photograph of the bite mark for comparison. Stereoscopic methods are also used these days for comparison.

SCARS

A scar is fibrous tissue covered with epithelium, resulting from healing process in an injury, involving dermis. There are no sweat glands or hair follicles present in the scar. A scar retains its shape throughout the life; however the size of the scar may change in the growing age group. In case of keloid formation the shape and size may increase. Scars can be removed by plastic surgery. Light or invisible scar can be made visible by application of heat or use of ultraviolet rays.

Medicolegal Importance

i. *Establish identity:* Scars are normally recorded as identification marks while preparing any medicolegal report. Shape, size, colour and location from any anatomical land mark are mentioned in the medicolegal reports so that the person can be identified in the court proceedings on a later date.

ii. *Weapon used:* Type of weapon used can be made out from the shape and size of the scar.

iii. *Grievous injury:* Any injury resulting in scar formation on the face is grievous injury as it leads to disfiguration of the head and face.

iv. *Drug addict:* A person having multiple scars in the antecubital region or of skin popping from needle pricks indicate that the person may be drug addict.

v. *Old pregnancy:* Presence of Striae gravidarum normally points toward earlier pregnancy in a female. Such scars may also be seen in ascites or large abdominal tumors.

vi. *Surgical scars:* Scars showing typical stitch marks are as a result of surgical intervention.

vii. *Age of the scar:* Scars are formed in about 10 to 12 days in case the healing is from primary intention. In case the healing is from secondary intention the scar formation takes longer time depending upon the severity of infection. If the infection is moderate it may take 2 to 3 weeks to form, but in severe infections the scar formation is delayed and may form after 4 to 6 weeks. Age of the scar can be made out from the appearance of the scar:

a. Fresh scars are soft, sensitive, reddish and tender for first few weeks.

b. Recent scars are soft, brownish or coppery red without any corrugations due to shrinkage in the next three months.

c. Old scars are white, glistening, contracted with corrugations and tough to feel after six months.

DEFORMITIES

Deformities present in a person can be used for identification purposes. They should be properly recorded and compared for identification of an individual. Deformities could be either congenital like hare lip, cleft palate, supernumerary fingers, etc. or acquired deformities like amputations, malunited fracture or circumcision, etc.

BIRTHMARKS

Birthmarks can also be used as one of the identification mark for identification. The size, shape, location and colour of the birthmark should be recorded for future identification purposes. Birthmark usually grows along with growth of a person and may also become lighter in colour.

TATTOO MARKS

Tattoo marks are the patterns produced by introducing pigments of various colours in the dermis by multiple puncture technique manually or by an electrical device (tattoo gun). Earlier days' simple patterns of name, god or ohm were tattooed but presently tattoo artists create beautiful multicoloured patterns. (Fig. 3.14).

Tattoo marks apart for identification of an individual also provide information about the religion, occupation, nationality, dug addition or mental makeup of the person.

Light or faded tattoo marks can be made visible by ultraviolet light, rubbing or applying heat to that area. In a dead body a tattoo mark can be seen by burning that area and removing the epidermis. Tattoo marks can be removed by surgical means, by applying corrosive agents or by electrolysis. In such cases pigment can be found at the local lymph nodes. Tattoo marks are of two types:

a. Voluntary: When the pigment is introduced in the dermis on his volition.
b. Involuntary: When the pigment get deposited in close range firearm injury.

Different types of pigments or dyes are used to produce tattoo marks like for black colour Indian ink, carbon dust or iron oxide; for brown colour silica, ochre; for red colour cinnabar or cadmium red; for orange colour cadmium seleno-sulfide; for yellow colour cadmium yellow or chrome yellow; for green colour chromium oxide, malachite or lead chromate; for white colour titanium dioxide, zinc oxide or lead carbonate and for blue colour, prussian blue or azure blue is used. In some cases allergic reaction may be seen to the pigment used.

Tattoo marks last for long time, they may fade if pigments are not introduced properly in the dermis or due to exposure to direct sunlight.

OCCUPATIONAL MARKS

Presence of callosities on various parts of the body depending upon the profession of the person can also help in the identification like linear callosities in the finger of a violinist, notch in the middle of upper incisors in carpenters from holding nails, stained finger and nails in photographers or presence of grease on the hands of a mechanic may reveal his occupation and indirectly help in identification of a person.

HANDWRITING

Handwriting in the form of signatures is commonly used for identification of a person in banks. Handwriting experts are made to analyze documents in question for identification of the author. There are natural variations or traits in the handwriting of a person:

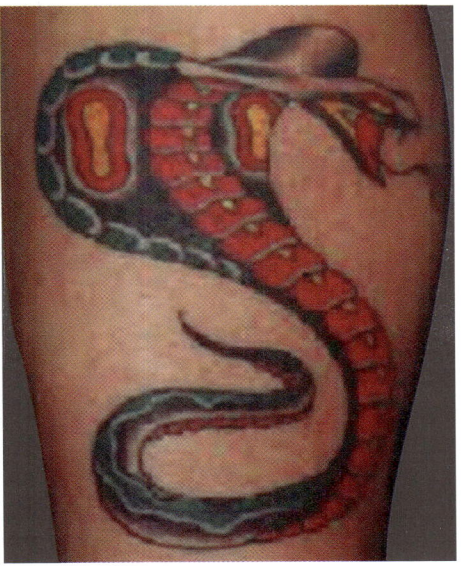

Fig. 3.14: Tattoo mark of a snake

a. *Letter form:* This includes curves, slants and proportional size of various letters used by an individual while writing.

b. *Line form:* This includes how smooth, light or dark lines are made, indicating the pressure applied by the writer.

c. *Formatting:* This includes spacing between the letters and words, placement of words in a line and the margin left on a paper while writing.

GAIT

The way in which a person walks can be used for identification of a person.

MANNER AND HABITS

It is possible to identify an individual from his habits like stammering, hand movements during talking or use of certain words.

MENTAL POWER AND MEMORY

In certain cases the mental power and memory are used for identification. The person in question may be able to recall some incidences from the past to establish his identity.

HEIGHT AND WEIGHT

Height and weight of a person can be helpful in identification especially when a dead body is recovered and the height and weight are matched with those of a missing person.

CLOTHS AND PERSONAL EFFECTS

These are helpful in identification especially in cases of advanced putrefaction. Laundry marks on the clothing, watch, identification cards and ornaments may establish the identity of a dead person in a mass disaster.

SUPERIMPOSITION TECHNIQUE

In criminal cases or mass disasters identification of the skeletal remains is frequently carried out by skull-photo superimposition. The photographs are enlarged to the same size as that of the skull. This is achieved through enlarging the photograph by measuring the bizygomatic skull width and the soft tissue thickness. It can also be done by visible teeth size or by mid pupillary distance measured from the skull. The skull is photographed in the same orientation as of the facial photograph for comparison. The superimposition can be done by "seeing through technique" by producing photographs of the person and of the skull on a transparent plate and comparing the two by placing them over each other. Appropriate anthropometric points are matched (Fig. 3.15). Presently "computer assisted superimposition" methods are used. Special software is used to digitize the photograph and the skull to compare them morphologically by image processing.

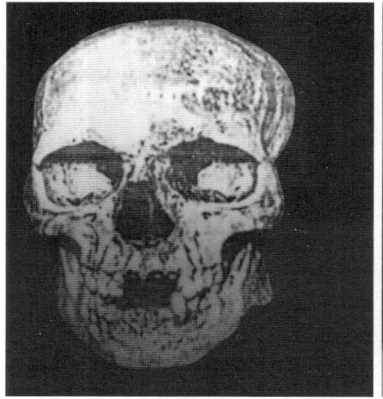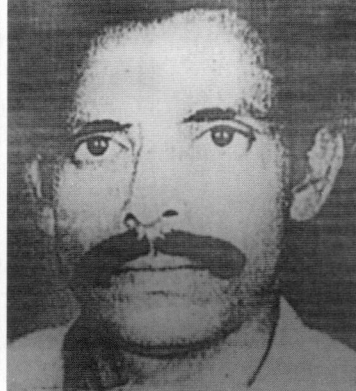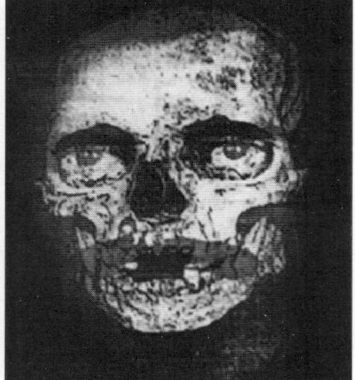

Superimposition (Curtsey Dr. DS Badkur, Director, MLI, Bhopal)

Fig. 3.15: Superimposition technique

DNA FINGERPRINTING

DNA (deoxyribonucleic acid) represents the blueprint of the human genetic makeup. It exists in every cell of the human body and differs in its sequence of nucleotides (adenine, thymine, guanine, and cytosine). The human genome is made up of 3 billion nucleotides, which are 99.9% identical from one person to the next. The 0.1% variation, therefore, can be used to distinguish one individual from another with a high level of certainty.

The complete DNA of each individual is unique, with the exception of identical twins. A DNA fingerprint, therefore, is a DNA pattern that has a unique sequence such that it can be distinguished from the DNA pattern of other individuals (Fig. 3.16).

Alec J. Jeffreys (1985) from the university of leicester in britain discovered that there are patterns of genetic material that are unique to almost every individual. DNA fingerprinting was originally used to identify genetic diseases. The two major uses for the information provided by DNA-fingerprinting analysis in forensic field are for (i) personal identification and (ii) determine genetic family relationships such as paternity, maternity, siblingship and other kinships.

DNA can be extracted from two different sources within the cell (i) nuclear DNA (nDNA) and (ii) Mitochondrial DNA (mtDNA). Nuclear DNA is analyzed in evidence containing blood, semen, saliva, body tissues, and hair follicles. DNA from the mitochondria, however, is usually analyzed in evidence containing hair fragments, bones, and teeth. Mitochondrial DNA analysis is typically performed in cases where there is an insufficient amount of sample, the nDNA is uninformative, or if supplementary information is necessary. Unlike nDNA, where one copy of a chromosome comes from the father and the other from the mother, mtDNA is exclusively inherited from the maternal side. Therefore, the maternal mtDNA should be the same as her offspring.

There are many methods that forensic scientists use to determine the sample's DNA fingerprint.

RFLP Analysis

The first method for finding out genetics used for DNA profiling involved "Restriction fragment length polymorphism" (**RFLP**) analysis. In case there is enough DNA, the DNA extracted from the sample can be cut or segmented using specific enzymes (proteins that speed up chemical reactions) called restriction endonucleases that act as molecular scissors by cutting specific sequences that they recognize. By cutting in the same sequence that is present in different locations throughout the genome, a pattern of fragments can be formed. Differences in the sequence patterns between two samples can be due to inherited variations in the DNA that can distinguish two different samples.

Once the DNA is cut, the separated fragments are then transferred to a nitrocellulose or nylon filter; this procedure is called southern blot. The DNA fragments within the blot are permanently fixed to the filter, and the DNA strands are denatured. Radio labeled probe molecules are then added that are complementary to sequences in the genome that contain repeat sequences the segments are arranged by size using a process called

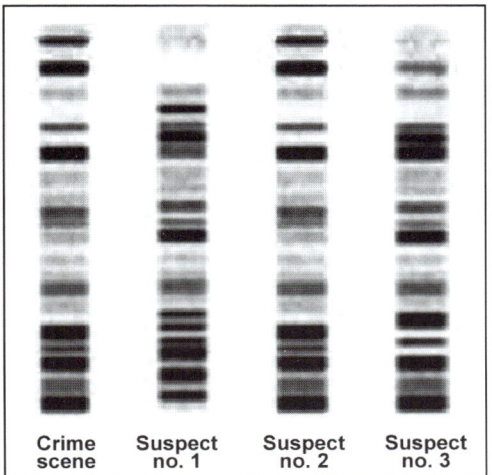

| Crime scene | Suspect no. 1 | Suspect no. 2 | Suspect no. 3 |

Fig. 3.16: DNA comparison

electrophoresis, whereby an electrical field is generated, pulling the negatively charged DNA toward the positively charged end through a gel-like matrix. The segments marked with radioactive probes are exposed on X-ray film, where they form a characteristic pattern of black bars. This pattern is called the DNA fingerprint. If the DNA fingerprints produced from two different samples match, the two samples are likely to have come from the same person.

PCR Analysis

In some cases, there is not enough DNA to directly evaluate it for RFLP analysis. If this occurs, a technique called the polymerase chain reaction (PCR) is used to amplify the genomic DNA from a sample. This procedure allows a scientist to amplify a specific sequence of DNA in the genome exponentially, so that it is in large enough quantities to be analyzed.

DNA analysis can be performed by sequencing the amplified DNA fragment using fluorescently labeled nucleotides and a laser that will recognize the nucleotide based on the fluorescent label to which it is attached. This technique is expensive, may not be informative, and is generally not the best approach to DNA fingerprint a sample.

Amplified Fragment Length Polymorphism (AmpFLP)

Amplified fragment length polymorphism was also put into practice during the early 1990s. This technique was also faster than RFLP analysis and used PCR to amplify DNA samples. It relied on variable number tandem repeat (VNTR) polymorphisms to distinguish various alleles, which were separated on a polyacrylamide gel using an allelic ladder (as opposed to a molecular weight ladder). Bands could be visualized by silver staining the gel. AmpFLP analysis can be highly automated, and allows for easy creation of phylogenetic trees based on comparing individual samples of DNA. Due to its relatively low cost and ease of set-up and operation, AmpFLP remains popular in lower income countries.

STR Analysis

The system of DNA profiling used today is based on PCR and uses short tandem repeats (STR). This method uses highly polymorphic regions that have short repeated sequences of DNA (the most common is 4 bases repeated, but there are other lengths in use, including 3 and 5 bases). Because unrelated people almost certainly have different numbers of repeat units, STRs can be used to discriminate between unrelated individuals.

The pattern of alleles can identify an individual quite accurately. Thus STR analysis provides an excellent identification tool. The more STR regions that are tested in an individual the more discriminating the test becomes.

Y-chromosome Analysis

Recent innovations have included the creation of primers targeting polymorphic regions on the Y-chromosome (Y-STR), which allows resolution of a mixed DNA sample from a male and female or cases in which a differential extraction is not possible. Y-chromosomes are paternally inherited, so Y-STR analysis can help in the identification of paternally related males. The analysis of the Y-chromosome yields weaker results than autosomal chromosome analysis. The Y male sex-determining chromosome, as it is inherited only by males from their fathers, is almost identical along the patrilineal line.

DNA Databases

There are now several DNA databases in existence around the world. Some are private, but most of the largest databases are government controlled. The United States maintains the largest DNA database, with the Combined DNA Index System (CODIS). The United Kingdom maintains the National DNA Database (NDNAD), which is of similar size.

Collection and Preservation of Samples

In forensics laboratories, DNA can be analyzed from a variety of human samples including, buccal smears, blood, semen, saliva, urine, hair, tissues, teeth, bones, other appropriate fluid and tissue from personal items, (e.g. a toothbrush, razor) or from stored samples, (e.g. banked sperm or biopsy tissue). DNA can be extracted from these samples and analyzed in a lab and results from these studies are compared to DNA analyzed from known samples. DNA extracted from a sample obtained from a crime scene then can be compared and possibly matched with DNA extracted from the victim or suspect.

1. *Blood samples:* About 5 to 10 ml of blood should be collected from a person or dead body in a plastic tube containing EDTA. The samples are frozen and transmitted to the laboratory using a cold chain.
2. *Bloodstains:* Stains on cloths are sent as such to the laboratory. Stains on hard surface can be scrapped and collected in a plastic container. Wet stains should be air dried. During transit they are kept cool.
3. *Buccal smears and other body fluids:* Buccal smears are collected on a sterilized cotton swab, which is air dried and frozen or kept cool as far as possible. Seminal or vaginal swabs are also air dried and transported in cool condition.
4. *Hair and teeth:* About 20 plucked hair are collected in a plastic bag and kept cool in a fridge. Bones and teeth in a dead body showing putrefaction are collected for DNA analysis from bone marrow or tooth pulp.
5. *Body tissues:* About 2 to 5 gm of the body tissues like muscles or organs are collected and kept in a frozen state.

Limitation of Use of DNA Fingerprints

1. *Coincidental match:* When using RFLP, the theoretical risk of a coincidental match is 1 in 100 billion (100,000,000,000), although the practical risk is actually 1 in 1000 because monozygotic twins are 0.2% of the human population. Due to the advent of more discriminating, sensitive and easier technologies; unrelated individuals with full matching DNA profiles, a match probability of 1 in a billion is considered statistically supportable.
2. *Laboratory error:* Error in matching DNA profile at the laboratory level could happen, especially when uniform standards are not used in various laboratories.
3. *Contamination:* Contamination of the sample is of great concern. Either material used to collect sample may be contaminated or the person collecting sample may contaminate with his body secretions.
4. *Fake DNA evidence:* The value of DNA evidence has to be seen in light of recent cases where criminals planted fake DNA samples at crime scenes.
5. *Time constrains:* Evaluating DNA profile is a time consuming process. It may take two to three months in some cases to give conclusive results.
6. *Ethical considerations:* Experts have doubts that DNA profile may be misused as DNA provides genetic information about that individual.

MISCELLANEOUS METHODS

1. *Facial reconstruction*: Facial reconstruction for identification has been tried with moderate success. Tissue depth at various points is accessed and reconstruction is done with the available skull.
2. *Lip prints (Cheiloscopy)*: Le Moyne Sunder in early 1950's postulated that lines, wrinkles or folds on the lips have individual characteristics. Lip prints were classified by Japanese Suzuki and Tsuchihashi in to five groups. Type-I, lips having long vertical lines; Type–I' Lips having short vertical lines; Type–II lips having branching pattern; Type-III Lips having intersecting lines with diamond grooves, Type-IV reticulate grooves, Type-V other types of grooves (Fig. 3.17). It was seen that even in uniovular twins the lip prints were different.

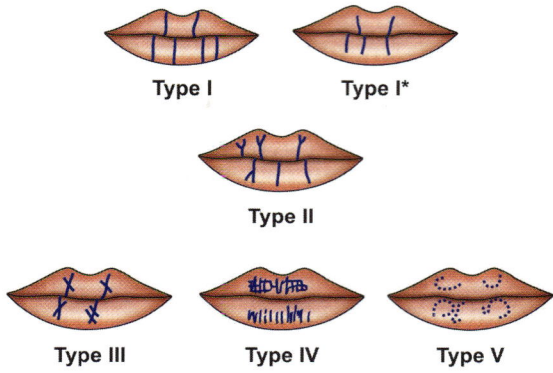

Type I Type I*

Type II

Type III Type IV Type V

Fig. 3.17: Lip prints

3. *Palato prints (Rugoscopy):* The folds present on the palate have been studied for identification. These folds are permanent and do not change with time. As availability of earlier palate prints for comparison is very less hence the role of palate prints is very much limited. This method was suggested by Harrison Allen.

4. *Venous pattern on back of hands:* Pattern of veins on the back of hands is different in different individuals, hence can be used for identification.

5. *Venous grooving pattern in skull:* Grooves created by the veins on the inner table of the skull can be used as an identification method provided earlier skull X-rays are available for comparison.

6. *Ear or nose prints:* Ears and nose shapes have also been tried for identification.

7. *Nasal sinuses:* Nasal air sinuses have different pattern in each individual, which can be utilized for identification. X-ray of the skull taken on different occasions can be matched for this purpose. Frontal sinuses are more commonly used for this purpose.

4 | Thanatology

Thanatology (Thanatos = death) is that branch of science which deals with various aspects of death like definition of death, causes, post-mortem changes and their medicolegal significance.

Death of an individual happens in two stages:

a. Somatic/clinical death
b. Molecular/cellular death.

SOMATIC DEATH

Complete and permanent cessation of vital functions of the body leads to somatic death. Earlier days only stoppage of respiration and circulation were considered to pronounce death of an individual, however, these days stoppage of 'Tripod' of life, i.e. stoppage in the functioning of respiration, circulation and brain are taken together to confirm death. Inclusion of brain death is as a result of following factors leading to uncertainty in confirming death.

Suspended Animation or Apparent Death

In suspended animation vital functions of the body are depressed to the minimal compatible with life. Vital functions like respiration and circulation cannot be appreciated in such a person, hence also known as apparent death. Such a person can be revived back with resuscitative measures. This stage between life and death is seen in following conditions:

a. *Involuntary:* Observed in hypothermia, drowning, electric shock or coma from drugs. Deep coma due to hypnotics or sedatives and hypothermia in elderly were of significance in including criteria of brain death.
b. *Voluntary:* Seen in yoga or trance.

Resuscitative Methods

Increasing use of the modern resuscitative methods which are used to maintain respiration and circulation has necessitated the inclusion of brain death.

Organ Transplantation

Demand for organs, which are suitable for transplantation has necessitated that these organs are removed almost immediately after death. Therefore, a person, if on respirator, can only be declared dead by following criteria of brain death.

Brain Death

Brain of a living individual has primarily two functions; (a) consciousness and related faculties and (b) maintaining vital functions of the body. When in a brain damage only the faculties of consciousness and communication are lost, the person is in deep coma but vital functions are maintained. Such an individual breaths spontaneously and his circulation is maintained, hence cannot be pronounced dead. Whereas, if the power to maintain vital functions is lost there is no spontaneous respiration or heart beats and the person is declared dead. If such a person is still maintained on the respirator or heart lung machine, due to edema, brain may undergo aseptic necrosis and liquefaction in 3 to 4 days' time known as *respirator brain*.

Criteria of Brain Death

The process for brain death certification includes:

1. Identification of history or physical examination findings that provide a clear etiology of brain dysfunction. Severe head injury, hypertensive intracerebral hemorrhage, aneurismal subarachnoid hemorrhage, hypoxic-ischemic brain and fulminant hepatic failure are potential causes of irreversible loss of brain function.

2. Exclusion of any condition that may confound clinical diagnosis of brain death.
   a. Shock/hypotension
   b. Hypothermia: Temperature < 32°C
   c. Drugs known to alter neurologic, neuromuscular function and electroencephalographic testing, like anesthetic agents, neuroparalytic drugs, methaqualone, barbiturates, benzodiazepines, high dose bretylium, amitryptiline, meprobamate, trichloroethylene or alcohols.
   d. Brainstem encephalitis.
   e. Guillain-Barre' syndrome.
   f. Encephalopathy associated with hepatic failure, uremia and hyperosmolar coma.
   g. Severe hypophosphatemia.

3. Performance of a complete neurological examination. Components of a complete neurological examination are:
   i. *Examination of the patient:* Absence of spontaneous movement, decerebrate or decorticate posturing, babinski reflex, response to verbal stimuli and response to noxious stimuli administered through a cranial nerve path way.

   ii. *Assessment of brainstem reflexes:*
   a. Pupils: No response to bright light (Size: mid-position from 4 mm to dilated state, i.e. 9 mm).
   b. Ocular movement: No deviation of the eyes to irrigation in each ear with 50 ml of cold water (tympanic membranes intact; allow 1 minute after injection and at least 5 minutes between testing on each side).
   c. No corneal reflex.
   d. No jaw reflex.
   e. No grimacing to deep pressure on nail bed, supraorbital ridge, or temporomandibular joint.
   f. No response after stimulation of the posterior pharynx.
   g. No cough response to tracheobronchial suctioning.
   h. Failure of the heart rate to increase by more than 5 beats per minute after 1–2 mg of atropine intravenously.

   iii. Absent respiratory efforts in the presence of hypercarbia. Generally, the **apnea test** is performed after the second examination of brainstem reflexes.
   The apnea test need only be performed once when its results are conclusive. Before performing the apnea test, the physician must determine that the patient meets the following conditions:
   a. Core temperature: ≥ 36.5°C or 97.7°F
   b. Euvolemia: Positive fluid balance in the previous 6 hours
   c. Normal PCO_2: Arterial PCO_2 ≥40 mm Hg
   d. Normal PO_2: Preoxygenation to arterial PO_2 ≥ 200 mm Hg.

After determining that the patient meets the above prerequisites, the physician should conduct the apnea test as follows:

1. Connect a pulse oximeter and disconnect the ventilator.
2. Deliver 100% O_2, 6 L/min, into the trachea by placing a cannula at the level of the carina.

3. Look closely for any respiratory movements (abdominal or chest excursions that produce adequate tidal volumes).
4. Measure arterial PO_2, PCO_2, and pH after approximately 8 minutes and reconnect the ventilator.
5. If respiratory movements are absent and arterial PCO_2 is ≥60 mm Hg, the apnea test result is positive, (i.e. it supports the diagnosis of brain death).
6. If respiratory movements are observed, the apnea test result is negative.
7. Connect the ventilator, if during testing:
   i. The systolic blood pressure becomes < 90 mm Hg or
   ii. The pulse oximeter indicates significant oxygen desaturation, or
   iii. Cardiac arrhythmias develop.

Immediately draw an arterial blood sample and analyze arterial blood gas.
a. If PCO_2 is ≥ 60 mm Hg or PCO_2 increase is ≥20 mm Hg over baseline normal PCO_2, the apnea test result is positive (it supports the clinical diagnosis of brain death).
b. If PCO_2 is <60 mm Hg and PCO_2 increase is <20 mm Hg over baseline normal PCO_2, the result is indeterminate and a confirmatory test can be considered.

Medical Certificate of Cause of Death

Medical certificate of cause of death is issued by a RMP mentioning immediate cause; antecedent cause; underlying condition along with other significant conditions contributing to the death (Fig. 4.1)

MOLECULAR DEATH

Molecular death means death of individual cells. Tissues take their own time to die. Vital centers of brain cells die in 5 minutes, muscles dies in about 3 hours, whereas, cornea takes still longer time to die and can be removed for transplantation within 12 hours.

MODES OF DEATH

Depends upon which system stops first french physician **Bichat** described three modes of death.

Coma
Coma is when brain damage leads to unconsciousness and there is failure of brain functions. Some of the reasons for death from coma are head injuries; hypnotic or sedative drug overdose; uremia or heat stroke.

Asphyxia
Death occurs as a failure of lung function. In such cases the respiration stops first. Some causes of asphyxia are lack of oxygen in

---

Medical certificate of cause of death:

Apart from mentioning the particulars of the individual who died in a hospital setup, cause of death is mentioned in the following manner.

I
A. Immediate cause: State the disease, Injury or complication which caused death and not the mode of death such as heart failure.   a. _____ (due to or as a consequence to)

B. Antecedent cause: Morbid condition, if any, giving rise to the above cause.   b. _____ (due to or as a consequence to)

C. Underlying conditions.   c. _____

II
Other significant conditions contributing to the death but not related to the disease or condition causing it.   _____

Fig. 4.1: Medical certificate of cause of death

the atmosphere, consolidation of lungs or mechanical asphyxia.

Syncope

Death in syncope is from stoppage of heart which usually results from hemorrhage, myocardial injuries, myocarditis, drugs affecting the heart or vagal inhibition.

CHANGES AFTER DEATH

Changes after death can be divided into three groups:

a. Immediate changes:
   i. Stoppage of respiration
   ii. Stoppage of circulation
   iii. Stoppage of brain functions
b. Early changes:
   i. Contact flattening and pallor and loss of elasticity
   ii. Eye changes
   iii. Cooling of body
   iv. Hypostasis
   v. Muscle changes
   vi. Biochemical changes.
c. Late changes:
   i. Putrefaction
   ii. Mummification
   iii. Adipocere formation
   iv. Entomology

Immediate Changes

These are the changes occurring at the time of death.

Stoppage of Respiration

Normally a person cannot hold breath for more than two minutes. Therefore, if a person is observed for 5 minutes, with no signs of respiration, is accepted as visible sign of death. Hearing breath sounds by placing a stethoscope over trachea is meant for medical practioners; however, (i) mirror in front of nostrils and looking for condensation of moisture, (ii) Winslow's test to see movement of reflected light from a plate filled with water placed over the chest or (iii) cotton or feather test by holding it in front of the nostrils and looking for any movement are meant only for lay persons.

Cessation of Circulation

In majority of cases, when heart stops functioning, then only the person is pronounced dead which may be there even when respiration has stopped. Hearing heart sounds by a stethoscope, feeling pulse and ECG showing a flat line confirms the stoppage of circulation. Other tests done to establish circulation are; (i) magnus test by tying a ligature around the base of a finger and observing the colour of the finger which remains white when circulation has stopped, (ii) diaphanous test by examining the web of fingers against bright light, which appears red when circulation is intact (iii) Icard's test by hypodermic infection of 1 ml of 20% fluorescein does not produce any yellowish discolouration to other parts of the body like conjunctiva.

Stoppage of Brain Functions

Which is observed when there is deep coma and the person does not responding to any stimuli, no cranial nerve reflexes, pupils are dilated and fixed with no EEG activity.

Early Changes

Pallor and Contact Flattening

Loss of muscle tone in the parts under pressures causes flattening, when the body is moved they remain as such. The area under pressure is pale and remains same when pressure is removed.

Changes in Eyes

After death (a) eyes seems to stare vacantly; (b) pupils assume a mid-position; (c) corneal reflexes disappear; (d) within minutes cornea becomes dry and hazy and then in about 10–12 hours becomes opaque, which cannot be removed by putting water; (e) sclera show triangular dark patches in about 3 hours, with base towards cornea due to dryness when the eyes are open (**Tache noire de la sclerotique** = French word for black patches on sclera); (f) ocular tension starts falling and becomes zero after 2 hours; (g) retinal vessels show fragmentation of blood column. In case chest is pressed these segments show movements known as **railroading phenomenon** and is seen immediately after stoppage of circulation; (h) optic disc becomes hazy in about 6 hours and (i) retinal colour changes to grayish yellow, starting from optic disc and reaches periphery in about 10–12 hours.

Postmortem Lividity or Hypostasis or Livor Mortis

Once the circulation has stopped, blood tends to pool gradually by the action of gravity, into the veins and venules of the dependent parts which produces a discolouration in that area. After about 1/2 hour of death, it appears as dull red patches, which coalesce and in about 6–12 hours an extensive area (dependent) is involved and colour becomes reddish purple. But this does not appear on parts where the body is in contact with hard surface like ground because of pressure, which prevents vessels from filling up. Hypostasis also occurs inside the body in various organs. Extent of lividity depends upon the volume of blood present in the body. Distribution of the hypostasis depends upon the position of the body, whenever hypostasis has fully developed and the position of the body is then changed, hypostasis will develop on now dependent portions but hypostasis already developed on earlier dependent areas does not fade or fades very slowly and incompletely. This is known as "**fixation of hypostasis**".

Surface tension and rigor mortis compressing the vessels not allowing blood to flow out are thought to be responsible for this.

Apart from knowing the position, sometimes from colour of hypostasis we can find out the cause of death like in mechanical asphyxia leaden hue is seen, cherry red hypostasis in carbon monoxide poisoning. Cold can also turn hypostasis pink, dark brown in phosphorus poisoning and cyanide poisoning produce brick red hypostasis.

Sometimes lividity on nondependent parts may be seen in small patches of 1 to 3 cm in diameter mostly present over upper front of the chest. They are caused by rigor mortis in the muscles of heart or vessels passing through muscles which are compressed in rigor mortis, causing the blood to move against gravity; these patches are known as antigravity hypostatic patches. Differences between hypostasis and bruise are mentioned in Table 4.1.

Muscle Changes

After death body muscles pass through three stages:
1. Primary relaxation
2. Rigor mortis
3. Secondary relaxation

1. Primary Relaxation

This stage is seen soon after death because of loss of muscle tone. All the body muscles are involved. No cellular death of the muscle cells

	True bruise	Hypostasis
Cause	Trauma	Gravity shifting of blood after death
Site	Anywhere	Present on dependent parts
Cuticle	May show abrasion	No damage
Swelling	Swelling present	No swelling
Edges	Not well defined	Well defined
Colour	Typical colour changes	Uniform in colour
Pressure effects	May be slightly lighter	Absent on pressure area
Extravasation of blood	Extravasation present and blood in the subcutaneous tissues cannot be washed away	No extravasation and blood can be washed away after giving a cut

Table 4.1: Differences between true bruise and hypostasis

has occurred during this stage hence they respond to electric stimuli. This stage lasts from 2–3 hours.

2. Rigor Mortis or Cadaveric Rigidity

This stage follows primary relaxation, when the muscles become stiff or rigid without any apparent shortening. During this stage molecular death of cells take place and involve all the muscles of the body, i.e. involuntary, cardiac and voluntary muscles. Because of rigidity of muscles, it requires some force to bend the joints, however, once broken rigidity never returns.

Mechanism of Rigor Mortis

Muscles are made up of long fibers which consist of myofibrils. These contain contractile proteins known as actin and myosin. Energy is provided by dephosphorylation of ATP (Adenosine triphosphate) which is required for contraction of muscles. Energy from ATP is also required for hydration and separation of myofibrils with the help of pumping calcium ions out of the cells. After death ATP is gradually destroyed, and this results in actin-myosin combination which is responsible for muscle rigidity with formation of gel like substance (Fig. 4.2). This stage persists till the protein complex is broken down by putrefaction.

Order of Appearance

It is initially seen in involuntary muscles and cardiac muscles followed by voluntary muscles. Small muscles are first to undergo rigor mortis in comparison with large muscles. Rigor mortis appear in following order, starting from jaw, head, elbow, arms, knee, hip and lower limbs.

Time of Appearance

Rigor mortis starts after 2–3 hours and takes 2–3 hours to spread to other areas of the body and is complete in 4 to 6 hours. In winter it lasts for 24–48 hours whereas in summer it normally of 18–36 hours duration.

Circumstances Modifying Onset and Duration of Rigor Mortis

a. *Age:* Rigor mortis is normally not seen below 7 months of intrauterine period. In children and old persons it sets in early and not well marked whereas, in healthy adults it is slow to develop and lasts for longer time.

b. *Conditions of muscles:* In exhausted muscles the onset is quick and of short duration.

c. *Manner of death:* In chronic debilitating diseases like Tuberculosis, Cancer or Uremia, onset is early and is of lesser duration. In asphyxia, apoplexy, paralyzing diseases onset of rigor mortis is delayed. In spinal poisons it appears early but last for longer duration.

d. *Atmospheric conditions:* In dry and cool climate it starts slowly and lasts longer. In warm and moist conditions it starts early but is of short duration. When the body is in water the rigor mortis starts early and is of longer duration.

Conditions Simulating Rigor Mortis

a. *Heat stiffening:* When body is exposed to high temperature more than 50°C or high voltage current passes through the muscles causes coagulation of muscle proteins. The body of the deceased may attain pugilistic attitude **(defensive or Boxer's posture).** Limbs are flexed at major joints. Heat stiffening may even be produced after death, in case the dead body is subjected to intense heat.

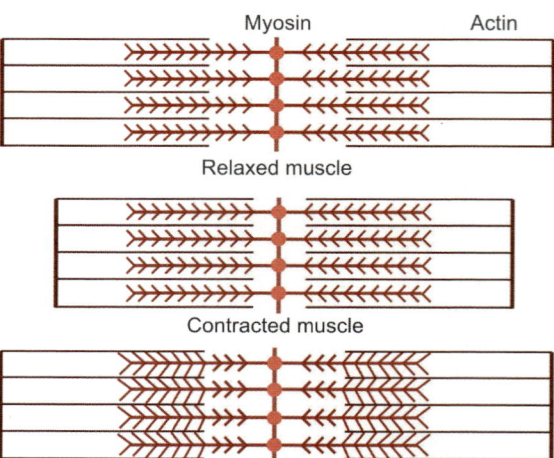

Fig. 4.2: Muscle fiber in stages of relaxation, contraction and rigor mortis

This stiffening cannot be broken easily, in case force is applied muscles gets torn. On postmortem examination affected muscles appears as cooked with extensive burns present over the body. Differences between heat stiffening and rigor mortis are mentioned in Table 4.2.

b. *Cold stiffening:* Seen when body is subjected to below freezing point temperature. Cold stiffening occurs because of solidification of body fats. This type of stiffness disappears when body is kept at warmer condition. This condition is followed by rigor mortis of shorter duration.

c. Gas *stiffening:* This type of stiffening is seen when gases of putrefaction collect in tissues making the body stiff. Such stiffening disappears when body cavities are opened to release gases of putrefaction during postmortem examination. All such cases show signs of advanced putrefaction.

d. *Cadaveric spasm or instantaneous rigor:* Muscles which are in contracted stage, becomes stiff without passing through primary relaxation phase. Only a group of muscles are involved. Mostly seen when the person before death was in mental tension or excitement or muscular exertion and death occurring suddenly. The attitude or posture remains same as just before death, which is helpful in finding out the nature of death like weeds in hand in drowning or gun held firmly in hand in suicide case. Great force is required to break cadaveric spasm. Differences between cadaveric spasm and rigor mortis are mentioned in Table 4.3.

Exact mechanism of cadaveric spasm is not known it is believed to be related to depletion of ATP present in those muscles. No molecular death of muscle cells has occurred but gradually passes onto the rigor mortis with death of the cells.

3. Secondary Relaxation

This is flaccidity of the muscles which follows rigor mortis. This is as a result of breakdown of protein complex formed during rigor mortis stage by putrefactive changes. The muscle cells are already dead hence they do not respond to electric stimuli as seen in primary relaxation. Muscle reaction is again alkaline whereas during rigor mortis it is acidic.

Cooling of Body

After death the body heat regulatory system does not function hence the body tries to attain the temperature of atmosphere. Invariably the atmospheric temperature is less than the body, except in extreme summers, therefore, the body starts loosing heat to the atmosphere. The heat loss is from the body surface. The temperature of the body for time since death

Table 4.2: Differences between rigor mortis and heat stiffening

Feature	Rigor mortis	Heat stiffening
Mechanism	Lowering of ATP below critical level	Heat coagulation of muscles
Onset	Takes 1 to 2 hour after death	Almost immediate when subjected to intense heat
Degree of stiffness	Moderate	High
When force is applied	It may break the stiffness	Muscles rupture
External appearance	Normal	Signs of extensive burns
Duration	Lasts from 12 to 24 hours depending on the weather	Till putrefaction
Medicolegal importance	Mainly indicates time since death	Only indicates exposure to intense heat and does not indicate whether burns are antemortem or postmortem.

Feature	Rigor mortis	Cadaveric spasm
Onset	Takes 1 to 2 hour after death	Immediate, no primary relaxation
Mechanism	Lowering of ATP below critical level	Exact mechanism not known
Degree of muscle stiffening	Less marked	More pronounced
Molecular death	Yes	No
Muscles affected	All body muscles	Only a group of voluntary muscles
Predisposing factors	Nil	Sudden death, exhaustion, tension, excitement or fear
Duration	Lasts from 12 to 24 hours depending on the weather	Gradually replaced by rigor mortis after few hours
Reaction to electric stimuli	No response	responds
Muscle reaction	Acidic	Alkaline
Medicolegal importance	Mainly indicates time since death	Indicates manner of death

Table 4.3: Rigor mortis and Cadaveric spasm

calculations is taken from the inner core of body.

How to Record Temperature?

To measure the inner core temperature of the body rectal thermometer (25 cm long) is inserted up to 10 cm into the rectum and left for at least 2 minutes. The temperature can also be measured by making a small cut below the right side ribs and placing the thermometer below the liver.

Frequent readings are taken approximately after each interval of one hour to measure the rate of cooling so as to calculate time since death.

Rate of Fall of Temperature

There is no fall in first 30 to 45 minutes; then a rapid fall at the rate of 1.4°C (2.5°F)/hour for next 6 hours, followed by a slow fall at the rate of 0.8°C (1.5°F)/hour during the next 6 hours.

Virtually Cooled Body

After body has cooled down to 85% of difference between atmosphere and the body is called virtually cooled as after that temperature fall is erratic and not predictable. Externally body reaches atmospheric temperature in 12–14 hours internal organs take 18–24 hours.

Factors Modifying Rate of Cooling

a. *Age:* Quick in children and old people.
b. *Sex and built:* Presence of fat in the body reduces heat loss, hence slightly slow in females.
c. *Atmospheric temperature:* If surroundings are of low temperature then rate of fall is quick.
d. *Cause of death:* It is rapid in wasting diseases.
e. *Exposed surface:* In mummy position 80% of the body surface loses heat, whereas in crouched up position only 60% of the body surface is exposed for heat loss hence the heat loss is slow.
f. *Clothing and breeze:* Clothing reduces loss of heat but breeze increases heat loss from the body.

Postmortem Caloricity

This is a rare condition when body temperature rises instead of falling after death. This condition is seen in following conditions:
1. Where heat regulating system was affected before death like in sunstroke or pontine hemorrhage.
2. Where there was great muscular activity before death like tetanus or strychnine poisoning.
3. Great bacterial infections like septicemia or cholera.

Biochemical and Enzymatic Changes

Various changes seen in the body fluids are helpful in estimating the time since death:

a. *Changes in CSF:* Potassium, inositol, NPN, creatinine and phosphorus show gradual increase after death.

b. *Blood:* After death there is decrease in the pH value of the blood due to increase in the carbon dioxide levels. There is increase in NPN to about 50 mg% during the initial 12 hours. Amino acid nitrogen and creatinine levels rise to more than 10 mg% in about 12 hours. Lactic acid, urea, potassium and magnesium also show increase, whereas there is decrease in chloride levels which is almost half after 72 hours.

In Indian conditions these changes are helpful in the initial period of 18 hours or so but after 24 hours their value decreases with the onset of putrefactive changes.

Various enzymes like phosphatase, transaminase, lactic dehydrogenase and amylase increase after death. They show rapid increase in the first few hours, after which there is linear rise for the next two days or till the putrefaction causes fall due to proteolysis.

c. *Eyes:* In vitreous fluid ascorbic acid and pyruvic acid decrease with time. NPN levels increase but is not reliable. Potassium levels increase show a linear relationship with time passed since death even up to 100 hours and can be relied for estimating time since death.

Late Changes

Putrefaction and Decomposition

After death tissues start undergoing decomposition by following methods:

a. *Autolysis or maceration:* Autolysis takes place in sterile conditions by tissue enzymes. There is softening and liquefaction of body tissues and is seen as maceration in dead born fetus or liquefaction of brain.

b. *Bacterial decomposition or putrefaction:* Bacteria present inside the body invades tissues and start their breakdown; Clostridium welchii plays a predominating role, along with streptococcus, staphylococcus, proteus and *E. coli.*

Externally putrefaction is observed as colour changes, gases formation and related changes.

In 6–12 hours during summer months and in 1 to 3 days during winter months there is appearance of greenish discolouration in right iliac fossa (formation of sulfmethemoglobin). Eyeballs become soft and cornea becomes hazy and white. There is nauseating smell coming from the body due to generation of Ammonia, H_2S, Methane, CO_2, Phosphorated hydrogen and mercaptans.

In 12–18 hours during summer months and in 3–5 days during winter months there is greenish discolouration that spreads all over abdomen, chest, neck and face. Superficial veins become prominent as degraded products of blood, stains vessel walls leading to "**Marbling of skin**". Fluid blood collects in serous cavities and there is increase in nauseating smell. The abdomen swells up due to formation of gases which may lead to escape of feces.

In 18 to 36 hours during summer months and in 6 to 10 days during winter months gases collect under pressure in tissues leading to bloating of features; eyes forced out from socket; tongue is protruded; bloodstained fluid comes out from mouth and nostrils; stomach contents may be seen coming out from mouth; scrotum is distended with blister formation. It becomes difficult to differentiate antemortem injury from postmortem injury. Maggots are seen over the body. Fliers lay their eggs almost immediately after death, which hatch in about 8 to 24 hours depending on the climatic conditions. Maggots migrate and get converted to pupa in 4 to 5 days and adult fly emerges from pupa after 3 to 5 days.

In 48 to 72 hours during summer months and in 10 to 20 days during winter months, rectum protrude out; gravid uterus expels its contents; hair becomes loose along with nails and brain gets liquefied.

In 3 to 5 days during summer months and in 20 to 30 days during winter months skull sutures in children separate and liquefied brain flows out. Teeth become loose and fallout from their sockets.

After this stage various body tissues start to liquefy and this is known as "**Colliquative putrefaction**" which is seen after 5 to 10 days in summer and after about 30 days in winter months. In this stage abdomen bursts open; chest may also burst open in children and gradually tissues become soft and loose seen as semi-liquid dark brown or black mass which separates from bones. Gradually cartilages become soft and ultimately bones may be left.

Internal findings: In the internal organs similar changes start from larynx, trachea, stomach, intestines, liver, brain, heart, lungs, kidneys and other organs whereas nongravid uterus and prostate putrefy in the end.

Putrefaction in water: Putrefaction changes are slow when the body is present in water in comparison to putrefaction in air. In deep buried bodies it is further delayed. This phenomenon is explained by "**Caspers law**" which states that if it takes 1 day in air, it takes 2 days in water and 6–8 days in deep soil for a body to reach similar stage of putrefaction.

Factors Modifying the Rate of Putrefaction
External
1. *Moisture:* Moisture enhances putrefaction.
2. *Temperature:* Maximum putrefaction changes occur between 21 to 38°C but below 0°C and above 48°C it is almost arrested.
3. *Air:* Free access increases whereas cold air retards putrefaction.
4. *Clothing:* Increase putrefaction in the early stages.
5. *Manner of burial:* Increases in damp and shallow graves.

Internal
1. *Age:* Retarded in newborn (lack of bacteria) and in old person.
2. *Cause of death:* Bacterial infections it is enhanced but retarded in anemic individuals and in some poisons.
3. *Mutilation:* Increases rate of putrefaction.

Adipocere Formation (Adipo = Fat; Cire = Wax) or Saponification

It the formation of waxy looking substance with greasy feeling; white or faint yellow in colour; having properties between wax and fat; melts on heating; floats on water; burns with yellowish flame; cheese like disagreeable smell (**rancid butter smell**) and becomes brittle when exposed to air.

Composition
It is formed of higher fatty acids like oleic acid, stearic acid, palmatic acid and hydrostrearic acid along with calcium soaps.

Mechanism of Formation
Due to gradual hydrogenation and hydrolysis of body fats, Adipocere is formed. Bacteria especially *clostridium welchii* producing lecithinase and body enzymes help in its formation. There is gradual increase from 0.5% in the free fatty acids to 60–70% when adipocere becomes visible to naked eye. Moisture and warmth enhance formation of adipocere, whereas the acidic media, running water, air flow causing dehydration of tissues retards its formation. Adipocere inhibits putrefaction due to dehydration of the tissues and increased acidity.

Therefore, it is mostly seen in bodies found in stagnant water or moist soil with little warmth.

Distribution
Seen mostly in areas where body fat is present like face, buttocks and abdominal wall. Mostly the changes are patchy but very rarely it may be seen involving the entire body. Even though the skin disappear but features are well preserved, which help in identification. Sometimes internal organs like liver may also show adipocere formation.

Time Required
It varies according to climate. In India, it may be seen as early as 15 to 21 days in summer months but in some rare cases it may be seen after a week. However microscopic changes have been noticed within few days. In western countries it usually seen after 3 months to one year.

Medicolegal Significance

a. Sometimes identification may be possible.
b. Antemortem and postmortem injuries can be differentiated.
c. Time since death can be ascertained
d. Place of burial could be made out.

Mummification

In this condition in place of putrefaction the body gets dehydrated and shriveled up due to evaporation of water from the body. The process starts from exposed portion of the body then gradually involve the rest.

Changes

Skin becomes dry, brown in colour and is adherent to the bones. Internal organs form a hard mass which gradually becomes dusty.

Predisposing Factors

a. Dry hot air or dry warm soil for a long period
b. Marked in deaths from dehydration
c. Chronic arsenic poisoning
d. Dry sandy soil
   Time required: 3 months to 1 year

Medicolegal Significance

1. Features retained to some extent
2. Injuries can be recognized
3. Time since death
4. Place of burial can be made out.

Entomological Changes

Forensic entomology deals with study of insects and other arthropods found on the dead body to determine the time since death and location of the body (Fig. 4.3).

a. **Using age and development of maggots:** This method is used within first few weeks after death. Maggots are the larvae or the immature developmental stages of the flies. Flies (order diptera) like blue bottle fly (calliphora), green bottle fly (lucilla) and common house fly (musca domestica) are initially attracted by the corpse. They lay their eggs usually in the wounds or moist area of the body soon after death. Depending upon the fly involved the eggs hatch into

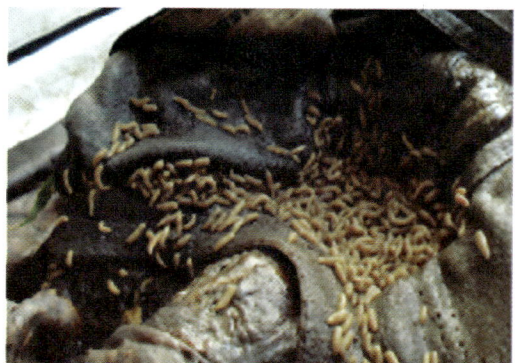

Fig. 4.3: Maggots

the first stage larva which then moults into second stage larva and subsequently into third stage larva. During larval stages they feed on the body and then migrate away from the body to pupate with hardened outer skin which gradually turns brown. Adult fly emerges from the pupa after number of days. Common house fly eggs which are white and about 1.2 mm in length hatch in about 12 to 24 hours depending on the season, first stage larvae moults in one to two days; same period is taken by the second stage larva to moults into third stage larva. Third stage larva takes about 3 to 4 days to convert into pupa and adult fly emerges from the pupa in another 3 to 5 days. Normally the complete cycle takes about 12 days or more depending on the weather conditions.

Collection of larvae: Larvae are collected after killing them in hot boiling water and preserved in a solution of 25% acetic acid and 75% alcohol. It may be difficult to differentiate maggots of different flies hence some larvae and pupae are kept alive till the adult fly emerges from the pupae. Maggots are kept in a corked glass tubes with a small piece of meat or muscle from the corpse. Care must be taken that too much food or too many larvae are not put in the test tube so that maggots may not drown in the moisture.

b. **Using successional waves of insects:** This method is used when the death has taken place few weeks back. During decomposition the body goes through rapid physical, biological and chemical changes which attract different types of insects at different intervals. Common house fly or blow fly are the first to get attracted by presence of body fluids or blood. Some insects arrive to feed on the other insects or larvae present on the body. Western literature reports that there may be eight different waves of insect invasion by different types of insects. However, due to fast rate of decomposition in Indian subcontinent all such waves are not possible. Literature may be referred for such interpretations.

TIME SINCE DEATH

It is the interval between death and postmortem examination to know the time when the crime was committed. Even though, in most of the cases it is difficult to give exact time of death. (Fig. 4.4)

Factor which help:

1. Cooling of the body
2. PM staining
3. Rigor mortis
4. Putrefaction
5. Forensic entomology
6. Biochemical and enzyme changes
7. Contents of stomach and rectum with reference to meal taken or defecation.
8. Bone marrow cells: WBC nuclei swell up in 1 hour becomes rounded in 4 hours and in about 10 hours the cell outline becomes obscure.
9. Growth of hair: Beard hairs grow at 0.4 mm/day after the last shave (1–3 mm/week) which may help in calculating the time of death.
10. Changes in bones: Green and smelling bones are recent whereas the dry and brittle bones are old bones.

Routine Method of Finding Postmortem Interval

a. Recently dead: Warm body with moist transparent cornea and no lividity.
b. 1 to 2 hours: Lividity just started and skin is cool to feel.
c. 2 to 3 hours: Rigor mortis has started and lividity patches are starting to coalesce.
d. 3 to 6 hours: Tache noir seen in the eyes, lividity fully developed.
e. 9–12 hours: Lividity and rigor mortis fully developed, optic disc margins obliterated
f. More than 12 hours: Signs of putrefaction with entomological studies.

EMBALMING

Embalming is done to preserve a dead body for transportation, wait for arrival of near relatives or anatomical dissection purposes in a medical college. Embalming has an ancient history. Egyptian used to preserve dead bodies of their pharos or kings. **Dr Thomas Holmes** is regarded as father of modern embalming. Contents of GIT, bladder and blood vessels are removed by suction apparatus and embalming fluid is injected in one of the major arteries either by gravity or by positive pressure. Some of the embalming fluid is also injected into body cavities, especially in autopsied bodies. Surface embalming may be required in burnt bodies.

Embalming fluids normally contains formalin (10%), methanol (55%), sodium borate and sodium citrate 15 gm each per liter, glycerin (20%), phenol (5%), eosin dye 5 ml per liter and perfuming agent oil of winter green 10 ml per liter of embalming fluid.

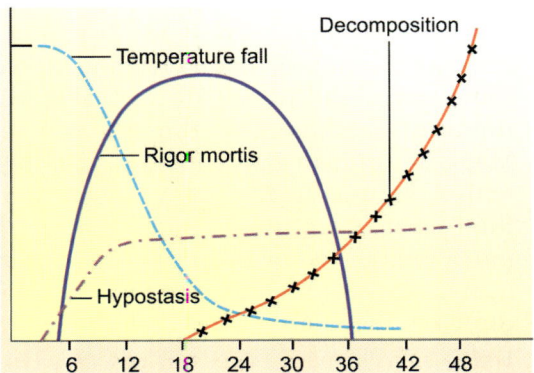

Fig. 4.4: Estimation of time since death

Before embalming dead body, consent from the relatives, death certificate and no objection from the area police and clearance in case of a foreigner from the concerned embassy are required.

EXHUMATION

Sometimes bodies are taken out from graves to find out the cause and manner of death. Therefore, such legal digging of a body from grave is known as exhumation. In criminal cases due to suspected foul play, injuries poisoning and abortions or in civil cases for identification or accident claims exhumation may be required. Some of the rules to be followed in exhumation cases are as follows:

   i. It is only done on the orders of a magistrate.
  ii. Should be done in the early morning time in presence of police and magistrate.
 iii. Spot should be identified by the relatives.
 iv. Earth from all sides of the body should be collected.
  v. One should stand in the windward direction.
 vi. There is no time limit in India to conduct an exhumation. Whereas in france it is up to 10 years and in Germany it is up to 30 years.
vii. Must preserve clothing, viscera, hair and other foreign objects.
viii. Autopsy at site but if it is possible, shift to the nearest mortuary.
 ix. Note the findings, people present and a rough sketch of the place.

Complete report is then prepared after completing the autopsy mentioning the magistrate's order, date and time of starting and completing the exhumation, person identifying the grave and the body, names of the person present, material collected including the earth samples and viscera. Sketch of the place is also enclosed with the report.

Presumption of Death

When an individual is missing for a considerable period of time and for inheritance, government service benefits to the family or for insurance purposes it is required to be established whether that person is alive or dead. Burden of proving him alive is dealt under *section 108 IEA* "the question whether a person is alive or dead and it is proved that he has not been heard for seven years by those who would normally have heard of him if he had been alive, the burden of proving that he is alive is shifted to the person who affirms it". Burden of proving that person is dead is dealt under *section 107 IEA* "when the question is whether a man is alive or dead and it is shown that he was alive within thirty years, the burden of proving that he is dead is on the person who affirms it".

Presumption of Survivorship

In case two persons of a family die under similar conditions simultaneously, it may be required to find out who died first and who died later for inheritance purposes. Mostly such cases are decided on the circumstances and other available evidence. It is presumed that adults survive for longer duration than young and elderly; males survive better than females; healthy individual will survive for a longer period than weak debilitated persons; Person with less severe injuries would survive for a longer duration than person with severe injuries or damage to vital organs.

THE TRANSPLANTATION OF HUMAN ORGANS ACT, 1994

This act was promulgated to provide for the regulation of removal, storage and transplantation of human organs for therapeutic purposes and for the prevention of commercial dealings in human organs.

Definitions

1. "Authorisation committee" means the committee constituted to evaluate norms as per THOA 1994.
2. "Brainstem death" means the stage at which all functions of the brainstem have permanently and irreversibly ceased and is so certified.

3. "Therapeutic purposes" means systematic treatment of any disease or the measures to improve health according to any particular method or modality.
4. "Donor" means any person, not less than eighteen years of age, who voluntarily authorizes the removal of any of his human organs for therapeutic purposes.
5. "Human organ" means any part of a human body consisting of a structured arrangement of tissues which, if wholly removed, cannot be replicated by the body.

Authority for Removal of Human Organs

1. Any donor may, in such manner and subject to such conditions as may be prescribed, authorize the removal, before his death, of any human organ of his body for therapeutic purposes.
2. If any donor had, in writing and in the presence of two or more witnesses (at least one of whom is a near relative of such person), unequivocally authorized at any time before his death, the removal of any human organ of his body, after his death, for therapeutic purposes, the person lawfully in possession of the dead body of the donor shall, unless he has any reason to believe that the donor had subsequently revoked the authority aforesaid, grant to a registered medical practitioner all reasonable facilities for the removal, for therapeutic purposes, of that human organ from the dead body of the donor.
3. Where no such authority was made by any person before his death but no objection was also expressed by such person to any of his human organs being used after his death for therapeutic purposes, the person lawfully in possession of the dead body of such person may, unless he has reason to believe that any near relative of the deceased person has objection to any of the decease person's human organs being used for therapeutic purposes, authorize the removal of any human organ of the deceased person for its use for therapeutic purposes.

4. The authority given shall be sufficient warrant for the removal, for therapeutic purposes, of the human organ; but no such removal shall be made by any person other than the registered medical practitioner.
5. Where any human organ is to be removed from the body of a deceased person, the registered medical practitioner shall satisfy himself, before such removal, by a personal examination of the body from which any human organ is to be removed, that life is extinct in such body or, where it appears to be a case of brainstem death, that such death has been certified by a Board of medical experts consisting of the following namely:
   i. The registered medical practitioner in charge of the hospital in which brainstem death has occurred.
   ii. An independent registered medical practitioner, being a specialist, to be nominated by the registered medical practitioner from the panel of names approved by the appropriate authority.
   iii. A neurologist or a neurosurgeon to be nominated by the registered medical practitioner from the panel of names approved by the appropriate authority.
   iv. The registered medical practitioner treating the person whose brainstem death has occurred.
6. Where brainstem death of any person, less than eighteen years of age, occurs and is certified, any of the parents of the deceased person may give authority, in such form and in such manner as may be prescribed, for the removal of any human organ from the body of the deceased person.

Removal of Human Organs not to be Authorised in Certain Cases

1. No facilities shall be granted for the removal of any human organ from the body of a deceased person, if the person required to grant such facilities, or empowered to

give such authority, has reason to believe that an inquest may be required to be held in relation to such body in pursuance of the provisions of any law for the time being in force.

2. No authority for the removal of any human organ from the body of a deceased person shall be given by a person to whom such body has been entrusted solely for the purpose of interment, cremation or other disposal.

Authority for removal of human organs in case of unclaimed bodies in hospital or prison:

1. In the case of a dead body lying in a hospital or prison and not claimed by any of the near relatives of the deceased person within forty-eight hours from the time of the death of the concerned person, the authority for the removal of any human organ from the dead body which so remains unclaimed may be given, in the prescribed form, by the person incharge, for the time being, of the management or control of the hospital or prison, or by an employee of such hospital or prison authorised in this behalf by the person incharge of the management.

2. No authority shall be given if the person empowered to give such authority has reason to believe that any near relative of the deceased person is likely to claim the dead body.

Authority for removal of human organs from bodies sent for postmortem examination for medicolegal or pathological purposes:

Where the body of a person has been sent for postmortem examination for medicolegal purposes by reason of the death of such person having been caused by accident or any other unnatural cause; for pathological purposes, the person competent under this Act to give authority for the removal of any human organ from such dead body may, if he has reason to believe that such human organ will not be required for the purpose for which such body has been sent for postmortem examination, authorize the removal, for therapeutic purposes, provided that he is satisfied that the deceased person had not expressed, before his death, any objection to any of his human organs being used, for therapeutic purposes after his death or, where he had granted an authority for the use of any of his human organs for therapeutic purposes after his death, such authority had not been revoked by him before his death.

Restrictions on removal and transplantation of human organs:

1. Save as otherwise provided, no human organ removed from the body of a donor before his death shall be transplanted into a recipient unless the donor is a near relative of the recipient.

2. Where any donor authorizes the removal of any of his human organs after his death, any person competent or empowered to give authority for the removal of any human organ from the body of any deceased person can authorize such removal, the human organ may be removed and transplanted into the body of any recipient who may be in need of such human organ.

3. If any donor authorizes the removal of any of his human organs before his death for transplantation into the body of such recipient, not being a near relative, as is specified by the donor by reason of affection or attachment towards the recipient or for any other special reasons, such human organ shall not be removed and transplanted without the prior approval of the authorisation committee.

Authorization Committees

1. The central government shall constitute, by notification, one or more authorisation committees consisting of such members as may be nominated by the central government on such terms and conditions as may be specified in the notification for each of the union territories.

The state government shall constitute, by notification, one or more authorisation committees consisting of such members as may be nominated by the state government on such terms and conditions as may be specified in the notification.

2. On an application jointly made, in such form and in such manner as may be prescribed, by the donor and the recipient, the Authorisation Committee shall, after holding an inquiry and after satisfying itself that the applicants have complied with all the requirements of this Act and the rules made thereunder, grant to the applicants approval for the removal and transplantation of the human organs.

3. If, after the inquiry and after giving an opportunity to the applicants of being heard, the authorisation committee is satisfied that the applicants have not complied with the requirements of this Act and the rules made thereunder, it shall, for reasons to be recorded in writing, reject the application for approval.

Regulation of hospitals conducting the removal, storage or transplantation of human organs:

1. On and from the commencement of this Act:
   a. No hospital, unless registered under this Act, shall conduct, or associate with, or help in, the removal, storage or transplantation of any human organ.
   b. No medical practitioner or any other person shall conduct, or cause to be conducted, or aid in conducting by himself or through any other person, any activity relating to the removal, storage or transplantation of any human organ at a place other than a place registered under this Act.
   c. No place including a hospital registered shall be used or cause to be used by any person for the removal, storage or transplantation of any human organ except for therapeutic purposes.

2. The eyes or the ears may be removed at any place from the dead body of any donor, for therapeutic purposes, by a registered medical practitioner.
   Explanation: For the purposes of this sub-section, "ears" includes ear drums and ear bones.

Prohibition of removal or transplantation of human organs for any purpose other than therapeutic purposes:

1. No donor and no person empowered to give authority for the removal of any human organ shall authorize the removal of any human organ for any purpose other than therapeutic purposes.

2. No registered medical practitioner shall undertake the removal or transplantation of any human organ unless he has explained, in such manner as may be prescribed, all possible effects, complications and hazards connected with the removal and transplantation to the donor and the recipient respectively.

Appropriate Authority

1. The central government shall appoint, by notification, one or more officers as appropriate authorities for each of the union territories for the purposes of this Act.

2. The state government shall appoint, by notification, one or more officers as appropriate authorities for the purposes of this Act.

3. The Appropriate Authority shall perform the following functions, namely:
   i. To grant registration or renew registration.
   ii. To suspend or cancel registration.
   iii. To enforce such standards as may be prescribed, for hospitals engaged in the removal, storage or transplantation of any human organ.
   iv. To investigate any complaint of breach of any of the provisions of this Act or any of the rules made thereunder and take appropriate action.

v. To inspect hospitals periodically for examination of the quality of transplantation and the follow-up medical care to persons who have undergone transplantation and persons from whom organs are removed.

vi. To undertake such other measures as may be prescribed.

Duties of the Medical Practitioner

1. A registered medical practitioner shall, before removing a human organ from the body of a donor before his death, satisfy himself:

   a. That the donor has given his authorization.

   b. That the donor is in proper state of health and is fit to donate the organ, and the registered medical practitioner shall sign a certificate as specified.

   c. That the donor is a near relative of the recipient and that the donor has submitted an application jointly with the recipient and that the proposed donation has been approved by the concerned competent authority and that the necessary documents as prescribed and medical tests, if required, to determine the factum of near relationship, have been examined to the satisfaction of the registered medical practitioner, i.e. incharge of transplant centre.

   d. That in case the recipient is spouse of the donor, the donor has given a statement to the effect that they are so related by signing a certificate and has submitted an application jointly with the recipient and that the proposed donation has been approved by the concerned competent authority.

   e. In case of a donor who is other than a near relative and has submitted an application jointly with the recipient, the permission from the authorisation committee for the said donation has been obtained.

2. A registered medical practitioner shall before removing a human organ from the body of a person after his death satisfy himself:

   a. That the donor had, in the presence of two or more witness (at least one of whom is a near relative of such person), unequivocally authorised before his death, the removal of the human organ of his body, after his death, for therapeutic purposes and there is no reason to believe that the donor had subsequently revoked the authority aforesaid.

   b. That then person lawfully in possession of the dead body has signed a certificate as specified.

3. A registered medical practitioner shall, before removing a human organ from the body of a person in the event of his brainstem death, satisfy himself:

   a. That a certificate has been signed by all the members of the Board of medical experts.

   b. That in the case of brainstem death of a person of less than eighteen years of age, a certificate has been signed by all the members of the Board of medical experts and an authority has been signed by either of the parents of such person.

   c. No facilities shall be granted for the removal of the human organs in the person required to grant such authority has reason to believe that an **inquest** may be required to be held in relation to such body in pursuance of the provisions of any law for the time being in force.

Duties as a Member of the Authorisation Committee

1. The medical practitioner who will be part of the organ transplantation team for carrying out transplantation operation shall not be a member of the authorisation committee constituted under the provisions of clauses (a) and (b) of sub-section (4) of section 9 of the Act.

2. Where the proposed transplantation is between a married couple, the registered medical practitioner, i.e. incharge of

transplant centre must evaluate the factum and duration of marriage and ensure that documents such as marriage certificate, marriage photograph, etc. are kept for records along with the information on the number and age of children and family photograph depicting the entire immediate family, birth certificate of children containing particulars of parents.

3. When the proposed donor or recipient or both are not Indian nationals/citizens whether 'near relatives' or otherwise, authorisation committees shall consider all such requests.

4. When the proposed donor and the recipient are not 'near relatives', as defined under the act, the authorisation committee shall evaluate that:

   i. There is no commercial transaction between the recipient and the donor and that no payment or money or money's worth as referred to the Act, has been made to the donor or promised to be made to the donor or any other person;

   ii. The following shall specifically be assessed by the authorisation committee:

      a. An explanation of the link between them and the circumstances which led to the offer being made.

      b. Reasons why the donor wishes to donate.

      c. Documentary evidence of the link, e.g. proof that they have lived together.

      d. Old photographs showing the donor and the recipient together.

   iii. That there is no middleman or tout involved.

   iv. That financial status of the donor and the recipient is probed by asking them to give appropriate evidence of their vocation and income for the previous three financial years. Any gross disparity between the statuses of the two must be evaluated in the backdrop of the objective of preventing commercial dealing.

   v. That the donor is not a drug addict or known person with criminal record.

   vi. That the next of the kin of the proposed unrelated donor is interviewed regarding awareness about his or her intention to donate an organ, the authenticity of the link between the donor and the recipient and the reasons for donation. Any strong views or disagreement or objection of such kin shall also be recorded and taken note of.

Punishment for Contravention of Any Provision of this Act

1. Whoever doctor removes the human organs without authority shall be punished with imprisonment for 5 years and fine up to 10000 ₹, along with removal of his name from state medical register for 2 years for first offence and permanently for subsequent offences.

2. Imprisonment for a minimum of 2 years, which may extend up to 7 years and fine for 10000 to 20000 ₹ for commercial dealing with human organs.

3. Whoever contravenes any provision of this Act or any rule made, or any condition of the registration granted, thereunder for which no punishment is separately provided in this act, shall be punishable with imprisonment for a term which may extend to three years or with fine which may extend to 5000 ₹.

5 | Sudden and Unexpected Death

When any person not known to be suffering from any serious disease or poisoning dies unexpectedly, such a case is subjected to medicolegal autopsy to establish cause of death. Forensic expert has to answer certain questions in such cases like whether the natural disease is the cause of death or an incidental finding or the cause of an accident.

All cases of sudden and unexpected deaths should be subjected to autopsy so as to confirm the cause of death. In case the autopsy surgeon is in doubt, he must take help of laboratory investigations at his command. These investigations may include histology, serology, bacteriology, virology, biochemistry and toxicology. There are few cases in which it may not be possible to assign a proper cause of death inspite of all investigations and are grouped under "**obscure or negative autopsy**". In about 10% of all autopsies the cause of death may not be ascertained to the full satisfaction of the forensic expert.

CAUSES OF SUDDEN AND UNEXPECTED DEATHS

The Cardiovascular System

Majority of sudden and unexpected deaths are as a result of involvement of CVS. Coronary artery disease, syphilitic aortitis, angina, myocarditis, valvular lesions of the heart, aneurism are some of the natural diseases causing unexpected deaths.

Coronary Artery Diseases

Heart attack as a result of coronary artery involvement is one of the reasons for sudden and unexpected deaths. Indians are quite susceptible to coronary artery diseases. Athromatus changes leading to blockage in the blood supply to heart involve various branches of the coronary arteries. Most frequently involved site is the Initial part of the left anterior descending (Anterior interventricular) from 45 to 64 per cent, followed by right main coronary artery from 24 to 46 per cent, left circumflex coronary artery from 3 to 10 per cent, main trunk of left coronary artery from 0 to 10 per cent and the least involved is right marginal and posterior descending artery (Fig. 5.1).

The occlusion of the coronary vessels may be from pure athromatus changes causing concentric or crescentric narrowing of the artery; thrombus formation on the athromatus patch due to ulceration; hemorrhage in the athromatus plaque (Sub-intimal hemorrhage) or very rarely periarteritis nodosa.

Sequence of events which may take place after coronary occlusion are (i) sudden death resulting from ventricular fibrillation by damage to the AV node or conduction system; (ii) myocardial infarction of the area supplied by the blocked coronary artery which may be full thickness, small satellite area in the heart muscles, sub-endocardial infarcts or papillary

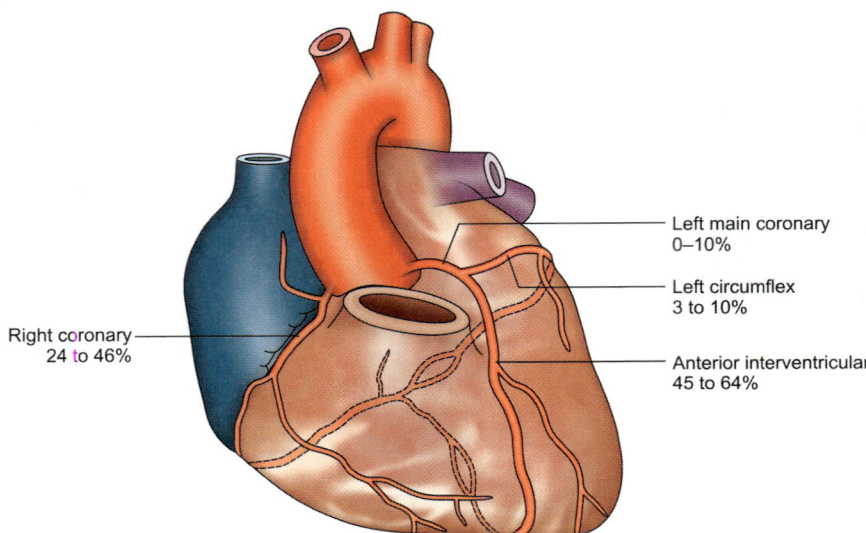

Left main coronary
0–10%

Left circumflex
3 to 10%

Right coronary
24 to 46%

Anterior interventricular
45 to 64%

Fig. 5.1: Coronary arteries atherosclerosis

muscles infarction; (iii) rupture of heart may take place after 2 to 3 days of the coronary occlusion due to necrosis leading to softening of the muscles, resulting in accumulation of blood in pericardial sac preventing heart to function properly and causing death from *Cardiac Temponade;* (iv) myocardial fibrosis occurs in the area having infarction which may be seen as grayish areas on postmortem indicating earlier infarction and (v) rarely myocardial aneurysm or pericarditis may be seen as a sequelae to coronary occlusion.

Demonstration of Myocardial Infarction on Postmortem Examination

Postmortem demonstration of myocardial infarction is of immense medicolegal importance, especially to rule out unnatural death and its role in traffic accidents. Unfortunately it becomes difficult to demonstrate changes due to myocardial infarction when the person dies immediately except for blockage in the coronary arteries:

a. Gross findings: There are no naked eye changes in the first eight hours of the coronary occlusion and in some cases very minimal changes may be noted even up to 18 hours. When the infarcted area is cut, it shows following changes:

i. *Edema:* Edema of the infarcted area is observed as the early change. The infracted muscles have coarsely fibrillar appearance, the muscles bundles appear separated showing grayish opaque sheen.

ii. *Colour changes:* Colour changes are observed after about eight hours of coronary occlusion. The infarcted area appears pale in comparison to the normal myocardium along with changes due to edema. This pale area gradually turns into brownish purple and to reddish. Sometimes, in about 24 hours, alternate bands of pale and reddish areas are seen in the infarcted region, known as *"tigroid appearance"*. By second day, with necrosis of the infarcted muscles the area assumes a yellowish discolouration with inflammatory reddish margins. Infarcted area becomes soft and gelatinous and is thus prone to rupture. Finally it is healed by formation of fibrous tissue in about a month.

b. Microscopic changes: Following changes are observed in histology slides stained with hematoxylin and eosin:

i. *Eosinophilia:* This is seen along with the swelling and granularity of the muscle fibers after 6 to 8 hours. There is increased reddening of the cells and is seen more clearly by using green filter.

ii. *Swelling of muscle fibers:* As a result of edema of the cells, intercellular space is reduced and intracellular partitions become indistinguishable. It is normally associated with eosinophilia.

iii. *Granularity of cytoplasm:* There is the typical cloudy swelling of the muscle fibers.

iv. *Blurring of cell membrane:* Cell membrane start to disintegrate due to necrosis.

v. *Corrugation:* Muscle fibers may show corrugation, in some cases the angulation may become sharp known as pinched appearance.

vi. *Increase in the interstitial cells:* Infiltration by macrophages may be observed after 8 hours of coronary occlusion. Polymorphs may be seen in the infarcted area after 18 to 24 hours.

C. **Histochemistry:** Many enzymes have been studied in frozen section. Some of them include lactate dehydrogenase, succinic dehydrogenase, and malate dehydrogenase.

Basic fuchsin technique: This technique of Lie and his colleagues used normal formalin fixed paraffin embedded sections to detect early changes due to myocardial infarction. This staining technique can detect hypoxic damage to myocardial muscles as early as half to one hour.

Periodic acid Schiff technique: By using this staining technique the infarcted myocardium can be stained purplish–pink.

Triphenyl tetrazolium chloride: This technique is also based on detection of dehydrogenases but is useful only after about 4 hour of the damage. Heart slice of 0.5 cm thick is incubated in 1% solution of TTC in phosphate buffer at pH 8 for about one hour. The normal myocardium takes up stain to become bright red whereas the damaged portion remains unstained.

D. **Ionic ratio:** Measurement of ionic ratio between potassium and sodium ions have been used for early detection of myocardial damage. Even Hydrogen ion exchange has been examined for the same purpose.

Myocardial Diseases

Lesions of myocardium may also result in sudden deaths. Apart from ischemic damage to the myocardium following conditions may be observed:

a. *Hypertrophy:* Thickness more than 1.5 cm of the left ventricular wall, 0.5 cm for right ventricular wall and 0.2 cm of arterial walls is taken as hypertrophy of the heart. This hypertrophy may result from hypertension, valvular diseases, and idiopathic cardiomegaly or associated with pulmonary diseases. Amyloidal changes are often found in hypertrophied hearts especially in elderly group. Heart may show hypertrophy of one side or both sides depending on the causative factor.

b. *Myocarditis:* It is the inflammation of the heart muscles indicated by exudative and inflammatory cellular reaction. Myocarditis may be of infective, toxic, autoimmune, metabolic, hypoxic or idiopathic in nature. Infective myocarditis from septicemia in rheumatic fever, streptococcal, meningococcal or in diphtheria may sometimes result in myocardial abscess formation.

c. *Alcoholic cardiomyopathy:* Consumption of alcohol can result in damage to the heart due to its direct toxic effects on the myocardium, nutritional deficiencies or beriberi heart disease. In toxic cardiomyopathy the heart is slightly hypertrophied, with scattered fibrosis in the ventricular wall mainly on the left side. There may be marked fatty degeneration of the heart.

d. *Neoplasm:* Primary tumor like rhabdomyoma, small fibromatoma causing pressure on the conduction system and rarely tumors of the AV node may be encountered. Secondary tumors are rare.

e. *Miscellaneous conditions:* Reflex vagal inhibition leading to cardiac arrest may be seen in trauma to vagal trigger areas, manipulation of internal organs, urethral dilatation, pleural puncture, intense fear or fright. There are no typical findings on post-mortem examination and the diagnosis is made on the basis of circumstantial evidence only. Drug induced anaphylactic shock with myocardial damage may sometimes result in sudden deaths. Hereditary conduction defects are rarely encountered.

Pericardium

Lesions of pericardium are (i) pericarditis following acute infection; (ii) hemopericardium from ruptured coronary, ruptured heart following myocardial infarction or adherent ruptured aortic aneurism and (iii) neoplasm from lungs may involve pericardium.

Endocardium

Subendocardial hemorrhages are mostly associated with sudden deaths when there is severe drop in blood pressure like in cases of head injury, obstetrical shock, arsenic poisoning, asphyxia, electric shock or bacterial endocarditis. Bacterial endocarditis may also be associated with formation of thrombus resulting in systemic thromboemboli. Fibroelastosis, a congenital anomaly may cause death in childhood.

Valvular Lesions

Congenital of rheumatic valvular diseases may contribute towards sudden deaths.

Aorta

Lesions of aorta commonly resulting in sudden deaths are coarctation of aorta, patent ductus arteriosis, hypoplastic aorta, and rupture of dissecting or atheromatous aneurism.

Respiratory System

Pulmonary embolism as a complication of the deep vein thrombosis is seen during pregnancy; intake of oral contraceptives or prolonged bedrest may cause sudden collapse and death. Massive hemoptysis in tuberculosis, anoxia due to obstruction in the respiratory passage from foreign objects, consolidation as a result of bronchopneumonia, acute respiratory infections especially in early childhood, diphtheria, acute pulmonary edema or status asthmaticus may be responsible for sudden death.

Central Nervous System

Majority of the deaths from CNS lesions are due to hemorrhages in the brain. Subarachnoid hemorrhages are mainly from; (i) ruptured aneurism in the circle of Willis; (ii) arterial malformations with weakness in the arterial walls; (iii) hypertension; (iv) blood dyscrasia.

Intracerebral hemorrhages are seen in the internal capsule region due to rupture of Charcot's artery a branch of middle meningeal artery. Hemorrhages may also be seen in pons or cerebellum. Primary pontine hemorrhage is mostly single, whereas secondary pontine hemorrhages are associated with head injury. Tumors like meningioma or glioblastoma normally lead to space occupying manifestations but fatal results are due to hemorrhage in these tumors. Infections like meningitis or encephalitis from bacterial, amebic or fungal origin may result in deaths. Falciparum malarial infections are a common cause of sudden death.

Digestive System

Haemorrhage, obstruction, perforation, peritonitis, herniation, appendicitis and tumors are some of the reasons of sudden death.

Blood

Deaths are frequently sudden and unexpected in most of the cases suffering from sickle cell anemia.

Metabolic

Hypoglycemia, Addison's disease involving adrenals, acute necrosis of pituitary gland in obstetric shock may result in sudden death.

Genitourinary

Hydronephrosis, pyonephrosis, chronic Nephritis, eclampsia and toxemia of pregnancy, ruptured ectopic pregnancy, twisted ovarian tumors and tumors are some of the lesions involving genitourinary system.

Miscellaneous

Death may occur from mismatched transfusion or anaphylactic reaction from drug usage.

6 Mechanical Injuries

INJURY

Injury (Section 44 IPC) denotes any harm whatever illegally caused to any person in body, mind, reputation or property.

Injuries bodily hurt can be classified on the basis of causative agents as:

Mechanical injuries:

a. Caused by blunt force impact/objects:
   1. Abrasions
   2. Contusions
   3. Lacerations
b. Caused by sharp weapon:
   1. Incised wounds
   2. Chop wounds
c. Caused by pointed objects:
   1. Stab wounds/punctured words
d. Caused by firearms:
   Firearm wounds
e. Fractures

Thermal injuries:

a. Caused by low temperature/cold:
   1. Generalized effect: Hypothermia
   2. Local effects: (i) Trench foot, (ii) Frost bite, and (iii) Immersion foot
b. Caused by high temperature:
   1. Generalized effects: (i) heat hyperpyrexia (sunstroke/heatstroke), (ii) heat exhaustion, (iii) heat cramps
   2. Local effects: (i) burns, (ii) scalds

Chemical injuries:

1. Corrosives (acids and alkalis)
2. Irritants (mercuric chloride)

Miscellaneous injuries:

This group includes injuries by:
a. Electricity
b. Lightening
c. X-ray radiation
d. Radioactive substances.

Injuries can also be classified according to legal provisions nature of injuries:

1. Simple
2. Grievous
3. Dangerous

They can also be classified according to manner of infliction:

1. Suicidal
2. Accidental
3. Homicidal

HURT: (SECTION 319 IPC)

"Whoever causes bodily pain, disease or infirmity to any person is said to cause hurt".

Wound

Wound from surgical point of view is any breach in the anatomical continuity of the skin or mucous membrane along with any other body issues as a result of mechanical force.

Mechanism of Wound Production

In the production of mechanical injuries the wounding force is supplied by the object striking the body or the body hitting an object (as in fall). This force produces traction or deformation strain which is resisted by the tissues depending upon their plasticity and elasticity.

Factors responsible for wound production: Wound production has a complex mechanism depending on variable factors, which may not be accurately assessed in each case. However following factors determine wound production:

1. **Nature of the object:** Shape of the object striking the body like sharpness, pointed or blunt object determine the area over which the energy is released. Therefore, in pointed or sharp objects the area over which the energy is released is very minimal.
2. **Amount of energy released:** Energy is released by a moving object when it strikes the body is equal to $1/2$ Mass $\times$ Velocity^2. Therefore the wounding power of a bullet is much more than a stone thrown at a person.
3. **Conditions under which energy is released:** Such factors include; (a) Pliability of area; (b) Time period over which the energy is released and (c) Whether body is free to move or not.
4. **Nature of affected tissues:** Tissues rupture when stretched beyond their elastic limits; hence, pliability and elasticity of the tissues modify wound production.

MECHANICAL INJURIES

Abrasion

Abrasions are injuries involving the superficial layers of the skin (epidermis), caused by friction or pressure between skin and some hard surface/object. Even though epidermis has no blood vessels, but tips of the dermal papillae projecting into the epidermis gets damaged in abrasion leading to oozing of blood. Hence, abrasions may bleed slightly but they heal without any scar formation.

Types of Abrasion

1. *Scratches:* These are caused by sharp object passing along the skin surface causing heaping of epidermis at the end, e.g. finger nails, pins, thorns, etc.
2. *Grazes:* These are caused by rough surface sliding over the skin and are mostly seen in a fall or being dragged on a rough surface. Show parallel lines with tags of epidermis. Brush burns are seen in traffic accident when body is dragged by a vehicle.
3. *Pressure abrasion:* These are caused by crushing of superficial layers of the skin associated with friction between the skin and the object with some movement; like patterned ligature mark reproduced in hanging or strangulation or bite marks.
4. *Impact abrasion:* These are produced by the direct pressure causing damage to the skin like radiator grill marks or tyre marks seen in road traffic accidents.

Age of Abrasions

1. Fresh abrasions are bright red covered with bleeding points.
2. In 12 to 24 hours lymph and blood dries up and form a scab which is soft and red.
3. In 2 to 3 days scab becomes hard and reddish brown.
4. In 4 to 7 days epithelium start growing inwards under the scab.
5. By 7th day the scab dries and falls off leaving a slight light coloured area which assumes normal colour in 10 to 12 days.

Medicolegal Aspects

Abrasions can provide valuable information in regards to following:
1. Site of impact
2. Possible object causing injury
3. Cause and manner of infliction of injuries like smothering or hanging, etc.
4. Direction of application of force.
5. Age of abrasion.

Abrasions are to be Dfferentiated from Following

1. *Postmortem abrasions:* These are mostly seen over bony prominences, yellowish and parchment like, exudation is less hence scab is thin and microscopic cellular reaction and enzymatic reactions are not observed.
2. *Erosion by ants:* There is characteristic brownish linear erosion with irregular margins, mostly seen on moist areas of the body like moist folds of the skin or mucocutaneous junctions and microscopic cellular reaction and enzymatic reactions are not observed.
3. *Excoriation by excreta:* Mostly seen in infants in the napkin area, pale yellow to deep coppery in colour and is parchment like.
4. *Pressure sores:* Mostly seen on the pressure points, coppery red in colour, infected at times and with relevant history of a person lying in same posture for days together.

BRUISE/CONTUSION

Contusion is extravasation of blood into tissues due to rupture of capillaries as a result of blunt force. It is normally seen in subcutaneous tissues without any breach in the continuity of the skin. Large collection of blood is known as hematoma.

Delayed bruising: Superficial contusions appear at once as a dark red discolouration, but deep seated bruises may take several hours to appear. It is advisable to have another examination after 48 hours to detect delayed bruising.

Patterned bruising: Shape and size of the bruise depends normally on the striking surface of the object, like rounded if caused by round end of a hammer or stick, elongated if caused by a stick. Cycle chain or belt causes specific pattern. A flexible cane or whip produces two parallel lines with intervening space equal to the width of the whip or cane. These two parallel lines are produced due to linear force causing break in the vessels along the edges of the stick. These parallel lines are called *"Rail track bruising".*

Gravity shifting of bruise: In certain areas of the body the bruise may not appear at the site of infliction of force but comes up at a different place. Deep seated extravasated blood gravitates to lower area and appears at a different place and is also known as *"Ectopic bruising"* like black eye in forehead injuries, or bruising around knee in thigh injury.

Factors Modifying the Appearance of Bruise

1. *Site of injury:* Bruising is more easily possible in those areas where the subcutaneous tissues are lax like face or genitalia and over those areas with bone underneath.
2. *Vascularity:* Vascularity of an area is directly proportionate to bruise production.
3. *Age:* Children and aged persons bruise easily.
4. *Colour of the skin:* Bruises are more evident in fair persons.
5. *Sex:* Female bruises easily especially if they are obese.
6. *Natural diseases:* Blood disorders, arteriosclerosis, clotting disorders, vitamin K deficiency, phosphorus poisoning may result in bruising with minimal force.
7. Gravity shifting of bruises and deep seated bruises.

Age of the Bruise

Age of a bruise can be determined by noting the colour changes due to degradation of blood pigments. Colour changes are noted on the periphery of the bruise as enzymatic action is visible at the periphery. Subconjunctival bruises do not show typical colour changes, they just turn yellowish and disappear.

a. *Fresh:* Red in colour
b. *Few hours to end of first day:* Bluish (reduced hemoglobin)
c. *2nd to 4th day:* Bluish black to brown (hemosiderin)
d. *5th to 6th day:* Green (hematoidin)
e. *7th to 12th day:* Yellow (bilirubin)
f. By end of 2nd week: Skin assumes normal colour

Healing of a Bruise Depends Upon

a. *Extent of bruising:* Bigger bruise takes more time to heal.
b. *Location of bruise:* Heals rapidly in more vascular area.
c. *Age of the person:* Delayed in aged person
d. *State of health:* Heals rapidly in healthy person.

Medicolegal Importance

Presence of a bruise in a person may provide following information:
   i. Site of impact
   ii. Degree of violence
   iii. Type of object
   iv. Manner of infliction or motive
   Bruises are of lesser importance than abrasions because:
a. Size does not correspond to the exact size of object
b. May appear after some time
c. May appear on some other site
d. Direction of force cannot be made out.

Bruises Are to be Differentiated from

1. *Postmortem bruise:* If considerable force is used within 2 hours of death slight bruising may be produced. However, other features of antemortem bruise are not present like:
   a. Swelling
   b. Typical colour changes
   c. Infiltration of blood in tissues
   d. Blood pigments are detected microscopically at site or in area lymph nodes which are seen after 12 hours of injury.
2. *Hypostasis:* After death sometimes the bruise has to be differentiated from hypostasis by noting the extravasation of blood in the tissues by giving a cut in that area and washing with water. Blood can be washed away in hypostasis but stain in the tissues cannot be removed in a bruise. Differences between hypostasis and true bruise have already been mentioned under hypostasis.
3. *Artificial bruise:* In case an artificial bruise is produced by applying some chemical agent or irritant substance, it can be differentiated by typical dark brown colour, irregular shape, vesicles at the margins, presence of itching and positive chemical tests from the site. Various differentiating features between a true bruise and artificial bruise are mentioned in Table 6.1.

LACERATIONS

Lacerations are tears in the skin, mucous membrane or parenchyma produced by the application of mechanical blunt force. They are caused when body tissues are stretched beyond their elastic limits.

Table 6.1: Differences between true bruise and artificial bruise		
	True bruise	*Artificial bruise*
Cause	Trauma	Application of irritant
Site	Anywhere	Accessible parts (self-inflicted)
Colour	Typical colour changes are seen	Dark brown
Shape	Mostly round or elongated	Irregular
Margins	Not well defined	Well defined
Vesicles	No vesicles are seen	Vesicles on the margins
Redness	At site	In surrounding area
Ecchymosis	Present	Absent
Contents	Extravasated blood	Acrid serum
Itching	Absent	Present
Finger tips	No changes seen	Tips may show discolouration with vesicles
Chemical tests	Negative	Positive for irritants.

Types of Lacerations

Split Lacerations

Split lacerations are seen when the skin splitting occurs between bone and the striking hard object, e.g. over scalp or shin of tibia. These injuries look like incised wounds; hence also called *"incised looking wounds"*. They can be differentiated from incised wounds by irregular edges, presence of bruising along the margins, hair bulb are crushed, tissue tags bridging the gap and less bleeding. Differences between incised wound and split lacerations are mentioned in Table 6.2.

Stretch Laceration

These injuries are caused by frictional impact resulting in overstretching and producing a flap. This flap indicates the direction of the force as seen in the glancing impact of the vehicle.

Avulsion Laceration

These are caused due to grinding compression of the tissues resulting in de-gloving of the skin by weight. The skin gets separated from the underlying tissues with bruising of the muscles underneath.

Tear Laceration

This is caused by impact against irregular objects like door handle of a vehicle which tears through the skin.

Cut Laceration

Caused by the blunt edged heavy weapon in which the skin is cut with bruising at the edges. Hair may be forced into the wound with involvement of the underlying bone.

Characteristics of Lacerated Injuries

1. Margins show irregular tearing at ends, diverging from the main laceration known as *"Swallow Tails"*.
2. Bruising and abrasion of the margins or of the surrounding skin.
3. Deeper tissues are unevenly divided.
4. Hair bulbs are crushed.
5. Less bleeding as vessels are crushed.
6. Shape and size may not correspond to the object causing the injury, like blunt end may cause stellate laceration, linear round object may cause Y shaped split at one end, linear object with an edge may produce Y shaped splits (swallow tails) at both ends.

Age of a Laceration

In uncomplicated wound, healing occurs by primary intention. Following features are noted to find out age of the lacerations:

a. *Fresh:* Bleeding is there.
b. *About 12 hours:* Blood is clotted, edges are red, swollen, if in approximation adhere with blood and lymph.
c. *24 hours:* Vascular bed start to form and the scab is formed.

	Incised wound	Incised looking wound
Fig. 6.2: Differences between incised wound and incised looking wound		
Location	Anywhere	Where bone is underneath
Edges	Regular edges	Edges are irregular if seen through magnifying lens
Bruising along the margins	No bruising is seen	Bruising or abrasions are present along the margins
Hair bulbs	Are cut	They are crushed
Tags bridging the gap	Not seen	Are present
Bleeding	Bleeding is more as vessels are cut	Bleeding is less as the vessels are crushed.
Foreign material	Not seen in the wound	May be present in the wound
Cause	Sharp cutting instrument	Blunt force

d. *By 2nd day:* Capillary network is complete (Granulation tissue).

e. *3 to 5 days:* Vessels show thickening, epithelium start growing.

f. 7th day onwards: Scab start separating and healing depending on the gap.

INCISED WOUND

These are produced by sharp edged weapons resulting in clean cut in the tissues. Incised wound is characterized by its length which is more than other dimensions, i.e. breadth and depth. Sometimes margins may be irregular due to "Rucking up" of the skin before the cutting edge especially where the skin is lax.

Characteristics of an Incised Wound

a. Clean cut edges.

b. Width is more than the cutting edge of the weapon.

c. Length is more than the depth and having no relationship with the length of the blade.

d. Shape is usually spindle shaped due to gaping.

e. Hemorrhage is more as vessels are cut.

f. From tailing of the wound (wound becomes increasingly shallower) the direction of application of force (direction in which the weapon has moved) can be made out.

g. In case the blade of the weapon is used obliquely there is "beveling" of the wound with overhanging margin.

Age of the Incised Wound

Age can be made out in the similar way in which the lacerated wounds are assessed.

Medicolegal Importance

Incised wounds provide following information:

1. Type of weapon used.
2. Site and direction of application of force.
3. Age of the wound.
4. Nature of death, i.e. suicidal (presence of hesitational/tentative cuts Fig. 6.1) or homicidal.

CHOP WOUNDS

Chop wounds are caused by heavy cutting weapons. These injuries mostly show abrasion or bruising of margins with deep cut reaching the underlying bone or even damaging the bone. Heel or toe of the axe may show typical *"signature fracture"* on the skull indicating relative position of the victim and assailant.

STAB WOUNDS

Stab wounds or punctured wounds are those injuries which are caused by sharp pointed weapons. Those stab wounds which enters body cavities are called "penetrating" wounds, whereas those stab wounds which pass through the body are called "perforating" wounds.

Characteristics of a Stab Wound

1. Length of the wound could be slightly less or more than the width of the weapon depending upon the relative movement between assailant and victim.
2. Depth is the greatest dimension, i.e. more than length and width.
3. Margins are clean cut if a knife is used. If the entire blade has entered there may be "hilt mark" at the entrance wound from the shoulder of the knife.
4. Both the ends are acute if caused by double edged weapon. In case the weapon is single

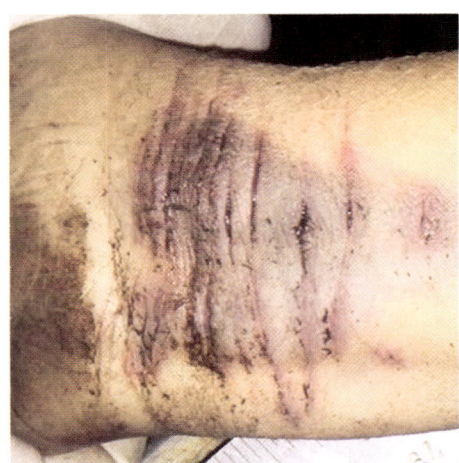

Fig. 6.1: Hesitational cuts

edged then only one end is acute and other end is round or triangular and may show some amount of bruising.
5. Direction can be made out by following the track of the wound.

Concealed Puncture Wounds

Punctured wounds are sometimes caused on the concealed parts of the body like nose, nape of the neck, fontanels, inner canthus of eye or natural orifices. While conducting autopsy on a small child, these areas must be carefully searched for concealed wounds inflicted for homicidal purposes.

Medicolegal Importance

1. Shape of the wound indicates type of weapon used.
2. Depth indicates the amount of force used.
3. Direction may indicate the relative position of assailant and victim.

4. Tentative cuts suggest suicidal wounds.
5. Tailing may suggest the direction in which the weapon was withdrawn.
6. Age of the injury form healing changes.

DEFENCE WOUNDS

These result from instinctive and immediate reaction of the victim to ward off an attack. These injuries are commonly seen on the hands and forearms.

FABRICATED INJURIES

Produced with some motive either to implicate some person or to pretending self-defence to avoid legal action:

1. *Self-inflicted:* Injuries are caused by the person himself
2. *Self-suffered:* When some other person produced those injuries with the consent of that individual.

7 | Firearm Injuries

Forensic ballistics is the science concerned with the investigation of firearm, their ammunition and problems arising from their use:

1. *Interior ballistic:* Study of various types of firearms, ammunition, projectiles and forces acting upon projectile while it is still inside the gun.
2. *Exterior ballistics:* Study of projectile while it is travelling though air or any other medium.
3. *Terminal ballistics:* Study of effects when projectile strikes the target. This also includes wound ballistics.

INTERIOR BALLISTIC

Firearm: Firearm is an instrument used for firing projectiles by the explosive force of the expanding gases produced by burning of explosive substance.

Construction of a Firearm

All firearms consist of a metal barrel. Barrel is a hollow metallic cylinder of variable length which is closed from one end by breech block and is called breech end. The open end of the barrel is called muzzle end. Inside of the barrel, at the breech end, is slightly bigger in size, where cartridge is loaded and is known as chamber. Leed or chamber cone joins the chamber with main barrel bore. Breech block contain the firing pin which is activated by pressing the trigger. To hold the firearm a handgrip or shoulder butt is provided.

TYPES OF FIREARM

Smooth Bore Firearm

Also known as shotguns. In these firearms the inside of the barrel is smooth. The barrel length may vary from 22 to 30 inches. They may be single barrel or double barrel (which may be side by side or on top of other barrel). These can also be classified as breech loader or muzzle loader. Projectiles fired from shotguns are called pellets or shots. Multiple pellets are fired in single shot from a shotgun.

"Bore" is the term used to describe the internal diameter of the barrel of a gun. This is denoted by number of lead balls of equal size having diameter equal to the internal diameter of that gun made from one pound of lead. Therefore, in 12 bore gun a lead ball of 1/12 pounds will fit in the barrel of that gun. This has no relationship with the pellets which are fired from that gun.

"Choking" of a gun indicate narrowing of the muzzle end of the barrel. Choking may be full choke, half choke, quarter choke or improved cylinder. Fortieth part of an inch (1 mm) of constriction is full choke, 20th part of an inch narrowing is half choke, 10th part of an inch of narrowing is quarter choke and 3rd to 5th part of an inch of narrowing is improved

cylinder. Choke attachments are available which can be attached to the barrel of the gun. Choking is done to reduce spread of pellets so as to increase the effective range of the gun.

Paradox gun: In paradox gun the terminal part of the shotgun show rifling.

Musket: It is a muzzle loader, smoothbore firearm, fired from shoulder used by armed forces and fires only single shot at one time. This gun is accurate to about 90 to 140 meters. This gun was primarily used from 14th century to late 18th century, eventually replaced by rifles.

Country made forearms: Very common in India and are mostly of 12 bore.

Rifled Firearm

In these firearms inside of the barrel has parallel spiral lands and grooves known as *"rifling"* (Fig. 7.1). These firearms have only one barrel and fires one shot at a time. These lands and grooves impart a spin to the projectile around its long-axis. This spin serves to gyroscopically stabilize the projectile so as to improve its aerodynamic stability thereby increasing accuracy of hitting the target along with increased range and penetration power of the projectile. Rifling is often described by the twist rate which is the distance rifling takes to complete one circle. Grooves are cut in the

barrel of the gun by broaching bit or forging the barrel over a madrel tool known as button. Projectile fired from rifled firearm are called bullets (Fig. 7.3).

Calibre of the firearm: Internal diameter disregarding depth of the grooves, i.e. distance between two diagonally opposite lands is known as "Calibre" of that gun. This is measured in thousandth of an inch or in millimeters (Fig. 7.2).

Rifled firearms are subdivided into two types:

   i. Hand-held, e.g. pistols and revolvers
   ii. Shoulder fired, e.g. rifles, light machine-guns, etc.

These rifles can also be classified depending on their firing mechanism:

1. *Single shot:* Slide action or bolt action is required to put the cartridge in the chamber and pull on the trigger fires the cartridge.
2. *Semiautomatic:* Only pull on the trigger fires the cartridge and empty cartridge is thrown or removed and a new cartridge is placed in the chamber and the gun is ready for the next fire.
3. *Fully automatic:* The gun keeps on firing till the trigger is pressed. In both semi-automatic and automatic guns the expanding force of the gun powder in the cartridge is used for actuation of the gun. Mechanisms used in fully automatic guns could be one of the following:
   i. Gas operated in which a hole is present near the muzzle end of the barrel connected

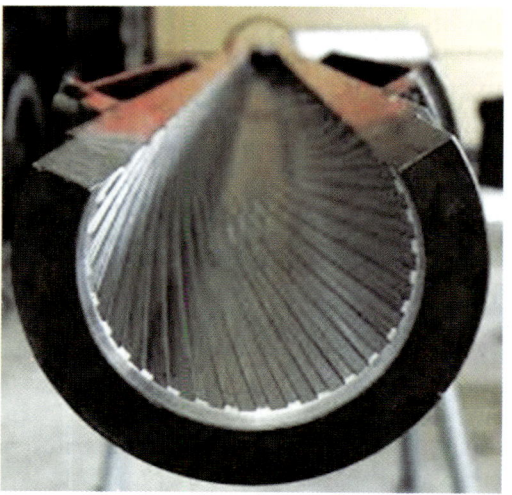

Fig. 7.1: Rifling inside the barrel

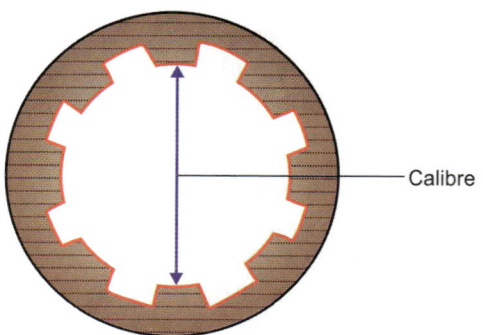

Fig. 7.2: Calibre of rifled forearm

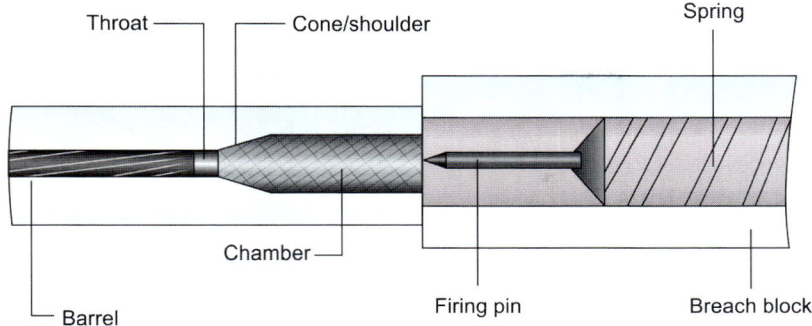

Fig. 7.3: Simplified model of a rifled firearm

with bolt mechanism. The expanding gases put pressure on the bolt for ejection of the spent cartridge case and cocking the gun for next fire.

ii. Recoil operated in which the barrel and the breech block moves backwards as a result of opposite action to firing of a bullet, which ejects the spent cartridge and compresses the spring for preparing the gun for next fire.

iii. Blowback operated in which the pressure in the chamber of the gun propels the breech bolt mechanism for ejection and cocking of the gun but is used in low chamber pressure weapons only.

These rifles can also be classified depending on the muzzle velocity of projectile fired:

1. Low velocity firearms: < 360 mtr/second
2. Medium velocity firearms: between 360 and 750 mtr/second
3. High velocity firearms: > 900 mtr/second.

Cycle of Firing a Cartridge

In order to fire a cartridge from a gun a chain of events take place so as to release a projectile from the gun:

1. *Feeding and chambering the cartridge:* This could be manual; in others magazine or clips may be provided for the same.
2. *Locking of breech bolt:* Breech bolt mechanism is locked before the firing pin is released.
3. *Release of firing pin:* Pull on the trigger releases the firing pin. The firing pin strikes the percussion cap. The primer ignites the powder charge resulting in intense high pressure from gases formed; cartridge case expands against the chamber walls and breech face. Increased pressure results in propelling the projectile.

4. *Unlocking of the breech bolt mechanism:* To help removal of the cartridge case.
5. *Extraction and ejection of the empty cartridge:* Every cartridge is having a rim or a groove (cannelure) at the base so that extractor or ejector can remove the spent cartridge from the chamber.

Ammunition Used in Firearms

One complete round of ammunition is called *Cartridge* (Fig. 7.4) or sometimes referred as shell or round, which consists of following parts:

a. Cartridge case
b. Percussion cap containing primer
c. Power charge
d. Projectile (bullet or pellets)
e. Wads and cards in shotgun cartridge.

Cartridge case

Cartridge case is completely metallic for rifled firearms whereas only the base is metallic for shotguns (high base or short base) and the rest is made of cardboard or plastic. Combustible cartridge cases are also available these days. Cartridge case maintain stability of various components of a cartridge.

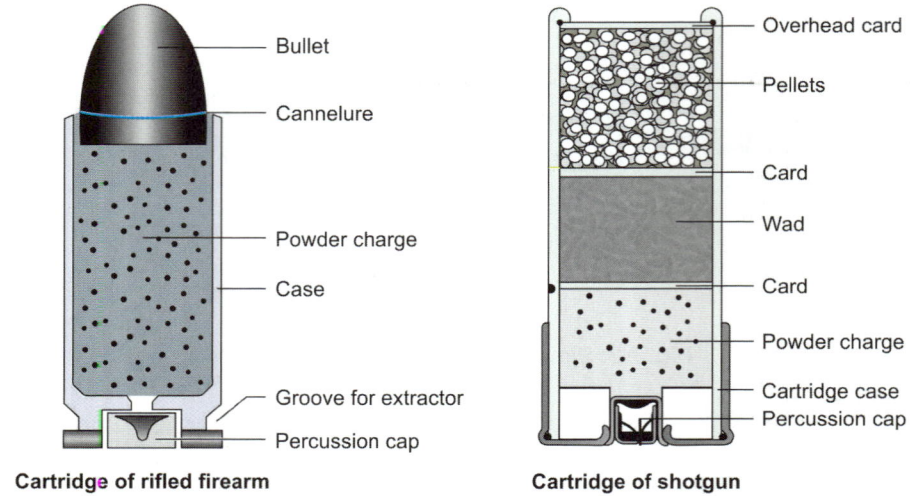

Cartridge of rifled firearm   **Cartridge of shotgun**

Fig. 7.4: Cartridges of shotgun and rifled firearm

Percussion caps

It is situated mostly in the center of the base of cartridge case. It contains primer, which ignites the powder charge when the firing pin strikes the percussion cap. Primer contains a mixture of potassium chlorate, antimony sulphide, barium nitrate, lead styphnate, mercury fulminate, tetrazine and lead per-oxide.

Powder charge

When it is ignited, form gases which in turn exert pressure over projectile and propels them. They are of following types:

1. *Black powder:* Consists of charcoal (15%), potassium nitrate (75%) and sulphur (10%). One gram on ignition produces about 3000 to 4500 ml of gases.
2. *Smokeless powder:* Mainly used in rifled firearms cartridges and consists of nitro-cellulose, nitroglycerin (high flame tem-perature) or nitroguanidine. When nitro-cellulose alone is used it is called "*single base*"; combination of nitrocellulose, nitro-glycerin is known as "*double base*" and when a mixture of nitrocellulose, nitroglycerin and nitroguanidine is used it is known as "*triple base*". Smokeless powder on ignition produces 12000 to 13000 ml of gases.

3. *Semi-smokeless powder:* It is the mixture of both types of powders, which commonly mixed in proportions of 20% of smokeless and 80% of black powder.

Projectiles

Projectiles of rifled firearms are known as bullets whereas the projectiles of shotguns are pellets.

Bullets

They are of various shapes and sizes. Mostly are made of lead in some cases it may be mixed with small amount of antimony to provide hardness, with or without copper and nickel or zinc jackets (*Semi-jacketed or full jacketed*). Tungsten bullets were also introduced with Teflon covering so that lands could grip the bullet. Nose of the bullet is normally rounded or pointed. They are fractionally bigger in size than the calibre of that gun so that they can grip the lands and rotate in the barrel. There are some special types of bullets:

a. *Dumdum bullet:* These bullets have hallowed point in front to cause more destruction at the target. Soft nose bullets are also of this category where the jacket is removed from the nose portion of the bullet. Ball mark III bullets have a small tube in the nose of the bullet.

b. *Frangible bullet:* These bullets disintegrate on impact.

c. *Gyro-jet bullets:* They have a rocket like mechanism so that the range can be increased.

d. *Tandem bullets:* When two bullets come out arranged one after the other are called *"tandem bullet"* or *"piggy back bullet"*. This may happen when weapon is defective and first bullet get struck inside the barrel, on subsequent firing, both bullets come out together. In some cases they may enter the body through single entrance wound but may come out separately making two exit wounds. Some military cartridges also contain two bullets; these strike the target at small distance from each other.

e. *Explosive bullets:* These have explosives in side them to explode on impact.

f. *Rubber baton rounds:* They are used to disperse the crowd. Initially they were made out of wood. These days they are made from rubber or PVC plastic. These are about 15 cm in length and 3 to 5 cm in diameter.

g. *Ricochet bullet:* Some cases the bullet before hitting the target is deflected from some surface or object. Such bullets produce irregular injuries. A bullet may ricochet even inside the body especially inside the skull and in rare cases may come out from the entrance hole.

h. *Souvenir bullets:* Sometime the bullet is not removed from a person and over a period of time thick fibrous tissue is formed around it.

Pellets

These are the projectiles fired from a shotgun and are mostly made out of lead Sometimes they are hardened by mixing antimony or by heating and cooling them. These types of pellets are called chilled pellets. The number of pellets in a cartridge varies depending on the purpose for which it is used. The number may vary from 6 pellets in LG (large game)

cartridge to dust. Slugs, even though fired from shotguns, have rifling marks or fins on them to provide stability in air.

Wads and cards

These are used in shotgun cartridges to keep various components in their place.

EXTERIOR BALLISTICS

Study of projectile after it comes out of the barrel and till it hits the target is done under exterior Ballistics. Following are some of the terms used in the exterior ballistics:

1. *Muzzle velocity:* Velocity of the projectile when it comes out of the muzzle end. In revolvers it is about 120 mtr/second (400 ft/second) to 370 mtr/second (1200 ft/second) and in case of rifles the muzzle velocity may be more than 1200 mtr/second (3900 ft/second).

2. *Tail wag/yawing:* Movement of the end of the bullet around the flight path (Fig. 7.5).

3. *Wobbling:* Entire bullet when fired at high speed may move in a circular manner around the longitudinal axis in the flight path. This may lead to release of high energy during this phase when the bullet strikes some object (Fig. 7.6).

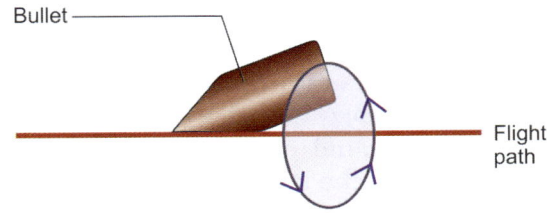

Fig. 7.5: Tail wag

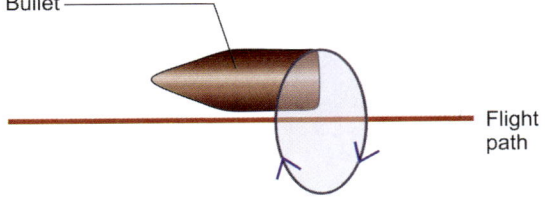

Fig. 7.6: Wobbling

4. *Tumbling:* During the last stages in the flight path the bullet may rotate and strike the target sideways is known as tumbling.

TERMINAL BALLISTICS

This relates to study of effects when projectile strikes the target.

Factors Modifying Wound Production in a Firearm Injury

1. *Velocity of the projectile:* The potential energy released is calculated by 1/2 mass × Velocity^2. Therefore, the velocity plays a greater role in wound production in firearm injuries.
2. *Shape and size of the projectile:* Pointed bullets cause less damage.
3. *Density of the tissues:* The energy is released proportionate to the density of the tissues:
4. *Hydrostatic forces in cavities:* In fluid filled organs/cavities the damage is more due to hydrostatic forces.

Firearms generally produce two wounds, one entrance wound and second exit wound. These are connected with track of the projectile. Entrance wound can be differentiated from exit wound by small size, inverted margins, presence of abrasion collar, blackening, singeing and tattooing. Detailed differentiating features are mentioned in Table 7.1.

Peculiar effects of firearms: In rare cases firearm injuries may not show typical injuries.
1. Entrance wound present but bullet not found inside the body: This may happen when the bullet comes out in feces, vomitus, coughed out or deflected through the same entrance hole (ricochet bullet).
2. Single entrance but multiple exit wounds: It may be seen when the bullet strike some hard object like bone and fragments into multiple pieces, or bone fragments act as missiles. In rare cases the tandem bullet may show this phenomenon.
3. Atypical wounds: Such wounds may be seen in ricochet bullet or when the bullet starts to tumble and strike sideways. Sometimes the bullet may graze the skin (Fig. 7.7).

Medicolegal Implications of Firearm Injuries

1. **Whether the injury is from firearm or not:**
   a. *By examining the injury:* Most of the times it is easy, but sometimes can be confused with stab wound. Sometimes surgical

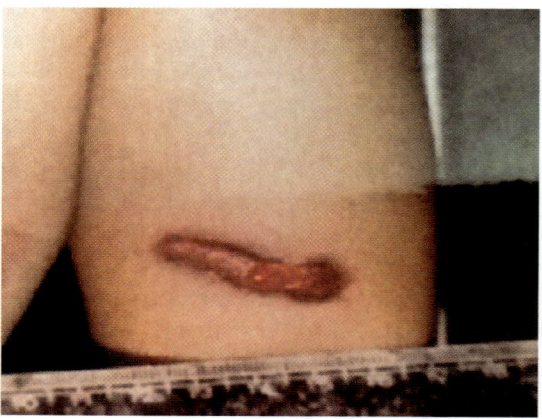

Fig. 7.7: Grazed injury by a bullet

Table 7.1: Differences between entrance and exit wounds		
Feature	*Entrance wound*	*Exit wound*
Size	Smaller except in contact range	Bigger in size
Margins	Inverted except in contact range	Everted
Blackening, singeing and tattooing	Present in close range	Absent
Fibers of cloth	May be seen going into the wound	Turned out
Tissues	May show cherry red discolouration	Not present
Abrasion collar	Present	Not seen
Muzzle impression	Seen in contact range	Not seen
Metallic ring	May be seen on radiological examination	Not seen

alteration or deliberately altering the wound may create confusion:

i. Kennedy phenomenon: Medicolegal evaluation of firearm injury made difficult by surgical suturing or alteration.

ii. Rayalaseema phenomenon: Medicolegal evaluation of a firearm injury made difficult by deliberate mutilation, e.g. cutting or stabbing through it or sometimes placing a fired bullet in a stab wound.

b. *By circumstantial evidence:* Someone hearing gunshot, presence of firearm, cartridge, bullet or pellets at the scene of crime may suggest use of firearm.

2. **Type of weapon used:** By examining the wounds the type of weapon used can be identified; whether caused by rifled firearm or shotgun. In case a gun is found at the scene it should not be touched unless fingerprints are taken.

3. **Type of projectile used:** Projectiles recovered from the scene of crime or from the body can help in deciding the type of firearm used. Projectile should be handled carefully while recovering them from the body. Try to avoid any damage or scratching to the projectile. The projectile should be removed with fingers or forceps covered with rubber tubing. Identification mark may be put only on the base of the bullet.

4. **Direction of fire:** It can be made out by examining the entrance wound and track of the projectile. When the bullet enters the skin perpendicularly the entrance wound is circular, but when it enters obliquely the entrance wound becomes oval and the abrasion collar is wider on the side from which the bullet has come. In near range the tattooing may also show the same findings. It can also be found out from the following:

a. *Bullet nose angle:* Angle made by the broad side of the abrasion collar from the length of the bullet.

b. *Sine Q functions:* Proportion of the minor line and major line distance of the entrance wound.

5. **Distance from which the gun was fired:** Distance from which the gun has been fired can be determined by examining the entrance wound. The distance from muzzle end and the target can be divided into three main groups (Fig. 7.8):

a. *Contact range:* When the weapon is held against the skin. In this the whole of the discharge containing gases along with bullet or pellets is blown in the track. Hence the entrance wound does not show any evidence of tattooing, blackening or singeing. The muzzle impression may be found around the entrance wound. The size of the entrance wound

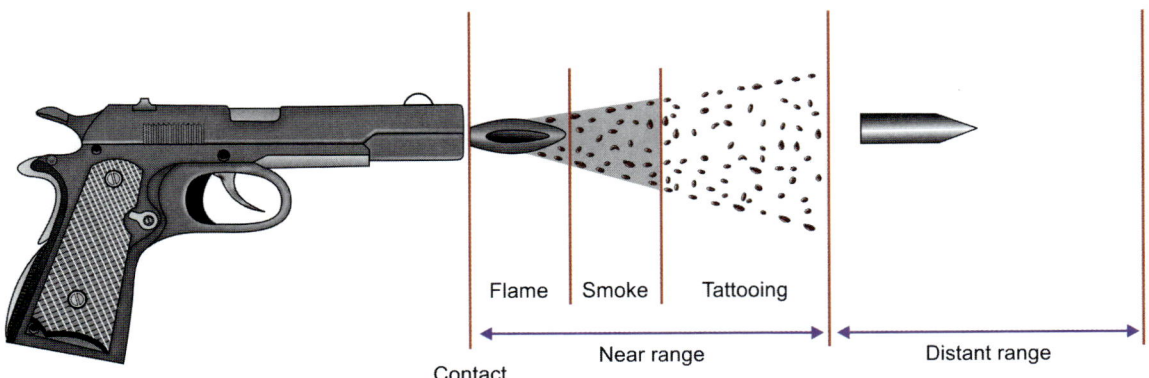

Flame | Smoke | Tattooing

Contact | Near range | Distant range

Fig. 7.8: Distance from which gun is fired

is large. In case there is bone underneath the entrance wound may show cruciate or elliptical splitting due to expanding gases (Fig. 7.9).

In cases the muzzle end is not in firm contact with skin, due to leakage of smoke and gases there is formation of *"corona"* around the entrance wound.

b. *Near range:* When the weapon is held away from the body but within the range of tattooing of that gun. In near range effects of smoke, flame and un-burnt powder particles are seen. Flame causes singeing of hair, blackening is produced from smoke and tattooing from un-burnt

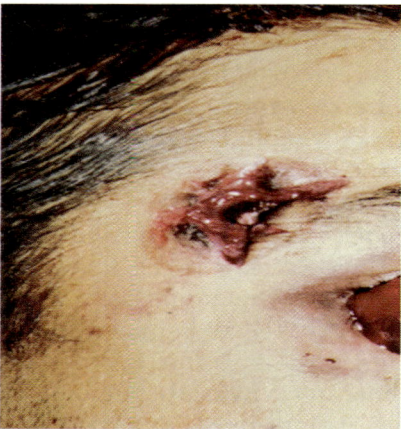

Fig. 7.9: Contact entry wound

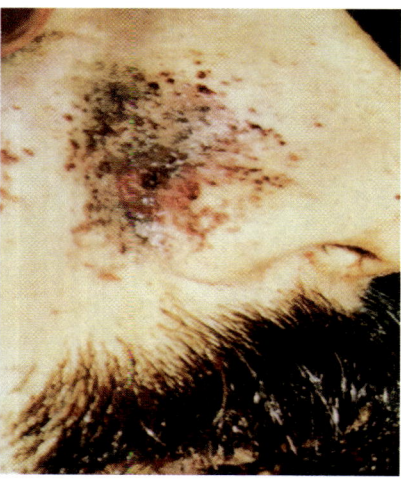

Fig. 7.10: Near range rifled firearm entrance wound

powder particles (Fig. 7.10). Distance up to which these changes can be seen depends upon the type of firearm and ammunition used.

When the body is covered with clothing the entrance wound may not show any singeing, blackening or tattooing as these things will present on the clothing.

Singeing or scorching is seen up to 7.5 cm in revolvers or pistols, up to 15 cm in case of rifles and up to 30 cm in case of shotguns. Blackening is seen up to 15 cm in revolvers or pistols, 30 cm in rifles and up to one meter in shotguns. Whereas tattooing is seen up to 45 to 60 cm in revolvers or pistols, up to 60 cm in rifles and 2 to 3 meters in shotguns.

Blackening can be removed by wiping the area with a wet cloth whereas tattooing cannot be removed and is permanent.

c. *Distant range:* When the distance is beyond the range of tattooing. It is difficult to find out the distance in case of rifled firearm beyond the range of tattooing from the entrance wound. Harrison and Gilroy test, Atomic absorption spectrometry and Neutron activation analysis for metallic ions like antimony in the metallic fouling at the entrance wound can be of some help in calculating the distance from which the rifled firearm was discharged.

In cases of shotguns the distance can be calculated by dispersion of pellets. After 2 meters the pellets start spreading and may show a large central hole surrounded by satellite small holes. After three meters the pellets enter individually and distance beyond this can be calculated by the spread of pellets.

Diameter of dispersion of pellets in cm/3 = distance in meters

However in choked gun spread in cm = {(distance-distance/4) −1} × 2.5

This way we can approximately have an idea about the distance from which the gun was fired. However, the definite opinion can only be given after test firing a particular weapon and noting down various effects at different distances.

Billiard ball ricochet effect: The spread of pellets may increase in case they hit some intermediary object like glass. Pellets which strike the glass show down and are hit by other pellets from behind to cause increased spreading.

6. **Number of shots fired:** In rifled firearms the number of shots can be calculated by noting the number of entrance wounds (Fig. 7.11). In some cases one shot may cause more than one entrance wound when it re-enters some other part of the body, e.g. a bullet piercing the arm may enter the chest. In shotguns mostly the shots are seen in groups. In case the person has been hit from quite a distance, counting the entrance wounds and comparing with the number of pellets in that cartridge or by finding different types of pellets if two different types of shotguns were used may give useful information regarding the number of shots fired. It becomes difficult to interpret which of the shot was fired first unless there is time gap between the fired projectiles. However, when bullets are fired into skull the radiating fractures caused by the second or subsequent fire normally terminate at the fracture lines of the first fire known as *"Puppe's Rule"*.

7. **Velocity of the projectile:** A bullet travelling at high speed causes clean, circular entrance wound and perforates the body. Whereas the low velocity bullets cause laceration at the entrance wound and can be easily deflected from some hard surface. A bullet coming out of rifle at high velocity show wobbling in the early part of the flight path for about 100 meters, therefore, on striking an object it liberates intense energy resulting in a form of explosion. This leads to gross lacerations and shattering of bones in a person hit from close distance.

8. **Time since fired:** Time since the gun has been fired can be calculated by examining the barrel of the gun for explosive gases like CO, H_2S, nitrates, sulphates and ferric salts. H_2S and CO are present for few hours whereas ferric, nitrate and sulphate salts increase in proportion to ferrous, nitrite and sulphide salts respectively, with time due to oxidation.

9. **Time between injury and death or the survival period:** This can be calculated from the age of the wound and also from the types of injuries sustained by the person. Always give a guarded reply regarding the volitional act in case of a firearm injury.

10. **Identification of the weapon used:** Weapon can be identified from the bullets or cartridges seen or recovered from the body of the victim or at the scene of crime.

Primary markings (class characteristics): Number of lands and their direction produces mark on the bullet and are known as primary markings. These help in finding out the type of gun used.

Secondary markings (individual characteristics): Irregularities in the barrel produces marking on the bullet known as secondary markings. They help in the identification of the firearm by comparing these markings with the test fired bullet.

Cartridges can also be identified by comparing it with test fired cartridge. Firing pin

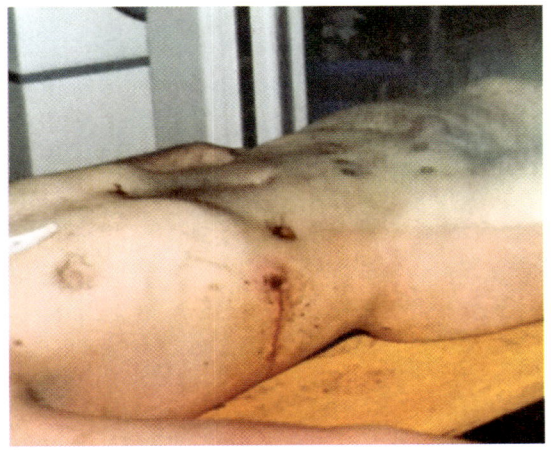

Fig. 7.11: Multiple firearm injuries from rifled firearm

mark, irregularities in the chamber, irregularities on the breech block or ejector may also help in identification of the weapon.

11. **Nature of injuries:** Circumstantial evidence, motive, type of gun used, distance of fire, number of shot fired site of injury, etc. are of great help in finding put whether the injuries are homicidal suicidal or accidental in nature.

12. **Dermal nitrate test (paraffin glove test):** It is done to find out whether a person has recently fired a gun or not. When the gun is fired there is breech flare (leakage from the breech end) which gets deposited on the hand. The test is done to detect nitrates or nitrites on hand by taking a paraffin mould of the hand and testing it with diphenylamine which gives blue discolouration.

8 | Blast Injuries

Blast or explosion injuries are traumatic injuries from direct or indirect exposure to the effects of blast. These injuries mainly depend upon the intensity of the explosion. Armed forces suffer injuries from the explosions in the wars; however, civilian population may also be affected from explosions at homes from blast of gas cylinders used for cooking, in mines from combustible gases, in factories from boilers or other combustible material and use of explosives by terrorists (Fig. 8.1). Injuries are more severe when blast occurs in a confined space.

High intensity blasts produces over pressure shock wave from rapidly expanding gases of explosion, which travels at supersonic speed for few milliseconds followed by negative

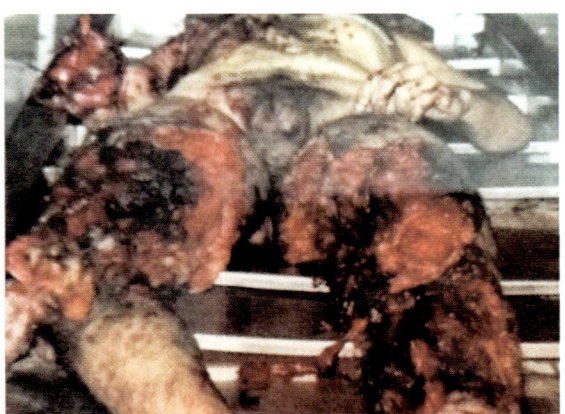

Fig. 8.1: Blast injuries

pressure wave. Degree of damage depends upon the following factors:

a. Distance from the point of explosion as the damage is indirectly proportional to the distance, hence more is the distance from blast less is the damage. A person present next to an explosion may be blown to pieces.
b. Medium in which explosion took place like water or air. As water is noncompressible so the pressure wave propagates rapidly with a slow rate of dissipation, hence there is greater potential for sustaining injuries in water than an explosion in air.
c. Presence of a person in a confined space. Shock waves may get reflected from solid surfaces like walls in confined space, resulting in greater damage.

INJURIES FROM EXPLOSION

Injuries produced from explosion are grouped under following four categories:

a. **Primary injuries:** Primary injuries are from the shock wave or over pressure wave. Main mechanisms of production of such injuries are pressure differential and implosion. Mostly there is absence of external injuries. Hollow organs, lungs and ears are primarily affected by the pressure wave. Ears most commonly show effects of the blast like ruptured tympanic membrane and damage to cochlea. Such a person may complaint of deafness which may be temporary or permanent and tinnitus. Ruptured tympanic membrane is indicative of other major organ damage in majority of cases. Lungs show severe damage with contusion, swelling, ruptured alveoli, vessels or even pneumothorax. The clinical picture of dyspnea, cough and hypoxia is referred to as "**blast lung syndrome**" and represents impaired gas exchange. Damage to gastrointestinal tract may be manifested as small petechial hemorrhages and contusions, however, perforations or ruptures are rarely encountered. These injuries are more frequently seen in under water explosions. Traumatic brain injury may also be as a result of primary blast effects. Death is mostly from blast shock initially followed by pulmonary edema and hemorrhages resulting in asphyxia or in some cases from air embolism.

b. **Secondary injuries:** These injuries are from the fragments or flying missiles propelled by the explosive forces. Material like fragments of container or metal shell shrapnel (antipersonnel bombs) and other materials like nails or metal pieces or nearby debris may act as flying missiles. Fragments may travel to many hundreds of meters to produce injuries. Sometimes the shattered windowpanes may act as shrapnel resulting in injuries. These fragments cause penetrating injuries resulting in blood loss or damage to vital organs. Sometimes the external bleeding is prevented by the impacted fragment but may lead to extensive internal hemorrhage in any of the body cavity. Amputation of limbs may be seen resulting in hemorrhage and death in some cases.

c. **Tertiary injuries:** Tertiary blast injuries are from the blast wind which may throw a person with great force against any solid object like a wall. The injuries are more severe in cases of children due to less body weight hence may be thrown to a greater distance. Resultant injuries are variable from contusions to fractures. Mostly blunt force injuries are seen in tertiary blast effects. Intracranial hemorrhages and contusions of brain substance may be seen and the person manifest loss of memory of events before and after explosion, confusion, headache, impaired sense of reality, reduced decision-making ability along with signs of concussion and post-traumatic stress disorder.

d. **Miscellaneous injuries:** Miscellaneous injuries are those which cannot be grouped under the first three categories like flash burns, injuries from falling masonry or toxic fumes. Temperature at the time of blast may reach 2000 to 3000°C resulting in burns directly from flames or from radiant heat. Psychological trauma can also be grouped under this category.

TREATMENT

Life support measures along with ventilatory help and fluids may be required at the site. Cases coming for treatment in secondary or tertiary treatment facilities require triage so that proper treatment to the serious patients could be expeditiously provided. Normally serious patient arrive late as they require ambulance services or buried person have to be excavated from debris and brought for treatment. Patient must be examined for any signs of poly trauma especially lung injuries and appropriate treatment including assisted respiration and oxygen inhalation, is initiated. Psychological help is equally important in all cases involved in blast effects.

POSTMORTEM FINDINGS

Aims of postmortem examination are identification of the dead body, to find out cause of death and ascertain cause of disaster as is done in mass disaster.

External Findings

Most of the cases show disruptive effects of the blast like amputation or lacerations. Body may be covered with dust, smoke or other debris. Typical features of traumatic asphyxia may be seen in person buried under debris.

Burns are frequently seen on the exposed portion of the body. Penetrating injuries from the flying missiles or shrapnel may be present on various parts of the body especially facing the blast.

Internal Findings

Lungs may show subpleural hemorrhages of different sizes. There may be pneumothorax. Lung parenchyma show hemorrhages. Mesentery and intestines show hemorrhages. Intestinal wall may be contused and edematous. Damage or perforations may be seen in the large and small intestines. Brain may show contusions, coup and contra coup injuries. Penetrating injuries from shrapnel may be observed along with damage to internal organs.

9 | Medicolegal Aspects of Injuries

On examining an injury case, a registered Medical Officer has to prepare an injury report. **Injury report** can be divided into three parts.

a. Preliminary information:
  i. Serial number of the report
  ii. Time, date and place of examination
  iii. Name, age, sex, occupation and address of the person
  iv. Details of the accompanying person and police
  v. Identification marks
  vi. Consent
  vii. History of the case.

b. Observations:
  i. *General physical examination (GPE):* Note down his conscious level, pulse and respiratory rate.
  ii. *Type of injury:* Whether injury is an abrasion, contusion, laceration, incised, stab or from a firearm.
  iii. *Location of injury:* Site of the injury, preferably in relation to any bony prominence.
  iv. *Size of injuries:* Exact dimension of each injury must be mentioned.
  v. *Any other information regarding injury:* Presence of any foreign article and age of injury related changes to be mentioned.

c. Opinion:
  i. Nature of injuries: Whether simple, grievous or dangerous.
  ii. Time since infliction of injuries or duration of injuries.
  iii. Type of weapon used and whether the weapon was dangerous or not.

NATURE OF INJURIES

Simple Injury

Simple injuries are those which are neither extensive nor serious and heal without leaving any disfiguration or deformity. Even though there is no clear cut definition of the simple injury in the law, hence those injuries which are not covered under grievous hurt are taken as simple injuries.

Section 323 IPC: Voluntarily causing hurt is punishable under this section for imprisonment up to one year or with fine which may extend to one thousand rupees or both.

Section 324 IPC: Voluntarily causing hurt by dangerous weapon or means is punished with imprisonment up to 3 years or fine or both.

Dangerous Weapon

Dangerous weapon is any instrument for cutting, stabbing, shooting or any instrument when used as a weapon of offence is likely to cause death.

Grievous Injuries

Under **Section 320 IPC**, following injuries are included under grievous hurt:

1. *Emasculation:* Deprivation of the masculine power by any injury is grievous injury.

Masculine power of a male could be related to potency or sterility. Therefore, any injury resulting in making a person sterile, (e.g. injury to testis or penis) or impotent, (e.g. injury to spinal cord) is labeled as grievous hurt.

2. *Permanent privation of the sight of either eye:* Any injury leading to permanent loss of the sight of either eye which may be complete or partial is a grievous hurt.

3. *Permanent privation of the hearing of either ear:* Any injury leading to permanent loss of the hearing of either ear which may be complete or partial is a grievous hurt.

4. *Privation of any member or joint:* Loss of any member capable of performing a distinct function or loss of a joint is grievous hurt.

5. *Destruction or permanent impairing of the powers of any member or joint:* Any injury even causing impairment of the powers of any member or joint is also grievous hurt.

6. *Permanent disfiguration of head and face:* Any injury which changes the personal appearance of a person provided it is permanent is a grievous hurt.

7. *Fracture or dislocation of a bone or tooth:* Any injury causing fracture or dislocation of bone or tooth is grievous hurt. However a superficial cut on the bone is not a fracture. Hairline fractures and loose tooth if proved to be as a result of injury are included under this clause.

8. Any hurt which endanger life or which causes the sufferer to be, during the space of twenty days in severe bodily pain or unable to follow his ordinary pursuits:

   a. Any injury which is likely to cause death as result of direct effects and can be ascertained by monitoring vital functions can be labeled as grievous hurt.

   b. Mostly it is difficult to prove that a person was in severe bodily pain for 20 days, but in case he was unable to perform day-to-day functions like taking bath, going to toilet taking food will render that injury as grievous. However mere stay in hospital or not attending office for more than 20 days will not render that person suffering from a grievous hurt.

Section 325 IPC: Any person voluntarily causing grievous hurt can be punished with imprisonment up to 7 years with or without fine.

Section 326 IPC: Any person voluntarily causing grievous hurt with dangerous weapon or means can be punished with imprisonment for life or imprisonment of either description up to 10 years and shall also be liable for fine.

Dangerous Injury

Any injury which causes imminent danger to the life of a person because of its direct effects is known as dangerous injury.

All injuries involving major blood vessels or vital organs of the body which normally prove fatal in absence of medical aid are grouped as dangerous injuries.

All dangerous injuries are grievous injuries, but all the grievous injuries are not dangerous injuries.

Section 299 IPC (Culpable Homicide): Whoever causes death by doing an act with the intention of causing death, or with the intention of causing such bodily injury as is likely to cause death, or with the knowledge that he is likely by that act to cause death commits the offence of culpable homicide.

a. *Explanation 1:* A person who causes bodily injury to another who is laboring under a disorder, disease or bodily infirmity, and thereby accelerate the death of that, other shall be deemed to have caused his death.

b. *Explanation 2:* where death is caused by bodily injury, the person who caused such injury shall be deemed to have caused his death, although by resorting to proper remedies and skillful treatment the death might have been prevented.

c. *Explanation 3:* The causing death of the child in mother's womb is not homicide, but it may amount to culpable homicide to cause the death of a living child, if any part of that child has been brought forth, though the child may not have breathed or been completely born.

Section 300 IPC (Murder): Culpable homicide is murder if the act by which the death is caused is done with the intention of causing death

or

Secondly: If it is done with the intention of causing such bodily injury as the offender knows to be likely to cause the death of the person to whom the harm is caused.

or

Thirdly: If it is done with the intention of causing bodily injury to any person and the bodily injury intended to be inflicted is sufficient in the ordinary course of nature to cause death.

or

Fourthly: If the person committing the act knows that it is so imminently dangerous that it must in all probabilities cause death or such bodily injury as is likely to cause death and commit such act without any excuse for incurring the risk of causing death or such injury as foresaid.

Exceptions when Culpable Homicide is Not Murder:

Exception 1: Culpable homicide is not murder if the offender whilst deprived of the power of self-control by grave and sudden provocation, causes the death of the person who gave the provocation or cause the death of any other person by mistake of accident.

Exception 2: Culpable homicide is not murder if the offender in the exercise in good faith of the right of private defense of person or property, exceeds the power given to him by law and causes death of the person against whom he is exercising such right of defense without premeditation and without any intention of doing more harm than is necessary for the purpose of such defense.

Exception 3: Culpable homicide is not murder if the offender, being a public servant or aiding public servant acting for the advancement of the public justice exceeds the powers given to him by law and causes death by doing an act which he, in good faith, believes to be lawful and necessary for due discharge of his duty as such public servant and without ill-will towards the person whose death is caused.

Exception 4: Culpable homicide is not murder if it is committed without premeditation in a sudden fight in the heat of passion upon a sudden quarrel and without the offenders having taken undue advantage or acted in a cruel or unusual manner.

Exception 5: Culpable homicide is not murder when the person whose death is caused being above the age of eighteen years suffers death or takes the risk of death with his own consent.

Section 302 IPC *(punishment for murder):* Whoever commits murder shall be punished with death or imprisonment for life and shall also be liable to fine. These days capital punishment is awarded in rare of rare cases.

Section 304 IPC *(punishment for culpable homicide not amounting to murder):* Whoever commits culpable homicide not amounting to murder if the act by which the death is caused is done with the intention of causing death or such bodily injury as is likely to cause death, shall be punished with imprisonment for life or imprisonment of either description which may extend to ten years and also liable to fine.

If the act is done without any intention of causing death or to cause such bodily injury as is likely to cause death the punishment is imprisonment of either description which may extend to ten years with or without fine.

Section 304-A IPC *(causing death by negligence):* Whoever causes death of any person by doing any rash or negligent act not amounting to culpable homicide shall be punished with imprisonment of either description for a term which may extend to two years with or without fine.

Section 307 IPC *(attempt to murder):* Whoever does an act with such intention or knowledge and under such circumstances that he by that act caused death, he would be guilty of murder, shall be punished with imprisonment of either description which may extend to 10 years and shall also be liable to fine; if hurt is caused by that act the offender shall be liable either to imprisonment for life or punishment as herein before mentioned.

Section 308 IPC (attempt to commit culpable homicide): Whoever does an act with such intention or knowledge and under such circumstances that if he by that act caused death, he would be guilty of culpable homicide not amounting to murder, shall be punished with imprisonment of either description which may extend to 3 years with or without fine; if hurt is caused by that act the offender shall be liable either to imprisonment of either description which may extend to 7 years with or without fine.

CAUSES OF DEATH FROM INJURIES

Causes of death from injuries can be divided into three groups:

1. Immediate causes of death:
   a. Hemorrhage
   b. Shock
   c. Injury to vital organs
2. Secondary causes of death:
   a. Infections
   b. Crush syndrome
   c. Thrombosis
   d. Embolism
3. Indirect causes of death.

Immediate Causes of Death

Hemorrhage

Hemorrhage can be external or internal. External blood loss mostly results in marked fall of blood pressure and death occurs from secondary shock. Amount of blood loss required to cause shock varies according to circumstances. Sudden loss of about 1/3 of circulating blood volume (total blood is 5–6% of the total body weight) is sufficient to cause death. But if the loss is slow, i.e. over a period of time then the person may be able to withstand this loss. Hemorrhage is often termed as primary, reactionary and secondary hemorrhage. Primary hemorrhage occurs from the injured blood vessels. But if the hemorrhage starts again after sometime up to 24–36 hours this is known as reactionary hemorrhage. Reactionary hemorrhage mostly results from rise in blood pressure in the recovery phase or loosening of a clot following muscular movements. Secondary hemorrhage results after infection has set in resulting in erosion of vessel wall, which normally takes place after a week or two.

Internal hemorrhage is more dangerous, sometimes even small amounts may cause death especially when takes place in brain substance. About 400 ml of blood in pericardial sac can result in death from cardiac temponade.

Shock

Shock is a form of circulatory disturbance characterized by reduction of blood flow in the peripheral vascular bed and inadequate tissue oxygenation. Perfusion pressure for oxygenation is dependent upon cardiac output and vascular resistance. Any factor affecting these two shall lead to shock:

1. **Primary shock:** Also known as neurogenic shock. Sudden death from neurogenic shock may occur when any receptor area of vagus nerve is stimulated, e.g. blow in the solar plexus, or in the genitals resulting in reflex vagal inhibition of the heart.

   Primary shock may also result from fear, fright or emotions. These cause sympathico-adrenal stimulation of the circulation resulting in sudden reduction in the venous blood flow back to heart due to peripheral pooling of the blood. There is yawing, sighing, dilatation of pupils, sweating rapid pulse followed by unconsciousness. In majority of such cases the person recovers in few minutes.

2. **Secondary shock:** In secondary shock the circulatory failure is gradual over a period of time therefore; it is also known as delayed shock. It can be subgrouped into cardiac, extracardiac and miscellaneous types.

Secondary shock is primarily due to hypovolemic conditions. Reduction of the blood volume is mainly as a result of the following factors:

a. Loss of blood or plasma following injury or burns.

b. Loss of body fluids by vomiting or diarrhea.

c. Increased capillary permeability leading to escape of fluids into the body tissues resulting from anoxic damage, bacterial sepsis or burn toxemia.

d. Failure of the pumping mechanism from damage to the heart.

Body tries to compensate this reduction in the blood volume by various means. With appropriate treatment in most of the cases of shock the circulation can be re-established and such type are known as *"reversible shock"*. But in cases were body compensatory mechanism fail and in spite of the best medical efforts condition of the patient gradually deteriorate leading to the death is called *"irreversible shock"*.

Postmortem Appearance

There may not be any postmortem findings in case of deaths from primary shock especially when the death is from vagal inhibition.

In cases of deaths from secondary shock the postmortem findings are of nonspecific nature. There is wide spread petechial hemorrhages, edema of various tissues with degeneration or necrosis of various organs:

a. *Gastrointestinal tract:* Mucosa is often congested, showing ulceration at places. Intravascular thrombosis may be seen as a result of blood stasis.

b. *Kidneys:* Kidneys are normal in size or slightly enlarged. There is severe tubular degeneration especially of the distal convoluted tubules, known as "shock kidney". However mostly lesion are scattered at random among nephrons and may be found in any part of the nephron. Casts are present. These changes are seen in about

24 hours and become marked in another 7 to 10 days.

c. *Heart:* Heart muscles show fatty degeneration in about 50% of cases.

d. *Liver:* Fatty degeneration is the main feature.

e. *Lungs:* Lungs are congested and edematous.

f. *Adrenals:* Lipid depletion from cortical area is seen after 24 hours along with focal necrosis.

Injury to Vital Organs

Severe injury to a vital organ or a major blood vessel can cause immediate death of a person.

Secondary Causes of Death

These include

Infection

Wound infection may take place from the organisms present:

i. On the skin, gastrointestinal tract or respiratory tract

ii. Organisms present in the environment, e.g. organism present in air, clothing or dressing.

These infections of the wound may result in septicemia or pyemia. In some cases death may result from infection reaching internal organs like meninges, lungs or abdominal cavity resulting in meningitis, pneumonia or peritonitis. In some cases tetanus or gas gangrene may supervene, especially in crush injuries resulting in death.

Crush Syndrome

In cases where severe damage of the muscles of the body occurs as a result of crushing of the limbs in an accident, damage is seen in the renal tubules leading to renal failure and death in such cases.

Acute tubular necrosis mainly in the distal convoluted tubules results from blockage of tubules by cellular and metabolic produces resulting from crushing of muscles but some are of the opinion that tubular necrosis result from renal ischemia.

Thrombosis

Thrombosis may develop at the site of the injuries when vessel wall is damaged or may occur in the leg veins when the person remains immobilized for some time.

Rarely thrombosis may occur in heart especially over valves, in dural venous sinuses or in aneurisms caused by trauma.

Death mostly occurs when a thrombus detaches from the vessel wall and block some important vessel, e.g. pulmonary trunk.

Main three factors responsible for the formation of the thrombus are known as "Virtue's Triad":

  i. Changes in the intima of the vessels
  ii. Changes in the velocity of the blood-stream.
  iii. Changes in the constitution of the blood mainly the platelets.

Embolism

Embolism is occlusion of blood vessel by any mass known as embolus, transported through the circulation, originating from within the body or from outside the body. They are classified as follows:

1. External embolism:
  a. Foreign body, e.g. bullet.
  b. Foreign material, e.g. air (100–200 ml is dangerous) or solid particles injected by drug addicts.

2. Internal embolism:
  a. Thromboembolism which is most common.
  b. Fat: Seen in soft tissue or skeletal injuries.
  c. Bone marrow: Seen in skeletal fractures.
  d. Body tissues: Muscle or liver particles.
  e. Amniotic fluid: May occur during delivery.

Depending upon the type of vessel occluded by an embolus, they can be classified into (a) arterial or (b) venous. In case the embolus originates from venous side and ends up blocking some artery then it is known as "paradoxical embolism" seen in a person with patent foramen ovale.

Indirect Causes

a. *Acceleration of the pre-existing disease:* Sometimes a pre-existing disease may be accelerated with even small amount of trauma, e.g. an aneurism may burst or a person with fatty degeneration of heart may have heart failure or rupture of the spleen or dissemination of a neoplasm. In such cases the assailant is usually not charged with culpable homicide but charged with simple or grievous hurt, provided he was not aware about this pre-existing disease and has not purposefully inflicted the injury in order to cause death of that individual.

b. *Supervening of new disease:* Fibrous scar tissue formation during healing of an injury may give rise to certain complication even resulting in death of that individual, e.g. healing abdominal injuries may result in intestinal obstruction or strangled hernia; in some cases of injuries to vessel wall may produce traumatic aneurism which may rupture later on.

In some rare cases even tumor may occur at the site of injury. However relationship between injury and tumor is guided by *"Ewing's postulate"*, which consists of following factors:

  i. There must be evidence to prove that the area was healthy before it was injured.
  ii. There must be sufficient proof to show the trauma to that part.
  iii. The tumor must arise at the site of the trauma.
  iv. The tumor must become apparent within the reasonable length of time, e.g. for meningioma it requires more than 1 year but less than 5 years to arise.
  v. Nature of the tumor has to be proved microscopically.

c. *Operational risks:* When death occurs after surgical operation performed by a competent surgeon with reasonable care and skill the assailant will be responsible for his death.

d. *Neglect of treatment:* Death may occur sometimes from the complications of the injuries resulting from negligence on the part of the injured person. Assaulted person is not bound to submit himself for treatment and if death occurs the assailant shall be held responsible.

AGE OF INJURIES

To find out age of an injury is of immense medicolegal importance so as to corroborate circumstantial evidence. Though it is not always possible to give exact time of infliction of injury but approximate age of an injury can be calculated from vital reactions occurring in an injury. Age of an injury can be made out by noting following changes.

Gross or Macroscopic Changes

Most of these changes have been described along with various types of mechanical injuries.

Histopathology of Wounds

Microscopy has an ever increasing role in forensic medicine. Based on the stages of inflammation and repair, the events in response to injury follow a well-defined pattern:

1. **Lag phase**
   a. *Phase of traumatic inflammation:* This is there during the 1 to 3 days with appearance of capillaries and fibrin.
   b. *Destructive phase:* Characterized between 4 to 6 days by appearance of leucocytes and macrophages.

2. **Progressive phase**
   a. *Proliferative stage:* Characterized by fibroblasts around the capillaries and some metachromasia of the tissue ground substance around 4 to 14 days.
   b. *Maturation phase:* Goes on for few months with collagen formation accompanied by decrease in the number of fibroblasts and increase in the tensile strength.

Process of inflammation can also be described under (1) Vascular changes; (2) Inflammatory exudates; and (3) tissue changes:

1. **Vascular changes:** There is dilatation of vessels resulting in increased vascularity manifested by redness and warmth. Pavementing of leukocytes takes place due to positive charge acquired by the endothelium. There is increased permeability of the vessel wall due to hypoxic damage and chemical stimuli from dead tissues or bacterial toxins.

2. **Inflammatory exudates:** As a result of increased permeability of vessel walls plasma passes out into the tissue spaces. Polymorphs and lymphocytes start migrating due to chemotaxis. Mast cells are responsible as they release heparin, histamine and permeability factor. In about half an hour leukocytes start migrating and in about 5 hours there is definite leukocytic reaction.

3. **Tissue changes:** Tissue changes were described by Raekallio (1961). He divided wound into two zones in about 16 hours. (a) central or degenerative zone of 200 to 500 micron showing decreased cellular as well enzymatic activity and (b) peripheral zone of 100 to 300 micron showing increased cellular and enzymatic activity (Fig. 9.1). There are early necrotic changes in the central zone by 32 hours. After about 64 hours advanced necrosis is seen in the center with mitotic activity at the periphery in connective tissues and epithelium. 5 days onwards collagen formation can be seen. Epithelial activity is seen in three phases; (i) lag phase; (ii) migration; and (iii) remodeling. Formation of poly bands by leukocyte migration defining dead tissue starts in about 18 to 24 hours. After 24 hours basal epithelial cells form wedge shaped masses between poly band and intact dermis which grows at the rate of 0.2 mm per day:
   a. *Mucopolysaccharides:* They disappear in the central zone but intensification is seen in the peripheral zone after about 32 hours, hence can be used to differentiate antemortem wounds from postmortem wounds. It is responsible for the formation of collagen with protein fraction derived from fibroblasts.

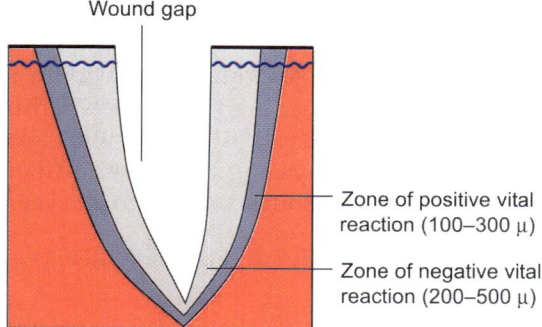

Fig. 9.1: Zones of vital enzymatic reaction in a wound

b. *Elastic tissue:* In antemortem injuries they get contracted and show wavy pattern whereas in postmortem injuries they remain straight.

c. *Fibrin:* Cook (1964) demonstrated that 4 to 12 hour old hemorrhages showed fine fibrin network: after 24 hours there is course fibrils in layers; after 4 days small contracted areas appear; after about 2 weeks solid areas predominate; after one month granular areas appear amongst solid areas and after 4 months only granular areas are seen. Martius scarlet blue stains fibrin yellow when fresh but stains red after about 16 hours. Immuno-fluorescence technique using fluorescent labeled rabbit ante-human antibodies is used for early detection of fibrin.

d. *Platelets:* Platelet changes are seen in four stages (i) platelet adherence; (ii) platelet aggression; (iii) platelet degranulation; and (iv) platelet disruption. First two stages are reversible to some extent but the last two stages are seen along with fibrin clot formation.

e. *Pigments:* Phagocytosis of red corpuscles is well marked after 48 hours. Formation of hemosiderin starts by 24 hours and is well developed in 2 to 5 days. Hematoidin formation is seen after 5 days and bilirubin is seen in the injured areas after 7 days.

Enzyme Histochemistry

Skin enzymes show increased activity in the peripheral zone and reduced enzymatic activity in the central zone:

i. *Esterases:* This enzyme is present in the basal and squamous layers of the skin in small quantities. It shows an increase in the peripheral zone in about 1 hour. On disc electrophoresis 8 constituents are observed out which 2 constituents show specific increase in antemortem injuries.

ii. *Adenosin triphosphate:* This enzyme also show increase in 1 hour along with esterases.

iii. *Aminopeptidase:* Increased activity is seen in the granular layer in about 2 hours. Initially for about 15 minutes there is decrease but increase starts after about 30 minutes.

iv. *Acid phosphatase:* A dense band of activity is seen at the junction of squamous and keratin layers in about 4 hours.

v. *Alkaline phosphatase:* Increase is seen in the regenerative cells, especially after collagen fibers formation starts in about 8 hours.

vi. *Dehydrogenases:* They are present in three metabolic pathways (a) Krebs cycle, like succinic, malic and isocitric dehydro genases; (b) glycolytic cycle like lactic dehydrogenase and NAD diaphoreses; and (c) pentose cycle like G-6-P dehydrogenase. In early re-generation there is increase in NAD diaphoreses and lactic dehydrogenase but when epithelium mature dehydrogenases increase in all three pathways.

Biochemical Changes

1. **Serotonin:** It is released early and is detectible in about 5 minutes and the maximum activity is seen in about 10 minutes.

2. **Histamine:** This also is released after the injury and is detectable in about 10 minutes. The peak levels are seen in 30 minutes.

These changes are seen only in antemortem injuries.

Bone Healing

Healing of fracture show following changes:

i. *Hemorrhage:* Hemorrhage in any fracture show fibrin network in few hours which get organized in about 48 hours.

ii. *Necrosis:* Necrosis occurs as a result of injury or ischemic damage and can be recognised by special stains in about 48 hours.

iii. *Traumatic inflammation:* This takes place in about few hours to several days. The gap is filled by highly eosinophilic fibrin in about 2 days followed by polymorphs and macrophages.

iv. *Osteogenic granulation tissue:* This is formed in about 3 to 14 days. Periosteum show mitotic features with formation of new vessels and by 7th day fibroblasts are in abundance with osteogenic cells.

v. *Medullary callus:* Fibroblast proliferation proceeds osteogenic activity. By 10th day fibroblasts lay down fibrin and then collagen and in 15 to 20 days damaged medulla is invaded by fibroblasts and osteogenic tissue. By 30 days the callus gap is obliterated and union is complete in about 6 weeks to 3 months. However, remodeling may go on for few months.

Healing of a tooth socket: When a tooth is lost, stoppage of bleeding takes place within 24 hours. The cavity is filled up with soft tissues by 7 to 14 days and the socket is filled with bony tissue in about six monts to one year.

WHETHER THE INJURIES ARE ANTEMORTEM OR POSTMORTEM

Antemortem injuries can be differentiated from postmortem injuries by noting the type and amount of hemorrhage, gaping, vital reactions histoenzyme and biochemical changes. Various differentiating features are mentioned in Table 9.1.

WHETHER INJURIES ARE SUICIDAL, ACCIDENTAL OR HOMICIDAL IN NATURE

To ascertain whether injuries are suicidal accidental or homicidal in nature following factors are taken into consideration:

1. **Scene of crime:** Findings at the scene of crime are extremely important:

   a. *Position of the body:* A concealed body in a gunny bag or in a trunk or buried in an

Table 9.1: Differences between antemortem and postmortem injuries

		Antemortem	Postmortem
1. Hemorrhage	i.	Copious	Slight
	ii.	Sprouting of blood seen	No sprouting as bleeding is venous
	iii.	Antemortem clots are seen	Only postmortem clots are seen
		a. Yellowish or grayish white	Yellow or red (chicken fat or currant jelly)
		b. Firm in consistency	Soft jelly like
		c. Laminated	Homogenous
		d. Firmly adherent to vessel wall	Not adherent
		e. Friable	Jelly like
2. Gaping of wound		Present because of elasticity of skin the edges retract	No gaping
3. Vital reactions		Signs of inflammation and repair present	Not seen
4. Histoenzyme changes		Present	Absent
5. Biochemical changes		Present	Absent

open land or forest indicate towards homicide.

b. *Place of occurrence:* Finding a body inside a room bolted from inside suggests suicide. Traffic accidents cases the body is present on the street or highways.

c. *Evidence of signs of struggle:* It points toward homicide.

d. *Distribution of bloodstains:* May help in deciding the nature of death.

e. *Footprints and fingerprints:* Their presence on the scene of crime or the weapon of offence can be of great importance:

f. *Suicide note:* Mostly indicate the suicidal nature of the death.

2. **Motive:** Almost always behind a murder there is a motive, e.g. revenge or to gain something.

3. **Weapon:** Recovery and examination of a weapon is of immense importance.

a. *Type:* Pistols revolvers or light sharp cutting weapons are usually used for committing suicide whereas any type of the weapon may be used in murders.

b. *Place where weapon was found:* In case of suicides the weapon is either held firmly in the hand as a result of cadaveric spasm or is found just by the side of the dead body. However in murders weapon is usually not seen at the scene of crime or is found concealed at some place.

c. *Fingerprints on the weapon:* Presence of fingerprints of the deceased on the weapon points towards suicide.

4. **Clothing:** A person committing suicide normally tries to avoid damage to his clothing. In case of murder signs of struggle in the form of tears or cuts are seen on the clothing.

5. **Injuries**

i. *Situation of the injuries:* Suicidal injuries are present in the accessible parts of the body, especially over vital organs. They are mostly incised, punctured or gunshot injuries. Any injury which is not present on the accessible area indicates murder.

ii. *Number of injuries:* Multiple injuries over different parts are suggestive of homicide. However single injury may be seen in suicidal, homicidal or accidental deaths.

iii. *Direction of the injuries:* Direction of injury in suicidal injury will coincide with movement of the hand. In cases of homicide, direction depends upon the relative position of the victim and assailant at the time of infliction of injuries.

iv. *Defence wounds:* Presence of defence wounds is indicative of homicidal nature of injuries.

v. *Hesitant cuts:* These are small, parallel, superficial cuts present in a group at the beginning of a major cut are indicative of suicide.

vi. *Trace evidence:* Hair, blood or any other trace evidence can also be of great help, e.g. presence of powder charge remnants on the hand of deceased in a case of suicide.

POWER OF VOLITIONAL ACTS AFTER SUSTAINING A FATAL INJURY

A medical witness should give a guarded reply in such cases, as there are recorded cases were the victims were able to perform certain acts after receiving severe or fatal injury.

WHICH OF THE SEVERAL INJURIES RESULTED IN DEATH?

In a case having multiple injuries it is essential to discover the injury which proved fatal. Injuries on the vital organs or involving major vessels can be held responsible for the death. However legally all the assailants are held responsible for the death of the victim if they all started with common object of intentionally causing such injuries as would be likely to result in death.

WHICH INJURY WAS RECEIVED FIRST?

It not easy to find out which injury was received first, however, minor injuries are presumed to be caused first than sever or fatal injury.

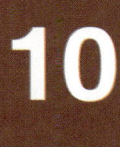

10 Regional Injuries

HEAD INJURIES

"Any type of craniocerebral injury can be caused by any kind of blow on any sort of head". **"Munro"**

Scalp Injuries

The outer covering over skull has five layers (i) skin, (ii) subcutaneous tissues, (iii) occipito-frontalis or its aponeurosis, (iv) loose areolar tissues, and (v) pericranium.

Mostly there are lacerated injuries seen on the scalp due to mechanical violence, vehicular accidents or fall from height. These lacerations look like incised wounds (split lacerations), bleed profusely but heal rapidly.

Bruising of the scalp may also happen with blunt force impact or fall from height. Marked edema may be present. These bruises are not visible at times but the swelling can be felt. In some cases there is hematoma formation known as cephalhematoma in newborn (the blood is located between the baby's bones of the skull and the lining pericranium), which has to be differentiated from skull fractures by X-ray examination.

Black eye apart from the direct injury may result from seepage of blood from an injury from the front of the scalp by gravitational force.

Veins of the scalp are connected to the Sagittal or lateral sinuses through emissary veins; hence infection or abscess present on the scalp may extend to intracranial sinuses.

Skull Fractures

Skull is formed by eight cranial bones that houses and protect the brain. There are three layers; the hard compact layer of the external table, the diploe in the middle, and the compact layer of the inner table of the skull. Break in the cranial bones is known as skull fracture.

Skull fractures may result from vehicular accidents, fall from height, blunt force impact or firearm injuries. Scalp injuries or brain damage need not be associated with skull fractures in all cases. Death from skull fractures normally happens from compression of the brain either from hemorrhage or brain edema in some cases fracture pieces may also damage brain substance.

Mechanism of Production Skull Fractures

Skull fracture may result from either direct force or indirect force applied to the skull.

a. *Direct force:* When any direct force is applied to the skull bones there is local deformation at the site of the application of the force which results in distortion of the skull bones. The area under impact bends inwards and there is compensatory out bulging of the adjacent areas. Depending upon the elastic limits of the bones the fracture may take place at both these places (struck hoop). When head is fixed the pressure applied on one side may result in fracture at the stress line running longitudinally between the pressure area where the force is applied and opposite fixed area of the skull. Linear fracture may happen due to stress area developing at some distance and the fracture line connect these two points, sometimes even running to the base of the skull.

b. *Indirect force:* When the force is not directly applied to the skull bone, e.g. fall on the buttocks or blow on the chin resulting in the fracture of the skull bones (ring fracture) as the force is transmitted through other body bones like vertebral column.

Skull Fractures Can be Classified in Following Manners:

a. *Classification based on clinical findings:* Clinically fractures of skull can be divided into following types:

i. Simple: Closed fracture without any other injury to the brain.

ii. Compound: Open fracture where some fractured portion of the bone is exposed to atmosphere.

iii. *Complicated:* When some damage to the brain or cranial nerves is also there.

b. *Classification based on physical findings:* On physical appearance or on X-ray examinations the fractures can be divided into:

i. Pond's fracture: These are seen in small children or infants when the skull bones are pliable. Force applied to the skull causes depression without any fracture. Gradually the skull assumes normal contour.

ii. Greenstick fracture: Incomplete fracture of skull bones.

iii. Fissured fracture or linear fracture: Fracture line is either straight or curved. May radiate from depressed fracture. These may radiate to the base of the skull.

iv. Punctured fracture: These are as a result of firearm injury or penetrating injury by appointed weapon.

v. Depressed fracture: Application of force in a limited area results in multiple fractures at the margin and the area gets depressed. In some cases the area resembles the shape of the weapon and is known as *"signature fracture"*.

vi. Elevated fracture: In some cases fractured fragments may be elevated.

vii. Comminuted fracture: When the skull bone fragments into multiple pieces.

viii. Gutter fracture: May be seen when a grazing bullet passes along the skull bone and removes the outer table of the skull forming a gutter. This may also be seen with a glancing blow to the skull by a sword.

ix. Ring fracture: Mostly caused by indirect force applied to the skull like fall on the feet or buttocks and blow to the chin. Fracture takes place around the foramen magnum.

x. Suture separation (diastasis): When the fracture line passes through the suture line with separation of the suture. It is more common in children.

Signs and symptoms of skull fractures are mainly from compression of brain and may also be associated in anterior cranial fossa with subconjunctival hemorrhage and blood or CSF coming from nose; in middle cranial fossa blood or CSF coming from ears and in

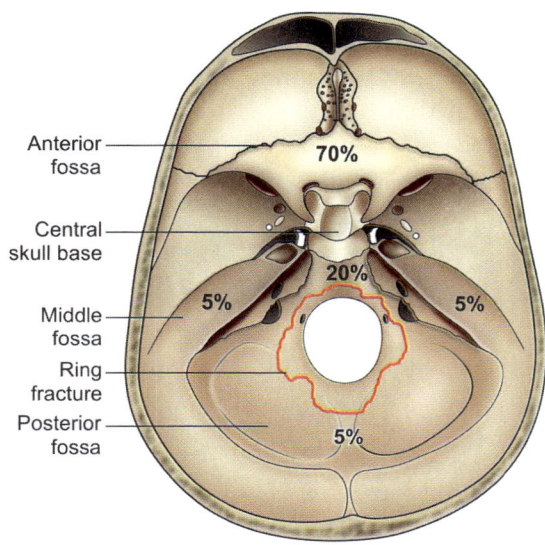

Fig. 10.1: Fractures of the base of skull

posterior cranial fossa formation of hematoma or bruising below mastoid region known as "Battle's sign" along with features of cranial nerve damage (Fig. 10.1).

Intracranial Injuries

Intracranial Hemorrhages: Mainly are divided into (1) extracerebral and (2) intracerebral.

Extracerebral

Can be divided into various types depending upon the location of the hemorrhage.

a. Extradural hemorrhage:
  i. Site: This hemorrhage is placed between skull and dura matter.
  ii. Cause: Mainly due to trauma, sometimes on postmortem it has to be differentiated from heat hematoma seen in burns.
  iii. Source of blood: Mainly from rupture of middle meningeal vessels with associated skull fracture but rarely could be from diploic veins or dural sinuses.
  iv. Location: Majority of hemorrhages take place in the temperoparietal region (Fig. 10.2).
  v. Signs and symptoms: Mainly due to compression of the brain. As this is a tight space the collection is slow hence the compression symptoms takes time to appear. These hemorrhages are not encapsulated.

b. Subdural: Commonest type of intracranial hemorrhage.
  i. Site: Located between dura matter and subarachnoid matter. Usually associated with fracture of skull and subarachnoid hemorrhage.
  ii. Cause: Mainly due to violence, but rarely could be from rupture of aneurisms with rupture of overlying arachnoid matter or from contrecoup effects.
  iii. Source of blood: Blood normally comes from veins entering dural sinuses or rarely from cortical veins if the arachnoid matter is torn.
  iv. Signs and symptoms are mainly of the cerebral compression like slowing of pulse rate, dilatation of one pupil. Death takes place due compression of midbrain due to herniation.
  v. Secondary subdural hemorrhages may be seen over grossly contused frontal or temporal lobes with blood coming to the subdural space through torn arachnoid membrane

c. Subarachnoid:
  i. Site: In the subarachnoid space, the blood is present in the sulci and the gyri are flattened.
  ii. Cause: Usually seen with external violence and is associated with subdural hemorrhage. In case it is present alone than usually it is due to; disease process like rupture of aneurism in the circle of willis, or of mycotic aneurism and in hypertensive athromatus changes in cerebral vessels or in some cases of asphyxia may lead to subarachnoid hemorrhage
  iii. Source of blood: From rupture of vessels crossing subarachnoid space or aneurism formation. Blood accumulation is seen mainly on the base of the brain. Commonly it is spread over a large area, but in some cases it may be patchy.
  iv. Symptoms are mainly of the compression of the brain.
  v. Secondary subarachnoid hemorrhages may be seen over the contusions or lacerations of the brain.

d. Intraventricular: Intraventricular hemorrhages come out into subarachnoid space

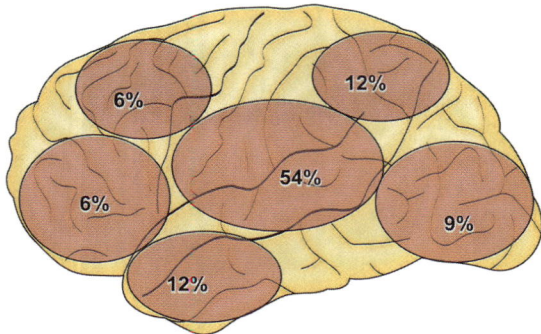

Fig. 10.2: Location of extradural hemorrhages

after sometime and Xanthochromia, i.e. yellow-tinged CSF is observed

Cause: May be traumatic or spontaneous.

Intracerebral

1. Causes:
   a. *Traumatic:* These are mostly associated with laceration of the brain. Traumatic hemorrhages are also seen as slit like collection in frontal or temporal regions.
   b. *Disease process:* Natural intracerebral hemorrhages may be seen in blood dyscrasia where small areas are involved at places, could be from rupture of aneurism or rupture of athromatus arteries or sometimes hemorrhage in the tumor may lead to intracerebral hemorrhage.
2. Spontaneous rupture of the charcot's artery a branch of lateral striate artery may cause hemorrhage in the internal capsule area.
3. Blood from intracerebral hemorrhage comes out in the lateral ventricles or subarachnoid space after about 6 to 8 hours. Which can be confirmed by doing a lumbar puncture.
4. Signs and symptoms depend upon the area involved along with features of compression.

Signs and Symptoms of Intracranial Hemorrhages Depend Upon

a. Type of hemorrhage.
b. Location or site.
c. Amount of blood collection: Few ml of blood in intracerebral hemorrhages and 100 ml of extracerebral hemorrhage can be dangerous.
d. Associated fracture of skull.
e. Associated brain damage.

Bruising or Laceration of Brain Substance

1. **Cerebral bruising:** The bruising of the brain substance may occur as a result of direct application of the force or indirectly by Contrecoup injuries. Contrecoup injuries are mostly seen in those areas where there are irregularities in the skull and the moving brain impinges upon these irregularities resulting in contusion of the frontal or temporal lobes. Mostly the crown part of the gyri are involved.
2. **Cerebral lacerations:** Lacerations of the brain may take place from blunt force impact; blow by an edged weapon or by intruding objects like fragments of the skull or projectile of a firearm.

Coup and Contrecoup Injuries

Cerebral lesions may be seen on the site of the blunt force impact which is known as coup injury and also on the diagonally opposite side in the line of force application, known as contrecoup injuries. Contrecoup injuries are seen when head in motion strikes a stationary object. These injuries are mostly hemorrhagic in nature like subdural hemorrhage, subarachnoid hemorrhage or contusions of the brain. Relatively these injuries are more severe than coup injuries in most of the cases. Other lesions seen in contrecoup injuries are decapitation of gyrus which on healing produces "hollow tooth gyrus" and hemorrhage in corpus collosum or floor of third ventricle or in reticular formation of the midbrain.

Fracture of the cribriform plate (orbital plate) may be observed in rare cases from the contrecoup forces.

Mechanism of Contrecoup Injuries

Damage resulting from contrecoup injuries involves complex mechanism. Some of the proposed theories explaining their production are mentioned below:

   i. *The struck hoop theory:* Flattening of the skull at the site of impact causing skull to assume momentarily ovoid shape, hence the opposite side of the skull impinges on the underlying brain.
   ii. *Russell's theory:* Sudden displacement of the brain towards impact site as a jelly mass and a potential space is formed on the opposite side rupturing vessels resulting in subdural and cortical damage.

iii. *Goggio's pressure gradient theory:* At the moment of injury there is positive pressure at the site and negative pressure on the opposite side causing bursting of vessels.

iv. *Rotational force theory:* Rotational forces taking place from the impact leads to shearing effects which results in the damage on the opposite side.

v. *Bony irregularity theory of rawling:* Brain in motion impinges upon the bony irregularities on the lesser wing of sphenoid bone or the orbital plate and thus gets damaged.

vi. *Moritz radiating wave theory:* Energy of impact in a hollow organ propagate by radiating waves along the meridional lines that diverge as they leave the site of the impact and converge as they approach the opposite side resulting in contrecoup injuries.

vii. *Cerebral edema:* Contrecoup injuries are thought to be due to direct effect of trauma as envisaged above or indirectly due to cerebral edema causing distortion of vulnerable vessels resulting in hypoxic damage to the brain.

Boxing Injuries

Boxers receive wide varieties of injuries to the head. Commonly there are subdural hematoma, pontine hemorrhages (known as boxers hemorrhage) and in some cases haemorrhage in the midbrain when severely beaten. "Punch drunk" is a condition seen in about 1% of all boxers resulting from small hemorrhages in brain especially in corpus stratum and thalamic region. There is deterioration of coordination, slurred speech, clumsy movements' tremors and even dementia. In few cases retinal detachment may be seen which is more common in myopic individuals. Very rarely there may be injury to pituitary gland resulting in diabetes insipidus or internal hydrocephalus.

Phases of Head Injury

Normally there are three phases seen in a head injury case.

a. Concussion
b. Lucid interval
c. Signs of compression.

a. Concussion

It is also known as stunning (commotio cerebri). A transient period of unconsciousness resulting from a blow on the head and may be followed with post-traumatic retrograde amnesia (forget things preceding head injury). Unconsciousness lasts from few seconds to few minutes with recovery in majority of cases.

This is seen in most of the head injury cases and is commonly observed when the head is free to move with striking speed of the object is more than 28 feet per second. Some cases this may be the only finding of head injury or is followed by compression features. Later on the person may complain of headache, fatigue, in-coordination, dizziness and intolerance to alcohol in few cases. The concussion was earlier thought to be functional damage to the brain but now it thought to be as a results of defuse axonal damage, damage to reticular formation or disruption of the white matter. There may not be any associated injury to the scalp or skull. On postmortem there may be capillary hemorrhages in the white matter or bruising of the brain.

Mechanism of Concussion

1. Concussion is more severe when the head is free to move than when it is fixed. Therefore, rotatory and swirling movements of the brain inside skull are responsible for concussion.

2. Damage to the reticular formation of the midbrain.

3. Defuse disruption of the nerve fibers of the white matter is related to the severity of the concussion and duration of the post-traumatic retrograde amnesia.

b. Lucid interval

This is a period when the person is free from all symptoms and signs in a head injury. This is seen between signs of concussion and compression in a head injury. This may last from few minutes to few hours.

c. Compression

Features of compression are seen after intracranial hemorrhage or cerebral edema which may be immediate or delayed. Features of compression are as follow:

i. Sever headache
ii. Projectile vomiting
iii. Neck stiffness due to meningeal irritation
iv. Pupils are dilated and eye may show conjugate deviation
v. Pulse is slow but in later stages it may be thready and fast
vi. Respiration is slow and labored
vii. Cranial nerve involvement
viii. Paralysis with head tilted towards the side of the lesion
ix. Temperature may be normal or raised
x. Planters are extensors
xi. Papilledema may be seen
xii. CSF may show blood in lumbar puncture
xiii. Glycosuria may be present
xiv. Followed by unconsciousness and death is from coma.

Medicolegal Questions in Case of a Head Injury

1. Was intracranial hemorrhage due to mechanical violence, disease or excitement?
   i. Extradural and subdural hemorrhages are always as a result of violence, either on the same side of the blow or opposite side from coup and contrecoup injuries.
   ii. Subarachnoid hemorrhage alone is common due to disease and less common from mechanical violence.
   iii. Combined subdural and subarachnoid hemorrhages are due to mechanical violence.
   iv. Deep intracerebral hemorrhage is mainly due to disease process.
   v. Associated injuries to scalp or fracture of skull are suggestive of mechanical violence
   vi. Aneurism or advanced athromatus changes suggest disease process.
   vii. Excitement cannot cause hemorrhage if the arteries are healthy, it may be possible in old age.
   viii. Ventricular hemorrhage alone or with deep intracerebral hemorrhages is mainly from disease process.

2. *Age of intracranial injuries:* How old is the intracranial injury can be found out from:
   a. Contents of the hemorrhage:
      i. Colour: During first 24 hours the contents are red in colour, for 3 to 4 days they are dark brown and after few weeks there is yellow tinge.
      ii. Consistency: Contents are solid for 3 weeks then they liquefy but formation of capsule may give firm feeling.
   b. Capsule formation: It takes 2 to 3 weeks for visible capsule formation. As the capsule becomes old the cellular contents is reduced.
   c. Microscopic examination of the brain tissue: Recent injury show foamy phagocytes and twined astrocytes, however after about 3 weeks the number of phagocytes is reduced with gliosis and microscopic shrinkage.
   d. Miscellaneous findings: Long standing hemorrhage cause deep impression on the brain substance. Associated external injuries are of great help in finding out the age of head injuries.

3. *Nature of injuries:* To decide whether the injury is simple, grievous or dangerous the person with head injury may have to be kept under observation for sometime.
   a. *Simple injury:* If the condition is not serious and full recovery is there after some rest.
   b. *Grievous injury:* When there is fracture of the skull or there is residual paralysis of limbs or injury endangers life or the person is not able to perform normal pursuits of life for a period more than 20 days.
   c. *Dangerous injury:* When there is imminent danger to the life of that person.

4. *Is it possible for a person to speak or give dying declaration after sustaining head injury:* It is possible in case the person is fully conscious.

Consciousness is lost early in subarachnoid hemorrhage than in intracerebral hemorrhage. Consciousness is lost late in extra-dural and subdural hemorrhages.

In crush injuries to head it may not be possible for a person to speak or give dying declaration.

In case a person suffers from concussion dying declaration should be corroborated with other witnesses as the individual may suffer from retrograde amnesia.

5. *Importance of lucid interval:* Lucid period is a phase of consciousness between two phases of unconsciousness due to concussion initially and later on due to compression of brain.

A person is held responsible for any act done during this period. However, in some cases, he may be disoriented during this phase due to retrograde amnesia and may give false statement.

6. *Volitional power after getting head injury:* No definite opinion can be given in such cases. In rare cases a person may walk some distance even after sustaining severe head injury. Death is almost instantaneous in cases where the head is completely crushed or compressed.

7. *Injury and disease:*
   i. *Development of new disease:* Some times after head injury the person may suffer from epilepsy, paralysis or psychomotor disturbance.
   ii. *Enhancement of pre-existing disease:* Rupture of pre-existing aneurism or hydrocephalous may get exaggerated from head injury.
   iii. Development of tumor at the site of injury: Some times after sustaining head injury tumor may develop in that area. Trauma and tumor development is assessed on the basis of Ewing's postulate consisting of following criteria.
      a. The tissue before the trauma was healthy.
      b. The trauma was focal involving that area.
      c. The tumor comes up in the same area.
      d. Tumor must come up in the period specified for that type of tumor, e.g. meningioma should come up after one year but within 7 years.
      e. Tumor must be histologically confirmed.

8. *Severity of the head injury:* Severity of the head injury sustained by a person can be assessed by Glasgow Coma Scale. The "**Glasgow Coma Scale**" or **GCS** is a neurological scale that aims to give a reliable, objective way of recording the conscious state of a person for initial as well as subsequent assessment. The patient is assessed on three criteria and score is given as mentioned below:
   a. **Eye opening:**

Spontaneous eye opening	4
Eye opening to loud voice	3
Eye opening to pain	2
No response	1

   b. **Verbal response:**

Oriented	5
Confused and disoriented	4
Inappropriate words	3
Incomprehensible sounds	2
None	1

   c. **Best motor response:**

Obeys	6
Move to localized pain	5
Withdraws (flexion)	4
Abnormal flexure posturing	3
Abnormal extension posturing	2
None	1

Generally, brain injury based on Glasgow Coma Scale is classified as:
   i. Severe when GCS is   < 8–9
   ii. Moderate when GCS is   8 or 9–12
   iii. Minor when GCS is   ≥ 13.

Head injury can also be assessed by period of "post-traumatic retrograde amnesia". If the period of amnesia is up to one hour to one day then head injury is mild, but in case it extends to one to seven days head injury is moderate and if it extends to more than a week the head injury is severe.

INJURIES TO OTHER PARTS OF THE BODY

Face

Injuries to face, because of high vascularity, bleed profusely but heal rapidly. Any injury causing permanent disfiguration of the face is grievous injury.

Neck Injuries

Mostly incised wounds are seen on the neck, which in most of the cases are homicidal in nature. Speech is possible if the incised wound is above the vocal cords. In traffic accidents "*Whiplash*" injuries may happen when the neck moves like a whip. It is more severe when the head moves back, i.e. when the vehicle is hit from the back. Therefore, modern vehicles are provided with head rests. When a vehicle hits some object in front then the head move to the front. Main features of whiplash injury are stiffness and pain in the neck, along with sympathetic disturbances and damage is seen between cervical 6th and 7th or 4th and 5th vertebrae. Rarely decapitation injuries may be seen (Fig. 10.3).

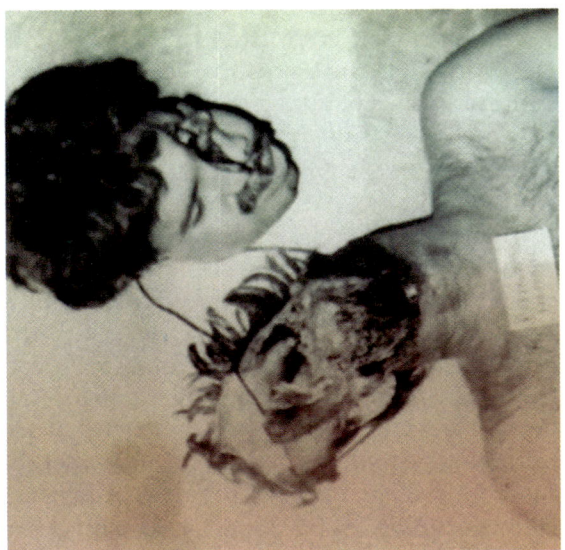

Fig. 10.3: Decapitation in traffic accident when head got transfixed on roadside railing

Spinal Cord and Spine Injuries

Fracture of the spinal column may be caused by a blow with a heavy object, fall from height, motor vehicular accidents or indirectly by forcible bending of the body. Death may occur immediately if the spinal cord is injured with damage to first four cervical vertebrae as phrenic nerve is involved. Death may be delayed for few hours if lower cervical vertebrae are involved. Death may be due to complications if lower vertebrae are damaged.

Compression fracture of the spine may occur as a result of transmitted force, most frequently at 12th thoracic or 1st lumbar vertebrae.

Concussion of spinal cord: Concussion of the spinal cord may take place in a fall from height or blow over the back. This is most commonly seen in railway accidents and is known as "*Railway Spine*". There is pain, paralysis of lower limbs, headache and loss of sexual power. Such a person may file a suit in the court of law for damages and surprisingly, in most of the cases, as soon as the case is decided the person recovers.

Chest Injuries

Injuries to the chest may be (a) nonpenetrating or (b) penetrating injuries.

a. *Nonpenetrating injuries:* Blunt force impact may result in fracture of ribs, sternum and injuries to lungs and heart. In some cases the blow may cause death from shock without any visceral injuries. There may be contusion and lacerations of the lungs and heart by fractured ends of ribs. Mediastinal injuries may be seen due to anteroposterior compression of the chest, resulting in rupture of the right auricle or ventricle, pulmonary vessels or even aorta. Compression of chest may also be seen in traumatic asphyxia with typical asphyxial findings. Blunt force can also cause multiple fractures of the ribs resulting in "*Flail chest*" which on examination show paradoxical respiration. Fractures of ribs are more common in the anterior or posterior axillary lines. Fracture of ribs may also take place during resuscitation. If lungs are penetrated by the fractured ribs there may be hemothorax, pneumothorax or even in some cases air embolism. There may be collapse of the lung with mediastinal shift due to hemothorax or tension pneumothorax.

b. *Penetrating chest injuries:* Majority of penetrating injuries are as a result of stabs or in some cases firearm injuries. These may damage the lung parenchyma, major blood vessels or heart. Cardiac temponade may result from collection of blood in the pericardial sac which does not allow the heart to function properly. Collection of about 400 ml of blood in the pericardial sac may prove to be fatal.

Abdominal Injuries

These injuries can also be nonpenetrative or penetrative injuries.

a. *Nonpenetrative injuries:* May take place from a blow to the abdomen, fall from height or traffic accidents. Blow to epigastric region may result in cardiac arrest and death due to vagal stimulation. In such cases abrasion or contusions may be seen on the abdominal wall. If the injury is severe then there may be laceration or contusion of the abdominal viscera. Liver is most commonly involved, spleen is less commonly involved unless diseased, kidneys are rarely involved. Stomach and intestines may sometimes show lacerations, intestinal lacerations are more common at the duodenojejunal junction.

b. *Penetrating Injuries:* May result from stabs, firearms or horns of the animals. Hara-kiri was used by Japanese to commit suicides by stabbing themselves or falling onto a ceremonial sword which was presumed to be an honourable death.

Pelvic Injuries

Fracture of pelvis is seen in traffic accidents or from fall from height. Common site of fractures are symphysis pubis, superior and inferior pubic rami or sacroiliac joint. Death is mostly from hemorrhage into surrounding tissues.

Injuries to Extremities

Injury to limbs are commonly seen in road traffic accidents or fall from height. They may be associated with fracture of bones. Femur fracture may in some cases result in fatalities due to hemorrhage in the thigh region.

FALL FROM HEIGHT

Fatal injuries as a result of fall from height are frequently seen in urban conditions due to high rise buildings. Construction workers, maintenance workers, workers employed for cleaning window panes or painters employed in such high rise buildings are frequently injured due to fall. In rural areas falls from trees are quite common. As majority of such activities are undertaken by males, hence majority of victims of fall are males. Even household accidental fall from stairs or ladders and while leaning from balconies may result in injuries. Sometimes person may commit suicide and rarely homicidal deaths from fall may be encountered.

Pattern of injuries present on the person normally depends on the; (i) height of fall; (ii) weight of the body; (iii) nature of the ground surface of impact; and (iv) the manner in which body hits the ground.

Kinetic energy with which the body strikes the ground from the momentum gained during fall under the influence of gravity, is mainly dependent on the height from which the person falls. This is clearly explained by a Chinese proverb; "the higher you climb the harder you fall". Hence falls from height can be grouped under; (a) low height falls like fall from stairs or fall at ground level from stumbling or slipping; and (b) great height falls when a person falls from higher levels.

At the time of impact with the ground, there is deceleration and the kinetic energy gained by the body during fall results in injury production. Factors responsible for fall from high rise buildings are mainly due to lack of proper training, failure to use protective harness, alcohol intoxication or dizziness.

Primary site of injuries is on the part of body which hits the ground first and such injuries are more severe in nature. Injuries present on primary impact site, in the form of external and internal injuries are of great importance in reconstruction of manner and cause of fall for medicolegal experts.

In majority of fatal fall accidents the primary site of impact is on the head and next in frequency is impact on the side of the body, buttocks and lower limbs.

Head injuries seen on the victim mostly include laceration of scalp, stellate or fissured fracture of skull. Such fractures may extend to the base of the skull. Subarachnoid hemorrhage and contusion laceration of the brain may also be seen. Cervical vertebral fractures may also be associated with head injuries in such a case.

Fall on the side of the body mostly result in rib fractures and spinal injuries along with damage to lungs and rarely to heart in some cases.

Fall on the buttock may result in fracture of pelvis and damage to abdominal visceral organs. Liver damage is most common, followed by spleen and sometimes it may involve kidneys. Ring fracture of the skull may be seen in some cases.

When a person lands on his feet, laceration of the heel along with fracture of calcaneum is seen. Fracture of lower limb bones may also be present. Transmitted force may result in indirect injuries to spine and even ring fracture of skull may be produced.

Medicolegal Aspects

Majority of the cases are accidental in nature. Body is recovered near the baseline of the building. This may be seen in some cases of suicidal deaths. In a case the person jumps or takes few running steps before jumping, the distance of body from the base of the building is more. Such a person may land on his feet resulting injuries to heel, leg bones and femur. In homicidal falls, when a person is pushed or thrown from the height, injuries due to struggle (defence wounds) may be observed along with injuries sustained from fall.

11 | Transportation Injuries

Transportation injuries are injuries sustained during road traffic, railways or aviation accidents. In our country most vulnerable group is the pedestrian.

ROAD TRAFFIC ACCIDENTS

A road traffic accident (RTA) can be defined as, "An event that occurs on a road open to public traffic; resulting in one or more persons being injured or killed, where at least one moving vehicle is involved". They involve high human suffering and socioeconomic costs in terms of premature deaths, injuries and loss of productivity.

Nearly 1.3 million people die every year on the world's roads and 20 to 50 million people suffer nonfatal injuries, with many sustaining a disability as a result of their injury. Road traffic injuries are one of the leading causes of death among young people aged between 15 to 29 years.

In India, the motor vehicle population is growing at a faster rate than the economic and population growth. According to the world health organization (WHO), road traffic injuries are the sixth leading cause of death in India with a greater share of hospitalization, deaths, disabilities and socioeconomic losses in the young and middle-aged population. Road traffic injuries also place a huge burden on the health sector in terms of prehospital management, acute care and rehabilitation.

Vehicular accidents can be grouped into two types: (a) elastic collision, where the kinetic energy is spent on distortion of the vehicle resulting in less injuries to the occupants; and (b) nonelastic collision where, kinetic energy is transferred to the victim resulting in more severe injuries.

Between 1970 and 2011, the number of accidents increased 4.4 times accompanied with 9.8 times increase in fatalities and 7.3 times increase in the number of persons injured. During 2011, a total of 497686 road accidents out of which 24.4% resulted in fatalities were reported in India.

Injuries to Pedestrians

Pedestrians are the most vulnerable individuals involved in the road traffic accidents. Such a person is required to be thoroughly examined so as to reconstruct the accident. It may also help the investigators to identify the vehicle involved, in case the vehicle has failed to stop. Injuries sustained by a pedestrian can be classified in the following manner.

1. *Primary impact injuries:* Caused by the part of the vehicle striking first like bumper of a vehicle. Depending on the relative position of the person he may receive injuries on the side facing the vehicle. Further whether the person is having one or both of the feet on the ground, point of impact in relation to the center of gravity of that individual,

height of the bumper, speed of the vehicle, types of footwear and the road surface are some of the factors which modify the injuries. Fracture of the tibia showing triangular fracture with apex towards the striking bumper is known as *"Bumper Fracture"*. Bruising of the calf muscles over the fracture site is commonly observed.

2. *Secondary impact injuries:* These injuries are caused by other parts of the vehicle. Mostly when a person is hit by a car, after sustaining injuries by the bumper he is thrown on the front of the car thereby sustaining secondary injuries from the windshield and other parts of the car. Run over injuries are sometimes seen in the form of the tyre tread marks, (Figs 11.1 and 11.2) crush injuries to chest and abdomen and avulsion lacerations over extremities.

3. *Secondary injuries:* Injuries received by the victim by striking other objects like ground.

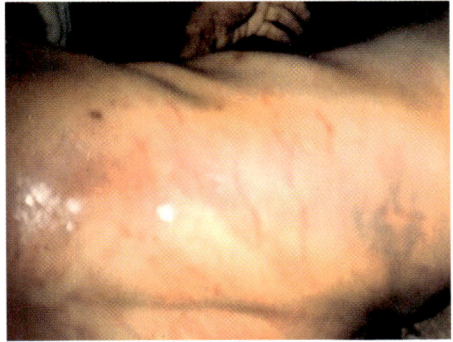

Fig. 11.1: Tyre tread mark

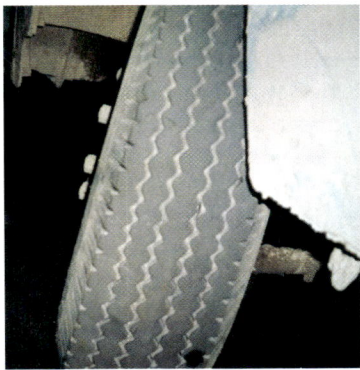

Fig. 11.2: Tyre responsible for tread mark

Injuries to the Occupants of the Vehicle

Occupants of the vehicle receive injuries from different parts of the vehicle depending upon their position in the vehicle. Hence, from the injuries received it may be possible to identify the position of various occupants of the vehicle. (Fig. 11.3)

1. The driver may sustain injuries from the steering wheel on his chest leading to fracture of sternum and ribs, wind screen injuries (spider web pattern) to his head, dashboard injuries to his knee, even causing "Plateau fracture of knee" in some cases (fracture line running through upper end tibia and lower end femur). Hip or femur fractures injuries may be seen due to transmitted force through his leg while applying brakes.

2. Front seat passenger will strike his head on the wind screen or window glass and sustain cut injuries from the shattered glass. Dashboard injuries to the knee are commonly seen. In case he also tries to apply brakes hip and femur fractures are seen. Whiplash injuries to neck with fracture dislocation of the cervical vertebrae may be seen. Front seat passenger is more prone to injuries than the driver of the car.

3. Back seat passengers may get injuries from the back of the front seat or striking the side

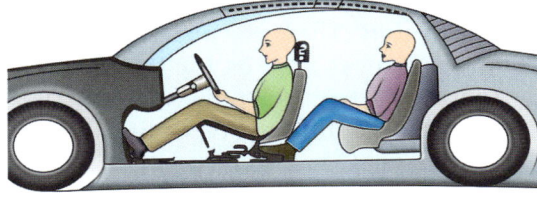

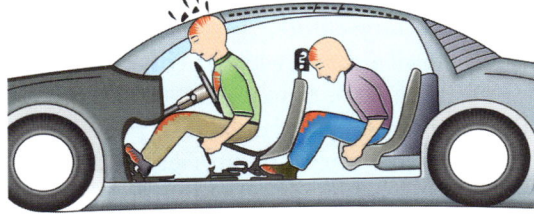

Fig. 11.3: Injuries of the occupants of a vehicle in frontal impact

doors. They normally get less severe injuries in comparison with the front seat occupants.

Safety Provisions (Prevention of Injuries)

These can be grouped under active safety provisions (primary prevention), passive safety provisions (secondary prevention) and tertiary prevention so as to reduce and mitigate the injuries received by the occupants of a vehicle.

Active Safety Provisions

Active safety provisions aim to prevent injuries before the actual accident. These include better road engineering, proper lighting on the road and crash avoidance system or devices. Crash avoidance system include driver alertness detection system (some cars will not start if the driver is drunk), automatic braking system, adaptive headlamps, reverse backup camera or sensors, lane departure warning to alert the driver, antilock braking system and obstacle detection sensors.

Passive Safety Devices in Modern Vehicles

These days with provision of safety designs morbidity and mortality has been reduced to a great extent, when a vehicle is involved in an accident. Modern vehicles have many safety devices as mentioned below:

i. *Safety belts:* These are provided both for front seat as well as for the back seat occupants with belt pretensioners. These belts are of different types like lap belts (airplanes), three point belts (car seat belts) or four point belts (racing car drivers) to seven point seat belts (acrobatic plane pilots)

ii. *Collapsible steering wheel:* This prevents or reduces damage to the chest of the driver.

iii. *Head rests:* Head rests are provided to prevent whiplash injuries to the neck when a vehicle is hit from the back.

iv. *Padding of dashboard and side doors:* Padding reduced injuries to the knee from the dashboard to the front seat occupants and padded doors reduces injuries to the side of the body.

v. *Airbags:* Airbags have reduced mortality and morbidity to a great extent. Modern vehicles have six airbags for this purpose.

vi. *Nonpenetrable wind screen:* These prevent cut injuries from the shattered wind screen.

vii. *Expulsion proof doors:* So that the occupants are not thrown out of the vehicle.

viii. *Crumple zone:* This absorb most of the impact force so as to minimize force transmitted to the occupants.

ix. *Side protection bars:* These reduce the force of impact from the side of the vehicle.

x. *Strengthening of cabins in the vehicles:* So that the occupants are safe on impact. Vehicles are tested these days for impact safety for safety of the occupants.

xi. *Fuel cut off switch:* Cut off switch prevent any chances of fire in an accident.

xii. *Electronic stabilising programme:* This prevents rolling of the vehicle on high speed or in an accident.

Injuries from Seat Belt and Air Bags in a Vehicular Accident

Injuries to the occupants may take place from the restrains actually used for the safety of passengers. Even though use of seat belts has been proved statistically to reduce mortality and morbidity in road accidents, however, sometimes they may result in some injuries in few cases. Lap belts are responsible for internal injuries to the abdomen and spinal cord, while shoulder belts often result in injuries to the shoulder, neck and sternum. The most severe injuries that can be caused by seat belts include fractures, dislocations, internal bleeding, abdominal organ damage like liver lacerations, myocardial contusion, spine injuries, and intestinal injuries leading to perforation are grouped under "**seat belt syndrome**".

Clinical presentation of seat belt syndrome in majority of cases is nonspecific, which leads to delays in diagnosis and therapy.

Typical features include contusions or abrasions on the chest and abdomen beneath the seat belt (seat belt mark) and the treating doctor should suspect and look for injuries mentioned under seat belt syndrome to the occupant.

The treatment of seat belt injuries is dependent on the severity of injured organ, as well as the general condition of the patient. Surgical intervention is normally required for perforation or damage to intestines, while parenchymal and vascular injuries can be treated conservatively or surgically. The prognosis is mainly related with the injured organ and its degree of damage.

Airbags can also result in various injuries to the occupants. Mostly these injuries are as a result of accidental deployment of airbags due to some defect. Some of the injuries seen with airbags are dependent on the rapidity with which the airbag gets deployed during an accident. Few of these injuries are mentioned below:

a. Contusion of the face, chest or upper extremities.
b. Strain, fracture or blunt trauma to the cervical spine.
c. Concussion and unconsciousness.
d. Fracture in the skull, rib cage, extremities or wrists.
e. Laceration of the liver or spleen.
f. Trauma to the fetus in a pregnant women or puncture in the placenta.
g. Wrist trauma and sprained fingers.
h. Airbag dermatitis or skin irritation.
i. Rare case of suffocation has been reported in children or small statured person.

Treatment of these injuries is also dependent on the severity of injuries and damage to internal organs.

Injuries Sustained by Rider of a Bicycle or Motorcycle

Injuries sustained by a rider would depend on the direction from which he is hit by another vehicle. Most of the injuries are like those sustained by a pedestrian, however the primary impact injuries are present lower on the body or on the bicycle or motorcycle. Secondary injuries may be more severe as the victim is thrown to a greater distance. Run over injuries with or without presence of tyre marks may be seen in case the other vehicle passes over the victim. Head injuries are most common in this group which can be prevented by the use of a helmet.

Investigation of a Road Traffic Accident

a. *Medical examination of the victim:* This is very important for reconstruction of the accident and should include (i) types of injuries sustained; (ii) severity of injuries; (iii) site of injuries; (iv) any characteristic pattern; (v) direction of application of force; (vi) height from heel of primary impact injury; (vii) any foreign material present; (viii) intoxication; and (ix) clothing should also be examined for tears, oil or grease marks. In fatal cases natural causes should be ruled out.

b. *Examination of the vehicle:* Vehicle if available should also be examined for (i) area of impact or damage and height from ground; (ii) direction of the impact; (iii) damage severity; (iv) foreign material or trace elements; (v) interior examination for damages; (vi) signs of attempt at cleaning or repairing; (vii) alcohol bottles in the car; and (viii) shoes of the driver for brake imprint.

c. Examination of the eye witnesses for detailed history of the accident.

d. Examination of the site for tyre marks broken parts of the vehicle and trace elements.

e. Interpretation and reconstruction of the accident from the above examinations.

RAILWAY INJURIES

Injuries sustained by a person would depend upon the position when hit by the train. Mostly the injuries are accidental or suicidal in nature. A simple decapitation normally suggests suicide by that individual.

i. *While crossing the line:* Primary impact is on the side involving shoulders and head and secondary injuries due to being thrown or run over by the train. Amputation of limbs is commonly observed in such cases.

ii. *While walking on the track:* Primary impact injuries from the front of the engine along with secondary injuries due to being thrown or run over are normally seen. On postmortem examination very minimal vital reactions are seen in secondary injuries.

iii. *While bending down (Platelayers injuries):* primary impact in these cases is normally seen on the buttocks along with secondary injuries as mentioned in above cases.

iv. *While walking along the track:* Any protruding object may cause injury to the side of the body or head. Height of this injury would depend on that protruding object. Trace elements on that object may be observed in such a case. Secondary injuries may also be seen due to body being thrown away.

v. *Jumping in front of the train:* Injuries are very severe and in most of the cases it may be difficult to interpret those injuries.

vi. *Falling from the train:* Amputation injuries may be seen in some cases when they come under the wheels otherwise abrasions contusions are present. Injuries from any object present along the track may also be seen.

vii. *While leaning out of the window:* mostly head injuries are observed when the victim hits some object present along the track.

viii. *When trains collide:* Mostly the injuries are similar to the back seat passenger of a vehicle. Secondary injuries may be as a result of falling overhead luggage. Compression fracture of the spine or concussion of the spine (*Railway spine*) may be observed in some cases.

ix. *When travelling on the roof of the train compartment:* A person standing on the roof may get electrocuted or sustain burn injuries when comes in contact or within arcing distance of overhead high tension wire. A victim may sustain injuries while the train is passing through a tunnel or overhead bridge. In such a case primary injuries are commonly seen on the head along with secondary injuries from falling down from the train roof.

AVIATION ACCIDENTS

Travel by an aircraft is safer in terms of passenger miles than the travel by a motor vehicle. About 80 % of the aviation accidents take place while taking off or landing. Midair accidents are few and mostly due to technical fault or terror related activities. Sudden deceleration forces on crashing may result in multiple injuries to the passengers and even breakup of the aircraft.

During landing and take off the passengers are normally secured by a lap seat belt. The deceleration at the time of crash may result in hyperflexion of the body with resultant injuries to the face when the head hits the back of the front seat, ring fracture of the skull and fracture of the spine. Multiple injuries take place in case the seat gets detached.

Internal injuries may include rupture of liver spleen, kidneys or abdominal aorta. Rupture of heart suggests sever vertical force. Flexion along with compression may cause lumbar spine fracture. A uniform pattern of injuries distributed amongst the fatalities may help in reconstruction of the accident.

Effects of the high altitude like hypoxia; decompression and escape from the aircraft by means of a parachute or ejection may sometimes result in incapacitation or injuries.

Role of a forensic pathologist in fatal accidents is primarily to identify the dead, reconstruction of the accident and if possible to help investigating agency regarding probable cause of the accident.

i. *Identification of the dead:* Identification may be difficult because of severity of injuries and associated conflagration.

Usual methods like visual identification, clothing, personal artifacts, dental examination, radiology and availability of the passenger manifest may help in the identification of passengers. Facial reconstruction may be of help in some cases.

ii. *Reconstruction of the accident:* Forensic pathologist may contribute to some extent in reconstruction of the accident by means of specific types of injuries, cause and manner of death and survivability of the victims.

iii. *Probable cause of accident:* This could be as a result of disease or incapacitation of the operator like in coronary insufficiency, hypoxia, hypoglycemia or carboxyhemoglobinemia. Alcoholic intoxication may be an associated factor in aviation accidents. These can be recognized on postmortem examination.

12 | Dysbarism and High Altitude Sickness

DYSBARISM

Dysbarism include various clinical features produced in a person due to the difference between the surrounding atmospheric pressure and the gas pressure in the body especially in the blood, body fluids, hollow viscera and body cavities. Dysbarism is mainly of two types; (a) hyperbaric: increasing pressure while diving under water or (b) hypobaric: decreasing pressure during rapid ascent from deep diving. Features of dysbarism are also seen at high altitudes however; high altitude sickness is mainly due to decrease in atmospheric oxygen.

These days' self-contained underwater breathing apparatus (SCUBA) is used for diving purposes. A scuba diver breathes from a compressed air source so as the loss of lung volume from pressure due to depth is negated.

Increasing pressure on diving affects compressible substances in the body, mainly on the gases in the body cavities, hollow visceral organs and gases dissolved in the body fluids like blood. According to **Boyle's law** volume of a perfect gas is inversely related with pressure. Temperature is also related directly to pressure; hence any decrease in temperature would reduce the pressure proportionately.

Decompression Syndrome (DCS)

This also known as *the bends, Divers' disease* or *Caisson's disease*. In this condition dissolved nitrogen gas comes out in bubbles inside the body due to decompression. Atmospheric air which we breathe is a mixture of many gases: predominantly being nitrogen (78%) and oxygen (21%). Nitrogen being an inert gas is not used by the body; however some amount is dissolved in the blood and other tissues. Compressed gas inhaled during a dive has nitrogen at high pressure hence more of nitrogen is absorbed into the circulation. When the diver ascends to the surface this gas is released in the form of bubbles in the blood and various tissues. Depending on the features, DCS is divided into two types; type-1 which has mild symptoms and type-2 having serious symptoms. Symptoms may be skin rashes, pain in joints, dyspnea, paralysis, neurological damage or even heart attacks and death. Helium gas is used in place of nitrogen in the breathing mixture to avoid these complications.

Features of Barotrauma

Features depend upon various organs or structures involved.

Ears: Dysbarism most commonly affect ears known as barotalgia. Eustachian tube is responsible to equalize atmospheric pressure with middle ear pressure. Failure to equalize pressure results in pain in the ears. Even when travelling in commercial planes the pressure inside the plane is almost three fourth of the pressure at sea level, hence person having sore throat or blockage of eustachian tube the pressure do not get equalized and such a person may feel pain in the ears. This can be relieved by valsalva's manoeuvre.

However, when there is rapid descent during diving pressure is exerted on the tympanic membrane which the diver is not able to compensate during breath holding dives. Deeper dives may result in barotrauma leading to damage to the tympanic membrane and middle ear ossicles. Similarly while ascending from deeper dives there is bulging of tympanic membrane leading to damage to the membrane and middle ear along with facial nerve damage in intramastoid portion resulting in facial nerve baroparesis. The diver complains of otalgia, tinnitus, hearing loss, vertigo, facial nerve paralysis or Bell's palsy.

Lungs: Lungs being one of the compressible organs in the body are affected by both increase as well as decrease in the pressure. When an individual dives in water without using any breathing apparatus, his lung volume goes on reducing depending on the depth from increase in pressure. During the descent, when the respiratory volume is reduced below residual volume; the pressure difference between the circulatory vessels in the lung and reduced pressure in lung tissues will lead to pulmonary edema and even rupture of vessels leading to hemoptysis. During ascent decreased pressure also causes lungs to expand leading to overinflation of lungs resulting in pulmonary edema, pneumothorax, subcutaneous emphysema and arterial gas embolism.

To avoid decompression while ascending from deep dives, it is recommended that the rate of ascent should not be more than a feet per second or even lower and make stops at 15 meters and 6 meters for about 5 minutes each. This help in release of nitrogen in the expired air.

Sinuses and teeth: Pressure in sinuses is also required to be equalized during deep dive or during ascent from deep dive. In case of any infection or any pre-existing disease which interfere with pressure equalization may result in pain initially and followed by rupture of vessels causing nasal bleeding. Similarly in tooth pulp disease, fillings or bridges present in divers may cause pain during ascend from deep dive. During descend the air due to pressure goes below the dental cavity fillings, but when such person is coming up from dive the air gets trapped and lead to pain known as **barodontalgia**.

Headache: Headache is normally associates with diving as a result of involvement of ear, sinuses or teeth. However inadequate ventilation may be the reason of headache in a diver. Apart from headache other neurological complications like paralysis or neurological damage may be observed in extreme cases.

Gastrointestinal: In rare cases abdominal distension may be seen with associated complications. Such complications are present due to excessive gas production due to fermentation of intestinal contents.

Joints and skin: Nitrogen which is released as bubbles during rapid ascend leads to joint pains commonly known as bends. Nitrogen can also lead to itching, skin rashes or erythematous patches.

Nitrogen narcosis: Release of nitrogen may produce features of narcosis.

Investigations of barotrauma complications: Complications in diving individuals may be due to running out of gas leading to asphyxia, equipment failure, sustaining injuries during a dive, rapid ascent and related complications.

Treatment

a. Remove the patient from the water.
b. Administer 100% oxygen, intubate if necessary. If possible hyperbaric oxygen administration which is the treatment of choice.
c. Administer saline or Ringer lactate solution.
d. Needle decompression of the chest for tension pneumothorax.
e. Administer aspirin for antiplatelet activity

f. Corticosteroids.

g. Bronchodilators and other symptomatic treatment.

Medicolegal Postmortem

In case of death from accidents during diving, postmortem examination should be carried out by a team lead by forensic expert and assisted by specialists experienced with such mishaps. Equipment used in the diving must be examined by the technical experts for any defect or malfunctioning. Details about the incident like depth of the dive, time the person was under water, place of dive and previous experience of the diver, etc. must be recorded.

Photographs of the body as recovered and condition of the body must be recorded. Postmortem if possible should be done in a well-equipped mortuary.

External Examination

Thorough examination must be done. Body should be examined for skin rashes, bulging or ruptured tympanic membrane, subcutaneous emphysema over chest wall of neck and presence of cyanosis. X-ray of the chest may reveal pneumothorax or fluids in the pleural cavity. X-ray of the joints especially knee may show air.

Internal Examination

In case of air embolism air sample should be taken with care and analysed for presence of nitrogen. Middle ear and chest must be examined for middle ear hemorrhage and hemothorax. Cerebral vessels should also be checked for air embolism. Heart chambers may also show bubbles. Viscera should also be examined for any drug or alcohol.

ALTITUDE SICKNESS

Altitude sickness or mountain sickness is due to respiration in decreasing amount of oxygen at high altitude. The person may complain of headache and fatigue initially. Gradually there may be pulmonary edema or cerebral edema, which may be life-threatening unless promptly treated. Mostly altitude sickness is seen above 1500 meters.

Moderate altitude is considered when the person goes above 1500 meters above sea level; high altitude is above 2000 meters, whereas very high altitude is considered when the altitude is more than 3500 meters.

Person may exhibit features which can be grouped under following three categories.

a. *Acute mountain sickness (AMS):* This is the most common form of sickness seen in persons travelling for recreational purposed like skiing, mountain climbing or hiking. They complain of headache and fatigue. However on second day they may have breathlessness due to fluid accumulation in the lungs.

b. *High altitude pulmonary edema (HAPE):* Life-threatening pulmonary edema may develop suddenly in a person. There is difficulty in breathing, leading to respiratory collapse and death. This condition requires immediate medical attention as mostly deaths are due to pulmonary edema.

c. *High-altitude cerebral edema (HACE):* Along with pulmonary edema, cerebral edema is also seen at very high altitudes. There is disturbed sensorium, loss of coordination, coma and death.

Treatment

In case a person is having mild symptoms of mountain sickness he should take rest and further climb must be avoided rather he should descend to lower altitude. He should not attempt to climb again unless he is free from all the symptoms. Normally it takes from two to three days for a person to get acclimatized. In case a person is having severe symptoms or the symptoms are not getting relived, he must get immediate medical help.

a. Oxygen treatment: Oxygen inhalation should be started immediately. Hyperbaric chambers or hyperbaric portable bags can temporarily reduce the symptoms to a great extent. However, such a person must be transported to lower altitude as early as possible.

b. Paracetamol or ibuprofen may be used in mild symptoms to relive headache.

c. Bronchodilators to open the respiratory passages.

d. Promethazine an antiemetic can be used to relive nausea, vomiting and giddiness.

e. Nifedipine an antihypertensive drug can be used to treat pulmonary edema due to high altitude.

f. Sildenafil which is a phosphodiesterase inhibitor can be administered to increase blood flow to the lungs.

13 | Role of Forensic Expert in Mass Disaster

Mass disaster is a catastrophe of severe magnitude causing damage to life and property. It is defined as an event which is natural or man-made, sudden or progressive in nature, which impact with such severity that community has to respond taking exceptional measures. Some of the major disasters which happened in India are gas tragedy in Bhopal (1984), earthquakes in Uttarakashi (1990), Bhuj in Gujrat (2001) and Sikkim (2011), Tsunami hitting east coast (2004) and bomb blasts in local trains of Mumbai. Mass disaster normally involves mortality of more than 10 individuals. As per WHO figures more than 2.6 billion people suffered from the effects of natural disasters like earthquakes, landslides cyclones or tsunamis in the last decade.

TYPES OF MASS DISASTERS

Mass disasters can be grouped under following categories:

a. *Natural:* These include floods, cyclones, earthquakes, tsunami, volcanic eruptions, forest fires, droughts, sunstrokes or cold waves, etc.
b. *Accidents:* Air crash, rail accidents, sinking ship or road traffic accidents.
c. *Industrial mishaps:* Explosions or gas leak.
d. *Man-made:* Wars, riots or terrorist attack.

Disaster Planning

Impact of disaster especially casualties from the disaster can be reduced by elaborate planning and preparedness for any such event. Many deaths following mass disasters can be prevented with immediate medical relief. In India there are disaster management authorities at national, state and district levels to develop strategies, for proper rescue or salvation response in case of a disaster, providing appropriate treatment to the injured cases and their rehabilitation apart from providing psychological support. Basic components of disaster plan should be based on following principles:

a. Disaster plan should be simple to follow and understood.
b. Different plans or flexible plan may be developed for different types of eventualities.
c. Different set of people must understand their responsibilities in mass disaster situations.
d. Fire brigade, police and hospital staff must be trained and go through regular drills.

These days' scientists can predict in some cases like tsunami or cyclones in advance so that proper precautions or proactive measures are possible including evacuating people from that area to reduce casualties. Risk from mass disasters can be minimized by taking measures like safe construction of buildings, evacuation plans and provision of shelters.

Role of Forensic Expert

Disaster relief work is the responsibility of the disaster management authority at the district level supported by the state and nations disaster management authorities. They are required to deploy trained team immediately at the site of disaster. The disaster relief team which arrives at the scene comprises of persons from various agencies like police, fire brigade, district administrative functionaries, doctors including forensic experts and volunteers. In massive disasters army may also be involved in relief work. Role of a forensic expert or a doctor is to provide help in first aid, triage, evacuation, transportation and treatment.

At the scene of disaster: First responsibility of the medical person at the scene of disaster is to rescue trapped persons and provide first aid treatment to the injured cases. Police should secure the area to avoid law and order problems. In order to optimize medical facilities triage by providing wrist bands is undertaken. Normally following colour bands are used for triage of casualties.

Priority 1: Red band is provided to serious patients.

Priority 2: Yellow band for persons requiring surgery.

Priority 3: Blue band requiring admission.

Priority 4: Green band for minor injuries.

Priority 5: Black band is used to identify dead.

If possible a sketch of the site may be prepared with location of dead persons. Photographs must be taken of all the dead, which help in reconstruction of the accident. Counselling of injured and their relatives is also responsibility of the medical team.

Transportation of injured must be done on the priority basis and available facilities to the nearest treatment center.

Treatment of injuries: Apart from the first aid which is provided at the site, treating major injuries or surgeries are undertaken at the referral Hospitals. Severe injuries especially head injuries may be referred to tertiary level health facilities.

Examination of dead: All dead bodies are shifted to the nearest mortuary for post-mortem examinations. Postmortem examinations of all the bodies of mass disaster are not required under Indian legal system. Police or magistrate may get sample postmortem done on few bodies and release the remaining bodies to their relatives.

PRIMARY AIMS OF THE POSTMORTEM EXAMINATIONS

Identification

Identification of all dead bodies must be carried out. This may be difficult in fragmented bodies and require detailed examination and investigations by fingerprint, dentition and DNA experts. All dead bodies or fragmentary remains must be photographed. Steps for identification of a body are taken in the following sequence:

i. *Visual identification:* When the body is intact it can be identified by a relative, friend or a colleague by visually identifying that dead body.

ii. *Personal effects:* Presence of personal effects like purse, rings, ornaments or watches recovered from body or clothing worn by the person may help in identification.

iii. *General features:* General features like age, sex, race, stature, deformities or other unique features like scars, tattoo marks, hair, stones in gallbladder or kidneys. These are of help even in fragmented bodies.

iv. *Dentition:* Help from the dentition experts may be obtained and proper dental charting is prepared along with any peculiar characteristic like caries, fillings, root canal treatment with capping, bridges, artificial dentures, etc.

v. *Fingerprints:* If possible fingerprints of the dead body are collected for further examination by the police.

vi. *Superimposition or reconstruction of facial features:* They are also used in exceptional cases for identification.

vii. *DNA fingerprinting:* DNA fingerprinting may be required in some cases for identification of fragmentary remains. They are compared with the relative claiming the body.

Cause of Death

Cause of death is equally important aspect of the postmortem examination. In earthquakes mostly crush injuries from the falling debris are recorded and death occurs from hemorrhage and shock, whereas in tsunami most of the deaths are from drowning.

Cause of Disaster

If possible cause of disaster should be found out from the injuries and manner of death. In transport accidents it is important to find whether any natural disease or firearm injuries or incapacitation of the pilot or driver due to intoxication is the cause of accident.

External Examination

Dead body received in the mortuary must be identified, photographed and identity tag placed on the body around the wrist. In case of fragmentary remains, they must be grouped according to colour of the skin and other features. Clothing are examined for any charring effects, bloodstains or tears. Identification of the dead body is done with the help of various features. Cadaveric changes like rigor mortis, cadaveric spasm, hypostasis and putrefactive changes are recorded. External injuries their type, location, dimensions and any special features are recorded.

Internal Examination

Internal examination is undertaken to record any injuries to internal organs or internal hemorrhage, evidence of any pre-existing diseases like coronary occlusion or ruptured cerebral aneurism, presence of foreign bodies or material inside the body and any evidence of poisoning.

Comparison of Records and Opinion

After conducting the autopsy and comparing records a final opinion is provided to the law enforcing agency for interpretation of the cause and manner of the disaster.

14 | Thermal Injuries

Thermal injuries or even death may result from prolonged exposure to extremes of temperature.

EFFECTS OF COLD

Effects from cold could be because of general or local effects.

Local Effects of Cold

Localized effects of cold are trench foot and frostbite:

1. **Frostbite:** These are normally seen on the exposed parts of the body due to freezing and localized necrosis of the tissues with inflammatory demarcation. During early stages there may be red itching lesions known as chilblains or *"Erythema Pernio"*. Later stages death of the peripheral nerves may also take place with deep gangrene. It is frequently seen over nose ears, face, fingers and even extremities. Treatment requires gradual warming of the part, preventing further damage and antibiotic cover.

2. **Trench foot:** This happens with exposure to severe cold along with dampness. It is mostly seen in soldiers deployed in cold and damp or wet conditions. This can be seen in prolonged immersion in cold water hence also known as immersion foot. Initially there is feeling of cold and loss of sensations gradually the area manifest burning sensation and becomes pale and finally leading to gangrene of the toes or of the entire foot. Treatment includes drying of the area, gradual re-warming at room temperature and preventing secondary infection by administering antibiotics. Precautions should be taken to prevent further damage to that area.

General Effects of Cold

Hypothermia occurs when the body loses heat faster than it produces. Hypothermia occurs when the body temperature falls below 35°C. Most common causes of hypothermia are:

1. Exposure to cold weather conditions, e.g. a person if not dressed properly for winter or inadequate heating in homes during winter months especially in old age or infancy.
2. Immersion in cold water, e.g. accidental fall in cold water or unable to get out of wet cloths. Waves in cold water can increase heat loss of a person up to 50%.

Certain medical conditions like diabetes, thyroid conditions, severe trauma, drugs or alcohol consumption increase the risk of hypothermia.

The body heat is lost in following manner:

i. *Radiated heat:* The heat from the exposed parts of the body loses heat by radiation.
ii. *By direct contact:* Body heat is lost much faster in cold water or when the cloths are wet by conduction and evaporation.

iii. _Wind:_ Wind carries away the warmth from the body by convection. Therefore, the wind chill factor is important in causing heat loss.

Signs and symptoms of hypothermia: Early stages of hypothermia as the temperature starts to drop there may be shivering, dizziness, nausea, slight confusion, fatigue and increase in the heart rate. In the moderate cases when the body temperature falls below 32°C the shivering stops, coordination worsens; drowsiness and weak pulse are observed. In severe cases when the inner core temperature of the body falls below 24–25°C, the person becomes unconscious and below 21°C death takes place as a result of failure of various organs from anoxic damage.

Postmortem findings: It may be difficult to ascertain death from exposure to cold because of very few diagnostic features.

External examination may show pink hypostasis as the oxygen dissociation is reduced. Pink or brownish pink patches may be seen especially over large joints. Extremities may be cyanosed or whitish in colour because of which hypothermic deaths are known as _"White Deaths"._

Internal examination may reveal dilatation of the heart, congestion of the organs, lungs are congested and edematous, gastric mucosa in majority of cases shows mucosal erosions or small submucosal gastric hemorrhages, congestion of internal organs, microembolism in small capillaries, focal myocardial necrosis and fat deposition in skeletal muscles.

Treatment: Includes removal of wet cloths, use of warm blankets, re-warming by only warm water, if required dry heat should be applied under proper precautions. Administer warm fluids. Try to preventing secondary infection by administering antibiotics. Precautions should be taken to prevent further damage to that area.

Neonatal Hypothermia

After delivery there is initial fall in temperature up to 2–3°C as the infant loose heat by convection, conduction, radiation and evaporation of surface water. In infants there is autoregulatory mechanism, without shivering the infant produces heat. This process may be depressed if the infant is in a hypoxic stage. Noradrenaline activates lipase, which metabolizes _"brown fat"_ present in the interscapular region, neck and also behind sternum and spine. Factors which predispose an infant are prematurity, congenital heart diseases, asphyxia, respiratory distress syndrome and intracranial injuries.

Moderate hypothermia is when the temperature does not fall below 32°C, whereas the severe hypothermia the temperature is below 32°C. _Severe hypothermia_ in infants is of two types.

i. Acute neonatal hypothermia is present, when the exposure is less than 6 hours.

ii. Neonatal cold injury is due to prolonged exposure to cold.

Presenting features: In most of the cases there is history of delivery at home in cold weather. The infant refuses feeds, swelling of extremities; apathy, cold to touch, anuria and face of the infant is red.

Treatment: Re-warming in warm water, fructose infusion, and preventing secondary infections by administering antibiotics.

HEAT INJURIES

Heat injuries could be because of general effects or local effects of application of heat.

General Effects

The human body functions best within a narrow range of internal temperature. This core temperature varies from 36 to 38°C. To remove excess body heat, following mechanisms are adopted by the body:

1. **Loss of Heat from skin:** The heart rate increases to move blood to the skin so as to increase heat loss along with cutaneous vasodilatation.

2. **Sweating:** Evaporation of sweat is the most important way the body gets rid of excess heat.

When exposed to direct sunlight and high temperature, the body can lose lot of water in the form of sweat. This dehydration also can interfere with the body's internal thermostat, leaving it vulnerable to heat-related illnesses such as heat cramps, heat exhaustion and heat-stroke.

Heat Cramps

Depletion of salt in sweat, while working in the hot environments but replacing only water leads to cramps in the calf muscles or other muscles of the extremities and abdominal wall. Someone with heat cramps should go immediately to a cooler location and lightly stretch and massage the affected muscles to relieve the spasms. Give sips of up to half a glass of cool water with salt every 15 minutes, and avoid drinks with alcohol and caffeine. Administration of intravenous saline brings about quick relief in such cases.

Heat Exhaustion

Heat exhaustion is a mild form of shock, marked by heavy sweating, weakness, cold, clammy skin, a weak pulse, dizziness, fainting, and vomiting. This usually occurs when people have been exercising heavily or working in a warm, humid place. Blood flow to the skin increases in an attempt to cool the body, causing blood flow to vital organs to decrease.

Victims should be moved to a cooler location, and their clothing should be loosened or removed if necessary. Apply cool, wet cloths and give sips of water if the victim is conscious, taking care to ensure the water is consumed slowly.

If left untreated, a victim's condition can worsen. The body temperature can keep rising, possibly leading to a heatstroke.

Heatstroke

Heatstroke is a life-threatening condition in which the body's internal thermostat has ceased to function. The ability to sweat often stops and the body's temperature can raise high enough that brain damage and death may occur in 10 to 15 minutes. Heatstroke may be seen in an individual suffering from prickly heat, whereby he is unable to lose heat by sweating known as *"anhidrotic heat illness"* and can lead to fatal heatstroke. Heatstroke is usually marked by a very high body temperature (41°C or above) as well as hot, red, dry skin, rapid and weak pulse and rapid, shallow breathing. The victim also may be having convulsions before becoming uncon-scious.

Try cooling the victim down with a cool bath and cool, wet sponging or a wet sheet to help lower body temperature. Watch for breathing problems and use fans and air conditioners as well.

Predisposing factors for heat related illness:

i. People over 60 years of age are most vulnerable.

ii. Fatal heatstroke occurs 3.5 times more frequently in overweight or obese adults than those of average body weight.

iii. Those with diabetes also have sharply higher rates of heat illness and death during heat waves.

iv. Heart disease may lead to fatality from heatstroke as for every one-degree celsius rise in core temperature, a person's heartbeat goes up by 30 beats per minute putting stress on the already weak heart.

v. Children under the age of 2 years do not have fully developed heat regulatory system to regulate body temperature.

Local Effects of Heat

These are the injuries produced by the application of heated substances or chemicals or radiation. Depending upon the causative factor they can be classified into following categories:

1. **Burns (dry heat injury):** Burns are caused by application of dry heat in the form of flame or heated objects like heated solids or molted metals leading to coagulative necrosis of the tissues. There is singeing of hair which may also be seen above the burnt

area in a case of flame burns. Blackening of skin with soot deposition may be seen in case the person is trapped in a place on fire, especially when kerosene or petrol is used. First degree burns may be seen with application of temperature around 44°C for some time. Second degree burns may be seen with application of 55°C temperature and destruction of tissues can occur with temperature exceding 72°C. Higher is the temperature lesser time it requires to produce burn effects.

2. **Scalds (wet heat injury):** These are produced by application of wet heat in the form of heated liquids or steam. Redness appears in the area immediately and within few minutes blister formation may take place. There is no singeing of the body hair. Scald may also be seen along the trickling marks or splashing of heated liquids. Scalds are to be differentiated from postmortem blisters. Scalds are accidental in majority of cases; however, sometimes boiling water may be thrown over a person to take revenge.

3. **Sunburns:** Radiant heat from the sun may cause burns on the exposed areas. Initially the skin may show redness and small blisters formation but later stages it becomes hard, light brown and leathery.

4. **Radiation burns:** Ionizing radiation like X-ray, gamma rays, radioisotopes and UV rays may produce damage to the skin over long exposure. Radiation injury occurs in various forms dependent on the ionizing radiation involved, its penetrating ability, the portion of the body exposed, the duration of exposure, and the total dose. Early signs and symptoms are itching, tingling, or a transient erythema or edema. Exposure to radiation can result in inflammation, erythema, and dry or moist desquamation. Radiation damage to hair follicles can cause epilation. Transient and inconsistent erythema can occur within a few hours of exposure and be followed by a latent, symptom-free phase lasting from a few days to several weeks. After the latent phase, intense reddening, blistering, and ulceration of the irradiated site are visible. Depending on the radiation dose, a third and even fourth wave of erythema are possible over the ensuing months or possibly years.

5. **Extreme cold:** Application of dry ice may also cause burn injuries. Initially the skin becomes red, with more exposure there is burning pain and skin turns white along with loss of sensations. Dry ice is cold enough to kill cells and cause serious injury and should be treated as burns.

6. **Explosive burns:** These may result in extensive burn injuries with tattooing and splinter injuries.

7. **Burns from electricity and lightening:** Electric burns show characteristic entry and exit injuries whereas lightening injuries produce fern like patterned marking known as "filigree burns" or "arborescent markings" as a result of staining of tissues from hemolysis.

8. **Chemicals burns:** These are as a result of application of corrosives or vesicants like acids, alkalis or blister forming substances like mustard gas. There may be ulceration or blister formation without any singeing of the hair or red line of demarcation. Discoloration depends on the chemical substance, e.g. yellow colour in nitric acid.

DEGREE OF BURNS

a. Dupuytren's classification: Dupuytren the famous 19th century French surgeon classified burns into six degrees, depending upon depth involved:
  i. *First degree burns:* Consist of an erythema of the skin without vesications.
  ii. *Second degree burns:* Result in injury to layers of epidermis with vesicle formation.
  iii. *Third degree burns:* There is destruction of full thickness of dermis along with epithelial glands and hair follicles.
  iv. *Fourth degree burns:* There is complete destruction of dermis extending into subcutaneous tissues.

v. *Fifth degree burns:* Complete destruction of subcutaneous tissue with involvement of muscles.

vi. *Sixth degree burns:* There is complete carbonization of the burnt parts with charring of bones.

b. Wilson's classification:

i. *Epidermal burns:* In this type of burns the lesion is confined to epidermis and takes the form of erythema with or without superficial vesications.

ii. *Dermoepidermal burns:* Epidermis as well as dermis is involved or we can say full thickness of the skin is involved including hair follicles, sweat and sebaceous glands. They are extremely painful as the sensory nerve endings are exposed and involved.

iii. *Deep burns:* Skin is totally destroyed and underlying structure burnt even up to bones. These burns are painless as nerve endings are damaged.

c. Therapeutic classification of burns:

i. *Slight burns:* First or second degree burns involving less than 10% body surface area (BSA) or third degree burns up to 2% of BSA.

ii. *Moderate burns:* First or second degree burns of 11–30% BSA or third degree burns up to 10% of BSA.

iii. *Severe burns:* First or second degree burns involving 31–50% of BSA or third degree burns of 11–20% of BSA. However in case the area is less than 31% can be grouped under severe buns provided one of the following is also present:
- Severe shock
- Complicated injury
- Moderate or severe inhalation injury

iv. *Extraordinary severe burns:* first or second degree burns above 51% of BSA or third degree burns above 21% of BSA.

BURNT AREA CALCULATIONS

1. **Wallace's rule of nine:** This describes the percentage of body surface burnt represented by various anatomical areas. Head and neck is 9%, both upper arms are 9% each, front and back of chest are 9% each, front and back of abdomen are 9% each, front and back of each lower leg are 9% each and perineum is 1%.

2. **Rule of palm of the hand:** A useful rule for estimating total surface area involved by a scattered burn injury is the "Palm of the hand rule" that is the surface area of the patient's palm is roughly 1% of the total body surface area.

Factors influencing the prognosis of burns:

1. *Degree of heat applied:* Severity of burns is proportionate to the degree of heat applied.

2. *Duration of exposure:* Duration of heat exposure increases the severity of burns.

3. *Area involved:* Prognosis of burn injuries are dependent on the area involved. In case of severe burns the prognosis is not good.

4. *Site of burn:* Burns on the head and face, genitals, perineum or front of abdomen are more dangerous.

5. *Inhalation burns:* Burns of the respiratory tract are dangerous due to respiratory distress or laryngeal edema.

6. *Age of the individual:* Extremes of age are more vulnerable to burn injuries.

7. *Sex of the person:* Females are more vulnerable to burns.

8. *Disease history:* Natural diseases may lead to poor prognosis.

Treatment of Burns

Treatment for burns depends on the severity of burns. Superficial and minor partial-thickness burns caused by heat can be treated at home. However, urgent medical help is required in cases having deep partial-thickness and full-thickness burns, chemical and electrical burns or such cases where inhalation burns are suspected.

In case medical help is not available immediately, keep cooling the burn with cool water for between 10 and 30 minutes for burns caused by heat. But avoid use of iced water. For burns caused by chemicals start cooling the burn immediately under cool or tepid water (unless instructed otherwise). Wear gloves if possible. Do not try to neutralize the chemical with another chemical. It is also important not to burst any blisters that form on burn because this makes them more likely to become infected. Cover the burn with cling film, it may reduce pain and prevent an infection. In case of severe burn protect damaged skin with dressings.

The initial stages of treatment at hospital are to evaluate burn injuries, treat fluid-loss and prevent infection by administering antibiotics. If the person has lost large amounts of fluid through skin having burns, give fluids through a drip, oxygen inhalation and maintain circulation.

"Parkland formula" is used to calculate fluid requirements in the first 24 hours, which is four times the product of body weight and burn percentage. Half of this calculated ringer lactate is given in the first 8 hours and the remaining in next 16 hours.

Fluids in ml = 4 × weight in Kg × % of burns

A person may need skin grafts to prevent or minimize scars. Physiotherapy can help an individual to regain movement in areas having thick scars.

CAUSES OF DEATH IN BURNS

a. *Shock:* It could be primary or neurogenic shock due to pain or fright initially or due to secondary or hypovolemic shock due to loss of fluids from the area having burns within 48 hours.
b. *Suffocation:* It may happen with inhalation of smoke and carbon monoxide gas.
c. *Traumatic asphyxia:* Traumatic asphyxia may take place with falling debris in conflagration.
d. *Accident/injuries:* Death may take place from injuries from falling masonry or while jumping from a height to escape from fire.
e. *Edema of larynx:* Glottis may get edematous in case there is inhalation injuries are sustained.

f. *Acute tubular necrosis:* Acute renal failure may take place due to damage to the lower nephrons on third or fourth day in severe burns of more than 30%.
g. *Toxemia:* Release of toxic substances from burnt area, which are absorbed leading to toxemic shock on third or fourth day.
h. *Complications:* Respiratory complications or biochemical disturbances may be responsible for death.
i. Gangrene or tetanus may cause death in some cases.

Postmortem Appearances

a. **External findings:** Clothing if present may give some idea about the manner of burning by showing the presence of stains, smell of combustible material such as kerosene oil, petrol or corrosives. Postmortem lividity is cherry red in colour due to formation of carboxyhemoglobin. Burnt area may show hyperemia or redness, blisters or even skin is charred. Hair is singed in flame burns. Vesicle has serous fluid containing albumin and chloride. When the vesicles burst it has red inflamed base with raised papillae.

Pugilistic attitude: Due to heat there is coagulation of albuminous material of the muscles because of which the body assumes a peculiar attitude in which the arms and knees are semi flexed and the fists are clenched, this attitude of the body is also known as boxers attitude or Fencing attitude. Due to heat stiffening there is no rigor mortis. This is a postmortem phenomenon.

Heat ruptures: When great degree of heat is applied skin contracts resulting in heat ruptures. They may resemble lacerations or incised wounds. Characteristics of heat ruptures are; (a) absence of bleeding; (b) nerves and vessels are seen bridging the gap; (c) margins are irregular; (d) absence of vital reactions like bruising, around the margins and severe burn injury.

For complete destruction of body, e.g. cremation purposes the body is subjected to temperature exceeding 1500°C.

b. Internal findings: All the internal organs are congested and blood is cherry red in colour due to inhalation of carbon monoxide. Brain and meninges are congested; skull bones show suture sepation in young or are fractured or may burst open due to intense heat, known as burst fractures. If death occurred due to suffocation by smoke, the nasopharynx, trachea and bronchial tube contain sooty carbon particles (Fig. 14.1). Numerous hemorrhagic spots are seen under the pericardium, the heart is dilated with both sides full of blood. Pleura are congested and inflamed and there may be serous fluid in the cavities, the mucous membrane of the stomach and duodenum is reddened and may show stress ulcers due to hypovolemia leading to ischemic necrosis of the mucosal cells known as *"curling's ulcer"*. Moreover soot particles may be found in the stomach. Liver shows congestion and necrosis of the cells. Kidneys are congested and show signs of nephritis. Spleen is congested, enlarged and softened.

"Heat Hematoma" may be seen when the head is exposed to intense heat. It consists of a soft friable mass, dark brown or chocolate in colour and is honey comb in appearance. The thickness of the clot is variable from few millimeters to fifteen millimeters. There is associated charring of the outer table of the skull. The source of blood is from the venous sinuses and diploic veins. Carboxyhemoglobin

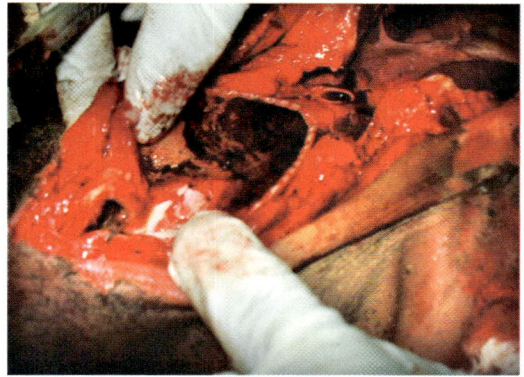

Fig. 14.1: Soot particles in trachea

is present in the clot, which is not there in extradural hematoma.

Medicolegal issues: In cases of burn deaths following medicolegal issues are of importance for a forensic pathologist.

a. Identification of the dead person: When the deceased is badly charred beyond physical recognition it is important to establish the identity of that individual. This may be possible by following means:

 i. *Age, sex and race:* These can be assessed by the external and internal sex organs, teeth, pelvis, ossification of bones and various bony indices.

 ii. *Dental identification:* By preparing dental charts and X-ray of the jaw. This can be compared with earlier data available.

 iii. *Personal effects:* Presence of watch, jewelry, spectacles, keys or even dentures are of great help in identification.

 iv. *Tattoos or scars:* In some cases where the epidermis is burnt but the scars and tattoos are still visible may be helpful.

 v. X–ray of the body; this may reveal some old fractures or deformities.

 vi. *DNA profiling:* This may be done from teeth or bones.

b. *Whether the burns are antemortem or postmortem*: Antemortem burns can be differentiated from postmortem burns by presence of red line of demarcation, (being vital reation may be seen where a person survives for some time after sustaining burns) soot particles in trachea and other changes as mentioned in Table 14.1. In cases the body is badly charred, presence of soot particles in trachea and cherry red coloured internal organs due to carboxy hemoglobin are of great importance.

c. *Estimation of time since burn (age of burn):*

 i. Redness— Immediate.

 ii. Vesications— Within 2–3 hours.

 iii. Pus formation— 36–72 hours.

 iv. Separation of slough:

  a. Superficial burns— 4–6 days.

  b. Deep burns— About 14 days.

 v. Scar formation— About 3 weeks or more.

Table 14.1: Differentiating features of antemortem and postmortem burns

Feature	Antemortem burns	Postmortem burns
Line of redness	Line of redness present around the burn, i.e. vital reaction	No line of redness
Vesications	True vesications: vesicle has serous fluid containing albumin and chloride. It has red inflamed base with raised papillae.	False vesications: vesicles contain air only, it may contain a small quantity of albumin but no chlorides, its base is hard, dry, horny and yellow
Reparative process	Reparative process such as inflammation, formation of granulation tissue, pus seen	Not seen
Soot particles	Soot particles in trachea and larynx seen	No soot particles seen
Carbon monoxide	Presence of carbon monoxide in blood	Carbon monoxide not present
Curling's ulcer	Curling's ulcer in stomach and duodenum seen	Not seen
Enzymatic activity	Peripheral zone show increase in enzyme activity	Not seen

d. **Whether the person was alive before sustaining burns or a dead body was burnt to conceal crime:** As mentioned under characteristic finding of antemortem burns, presence of soot particles in trachea and cherry red discolouration are important features to ascertain that the person was alive before sustaining burns. Carbon monoxide is more than 10% in the blood of such persons as heavy smoking before death can result in carboxyhemoglobin levels but not beyond 10%. Dead body must be thoroughly examined to rule out any other cause of death especially homicidal in nature.

e. **Whether the burns are accidental, suicidal or homicidal in nature:** Accidental burns are commonly seen in children and women while playing with fire or cooking respectively. Smoking in bed may result in accidental fire, where the individual may be incapacitated by intoxication or inhalation of carbon monoxide. Suicidal burns may be seen in females, committing suicide by pouring kerosene and setting themselves on fire. Homicidal burns are also common in India. Dowry deaths (bride burning) of newly-wed girls by the in-laws are quite common. Dowry deaths are punishable under section 304B of IPC; where death of a woman is caused within 7 years of marriage.

15 | Electricity and Lightning

Cases of injury or death from electricity are commonly encountered in big cities or places where electricity is used for lighting or electromotive purposes.

Injuries sustained from electric current can be divided into two groups:

a. *Domestic (low voltage):* The voltage of domestic current varies from country to country. Standard domestic voltage in Great Britain and India is 220–240 volts at 50 cycles, whereas in United States it is supplied at 110 volts at 60 cycles.

b. *Industrial (high voltage):* Electricity is supplied at very high voltage which also includes railways and electric grid stations. There may not be any physical contact with the live wire; the victim only has to come within the "arcing distance".

FACTORS RESPONSIBLE FOR THE PRODUCTION OF ELECTRIC INJURIES

a. **Types of current**

   i. *Alternating current (AC):* It reverses its direction at regular intervals (25–60 cycles per second).
   ii. *Direct current (DC):* In which current flows in the same direction.

   Alternating current is more dangerous as current can enter and exit the body without a close loop and heart can also be influenced by way of ventricular fibrillations. However, it may throw the person away in some cases due to muscular convulsions, whereas direct current causes violent muscular contractions which are responsible for "hold on" phenomenon.

b. **Path of current through the body:** The passage of current through the region of heart is most dangerous. Therefore, mortality is more when current flows from left hand to right leg or from one hand to other hand. When head comes directly in contact, brainstem may be directly involved leading to paralysis of cardiac and respiratory centers.

c. **Duration of contact:** Longer the contact, greater will be the damage.

d. **Properties of the electric current:**

   i. *Voltage:* Volt is the unit of electromotive force or difference in electrical potential between two points. Usually deaths are not reported from contact with the low voltages of less than 50 volts. Most of fatalities take place when the current is above 200 volts. High voltage current is dangerous but chances of victim being thrown away are very many.

   ii. *Amperage:* Current, expressed in amperes, is a measure of the amount of energy that flows through an object. As defined by Joule's law, the heat generated is proportional to the amperage. Amperage is dependent on the source voltage and the resistance of the conductor. Current of

10 mA causes pain and muscle contractions, over 60 mA current are dangerous and over 100 mA current are mostly fatal. Current over 4A is less dangerous hence used in defibrillators.

Amperage = Voltage/Resistance.

iii. *Resistance:* Resistance is the tendency of a material to resist the flow of electric current. It is specific for a given tissue, depending on its moisture content, temperature, and other physical properties. The higher the resistance of a tissue to the flow of current the greater is the potential for transformation of electrical energy to thermal energy. Bone, tendon, and fat, which all contain a large amount of inert matrix, have a very high resistance and tend to heat up and coagulate. Dry skin offers up to 2000 to 3000 ohms of resistance. Heat generated due to resistance in gram calories = $C^2 R/4.187$.

e. **Earthing:** Unless earthing is present or both positive and negative wires are touching the body the current cannot flow through. Therefore, rubber soled shoes reduces the risk.

f. **Arc current:** Body injuries in high voltage current may take place without direct contact with the conductor of electric current. The Arcing distance for 1000 volts is few mm, 5000 volts it is 1 cm, 20000 volts it is 6 cm whereas current of 100,000 volts it is 35 cm.

g. **Preparedness for shock:** Preparedness reduces the amount of damage.

ELECTROCUTION INJURIES

Injuries from Direct Contact

i. *Electrothermal heating:* The primary electrical injury is burns. Secondary blunt trauma results from falls or being thrown from the electrical source by an intense contraction of muscles. Heating of tissues secondary to current causes electrothermal burns. A characteristic injury is usually present at the point of entry and exit. It may however be absent. The point where the electricity enters the body heat is generated from the skin resistance to the current leading to *endogenous burns,* known as *"electric mark"* or *"joule burn"*. The lesion at the point of entry is a raised blister containing either gas or a little fluid. In some cases small area of pale hardened skin with round or oval mark having shallow crater of 1–3 mm ridge of skin may be seen. The lesion is often seen at the pads of the fingers and thumb. Occasionally the mark may have a distinct shape of the conductor surface. Microscopically there may be separation of cells with slits, skin papillae are flattened and lace like honey comb appearance of dermal cells. At the entry point because of metallization of the conductor different colours may be seen like silvery in case of aluminium, brown with iron and reddish brown in copper. Metal can also be detected by spectroscope or by histochemistry. At the point of exit the tissue usually split in the form of punctured or lacerated wound. Severe electrothermal burns can occur, if a person comes in contact with high voltage conductor. The prolonged flow of current can result in significant burns anywhere along the current path. Typically the skin lesions of electrothermal burns are well-demarcated varying from partial to full-thickness deep burns.

ii. *Spark burn:* It is due to poor or intermittent contact with the electrical equipment and the resistance of the dry skin. The damaged area shows a dry pitted lesion (often very tiny) due to arc injury or spark produced due to passage of the current from the conductor to the skin. A yellowish parchment like scab may form with a pale halo around it due to capillary contraction. These lesions may be multiple but hard to find on calloused hands of a workman and microscopic examination may be necessary to establish their nature. Similar lesions may be found on the soles of the feet where the current from metal studs on the shoes have produced a spark injury to the skin.

Injuries from Indirect Contact

i. *Arc injuries:* The most destructive indirect injury occurs when a victim becomes part of an electrical arc. An electrical arc is a current spark formed between two objects of differing potential that are not in contact with each other, usually a highly charges source and a ground. Because the temperature of an electrical arc is approximately 2500° C, it causes very deep thermal burns at the point where it contacts the skin. The man may be hurled from the vicinity by the force of the discharge. All types of burns may occur. Actual charring of the tissue with carbonization is common but depending on the degree there may be brownish discolouration of large areas of skin apart from actual burning. Violent contractions may result in fractures of bones. High current may cause melting of bones and bone pearls of calcium phosphate may be seen on the surface of injured bone. Coagulative necrosis of muscles may lead to myoglobin urea resulting in renal failure.

ii. *Flame injuries:* By flames that result from the ignition of clothing.

iii. *Flash injuries:* Instead of jumping in the form of a discrete arc causing contact point burns, current may jump the gap by splashing across the entire body. These splash burns may cover a large portion of the body but are generally only partial thickness lesions. Skin in this area is known as *"crocodile skin"*.

Causes of Death from Electrocution

Ventricular Fibrillation

Passage of AC current through the body could cause ventricular fibrillations. Passage of current from one arm to opposite side leg is most dangerous. This also depends on the strength of the current and the duration of contact.

Spasm of Respiratory Muscles

The current causes muscular spasm leading to respiratory paralysis. Death is due to asphyxia and the heart may continue to beat for some time till death takes place. There are signs of asphyxia like, cyanosis and petechial hemorrhages on the face and conjunctiva.

Paralysis of Respiratory Center

When the current passes through the respiratory center in the brain, it results in respiratory paralysis. Prolonged artificial respiration may save some of the victims.

Secondary Causes

Such as fall from height, head injuries, severe burns may cause death in cases of electric injuries.

Mostly deaths from electrocution are accidental in nature; while handling some faulty electrical equipment, without proper precautions. Electrocution may also result from damaged overhead electric wires. Proper earthing, protective gloves and use of circuit breakers reduce the chances of lethal electrocution.

Homicidal or suicidal cases from electrocution are very few. Capital punishment in United States is awarded by means of electric chair, where electrodes are placed on the legs and the head. A current of 500 to 2000 volts for 30 seconds is applied to cause the death of the condemned prisoner. Use of this method is on decline as lethal injections are preferred for execution these days.

POSTMORTEM FINDINGS

External Features

There will be local lesions as mentioned under electrocution injuries, at entrance and exit of current. Along with appearances of shock, e.g. pale face, congested eyes, dilated pupils, dry cuticle, insignificant wheal with little burning. Microscopic examination of the entrance wound may show shrinkage of epidermis, vacuolation in deeper layers of skin from steam generation and local capillary contraction causing white pallor. Metallization from conductor can be detected by specific stains.

In case or arcing injuries deep thermal burns (*exogenous burns*) at the point where it contacts the skin along with charring of the tissue with carbonization may be seen. Crocodile skin may be seen in flash burns from high voltage current.

Internal Findings

These are not characteristic, however, organs are congested, lungs are edematous, minute hemorrhages in meninges, and Tardieu's spots in pleura are normally present.

LIGHTNING INJURIES

Lightning is a natural atmospheric electrical discharge that occurs between regions of net positive and net negative electrical charges. The power of lightning is awesome, an estimated 10,000–200,000 amperes of current and 20 million to 1 billion volts.

Updrafts of air drawing moisture from the upper atmosphere result in rapid cooling and formation of ice particles. Complex updrafts and downdrafts associated with storm formation cause these particles to collide rapidly, building up static electrical energy. When the potential difference exceeds the insulating properties of air, a lightning flash occurs. Its passage through air, the lightning flash liberates tremendous amount of energy in the form of heat, this cause explosive expansion of the air. When the flash approaches earth it splits into a number of subsidiary flashes. Lightning with high potential tends to pass along the surface of a conductor rather than through it, therefore, persons inside a building are rarely injured. Lightning injuries are as a result of passage of high potential current and also due to blast effects of rapidly expanding air. A bolt of lightning can reach temperatures approaching 28,000°C in a split second and the intense heat generated by a lightning strike can burn tissue, and cause lung damage, and the chest can be damaged by the mechanical force of rapidly expanding heated air.

Manner in which Lightning Can Strike or Injure Humans

a. *Direct hit* is when the electrical charge strikes the person first.

b. *Splash* hits occur when lightning jumps to a person (lower resistance path) from a nearby object that has more resistance, striking the person on its way to the ground.

c. In *ground* strikes, the bolt lands near the person and is conducted by a connection to the ground (usually the feet), due to the voltage gradient in the earth. This can still cause substantial injury. Lightning is attracted to metallic objects present on the victim. Metal at the point of entrance and exit often gets melted.

d. Explosive expansion of the atmospheric gases and the compression of return wave may also produce substantial damage to a person in the vicinity of the lightning strike.

Classification of Lightning Injuries

Because a lightning strike can be variable and diffusely spread over the body, the lightning injuries can be categorized as mild, moderate, or severe.

Mild lightning injury is rarely associated with superficial burns, but persons struck often report loss of consciousness, amnesia, confusion, tingling, and numerous other nonspecific symptoms. Lightning burns are invariably superficial and have little or no deep-tissue damaging effects. Skin marks often form a characteristic fern like pattern known as *"Arborescent Markings"* or *"Filigree Burns"* or *"Lightning Flowers"*; they may persist for hours or days. Pattern is due to local erythema, rupture of small capillaries under the skin and some amount of hemolysis staining the vessel walls. A burn mark at the exit point is more severe than injuries seen along the passage of the lightning.

Moderate lightning injury may cause seizures, respiratory arrest, or cardiac standstill, which spontaneously resolves with resumption of normal cardiac activity; superficial burns are much more common.

Patients with severe lightning injury usually present with cardiopulmonary arrest. Survival is rare in this group unless CPR is administered expeditiously.

Medicolegal Aspects

Death from lightning is accidental in nature; however the presence of a thunder storm during the relevant period is invariably helpful in the predicting death from lightning. Examination of the scene may show blast effect and scorched grass or leaves. Metallic objects are fused or magnetized with burns on the underlying skin. Cloths and shoes worn by that person may be damaged. Body hair may be singed along the passage of the lightning current.

16 | Clinical Forensic Medicine

Clinical forensic medicine is mainly centered on examination of medicolegal cases (MLC), reporting and giving evidence in the court of law. A doctor working in casualty of government hospital has legal responsibility to examine and report all medicolegal cases coming to that hospital. Even though a doctor has the right to choose his patient while working in private sector but is duty bound to provide medical care in emergency situations and undertake medicolegal responsibilities. Supreme court has categorically directed in case of Parmanand Katara vs Union of India that "**Every medical doctor is bound to provide medical care to the victims irrespective the cause of injury; he cannot take any excuse of allowing the law to take its course**".

Therefore, priority is always given to save the life of the patient. In an emergency resuscitation of the patient is undertaken before medicolegal formalities are completed.

According to Clinical Establishment Act 2010 it is mandatory that clinical establishments shall undertake to provide such medical examination and treatment as is required to stabilize emergency conditions.

MEDICOLEGAL CASE

A medicolegal case is any case of injury or ailment where the doctor attending such a case after detailed history and examination is of the opinion that investigation by law enforcement agency is required to fix responsibility regarding causation of that injury or ailment and also any case (whether accused or victim), involved in any offence is brought by police for medical examination or age estimation.

A medicolegal case is usually encountered by a medical practitioner when such a case is brought by police; or ordered by a magistrate for medical examination; or when a doctor after examining the case label it to be a medicolegal case; or when a patient report some crime committed resulting in injuries or ailments.

However, request of the patient or relatives of the patient to make the case MLC or not should not influence the decision of the treating doctor.

RESPONSIBILITIES OF A DOCTOR IN MEDICO-LEGAL CASE

Whenever a doctor after taking history and examination of a case is of the opinion that the case should be labelled medicolegal then concerned police station or the police post located in the hospital premises must be informed.

Under section 39 CrPC every person (including a doctor) aware of the commission of or intension of any other person to commit any offence punishable under any of the sections of the IPC as mentioned in this section is duty bound to report the same to the nearest magistrate or police officer. His failure to report such crimes is punishable under section 176 IPC with simple imprisonment up to six months or fine up to one thousand or both.

Causing disappearance of evidence of offence or giving false information to screen offender is punishable under section 201 IPC.

All cases coming to the casualty of a hospital are entered in the casualty register. When MLC report in not prepared, detailed findings and treatment provided is recorded in the casualty register.

Medicolegal case report is prepared by the concerned doctor in the casualty completing the three components of the MLC report:

a. Preliminary information component include the MLC number, name, age, sex, occupation, address, place, date and time of examination, details of accompanying person, informed consent, name of the police personal, his belt number and police station, minimum two identification marks, brief history of the incident and findings of general physical examination.

b. Observations regarding type, location, dimensions and any other information about injuries present. In case of poisoning signs and symptoms are recorded in detail.

c. Opinion on the base of observations mentioned in the second part are expressed in this section. In an injury case nature, age of injuries, type of weapon used and whether weapon used is dangerous or not are mentioned. Any object like clothing, any weapon recovered and gastric lavage, etc. are preserved and handed over to the police. Treatment provided, investigations advised and results should also be mentioned in the report. Report is signed by the doctor with full name in capital letters.

Consent may not be required in case a person is arrested by police under section 53 CrPC. On the request of a police officer not below the rank of Sub-inspector an accused person can be examined by a doctor using reasonable force. However, a female should be examined only by a female medical practioner. In all other cases doctor should not examine a case without the consent of that individual. In a case where patient refuses to give consent, a doctor must mention the same on the MLC report.

Medicolegal reports are prepared in duplicate. Original is handed over to the police and duplicate copy is retained. In poisoning case the report is prepared in triplicate so that a copy is sent to forensic laboratory along with sealed vomitus or gastric lavage.

In medicolegal reports a doctor should use simple language and legible handwriting so that it can be easily understood by the lawyers and the judges. Preferably no abbreviations should be used.

In case the patient is admitted in the hospital or report of any investigation requested is awaited, the medicolegal report is handed over to police with "under observation" comment on the report. Police officer gets the report completed later on from the concerned doctor.

MLC reports are confidential documents and are handed over to the police only and a receipt obtained. Copy of the report is not handed over to the patient or his relatives unless a no objection is given by the police in writing.

When patient require specialized treatment from some other hospital the patient is referred to that hospital with detailed history and treatment provided along with mentioning the preparation of the MLC report. No new MLC report is required to be prepared at the referred hospital for the same patient.

It is the responsibility of the doctor preparing the report initially to complete the same after collecting all relevant information from the other treating doctors and results of the investigations requested.

Whenever, a medicolegal case is to be discharged or he absconds from the hospital the police must be informed immediately. Similarly when death of such a case takes place apart from informing the police, body is also handed over only to the police.

LATE MLC

Medical practitioner must register a medico-legal case as early as possible and inform the police. In some cases proper history is not provided by the patient or misleading history is provided so as to avoid legal complications. In such a case MLC report is required to be prepared as soon as the facts of the case are brought to the knowledge of the treating doctor. Indoor treating doctor can also make a case MLC if he thinks that it should have been made initially. Late MLC is some time prepared on the request of the police when some crime is committed but the doctor examining the case did not suspect the same on the basis of misleading history provided. In such cases MLC is prepared from the detailed findings recorded in the casualty register. However, avoid making back dated MLC reports.

Fitness for Statement

Whenever a police officer request for the fitness of the patient for obtaining a statement, the patient is fit or not is certified by the doctor on the original MLC report sheet with date, time, signature and full name of the doctor.

CASES REQUIRED TO BE LABELLED AS MLC

A doctor is required to make an MLC report in following cases:

1. All unnatural and vehicular accidents.
2. Accidents in a factory.
3. Attempted homicidal acts.
4. All trauma or burn cases, when foul play is suspected.
5. All suspected poisoning or intoxication cases.
6. Electrocution cases.
7. Sexual offence cases.
8. Criminal abortion cases.
9. Case with history of foul play.
10. Cases brought by police or referred by court including age estimation.
11. Brought dead cases (except when the patient was under treatment with proper medical records) including dowry deaths.
12. Private practitioner may not inform the police in attempted suicidal cases (not covered under Section 39 CrPC) but if the person dies then the case has to be informed to the police. However, doctors working in government hospitals are instructed to inform the police and make all suicidal cases medicolegal (attempted suicides are going to be decriminalized with enactment of Mental Healthcare Act).
13. Comatosed patients where cause is not ascertained.
14. Starvation cases including cases on hunger strike.
15. Medical negligence cases.

RECORD MAINTENANCE

All medicolegal reports, investigations and related documents are marked with bold MLC letters on the top or are stamped MLC and are kept under safe custody under lock and key. After the MLC register is complete it is sent to the Medical Record Section for safe keeping.

As there is no specific time limit for their safe keeping hence they are preserved as per the hospital policy or for at least 10 years or till disposal of the case by the court.

Case file is retrieved from the medical record section for production in the court, whenever summon is received by the doctor in such a case.

17 | Asphyxial Deaths

Two terms are commonly used to signify lack of oxygen in the body (a) hypoxia or anoxia, and (b) asphyxia.

HYPOXIA OR ANOXIA

Hypoxia or anoxia is used to denote either "failure of oxygen to reach cells or failure of cells to take up oxygen". Hypoxia means low oxygen, whereas anoxia denotes without oxygen (Fig. 17.1). **Gordon** classified this condition into four types:

a. *Anoxic-anoxia:* Defective oxygenation in the lungs, which may result from; (i) lack of oxygen in the inspired air like high altitude or confined space; (ii) obstruction of external respiratory passages to prevent entry of air into respiratory passages like smothering or suffocation; (iii) blockage of respiratory passage like chocking, strangulation or laryngeal spasm; (iv) compression of chest walls so that the chest cannot expand like in traumatic asphyxia; and (v) paralysis of respiratory muscles like in narcotic poisoning.

b. *Anemic-anoxia:* Oxygen carrying capacity of the blood is reduced like in severe anemia or carbon monoxide poisoning.

c. *Stagnant-anoxia:* Oxygen does not reach cells because of circulatory failure mainly seen in shock.

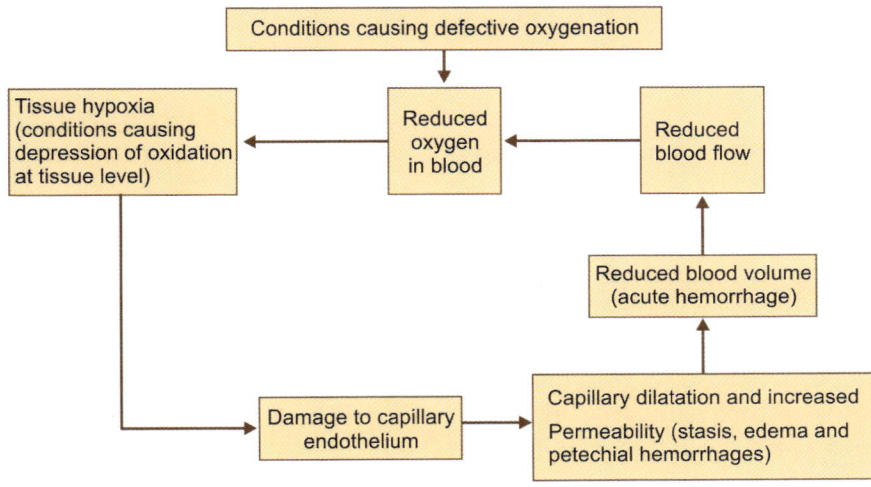

Fig. 17.1: Hypoxia cycle

d. *Histotoxic-anoxia:* Cells are not able to utilize oxygen for oxidative metabolism; this can be further subdivided into four groups:

1. *Extracellular:* Due to depressed tissue oxygen enzyme system, like in cyanide poisoning or hypnotic drugs.
2. *Pericellular:* Oxygen cannot enter into cells as the permeability of the cell wall is reduced, like in chloroform or carbon tetrachloride poisoning.
3. *Substrate:* Lack of food material for oxidation, like hypoglycemia.
4. *Metabolic:* Metabolites are not removed which interfere in further metabolism, like carbon dioxide poisoning or uremia.

ASPHYXIA

Asphyxia term is derived from Greek, meaning *"absence of pulsation"*. It can be defined as *"impaired exchange of respiratory gases"*. Asphyxia may result from; (a) high altitude or lack of oxygen in the atmosphere; (b) mechanical obstruction to respiratory passage; (c) stoppage of respiratory movements or (d) collapse of lungs as in pneumothorax.

In medicolegal practice, forensic pathologists are primarily concerned about deaths from mechanical asphyxia. Therefore, asphyxia can also be defined for medicolegal practice as *"a condition of oxygen lack arising from mechanical interference with respiration"*.

Phases of Asphyxia

Oxygen lack in the body is manifested in three stages:

a. *Inspiratory phase (reduced oxygen):* Deep and laboured inspiration effort, anxious look, heavy head, ringing in the ears, prominent eyes, raised blood pressure and slow pulse.
b. *Expiratory phase (increased carbon dioxide):* Pronounced expiratory efforts, constricted pupils, convulsions, exudation of fluid from mouth, gradually loses consciousness, tongue is protruded and sphincters may get relaxed.
c. *Apneic phase (exhaustion with damage to brain):* Unconscious, reflexes are lost, low blood pressure, dilated pupils and heart may continue to beat for some time after the respiration has stopped.

Findings in Asphyxia Case

Findings of asphyxia are nonspecific in nature and except cyanosis other findings are not consistent in all asphyxial cases.

External Findings

1. *Cyanosis:* Cyanosis is present in asphyxial deaths. However it should be critically evaluated as intense cyanosis within few hours of death is significant. Cyanosis can also be present in other conditions. Presence of cyanosis after a day may be due to postmortem change. Postmortem lividity in a case of cyanosed body may turn pink if kept in cold storage.
2. *Protruded tongue:* It is seen in most of the mechanical asphyxial deaths, however it is not pathognomus.
3. *Bloodstained froth:* Typical froth may be seen in drowning. In other asphyxial deaths bloodstained froth is seen. It may also be seen in other conditions especially in opium or barbiturate poisoning causing respiratory depression.
4. *Petechial hemorrhage:* These are capillary hemorrhages of pin head size occurring where skin is lax, commonly seen over face and conjunctiva. It also occurs internally over visceral surfaces of organs like lungs and heart. These small hemorrhages are known as "Tardieu's Spots". There are two theories regarding their causation.
   a. Increased intracapillary pressure causing rupture of vessel walls leading to hemorrhagic spots.
   b. Hypoxia causes damage to capillary endothelium leading to increased capillary permeability.

It is thought that these mechanisms act together to produce tardieu's spots. Large hemorrhages over lungs especially in drowning are known as "Peltauff's hemorrhages".

These petechial hemorrhages are not only confined to asphyxial deaths and are present in many other conditions as mentioned below.

a. Blood dyscrasia
b. Electric shock
c. Convulsions
d. Acute heart failure
e. Bacterial endocarditis
f. Neurotic poisonings
g. Some times these spots are seen in dependent parts of the body especially over face when the head is below the level of the rest of the body.

Internal Findings

1. *Congestion:* Systemic congestion with dilatation of the right side of the heart is commonly seen in asphyxial deaths, but is in no way specific for asphyxial deaths.

2. *Pulmonary edema:* Some amount of pulmonary edema is common in asphyxial deaths, but is of no diagnostic value as it is present in many other conditions.

3. *Internal petechial hemorrhages:* Petechial hemorrhages are also seen over visceral surfaces.

4. *Fluidity of blood:* It was earlier thought that fluid blood in vessels indicates asphyxia. However, **Mole** in 1948 studied the fluidity of blood and concluded that fluidity of blood after death depends on enzyme "Fibrinolysin" released from endothelium and the amount of this enzyme is related to the rapidity of death rather than the cause of death.

5. *Hyoid larynx complex damage:*

   i. *Hyoid bone:* Fractures of hyoid bones are more common after 40 years of age. There are three types of hyoid bone fractures seen depending upon the mode in which pressure is applied and can be identified from which side the periosteum is torn (Fig. 17.2).

   a. *Abduction fracture:* Results from anteroposterior compression, the hyoid bone is pushed backwards causing outward movement and fracture of the greater cornu of the hyoid bone. The fractured segment can move outwards but the inward movement is restricted due to intact periosteum on the outer surface. This type of hyoid bone fractures are seen in hanging or ligature strangulation deaths.

   b. *Adduction fracture:* Fracture results from inward compression of greater cornu of hyoid bone. The fractured segment in this case can move inwards but the outward movement is restricted as in this case the periosteum is intact on the inner side. This type of hyoid bone fracture is seen in manual strangulation.

   c. *Avulsion fracture:* Due to indirect force through muscular activity. The hyoid

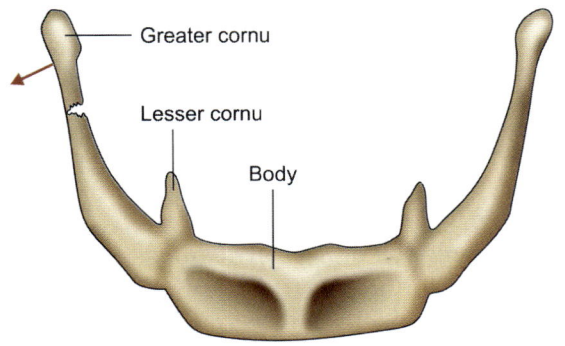

Abduction fracture of hyoid bone

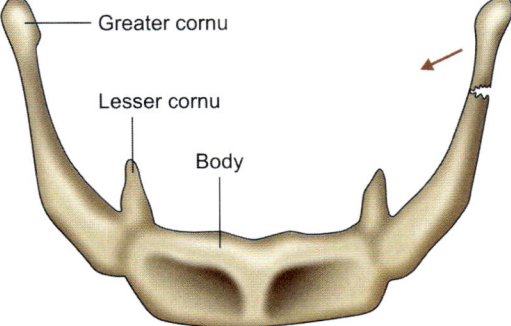

Adduction fracture of hyoid bone

Fig. 17.2: Hyoid bone fractures

bone is drawn up and held rigid by muscles attached to upper border and the traction is applied through thyro-hyoid ligament.

ii. *Thyroid and cricoid cartilages:* Fracture of the superior cornu of the thyroid carti-lage is commonly seen and is also known as traction fracture. The traction is applied through thyrohyoid ligament. Fracture through the middle of the body of thyroid cartilage is due to direct force and is less commonly seen.

6. *Pharyngeal hemorrhages:* Large submucosal hemorrhages in pharynx especially over dorsum of cricoid are commonly seen as a result of direct trauma in asphyxia. This may also be seen in deaths unconnected with asphyxia or trauma.

Dissection of neck: In asphyxial deaths before dissecting neck structures, neck vessels should be drained by opening the skull and the chest cavities so as to avoid artifacts from seepage of blood. Midline or Y shaped incision are made to reflect the skin and *in situ* dissection of the neck structures is preferred. Sub-cutaneous tissues and neck muscles are examined in layers. After removing the thyroid gland thyroid cartilage and hyoid bone are examined. Neck vessels are dissected and examined for any tear in the intima.

Mechanical Asphyxia

Mechanical asphyxial deaths may result from hanging, strangulation, suffocation or drowning.

DEATH BY HANGING

Deaths from hanging are produced by "sus-pending the body with a ligature around the neck and the constricting force being the weight of the body".

Types of Hanging

Hanging can be classified depending on (a) weight of the body or (b) position of the knot.

1. **Weight of the body**
   a. *Complete hanging:* Full weight of the body acts as the constricting force.
   b. *Incomplete hanging:* When partial weight of the body is acting as constricting force with some part of the body resting on the ground or some other object.

2. **Position of the knot**
   a. *Typical hanging:* Knot is positioned at midline of occipital region on the back of the neck.
   b. *Atypical hanging:* Position of the knot is anywhere else other than midline of the occipital region.

Nature of the ligature: As hanging is mostly done for suicidal purposes, hence whatever material is available at that time can be used, like rope, wire, belt, dupatta, sari, turban, bed sheet or any cloth twisted to make a rope like structure.

Preservation of the ligature material: When a body is sent for postmortem examination, it is duty of the doctor to remove ligature material in the following manner. After securing the knot in case it is noose type, ligature material is divided away from the knot and both ends are tied. After measuring the length of the loop around the neck, texture and strength of the material should be noted after which the material is sealed and handed over to police.

Symptoms: Individuals who recovered after an attempted hanging enumerated following symptoms:
a. Loss of power: Individual is not able to save himself, even when they change their mind, because of loss of muscular power.
b. Flashes before the eyes.
c. Ringing in the ears.
d. Old memories may flash before the eyes before the loss of consciousness.

Various Causes of Death

a. *Compression of neck structures*
   i. *Respiratory passage:* Compression of neck causes blockage of respiratory passage. This requires about 15 kg of weight acting on the noose to block respiratory passage.

ii. *Veins:* Compression of neck veins causes congestion of brain (apoplexy) resulting in stoppage of cerebral circulation. Jugular veins are blocked with about 2 kg of weight.

iii. *Arteries:* It results in cerebral ischemia. About 3.5 Kg of weight can block carotid arteries and about 16 Kg of weight can block vertebral arteries. Consciousness is immediately lost when the arteries are blocked.

b. *Damage to spinal cord:* This is mostly seen in judicial hanging cases. Fracture dislocation occurs between cervical 2nd and 3rd or between cervical 3rd and 4th vertebrae. This results in compression of spinal cord or even separation of Pons and Medulla. Transverse tear in the intima of carotid arteries may be seen at the bifurcation of common carotid artery.

c. *Cardiac arrest (vagal inhibition):* Carotid bodies may be stimulated by the ligature, resulting in vagal inhibition of the heart.

Fatal Period

Depends upon the damage or blockage of various neck structures. Vagal inhibition causes immediate death, arterial blockage also result in early death. Usually death occurs in about 5 to 10 minutes in majority of cases.

Treatment

In case the person is rescued, immediately remove the constricting object. Give him artificial respiration and respiratory stimulants. Treat late complications, if required.

Complications

If a person survives he may suffer from convulsions, amnesia, infection in throat, parotitis, epilepsy and some times even hemiplegia.

Postmortem Findings

External Findings

These are due to either ligature mark or asphyxia:

1. **Ligature mark:** Ligature mark follows the position of the ligature material around the neck. It is interrupted at the point of suspension or shows an irregular mark of the knot. Hanging ligature mark is situated above thyroid cartilage and is directed obliquely upwards along the mandibular line, whereas at the point of suspension it is present in an inverted V shape. Along the margins of the ligature mark some amount of abrasions and ecchymosis may be seen in few cases, if present are suggestive of antemortem hanging. Presence of clothing or hair below the ligature material may not allow the mark to develop in those areas. Margins may be slightly red and congested. The base is pale initially but after few hours it becomes hard, reddish brown or chocolate brown, leathery and parchment like. The mark of hanging depends on following factors:

a. *Type of the material used:* In case abroad and soft ligature material is used there may be a very faint and broad ligature mark on the neck. If ligature is patterned, similar pattern may be produced on the neck. The mark will be deep and narrow when a thin and hard ligature is used. When ligature is having two loops, two distinct marks are seen, one may be circular and the other oblique or some times parallel to each other.

b. *Weight of the suspended body:* Mark becomes more distinct when there is complete hanging. In partial hanging cases, the impression may not be so marked.

c. *Length of the time of suspension:* The mark becomes more distinct with prolonged duration of suspension.

d. *Position of the knot:* The ligature mark is more prominent on the opposite side of the knot. In case of slipknot is applied, which tightens with application of constricting force, the mark may be seen completely encircling the neck.

e. *Slipping of ligature:* Slipping of the ligature may produce double mark interconnected with some amount of abrasions.

2. **Asphyxial and other findings:** Postmortem findings depend on the occlusion of the arteries of the neck, in case they are occluded then the face would be pale with hardly any petechial hemorrhages. If there is occlusion of neck veins with respiratory passage, asphyxial finding are much more pronounced.

   a. *Tardieu's spots:* Petechial hemorrhages may be seen in the skin and conjunctiva along with congestion of the head. They may be completely absent in case arteries are blocked. Congestion of the head may disappear after some time, which is thought to be due to drainage of blood through vertebral venous plexus.

   b. Saliva trickling from the angle of the mouth is diagnostic of antemortem death from hanging due to stimulation of salivary gland by the ligature material. Froth may be seen at the mouth in some cases. Front of the shirt of deceased should be routinely examined for saliva stains.

   c. Neck is found stretched and elongated with head tilted opposite to the side to the knot.

   d. Postmortem staining may appear over legs and arms.

   e. Open eye with dilated pupil on the side of the knot is known as "Le facie sympathique".

   f. Seminal fluid at the urethral opening.

   g. Feces and urine may escape.

Internal Findings

a. On dissecting the neck subcutaneous tissues under the ligature mark are dry white and glistening.

b. Usually no effusion is seen in the neck structures; however in 5 to 10% cases platysma may be lacerated.

c. Carotid arteries intima may show horizontal tear near the bifurcation in judicial hanging due to stretching. Vertebral and spinal cord damage may also be seen in judicial hanging.

d. Abduction fracture of hyoid bone may be seen in about 15 to 20% cases especially in old age. Traction fracture (Tua fracture) of the greater horn of the thyroid cartilage may be present.

e. Lungs and abdominal organs are congested and edematous.

f. Brain may be pale if arterial flow is blocked or congested if only veins are blocked. Subarachnoid effusions may be seen in some cases.

Medicolegal Problems

1. **Whether death is from hanging:** To ascertain whether hanging is antemortem or postmortem following features are considered:

   i. *Vital reactions:* These are suggestive of antemortem hanging:
      a. Saliva trickling marks from the angle of the mouth.
      b. Ecchymosis or slight abrasions along the margins of the ligature marks.
      c. Laceration of the intima of carotid arteries.
      d. Fracture dislocation with associated damage to the spinal cord.

   ii. *Ligature material:*
      a. If a rope is used, fibers from that rope may be found on the hands of the deceased.
      b. In few cases, from the direction of the fibers on the beam where the rope is tied it can be observed whether the rope was tied first and then the person jumped or he was pulled up and the knot was tied.

   iii. No evidence of struggle marks on the body or absence of any other cause of death also suggests that the person committed suicide from hanging.

2. **Whether hanging was suicidal, homicidal or accidental:**

   a. Hanging is always presumed to be suicidal unless proved otherwise as hanging is a common method of committing suicide.

b. Homicidal hanging is rare, unless the person is unconscious or is held by many assailants. **"Lynching"** is a form of homicidal hanging by a mob. Lynching was initially done by a mob of white people, when they hanged a black person accused of sexually assaulting a white female.

c. Accidental hanging is rare but may occur in children or during sexual asphyxia.

DEATH BY STRANGULATION

Strangulation is a violent form of asphyxial death which results from constriction of the neck but the constricting force is other than that of body weight.

Types of Strangulations

a. *Ligature strangulation:* Neck is compressed with a ligature around the neck (Figs 17.3 and 17.4).

b. *Manual strangulation (throttling):* Neck is compressed manually with hands.

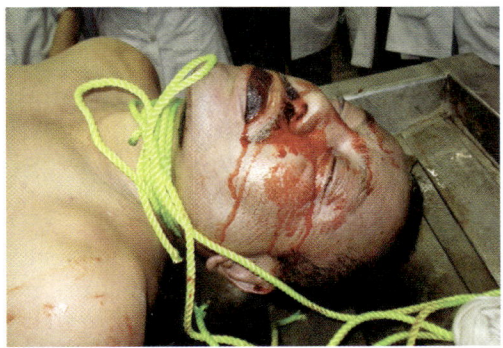

Fig. 17.3: Strangulation with plastic rope

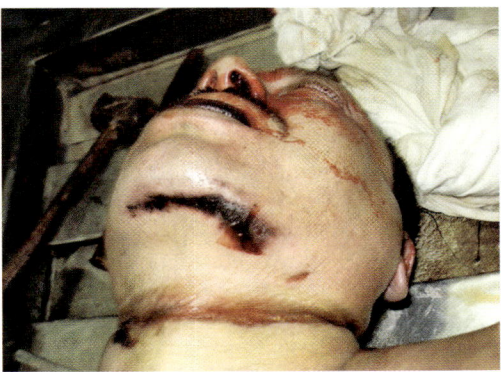

Fig. 17.4: Ligature mark in strangulation

c. *Mugging:* Neck is held in the elbow or knee bend.

d. *Bansdola:* Two bamboos or sticks are placed across the neck and pressed together.

e. *Garroting:* A thin ligature is thrown over the head from back onto the neck and pulled back with force.

Signs and Symptoms

These depend upon the mode of death. In case the death is from vagal inhibition the death takes place immediately. If wind pipe is closed, individual becomes powerless and becomes insensible rapidly. With venous blockage there is ringing in the ears, vertigo, muscle weakness, cyanosis, bleeding from mouth and nostrils, convulsions may be there before death.

Causes of Death

Mostly death occurs due to asphyxia but can also take place from vagal inhibition, venous congestion or cerebral ischemia.

Treatment

As strangulation is mostly done for homicidal purposes, treatment is hardly required. If required, artificial respiration and respiratory stimulants can be used.

Postmortem Findings

External Appearances

1. **Changes due to constricting force:** Depends upon the means adopted to constrict neck.
   i. *Ligature strangulation:* In case a ligature material is used to constrict neck, the ligature mark or depression will be present corresponding to the form, texture and width of the ligature material.
      a. The ligature mark of strangulation is situated low down on the neck, below the thyroid cartilage, circulating the neck horizontally and completely.
      b. Base of the ligature mark is usually reddish, soft to feel with ecchymosed margins. Sometime the ligature mark

may become parchment like if the skin is excoriated. In putrefied bodies the neck should be examined carefully as skin fold may be preserved for longer duration and may resemble ligature mark.

c. There may be multiple marks in case the ligature material is twisted many times around the neck. In case soft material is used, the ligature mark may not be visible on the neck or a very faint mark may be seen.

ii. *Throttling or manual strangulation:* In such cases marks of fingers and thumb are seen on either side of the neck in the form of red bruises and nail marks. Position of these marks varies upon the hold applied. If one hand is applied from front the finger marks are seen on one side and thumb impression on the other side of the neck. In case both hands are used from front both thumb marks are seen in front of the neck and faint finger marks are present on the posterior side of the neck. However if the neck is held by both hands from the back finger marks are seen on both sides of the neck in front. These marks may become parchment like after some time with drying of the skin.

iii. *Bansdola:* Linear and horizontally placed bruise is seen on the front of the neck, corresponding to the stick applied.

iv. *Garroting:* Ligature mark may resemble the ligature mark seen in hanging as it is placed obliquely and high on the neck. However the base is red and show ecchymosis with prominent signs of asphyxia.

2. **Asphyxial findings:** Face is congested and cyanosed with petechial hemorrhages; eyes are prominent and open and conjunctiva is congested. Froth is seen coming from mouth and nostrils mixed with blood. Tongue is protruded. Marks of struggle are also present on the body.

Internal Examination

There is extravasation of blood into the subcutaneous tissues under the ligature mark or finger marks. Neck muscles may show effusion and lacerations. Hyoid bone may show fracture, carotid sheath may be lacerated. Larynx and trachea are congested with presence of froth. Lungs are congested and may show emphysematous bullae over the surface due to excessive effort to breath. Right side of the heart is dilated. Other internal organs are also congested. Differentiating features between ligature strangulation and hanging are mentioned in Table 17.1.

Medicolegal Issues

a. *Whether death is by strangulation or not:* It cannot be decided from the ligature mark alone, as some times the ligature mark is faint if produced by soft and broad material.

Table 17.1: Differentiating points between hanging and ligature strangulation		
Differentiating point	*Hanging*	*Strangulation*
Motive	Mostly suicidal	Mostly homicidal
Marks of violence	Not seen	Present as scratches bruises over face neck and other parts
Sexual assault	No evidence of sexual assault	May be present
Ligature mark	a. Obliquely placed	a. Horizontally placed
	b. Above thyroid cartilage	b. Below thyroid cartilage
	c. Hard, yellow and parchment like	c. Soft and reddish mostly
	d. Abrasions around are rare	d. Abrasions and ecchymosis present around the mark

Contd.

Table 17.1: Differentiating points between hanging and ligature strangulation *(Contd.)*		
Differentiating point	*Hanging*	*Strangulation*
External findings	a. Saliva trickling marks present	a. Not seen
	b. Face usually pale, petechial hemorrhages are rare	b. Face congested with marked petechial hemorrhages
	c. Neck is stretched	c. Not seen
	d. External signs of asphyxia not marked	d. Well marked
	e. Bleeding from nose rare	e. Commonly seen
	f. Escape of feces rare	f. More commonly seen
	g. Seminal fluid may be seen at glance	g. Seen very rarely
Internal findings	a. Subcutaneous tissues under the ligature mark are white, hard and glistening	a. Tissues show ecchymosis
	b. Neck muscles are rarely damaged	b. It is commonly seen
	c. Fracture of hyoid bone and thyroid cartilage is rare	c. More frequent
	d. Fracture dislocation of cervical vertebrae common in judicial hanging	d. Rare
	e. Carotid artery intima may be lacerated in judicial hanging	e. Commonly carotid sheath is lacerated
	f. Lungs do not show emphysematous bullae	f. Commonly seen

It is important to note the effusion and damage in the underlying tissues along with the ligature mark. Other causes of asphyxia have to be ruled out in view of the prominent asphyxial findings.

b. *Whether suicidal, accidental or homicidal in nature:* Death from strangulation is commonly homicidal in nature. Suicidal deaths are rare, as manual strangulation is not possible. Sometimes the person committing suicide may apply a ligature around the neck with a stick in the loop. This stick is twisted to tighten the loop and held against the chin or any other object. Accidental deaths may take place when some ligature material suddenly tightens around the neck, like tie or duppata which may get caught in some moving parts of a machine or a motor vehicle.

DEATH BY SUFFOCATION

Suffocation is a form of death in which there is mechanical obstruction to respiration by means other than compression of neck or drowning.

Types of Suffocation Deaths

1. **Smothering:** Closure of mouth and nostrils by (a) pillow or any soft material; (b) pulling a plastic bag over head and face; (c) pressing infant against breast while feeding; (d) by hands or (e) falling face down in sand, mud, flour or ashes in intoxicated state.

2. **Gagging:** By putting some substance in mouth and oropharynx like cloth, stone, etc. A person may be able to breathe for some time with cloth inside the mouth till it gets soaked with saliva and blocks the respiration.

3. **Chocking:** Some foreign material getting into the larynx or trachea to block the respiration like buttons food article, coin or artificial teeth. Even a small object can cause death from chocking due to "laryngeal spasm".

"**Café coronary**" is a condition when a drunken person, while eating his food, suddenly complains of chest pain and respiratory problem collapses and dies.

Features are those of sudden heart attack, but actually he dies from chocking. Predisposing factors are primarily based on suppressed gag reflex like old age, consumption of alcohol or narcotic drugs.

In such a case give 5 back blows between the shoulder blades or 5 abdominal thrusts. In case of a pregnant woman or obese person give high abdominal thrusts by standing behind the person and quickly pulling inwards and upwards with hands placed at the epigastric region **(Heimlich maneuver).** If not successful emergency tracheostomy may have to be performed or foreign body removed with the help of a laryngoscope.

4. **Pressure on the chest:** Pressure on the chest may result in asphyxial deaths like *"overlaying"* when a mother during sleep turn over and presses the chest of the child sleeping next to her, *"traumatic asphyxia"* where the chest is compressed by some heavy object falling over the chest like house collapse, vehicular accident or trench collapse and when chest is compressed between two bamboo sticks it is known as *"Bansdola"*.

Mode of Death

Mostly due to asphyxia but may occur due to vagal inhibition of the heart.

Postmortem Appearances

External Features

External findings could be as a result of (a) reason causing suffocation and (b) due to asphyxia.

a. *Cause producing suffocation:* In smothering bruises and abrasions are seen over the face especially over nostrils and lips. Lips may be lacerated along the margins of the teeth. Gums may show effusion and nose may be flattened. There may not be any finding in case a soft material is used. In traumatic asphyxia congestion above the level of compression is present. Ribs may be fractured on both sides due to compression of the chest.

b. *Asphyxial findings:* Face is congested, eyes are open and prominent, conjunctiva congested, petechial hemorrhages are present, and blood tinged froth may be seen coming from nostrils.

Internal Findings

In gagging foreign material may be seen inside oral cavity. In chocking foreign material will be seen in trachea or larynx. Trachea is congested and covered with bloodstained froth. Tardieu's spots are seen over visceral surfaces. Right side of the heart is dilated and full of blood. Other organs are congested.

Medicolegal Issues

a. *Whether death is from suffocation or not:* Apart from prominent asphyxial findings marks of violence are helpful to ascertain death from suffocation. Circumstantial evidence is equally important in such cases.

b. *Whether death is suicidal homicidal or accidental:* Death from suffocation is mostly homicidal in nature especially in small children or infants. Sometimes combinations of methods are used like employed by "Burke and Hare". They used to kill people to supply dead bodies to a medical school. After offering drinks to a victim, one used to close his mouth and sit on his chest while the other used to drag him across the room by holding his feet.

Suicidal suffocation may be seen especially using plastic bags over the head and face or rarely gagging oneself. Accidental deaths from suffocation may occur when a person is buried alive; from masochistic procedure like putting a plastic bag over head or getting chocked while eating especially in small children or aged person.

DEATH BY DROWNING

Drowning is a form of death in which fluid medium prevents the entry of air into the lungs. Some authors define it as an asphyxial death due to submersion in a fluid medium.

For drowning death to take place, it is not required that the complete body should be submerged in water. If only nostrils and mouth are submerged, even then drowning may be caused, e.g. an intoxicated person falling face down in a small pit containing water. Therefore, it is literally possible for a person to drown in "chulu bhar pani".

Types of Drowning

1. **Wet drowning:** Due to submersion in water also known as "primary drowning". The water enters trachea and lungs, which is churned with mucus due to violent respiratory efforts into froth. This froth blocks the entry of air into the lungs. Wet drowning can be subdivided depending upon the type of fluid medium in which a person has drowned.

   a. *Fresh water drowning:* When drowning occurs in fresh water, the water in the lungs gets absorbed into the circulation and causes hemodilution and hemolysis which increases the potassium level resulting in ventricular fibrillation.

   b. *Sea water drowning:* Whereas, in salt water drowning water from the circulation is absorbed into the lungs causing pulmonary edema and hemoconcentration, resulting in myocardial anoxia and death in about 8 to 10 minutes.

2. **Dry drowning:** Some times when a body is recovered from water after drowning, no water is present in the trachea and lungs. The cause of death is asphyxia due to water entering larynx causing laryngospasm, which in turn prevent water from entering larynx and trachea. However, in such cases before labelling it to be a death from dry drowning, other causes of death must be ruled out.

3. **Immersion syndrome (hydrocution or submersion inhibition):** In some cases where drowning occur in cold water (about 1–2%), death takes place without any struggle. It has been observed that a sailor after consuming alcohol and heavy meals when fall down in cold water do not show any struggle and just goes down. It is postulated that cold receptors in skin and especially in the nasal cavity or ear drums cause vagal inhibition of the heart. Most of such cases the person enters water feet first, which allows water to rush up into the nose. Some times, when a person enters water horizontally (duck diving), the water sticking epigastrium may stimulate solar plexus, resulting in vagal inhibition of the heart.

4. **Secondary drowning (postimmersion syndrome or near drowning):** When a person is rescued from submersion in water, he may still die anytime from 20 minutes to 4 days due to complications like pulmonary edema, circulatory failure, from disturbed acid base balance or anoxic damage to brain is known as secondary drowning.

Stages of drowning: When a person falls into water he sinks to a depth proportional to the momentum gained then rises to the surface because of buoyancy of the body, air trapped in clothing and struggling movements. As soon as his eyes are above water level he tries to shout for help, he draws water into respiratory passage which causes him to cough. By coughing he expels more air from the lungs and draws more water. He sinks again but because of struggling movements comes up to the surface again, draws more water into the respiratory passage and sinks once again. Normally the drowning individual comes to the surface for three times. After which he becomes insensible and sinks to the bottom.

Symptoms: Mostly persons recovered from drowning have narrated auditory or visual hallucinations or mental confusion during drowning. Some persons have reported flashes of the past events before their eyes.

Cause of Death

a. *Asphyxia:* Water entering respiratory passage is churned with air and mucous thus producing fine thick froth which obstructs air entry into lungs resulting in asphyxia. In cases of dry drowning, asphyxia is produced due to laryngeal spasm.

b. *Vagal inhibition:* In Immersion syndrome or even in some cases due to fright or terror of suddenly falling into water can produce vagal inhibition of heart.

c. *Injuries:* In some cases injuries sustained during fall in water and striking any object in water may result in death of the individual.

d. *Ventricular fibrillation or myocardial anoxia:* It depends upon the fluid medium in which a person drowns. Ventricular fibrillation is seen in fresh water drowning and myocardial anoxia in sea water drowning.

e. *Apoplexy:* May be seen in old aged person.

f. *Exhaustion:* Due to continued efforts a person may suddenly collapse.

g. *Other complications:* As observed in secondary drowning.

Fatal Period

Asphyxia occurs in 2–3 minutes and death takes place in 5 to 10 minutes.

Treatment

1. Remove the person from water.
2. Clear respiratory passage.
3. Artificial respiration by Schafer's or Holger Neilsen method or even mouth to mouth.
4. Apply warmth to the body by blankets and hot drinks.
5. Stimulants may be given.
6. Antibiotics to prevent pneumonia.
7. Electrolyte imbalance to be corrected.

Postmortem Findings

External findings

a. Due to presence of body in the water:
1. Cloths are wet sand or mud may be present over the body.
2. Rigor mortis sets in early because of struggle for life.
3. Cutis anserina: Also known as "Goose Skin" which is produced by contraction of arrector pili muscles of the skin in cold water and later on due to rigor mortis.
4. Face is pale and eyes are half open.
5. Penis and scrotum are found retracted in cold water.
6. Washer woman's hands: Skin of the hands and feet becomes bleached and corrugated in 12 to 24 hours of body in water.

b. Those due to drowning process:
1. Fine, leathery (shaving leather like), white and tenacious froth present around mouth and nostrils. Froth is rarely tinged with blood. If chest is pressed more froth may come out.
2. Gravels, sand, weeds or grass may be grasped firmly in hands as a result of cadaveric spasm. Sand may be present under the fingernails or nails may be damaged due to efforts in catching something.

Internal Findings

1. *Larynx:* Trachea, bronchi and larynx are filled with white fine froth which may contain sand or mud particles.
2. *Lungs:* Lungs are voluminous, overdistended and cover the heart and is known as "Emphysema equosum". They bulge out of chest on dissection of the chest. Lungs show indentation of ribs, have doughy feeling and pits on pressure. They show mottling due to rupture of vascular bed known as Paltauf's hemorrhages.
3. *Brain and meninges:* They are congested.
4. *Heart:* Right side of the heart is distended and filled with blood.
5. *Stomach:* May contain similar water with mud sand or plants, in about 70% of drowning cases. It was postulated by Rushton that water may enter stomach in postmortem drowning cases but not into the lungs. However it is seen that due to hydrostatic pressure some amount of water may enter lungs of a dead body (hydrostatic lung) but typical froth is not seen.

6. *Small intestines:* May show water in few cases along with mud, sand, etc. especially in the duodenum.
7. *Middle ear:* Water may enter middle ear due to violent respiratory efforts.
8. *Nasal sinuses:* Water may be seen in the nasal sinuses in drowning cases.
9. *Temporal bone hemorrhage:* In some cases temporal bone hemorrhages may be seen but these hemorrhages are also present in hanging, head injury and carbon monoxide poisoning.
10. *Chemical changes in blood:* Gettler suggested that the chloride concentration of blood (96–106 mEq/L) may differ from right side and left side of the heart. It was thought that 25% difference was diagnostic of drowning. In fresh water drowning the chloride concentration will be more on the right side of heart as dilution occur on the left side, whereas in salt water drowning the chloride concentration is more on the left side of heart. However, these days it is not relied upon, as the surfactant a lipoprotein present in lung alveoli, gets diluted as soon as fresh or sea water enters the alveoli, resulting in collapse of the alveoli hence exchange of fluid or electrolytes is minimised. Magnesium levels have also been studied (Moritz) in drowning.
11. *Adrenal preservation:* It putrefies late in drowning cases.
12. *Diatoms:* Diatoms are unicellular algae of different shapes and sizes found in water (Fig. 17.5). They have hard siliceous covering known as "frustules". They pass through alveolar wall into the blood and get deposited at various places. Presence of diatoms by microscopic examination of bone marrow, brain and liver may help in diagnosing death from drowning. Water sample from the place of drowning is also taken and the diatoms present are matched with the diatoms found in the body organs. They are mainly helpful in putrefied bodies but not highly reliable in other cases unless they are matched with the diatoms present in water from where the body was recovered.

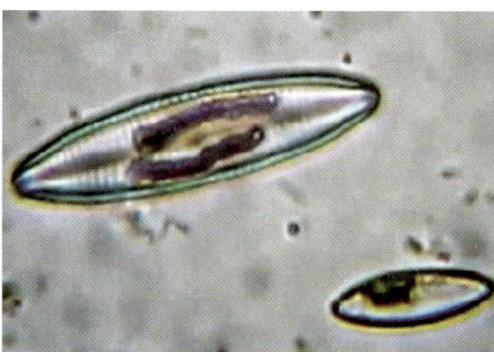

Fig. 17.5: Diatoms

Medicolegal Issues

1. **Whether death is from drowning:** In case a person is killed and thrown in water then such a case has to be differentiated from antemortem drowning by noting following features:
   a. White, fine, lathery froth at the mouth and nostrils.
   b. Grass or weeds held in hands due to cadaveric spasm.
   c. Fine froth in the respiratory passages.
   d. Voluminous, water lodged lungs (emphysema equosum).
   e. Presence of water containing weeds, sand or mud in stomach and small intestines.
   f. Diatoms are helpful in putrefied bodies.
   g. Adrenal preservation can also be of some help in early putrefaction.
   In decomposed bodies it may be difficult to determine death from drowning. It can be decided by circumstantial evidence, absence of any other cause of death and presence of diatoms. In immersion syndrome presence of large quantities of alcohol may be significant.
2. **Drowning is homicidal, accidental or suicidal in nature:** Death from drowning is mostly accidental, sometimes suicidal and rarely homicidal.
   Accidental deaths from drowning occur in non-swimmers, when they accidentally fall in water. Sometimes expert swimmers may also drown as they take deep breaths before diving

for a longer distance. Once they dive, are not seen on the surface again and drown. Such a condition is known as "*Hyperventilation Syndrome*". By hyperventilating before the dive they take in oxygen but washes away more of carbon dioxide. While diving oxygen level goes down but the carbon dioxide level does not rise to that level which can trigger signals to the brain so that a person can come to surface for breathing.

Suicidal drowning deaths are mostly seen in females. Before committing suicide they tie up their cloths so that the body is not exposed. Sometimes they even tie their hands, which can be made out by the manner in which they are tied.

Homicidal deaths are rare except in infants or small children. They are robbed and thrown in wells or ponds. Female infants are also killed by drowning them in milk, so as to avoid any suspicion in north India, known as "Doodh peeta Karna".

SEXUAL ASPHYXIA

Some times death occurs in a person while he is producing partial asphyxia for sexual gratification. Deaths in such cases are due to failure of some safety mechanism. Following factors are considered to ascertain death from sexual asphyxia:

a. *Scene of death:* It is some quite place where no one can disturb them. Rest of the family members are away. Pornographic material is present around. Some mechanism to produce partial asphyxia is present.

b. *Clothing:* Invariably the body is found naked or dressed in female attire.

c. *Age and sex:* Males are all most exclusively involved in such cases; females rarely indulge in such practices. Age group of such persons is between 12 to 23 years. White color workers and artistic class of people are mostly seen to practice sexual asphyxia.

d. *Mode of asphyxia:* Most of the times partial asphyxia is produced by constricting neck, which may be augmented by some chemical substances. There is some safety mechanism which releases the pressure once the aim to produce partial asphyxia is achieved. Death is due to failure of this mechanism.

18 | Operation Theater Mishaps

Any death occurring inside the operation theater is a matter of great distress to the relatives and the surgical team including anesthetist. Type of anesthesia, nature of operation and clinical condition of the patient prior to surgery determine the anesthetic risks. Death and complications occurring during anesthesia are on the decline with advent of safer drugs, equipment and monitoring procedures. In majority of cases anesthesia may be a contributory factor in the morbidity and mortality during surgical procedure whereas the fatalities from purely anesthetic mishaps are very few, even less than 0.1% of cases.

COMMON CAUSES OF SURGICAL OPERATION RELATED MISHAPS

a. *Death from disease or injury for which the surgical procedure was required:* In certain critical conditions the surgeries are performed to save the life of the patient like severe head injuries or penetrating injuries to heart and lungs. Relatives are well aware in such a situation that the patient may or may not survive the operative process. In such cases the morbid condition is mentioned as the cause of death, which may be challenged by the relative demanding an inquiry to determine the cause of death.

b. *Comorbid conditions resulting in death of the patient:* In certain situations the death of the patient may take place from some other condition which existed prior to the operation. Hence all the patients must be evaluated for any comorbid conditions like hypertension, myocardial infarction, corpulmonale before the operative procedure and anesthesia.

c. *Anesthetic mishaps:* In rare cases anesthetic mishap may be the cause of death during surgical procedures. Deaths due to purely anesthetic reasons are very few:

   i. *Anoxia:* It could be as a result of hypoventilation, inadvertent mixing of cylinders, failed intubation, aspiration of vomitus or overhydration leading to pulmonary edema.

   ii. *Cerebral ischemia:* There may be cerebral ischemia resulting from hypotension or excessive hemorrhage.

   iii. *Cardiac arrest:* This may take place from coronary insufficiency due to hypotension or ectopic resulting from anesthetic drugs.

   iv. *Equipment failure:* Malfunctioning equipment may some time leads to the death of a patient.

   v. *Overdose of drugs:* Drug overdose may result from use of multiple drugs, accidental intravascular injection, injection of concentrated stock solution or use of drugs with narrow safety margin.

vi. Inadequate resuscitation or crisis management may be due to inexperience in handling such situations.

vii. Inadequate reversal or inadequate post-operative management

Reasons for anesthetic mishaps purely based on anesthetist:

i. *Technical:* Deficiency of technical skills and poor understanding of the equipment.

ii. *Judgmental:* Bad decision due to poor training or anxiety.

iii. *Monitoring and vigilance failure:* Failure to recognize a problem and delayed response.

d. *Surgical mishaps:* Inexperienced surgeon may some times causes death of the patient from excessive bleeding or cardiac arrest due to vagal inhibition.

e. *Miscellaneous:* This group includes certain unexpected events occurring during the surgical procedure like mismatched transfusion or embolism.

Preventive Aspects

1. *Consent:* Before any procedure of anesthesia, proper informed consent must be obtained from the patient. Individual should be informed about the risks of the procedure and alternatives available for his condition.

2. *Record maintenance:* Proper records must be maintained including history of the ailment, old medical history, details of the procedure and the details of the adverse events if any. Records must not be altered by overwriting.

3. *Attending the patient:* Patient to be operated must be visited frequently by the surgeon as well as by the anesthetist to explain the procedure and risks involved. Patient must be clearly identified along with the type of surgery and the side on which it is to be performed must be recorded.

4. *Proper investigations:* All required investigations must be carried out to make sure that the person is fit for operation and anesthesia.

5. *High-risk cases:* If required consult the concerned specialist for any heart or chest ailment regarding fitness for the procedure. Proper preoperative assessment must be carried out.

6. *No guarantee:* Never give any guarantee for the cure.

7. *Nothing against the will:* Patient must be aware of all the anesthetic and surgical procedure and nothing should be done against the will of the patient.

8. *Equipment maintenance:* Anesthetic or surgical equipment must be periodically checked by the trained technicians. Anesthetist must see that they are fully functional before the start of the operation.

9. *Training:* All members of the surgical and anesthetic team must be trained and knowledgeable. They must attend relevant CME's to keep them fully trained to handle any eventuality.

10. *Proper protocols:* All the procedures must be performed following proper protocols.

11. Monitoring: Supervision by senior experienced staff is desirable. Monitoring of the patient by various equipment to keep a check on the vitals of the patient must be done. Patient must never be left with an inexperienced junior staff for monitoring. Always keep a watch during reversal of the anesthesia.

Medicolegal Autopsy

Proper investigations including an autopsy should be carried out in all deaths occurring, during or just after the operative procedure. Autopsy surgeon may have to answer certain questions after the autopsy procedure.

a. Whether surgery was required or justified for the ailment.

b. Whether the surgeon and anesthetist were competent, experienced and skilled to perform the procedure.

c. Whether the death was from the operative or anesthetic misadventure or from the pre-existing disease or injury.

d. Whether the procedures adopted were as per the routine practice or protocols.

e. Whether proper preoperative investigations/preanesthetic checkup was done along with investigating comorbid conditions if any.

f. Whether death was from some unexpected event.

g. Whether proper monitoring facilities were available during the operation.

h. Cause of death.

Autopsy surgeon is not competent to answer some of the above quarries; hence he should involve independent anesthetist and surgeon in the investigations. In majority of cases of anesthetic mishaps, it may not be possible to pinpoint cause of death. The investigative team should proceed in following manner:

a. *History:* Detailed history must be obtained from the surgical team and the anesthetist about the event. Medical history must be enquired from the relatives. It may be possible that patient might not have disclosed certain medical conditions to the operating surgeon like asthma or diabetes.

b. *Records verification:* All the hospital records like preoperative details including clinical status of the patient, radiographs, PAC documents, consent form, nursing notes, operation and anesthesia notes, resuscitative measures records must be checked for any discrepancy in required investigations, drug doses, monitoring procedure, etc.

c. *Surgical and anesthetic equipment:* These must be examined along with experts from the concerned specialty and the technicians form the equipment supplying firm. Monitoring equipment must also be tested for their functioning as well as any leakage of current. Intravenous fluid bags or blood bags must be collected, sealed and handed over to investigating officer.

d. *External examination of the body:* Body should be properly examined for signs of asphyxia like cyanosis, pale colour indication blood loss, any swelling or edema present. Signs of injection prick marks, their number and location must be recorded. Presence of any cannula, catheters, endotracheal tubes and drainage tubes must be mentioned in the report.

e. *Internal examination:* Autopsy surgeon must be careful while dissecting the body. Check the location and position of the endotracheal or any other tube before collecting and preserving them. X-ray before the autopsy may be of help to check the position of the endotracheal tube. Check for any pneumothorax or hemothorax before opening the chest. Mouth, larynx and trachea must be examined for any signs of aspiration from vomitus after ruling out terminal regurgitation. Larynx must be examined for presence of any laryngeal edema. Brain must be preserved for histopathology for the possibility of anoxic damage. All other visceral organs must be examined and samples preserved. Bladder must be examined for any residue urine.

f. *Operative procedure:* Literature must be studied regarding the surgical procedure carried out before the surgical site is explored. Note any deviation from the normal. Any excessive bleeding at the site from any loose bleeder or slippage of the knot must be recorded.

g. *Preservation of samples:* Various samples are collected from the body to ascertain the cause of the death.

  i. Blood, urine, CSF and vitreous samples: These samples are collected and preserved for toxicological analysis to find out any overdose. However the drugs used in anesthesia are metabolised very fast in the liver hence the tests may not be reliable in most of the cases. Blood may also be sent for creatinine phosphokinase.

  ii. Brain to find out any anoxic changes on histopathology.

  iii. Lung may be preserved in a water tight plastic bag for respiratory gases used during anesthesia.

  iv. Visceral organs: About 100 grams of each should be preserved.

  v. Skeletal muscles: Sample is collected for enzymatic studies for hyperpyrexia.

19 | Forensic Osteology

Forensic osteology mainly deals with the forensic assessment of human skeletonised remains. Whenever, a forensic expert encounters a complete or a partial skeleton, it is always a challenge to answer many questions posed by the law enforcement agencies. Problem becomes more serious when fragmented bone pieces are brought for examination.

When skeletonised structures are brought for examination, details about their condition and numbers are noted. Presence of maggots and their development stages are recorded apart from preserving maggot samples in acetic-alcohol and another sample with soft tissues in a corked test tube. Bones are then cleaned and prepared for further examination. There are different ways to prepare the bones to be examined. In quick method the stock solution known as "*Antiformin*" is prepared by dissolving 150 gm of sodium carbonate in 250 ml of water and 100 gm of bleaching powder (CaOCl) in 750 ml of water and the mixing the two solutions. This solution is mixed with 1 liter of 15% sodium hydroxide solution. The solution is diluted by adding 10 times water before boiling the bones in this solution. This is a fast process and may clean the bones in about one hour. There are number of other methods for cleaning the bones. Second commonest method is by mixing bleach solution with sodium hydroxide for removing fat and soft tissues.

HUMAN OR ANIMAL BONES

1. *Anatomical features:* To answer whether the bones are of human origin or not, forensic experts mostly depend on the anatomical characteristics. However in fragmented bones it may be difficult to predict the source. There are similarities in the human bones and the closely related species like great apes. Similarities have been observed in the bones of hand and feet of humans and bears. Anatomical features present in skull like facial features in a vertical plane except in negroid race where some protrusion of the jaw bones is present, large skull capacity, location of foramen magnum anteriorly than in animals, at the junction of posterior and middle one-third are some of the differentiating features. Linea aspera in femur is present in humans. Ossification of costal cartilage takes place on the surface of the cartilage in humans whereas in animals the entire cartilage is ossified.

2. *Precipitin test:* Bone fragments which are relatively fresh can be easily identified as human or animal by performing precipitin test. In case bones are subjected to heat or chemicals, precipitin test may not give proper results.

3. *Microscopic examination:* Microscopy may be of little help in the identification of human bones as the bone structure is similar in mammalian species. However haversian

canal system has been studied and differences were observed in the micrometric data of skeletons from different sources.

4. *Corticomedullary index:* Cortical thickness comparison with medullary diameter of femoral bones has been used to differentiate human bone from animal bones with some success.

TIME SINCE DEATH

Interpretation of time since death depends on circumstances and conditions in which the dead body was subjected after death. Time since death can be determined in skeletonised body by means of (1) physical observations; (2) using dating techniques, and (3) deterioration of the articles present on the body like cloths or shoes.

1. **Physical observations**
   i. *Putrefactive changes:* Whether exposed to atmosphere; buried in soil or presence of body in water; cold or hot season or climate may enhance or decrease rate of putrefaction leading to skeletonisation. Factors which also affect the rate of putrefaction are circumstances of death, pre-existing condition of the body, environment, temperature, humidity, invasion by insects; and mutilation by animals.

      After the loss of soft tissues of the body ligaments take longer time to disappear. Skeletonisation of the body, depending upon the factors mentioned above, may take place from few months to few years. Bodies buried under snow are sometimes recovered intact even after many years.
   ii. *Odor of decay:* It is one of the indicators suggesting the bones are fresh; therefore, Green and smelling bones are recent whereas the dry, odorless and brittle bones are old bones.
   iii. *Invasion by insects:* It is helpful in determination of time since death in two ways:
   a. *Using maggot age and development:* This method is used within first few weeks after death. Maggots are the larvae or the immature developmental stages of the flies which are attracted first to the corpse. Flies (class deptera) like, blue bottle fly (calliphora), green bottle fly (lucilla) and common house fly (musca domestica) are initially attracted by the corpse. They lay their eggs usually in the wounds or moist area of the body soon after death. Depending upon the fly involved the eggs hatch into the first stage larva which then moults into second stage larva and subsequently into third stage larva. During larval stages they feed on the body and then migrate away from the body to pupate with hardened outer skin which gradually turns brown. Adult fly emerges from the pupa after number of days. Details mentioned in chapter on changes after death under time since death from putrefaction.
   b. *Using successional waves of insects:* This method is used when the death has taken place few weeks back. Western literature reports that there may be eight different waves of insect invasion by different types of insects. However, due to fast rate of decomposition in Indian subcontinent all such waves are not possible. Literature may be referred for such interpretations.

2. **Dating techniques:** These methods are primarily used by anthropologists to date old bones. Some of the tests done for this purpose are mentioned below:
   i. *Total nitrogen content of bone:* It decreases with time; in dry fresh bones nitrogen content is about 4% if nitrogen content is more than 3.5 gm then the bones are less than 50 years old and when the nitrogen content goes below 2.5 gm by weight the age is more than 350 years.
   ii. *Amino acids:* There is selective loss of amino acids from bone protein after death. There are 17 amino acids in bones, if the number goes below 7 the bones are more than 100 years old.

iii. *Fluorescent studies:* These are done with ultraviolet rays from the freshly cut surface of the bone. Full fluorescence is present up to 100 years, half up to 400 years and residual fluorescence up to 1800 years.

iv. *Immunological studies:* These are done with anti-human serum and are possible up to 5 to 10 years.

v. *Radioactive C_{14} studies:* Carbon dating have been of use in dating old bones.

vi. *Dipartite crystal:* Studies are done to measure the increasing size with increased time interval by stereo-scan electron microscope.

vii. *Benzidine test:* Benzidine test is positive up to 5 to 10 years but may show some residual positivity up to 150 years.

viii. *Specific gravity:* In recent bones the specific gravity is 1.7 to 2.2, whereas, fossil bones have lower specific gravity of less than 1.7.

ix. *Conductivity* of supersonic oscillations gives higher figures in recent bones in comparison to older bones.

x. Some studies have been done to measure fat content of the bone, urea levels, potassium contents and sulphur concentration in the bone to estimate time since death.

3. **Deterioration of the articles present on the body like cloths or shoes:** Preservation of clothing and other artifacts present on the body deteriorate at a very slow rate depending on the material from which they are made. Things made of synthetic fiber show slow degradation in comparison with the natural fibers.

SEX DETERMINATION

Sex differentiating features appear only after the onset of puberty. It is advisable to determine the sex from the bones before, assessing the age in case the bones are of post-adolescent period.

Subjective Sex Determination

Differentiating features are apparent after the secondary sex characteristics have made their appearance. Changes due to old age may sometimes interfere in the interpretation; hence sex features are best assessed between 20 to 55 years of age. In case a complete skeleton is available the sex can be determined easily and accurately. If only the pelvis is available the sex prediction is accurate up to 95% of cases; from skull it is possible up to 90%. However if both skull and pelvis are available sex can be predicted up to 98% of cases. When whole skeleton is available sex can be accurately predicted in an adult. (Fig. 19.1).

In general male bones are larger, ridges are prominent, rough in comparison and long bones are larger in size when compared to the female bones. (Tables 19.1, 19.2 and 19.3).

Objective Sex Determination

Objective sex determination is done by using ratio between two measurements in a bone.

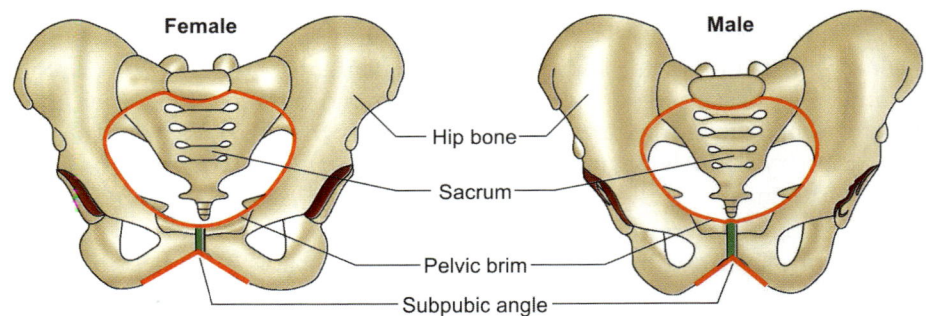

Fig. 19.1: Pelvis sex differentiation

Table 19.1: Sex differences in mandible

Feature	Male	Female
1. General appearance	Larger, thicker	Smaller, thinner
2. Body height at symphysis	More	Less
3. Ascending ramus	Broad	Less broad
4. Chin	Square	Rounded
5. Angle between body and ramus (Gonial)	Less obtuse (<125)	More obtuse (>125)
6. Mandible angle	Everted	Inverted
7. Condyles	Larger, more articular area	Smaller

Table 19.2: Sex Differences in Pelvis

Feature	Male	Female
1. Pelvis framework	Rough, heavy with prominent muscle marking	Smoother with less muscular markings
2. Brim	Heart shaped	Circular or oval
3. True pelvis	Smaller	Spacious, more oblique
4. Body of pubis	Triangular	Quadrangular
5. Subpubic arch	V shaped	U shaped, broader
6. Symphysis	High	Low, may show parturition scars on dorsal surface.
7. Preauricular sulcus	Infrequent	More common and deep
8. Ischiopubic rami	Slightly everted, convex above	More everted and concave above
9. Acetabulum	Large	Smaller
10. Greater sciatic notch	Smaller, narrow and deep	Large, wide and shallow
11. Ilia	High, more upright	Lower, more flaring in upper portion
12. Sacroiliac articulation	Large	Smaller, more oblique
13. Sacrum	High and narrow	Shorter and broader, less curved in upper segments
14. Ischial tuberosity	Inverted	Everted
15. Obturator foramen	Large oval with base upwards	Small, triangular, apex forwards
16. Pelvic outlet	Smaller	Larger

Table 19.3: Sex differences in skull

Feature	Male	Female
1. General appearance	Larger, heavier, rough	Smaller, lighter, smoother
2. Frontal eminences	Less prominent	More prominent
3. Cranial capacity	more 8 to 12% (>1450 ml)	Less (< 1350 ml)
4. Glabella	More prominent	Less prominent
5. Supraorbital ridges	More prominent	Less prominent
6. Frontonasal angle	Show angulation	Smoothly curved
7. Orbits	Square, rounded margins	Rounded, sharp margins
8. Zygomatic arches	Prominent	Less prominent
9. Parietal eminences	Less prominent	More prominent
10. Mastoid process	Large, pointing downwards	Small, medially pointing

Contd.

Table 19.3: Sex differences in skull *(Contd.)*		
Feature	*Male*	*Female*
11. Occipital area	Prominent muscular markings	Muscular markings not prominent
12. Foramen magnum	Opening area is large	Small, rounded
13. Palate	Larger, U shaped	Smaller, parabolic
14. Occipital condyles	Large	Small
15. Nasal aperture	Higher, narrower	Lower, broader
16. Forehead contour	Irregular, less rounded	Rounded, infantile
17. Sphenoid body	Longer	Smaller

1. **Fetal sex**
   a. *Sciatic notch index (Boucher, 1955):* Sciatic notch width/by sciatic depth × 100 is more in females, i.e. between 5 and 6 whereas it is between 4 and 5 in males and can give positive results in about 85% of cases.
   b. *Chilotic index:* Ilium posterior height/ ilium anterior height × 100 has been used for sex determination. The index is more in males.
2. **Sex determination during infancy:** Boys lead in pelvic height, breadth, iliac breadth and length of femoral neck. Whereas girls lead in bi-ischial breadth, pubic length, breadth of greater sciatic notch, relative inlet breadth and inter pubic breadth.
3. **Adults**
   a. *Pelvic indices:*
      i. *Ischium pubis index:* Pubic length/ ischium length × 100 which is less in males and more in females.
      ii. *Angle of sciatic notch:* Angle formed at the sciatic notch is more in females and give 75% positive results. In combination with ischium pubic index the prediction rate goes up to 95%.
      iii. *Pelvic index:* This index has been used for sexual differentiation. It is calculated in the following manner.
      Anteroposterior diameter/transverse diameter × 100.
      iv. *Cotylo-sciatic index:* Distance from the edge of acetabulum to sciatic notch/ sciatic height perpendicular to same

boarder to posterior iliac spine × 100. In females on an average it is 141.0 whereas average in males it is 104.6.
   v. *Chilotic line:* Point on the iliopectineal line at the union of pubis and iliac bone, and point on the anterior margin of the auricular surface nearest the earlier point are joined and the line is extended up to iliac rest. The sacral part of this line is less and pelvic part is more in females, however the combined length is more in males (Fig. 19.2).
   vi. *Ilium indices:* (a) upper iliac height/ lower iliac height and (b) iliac breadth/ direct iliac height are used for sexual differentiation.
   vii. Phenice (1969) use three criteria to find the sex (a) triangular area on the ventral surface of the pubic body at the inferior medial angle: (b) convexity of the medial boarder of inferior ramus

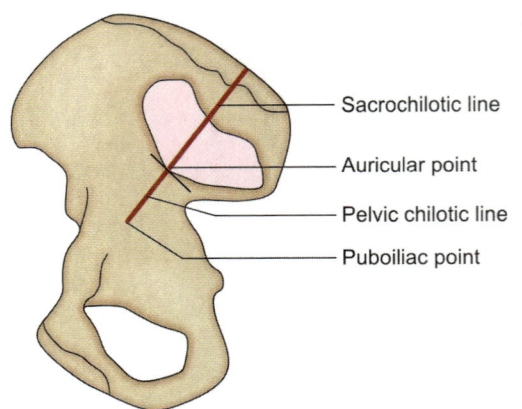

Fig. 19.2: Chilotic line

near pubic arch and (c) ridge extending from inferior end of articular surface ventromedially into inferior ramus.

viii. *Parturition pits:* These scars may be seen on the dorsal surface of the pubis in the form of irregularities and pits in females who had babies.

ix. *Sacral index:* Out of the sacral measurements, mean maximum length of sacrum is more in males.

b. *Skull and mandible indices:*

i. *Discriminant function studies:* Various cranial measurements have been used to devise discriminant function sexing like maximum cranial length, maximum cranial breadth, basion bregma height, basion to nasion height, facial height and facial breadth. Discriminant function scores less than the sectioning points classify that bone as female.

ii. *Mastoid process:*

- Mastoid process has been divided depending on the direction and the concavity above the base of the process into M, N and F types. M type; the mastoid process is directed downwards and there is concavity above the base of the process. N type; the mastoid process points downwards but without concavity. F type; the mastoid is medially directed. M type is seen in majority of male skulls whereas F type is predominantly seen in female skulls. (Fig. 19.3).
- Mastoid module may be of some help in differentiating sex. This is achieved by multiplying mastoid height (vertical height up to porion) with mastoid length (asterion to porion length).

iii. Foramen magnum area is more in males than in females.

Sternum and Ribs

Various measurements of sternum are used for sexual dimorphism like; (i) manubrium

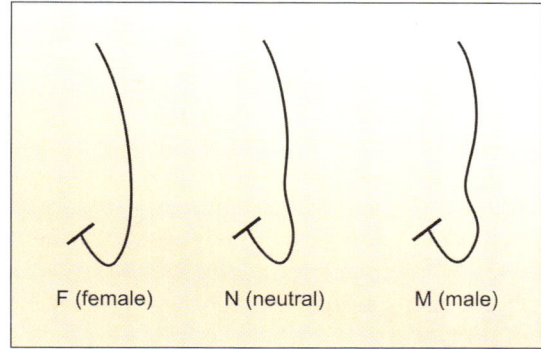

F (female)   N (neutral)   M (male)

Fig. 19.3: Sexual differences in mastoid bone

length; (ii) body length of sternum; (iii) manubrium-corpus index: manubrium length to body length of sternum gives lower figures for male in comparison to females; (iv) combined length of manubrium and body length, which according to *Ashley's rule (the 149 rule)* is more than 149 mm in males and (v) Relative width index: first sternebral width to third sternebral width of sternum.

Fourth rib has also been studied for the sexual differentiation.

Scapula

Scapular measurements like scapular height, scapular breadth, total length of spine, width of glenoid cavity and maximum length of the glenoid cavity have been used to find out sex of scapula.

Long Bones

1. *Medullary index:* Humerus, radius ulna and tibia are most suited for estimating medullary index for sex determination.

2. *Other parameters of femur bone:* Some dimensions have been used in femur to differentiate sex like (a) vertical diameter of the head; (b) popliteal length; (c) trochanteric oblique length, all these lengths are more in males.

3. *Humeral mid shaft circumference:* Radial length, mid shaft and head circumference; Ulnar length and mid shaft circumference have given good results in sex differentiation.

AGE DETERMINATION

Determination of age from skeletal remains is of great importance in crime detection. Cases can be included or excluded on the basis of age of the skeletal remains. Various factors influence appearance and union of various centers and growth of bones. Sex, race, environment and nutrition are some of them:

a. *Size of the bones:* With age the bones of the body goes on growing till the growth stops. In the long bones the growth takes place at the epiphyseal plate and continues till the epiphysis unites with diaphysis.

   Out of the long bones femur diaphyseal length (shaft) has been examined against the crown-rump length during intrauterine period and stature during childhood, which is considered as the best indicator of age. The results were comparable to the eruption time of teeth. Average length calculations were done separately for males and females. Many such studies have also been done by radiographic methods.

b. *Appearance of ossification centers:* Even though adult person has 206 bones but these bones develop from multiple ossification centers. First ossification centers are seen in the clavicle bone between 4 and 5 weeks of intrauterine period. Most of the long bone shafts have ossification centers by 8th week of intrauterine (IU) period which are known as primary centers. At birth there are about 450 ossification centers out of which there are only six centers for epiphysis; head of humerus; condyles of femur and tibia; talus; cuboid and calcaneus bones of the foot. Secondary ossification centers appear after birth. Appearance of ossification centers is a very good indicator of the age of a person.

c. *Epiphyseal union:* Most of the long bone shafts are ossified before birth however ends of the bones, i.e. epiphyses ossify after birth. Long bones have epiphysis at either ends with single or multiple ossification centers, whereas, metacarpals metatarsals, phalanges, ribs and clavicle have only one epiphyseal end. These centers join with the diaphysis at different time intervals by which the age of an individual can be determined (Fig. 19.4 and Table 19.4). Bones

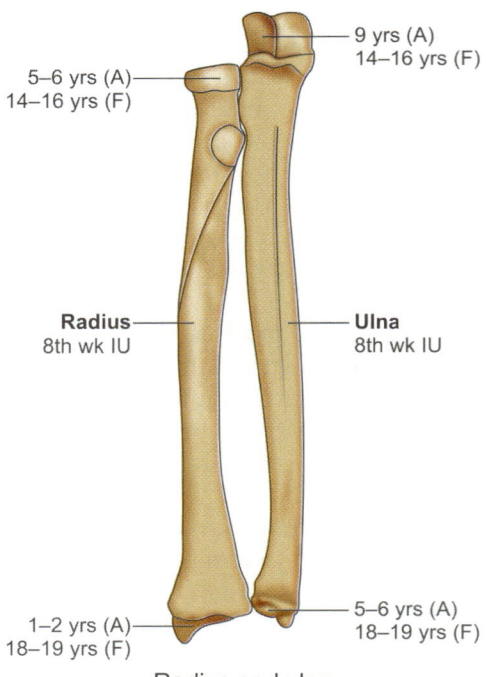

1 yr (A)
3 yrs (A)
5 yrs (A)

Centers fuse by 8 yrs and fuses with shaft at 18–19 yrs

8th wk IU

Conjoint epiphysis formed at 12–14 yrs

5–7 yrs (A)
14–16 yrs (F) fuses separately

11 yrs (A)
1 yr (A)

9–11 yrs (A)

Conjoint epiphysis 14–16 yrs (F)

Humerus

9 yrs (A)
14–16 yrs (F)

5–6 yrs (A)
14–16 yrs (F)

Radius
8th wk IU

Ulna
8th wk IU

1–2 yrs (A)
18–19 yrs (F)

5–6 yrs (A)
18–19 yrs (F)

Radius and ulna

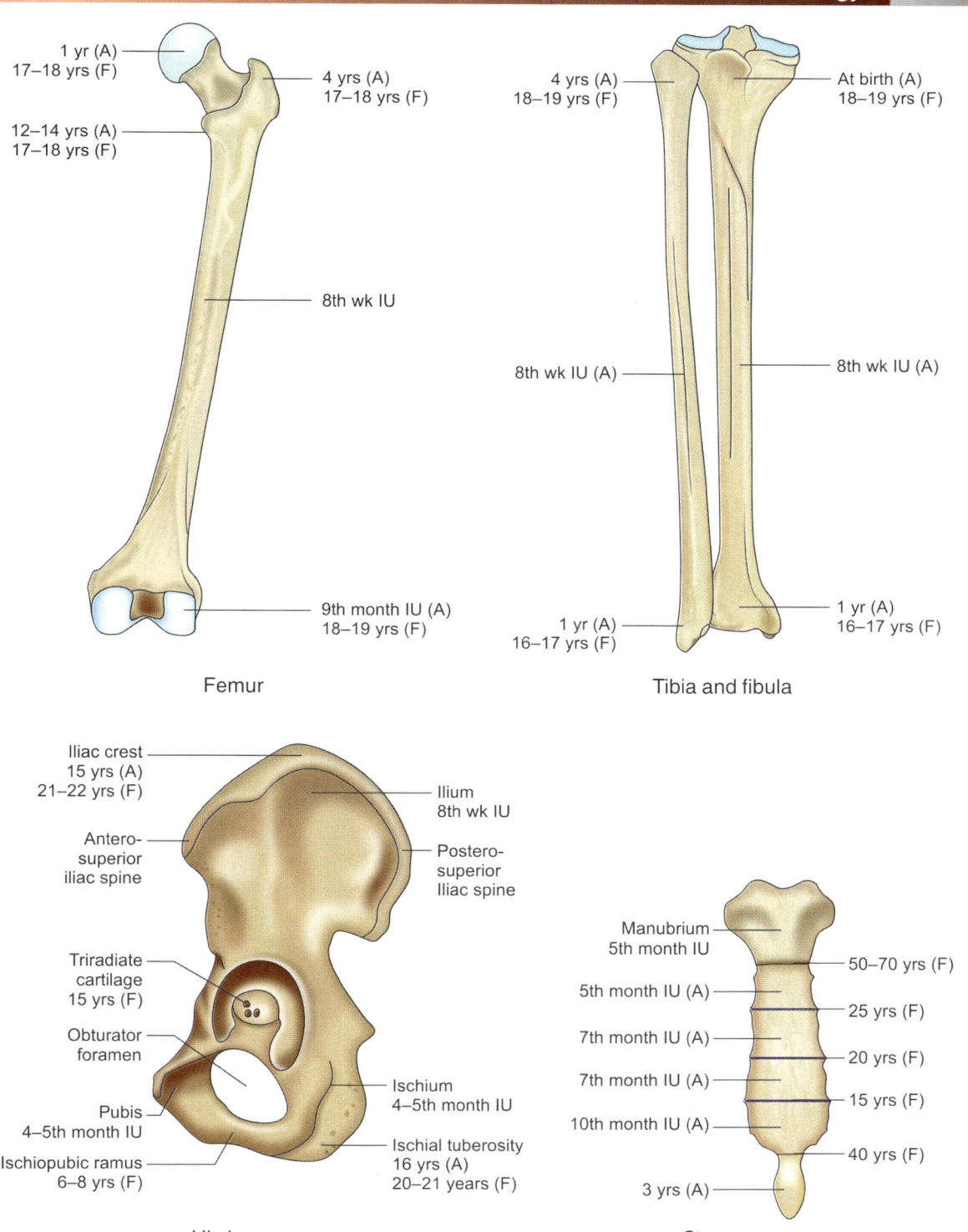

Fig. 19.4: Appearance (A) and Fusion (F) of ossification centers

Table 19.4: Ossification centers their appearance and fusion			
Bone	*Center of ossification*	*Age of appearance*	*Age of fusion*
Sternum	Manubrium	5th month IU	60–70 years
	First body segment	5th month IU	
	2nd body segment	7th month IU	15 yrs to 25 yrs from below upwards
	3rd body segment	7th month IU	
	4th body segment	10th month IU	
	Xiphisternum	3 yrs	> 40 years
Clavicle	Medial end	18–19 yrs	20–22 yrs
Humerus	**Upper end:**		Composite epiphysis at upper end is
	Head	1 yr	formed by 6 yrs, which joins with shaft
	Greater tubercle	3 yrs	at 18–19 yrs.
	Lesser tubercle	5 yrs	
	Lower end:		
	Medial epicondyle	6–7 yrs	15–16 yrs
	Lateral epicondyle	12 yrs	Conjoint epiphysis is formed by 14 yrs
	Trochlea	9–11 yrs	and fuses with shaft at 15–16 yrs
	Capitulum	1–2 yrs	
Radius	Upper end	5–6 yrs	14–16 yrs
	Lower end	1–2 yrs	18–19 yrs
Ulna	Upper end	8–9 yrs	16–17 yrs
	Lower end	5–6 yrs	18–19 yrs
Femur	**Upper end:**		
	Head	1 yr	17–18 yrs
	Greater trochanter	4 yrs	17–18 yrs
	Lesser trochanter	12–14 yrs	17–18 yrs
	Lower end	9th month IU	18–19 yrs
Tibia	Upper end	At birth	18–19 yrs
	Lower end	1 yr	16–17 yrs
Fibula	Upper end	4 yrs	18–19 yrs
	Lower end	1 yr	16–17 yrs
Hip bone	Ischiopubic ramus	–	6 yrs
	Triradiate cartilage	–	15 yrs
	Iliac crest	15–16 yrs	20–21 yrs
	Ischial tuberosity	16 yrs	20–21 yrs
Carpal bones	Capitate	1 yr	–
	Hamate	1 yr	–
	Triquetral	2–3 yrs	–
	Lunate	4–5 yrs	–
	Trapezium	5 yrs	–
	Scaphoid	5–6 yrs	–
	Trapezoid	6 yrs	–
	Pisiform	9–11 yrs	–
Tarsal bones	Calcaneum	5th month IU	–
	Tuberosity of calcaneum	6–8 yrs	14–16 yrs
	Talus	7th month IU	–
	Cuboid	9th month IU	–
	Lateral cuneiform	1 yr	–
	Medial cuneiform	2 yrs	–
	Middle cuneiform	3 yrs	–
	Navicular	3 yrs	–
First metacarpal	Base	2–3 yrs	15–16 yrs

are examined for union at the metaphysis by noting changes of union. **McKern and Stewart** carried out evaluation of Korean skeletal remains by dividing the changes into five stages from 0–4. For non-union stage 0; for 1/4 union stage 1; for 1/2 union stage 2; for 3/4 union stage 3 and for complete union stage 4 was assigned. Four stages recognized by **Stevenson** were no union, beginning of union, recent union and complete union. However based on radiological examination **Todd** divided these changes into nine stages:

Stage 1: Diaphysis and epiphysis are in approximate to each other without any intimate relation.

Stage 2: Obscuration of adjacent bony surfaces by transformation into thick hazy zone.

Stage 3: Clearing of haze with appearance of fine delimiting surface as fine white line.

Stage 4: Adjacent surfaces show billowing.

Stage 5: Adjacent surfaces show reciprocal outline parallel to each other.

Stage 6: Gap between adjacent surfaces becomes narrow.

Stage 7: Commencement of union with breakup of fine bellowed outline.

Stage 8: Union is complete showing as red line on the bone.

Stage 9: Complete union with continuity of the trabeculae from shaft to epiphysis.

d. *Suture closure:* Suture closure has also been used to determine the age of an individual. There is wide variation in the suture closure and it may best be used as corroborative evidence. Suture closures are mainly used after long bones show complete epiphyseal union. There are no significant race or sex differences in the skull sutures closure.

i. *Immature skull:* Posterior fontanel closes within 6 months of life. Anterior fontanelle closes between one and half years to two years. Metopic suture closes by 2 to 4 years, however, it may persist in 5 to 10% cases. Occipital bones show fusion of squamous part with lateral

parts at about 3 years and the lateral parts join with basilar part around 6 years. Basilar part joins with base of sphenoid bone at about 18 to 25 years of age.

ii. *Adult skull:* The sutures start closing from inside first (endocranially). *Brocha* described skull suture closure in five stages:
Stage 0: Open suture with well demarcated margins.
Stage 1: Suture show initial stages of closure with suture as clear zigzag line.
Stage 2: Thin suture line may be interrupted at places.
Stage 3: Small remnants of suture are seen as pits at places.
Stage 4: Suture is completely obliterated.
Posterior one-third of the sagittal suture fuses between 30 and 40 years, anterior one third between 40 and 50 years and the middle portion gets united by 50 to 60 years. Outer half of the coronal suture joins first between 40 and 50 years followed by the inner half between 50 and 60 years. Medial half of the lambdoid suture joins first by 50 to 60 years and outer half by 60 to 70 years. Last to close is the temporal suture, which closes by 70 to 80 years.

e. *Changes at pubic symphysis:* Pubic symphysis also show various changes related to the age of a person. **McKern and Stewart** (1957) divided the pubic surface into three components and each component showing 6 stages (0 to 5) to access the age.

Component I: It is the dorsal half of the pubic joint surface showing following changes:
Stage 0: Dorsal margin is absent.
Stage 1: Slight margin formation in the middle one-third.
Stage 2: Margin formation along the entire dorsal boarder.
Stage 3: Resorption of ridges and formation of plateau in the middle one-third of the dorsal surface.
Stage 4: Plateau with remnants of billowing extends to entire dorsal surface.
Stage 5: Billowing disappears completely.

Component II: It is the ventral half of the joint surface showing changes in following stages:

Stage 0: Ventral beveling is absent.

Stage 1: Ventral beveling present in the upper part.

Stage 2: Ventral beveling present along the entire boarder

Stage 3: The ventral rampart begins from either or both extremities.

Stage 4: Rampart is complete except gaps in the upper two-third.

Stage 5: Rampart is complete.

Component III: It is the entire surface of the joint observed after the other changes have taken place:

Stage 0: Symphysial rim is absent.

Stage 1: Partial dorsal rim is present.

Stage 2: Dorsal rim is complete.

Stage 3: Entire symphysial rim is complete.

Stage 4: The rim begins to breakdown with some evidence of lipping on the ventral edge.

Stage 5: Further breakdown of the rim and rarefaction of the symphysial surface.

The score from the three components is totaled and compared against the known scores for various age groups (Fig. 19.5). Parturition scars in females may interfere in the calculation of age in this method.

f. *Scapular changes:* Scapular changes have also been studied in relation to the age of a person. Lipping of the glenoid cavity and the clavicular facet may be seen after 35 or 40 years. There is increasing demarcation of the triangular area at the base of scapular spine which is seen after 50 years. Cristae Scapulae start appearing after 50 years and becomes more roughened or serrated with advancing years.

g. *Sternum:* Four segments of sternal body fuses from below upwards between 14 and 25 years and xiphoid process joins at 40 years with the body.

h. *Hyoid bone:* Greater cornua of hyoid bone joins with body at about 40 to 60 years.

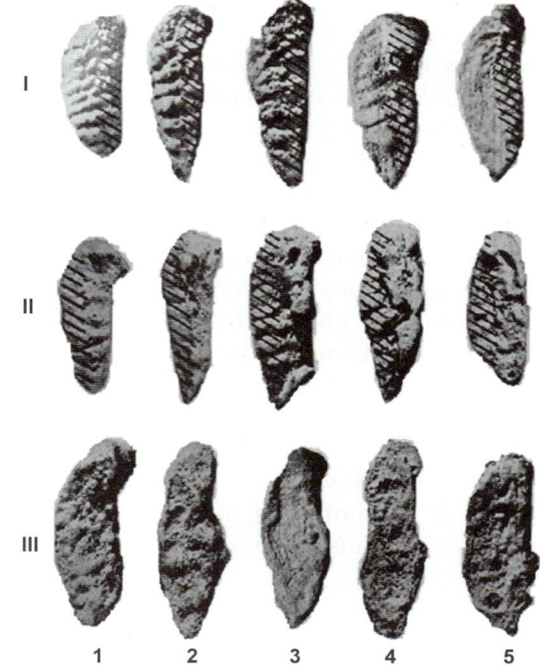

Fig. 19.5: Age related changes in pubic symphysis. Component I; Changes in dorsal half, Component II; Changes in ventral half, and Component III; Changes in the lip. Each component showing changes from stage 1 to stage 5. (McKern and Steward, 1957)

i. *Mandible:* Age related changes are observed in mandible with growth and appearance of teeth till adult age. With loss of teeth in old age there is shrinkage of the body with upward placement of mental foramen (Fig. 19.6).

RACE

Skeletal examination especially the skull may provide some information about the race of the individual.

1. **Skull:** Race can be determined from cephalic index. **Cephalic index** = maximum transverse breadth/maximum anteroposterior length × 100.

Based on the cephalic index the skulls can be classified into following types:

a. *Dolichocephalic:* They are also called long headed with the cephalic index from

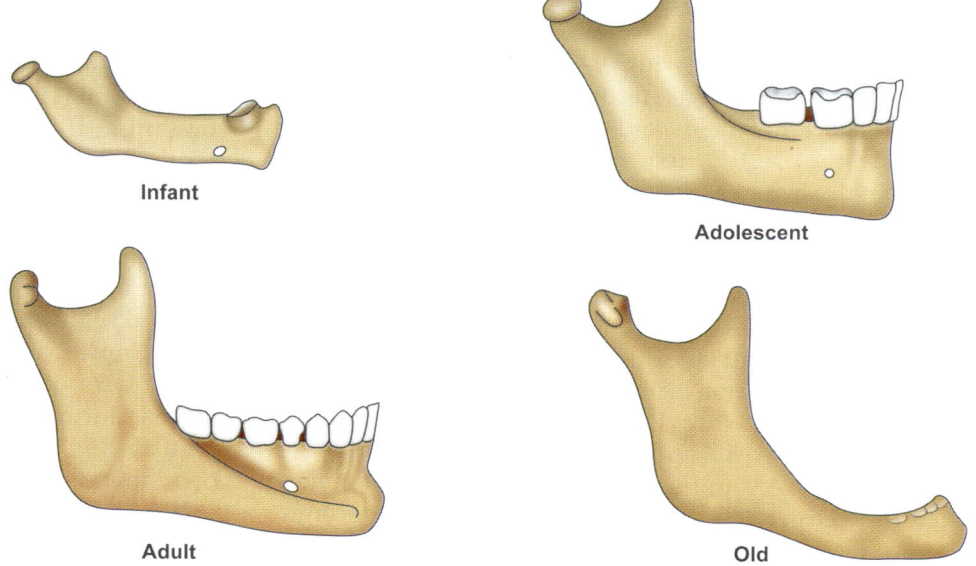

Infant

Adolescent

Adult

Old

Fig. 19.6: Age related changes in mandible

70 to 74.9 and mostly seen in negroid or Aryan race.

b. *Mesaticephalic:* They are medium headed with cephalic index between 75 and 79.9 are present in Europeans.

c. *Brachycephalic*: They are short headed with cephalic index varying from 80 to 84.9. Indians are mostly covered under this category.

Zygomatic arch, which determine the width of the face is more prominent and may exceed head width in mongoloid race. Nasal opening width is more in negroid in comparison with caucasian race.

2. **Long bones:** Femur is slightly straighter in negroid race. Some indices of long bones like brachial index (length of radius/length of humerus × 100) or crural index (length of tibia/length of femur × 100) may be of some help but are not reliable.

3. **Teeth:** Shovel shaped upper medial incisors are seen in mongoloid race. Negroid race have bigger teeth with thicker enamel in comparison with caucasoid race; however, largest teeth are seen in Australians.

STATURE

Estimation of stature from skeletal remains has been tried by various anthropologists. Measurements of the long bones especially of the lower limbs provide better estimates. After calculating stature from the skeleton 2.5 to 4 cm are added for the soft tissues. To get better results stature must be calculated from two or more bones. Race, sex and age of the person at the time of death must be taken into consideration as they modify the stature estimation. A person attains maximum height at the age of 20 to 25 years and progressive loss in stature starts after 25 to 30 years at the rate of 0.6 to 1.0 cm for every decade.

Stature from long bones: Estimation of stature from long bones is done by measuring the maximum length by means of Hepburn type of osteometric board.

i. *Multiplication factor:* The length of the bone is multiplied by a given multiplication factor to calculate the stature. The multiplication factor varies depending upon the sex of the individual.

Pan (1924) worked on the east Indian (Bihar, West Bengal, and Odisha) population and formulated multiplication factors for humerus were 3.82 for males and 3.8 for female; for tibia these were 4.49 for males and 4.46 for females; for humerus it was 5.31 both for males and females; Radius these were 6.78 for males and 6.7 for females whereas for ulna it was 6.0 both for males and females.

Nat (1931) worked on male bones from Uttar Pradesh whereas Siddiqui and Shah worked on male bones from Punjab and devised multiplication factors. Femur the multiplication factors were 3.7 and 3.6; tibia they were 4.48 and 4.2; Humerus they were 5.3 and 5.0 and for radius they were 6.9 and 6.3 for UP and Punjab respectively.

ii. *Relative proportion:* Hardlicka (1939) calculated relative proportion of the length of the femur and humerus in American whites and black population. Humerus to stature index was 19.31 and 18.97 in white males and females whereas it was 19.8 and 20.34 in black males and females respectively. Femur to stature index was 26.6 both for white males and females whereas it was 27.27 and 27.29 in black males and females respectively.

iii. *Regression equations:* For better accuracy regression equations were devised either from a single bone or combination of two bones.

   a. *Pearson formula:* Karl Pearson (1899) calculated stature from long bones of European origin by multiplying with a multiplication factor and adding a constant as additive factor specific for each bone. He devised separate formulae for wet and dry bones. Stature from male dry femur was calculated by multiplying the length of the femur with 1.88 and adding 81.306 cm, whereas stature from dry female femur was calculated by multiplying

the length of the femur by 1.945 and adding 72.884 cm.

   b. *Trotter and Glesser's formula:* They improved upon the formula devised by Pearson by combining the length of two bones or more, like combined length of femur and tibia multiplied with a multiplication factor and then adding a constant specific for that bone and sex of the person, e.g. stature of white male was calculated by adding length of femur and tibia, multiplying with 1.26 and adding 67.09 cm, whereas stature of white female was calculated in the similar manner by taking the combined length of femur and tibia, multiplying with 1.39 and adding 53.20 cm.

   Similar studies have been carried out by various authors in different populations and devised different formulae based on the regional variations.

iv. *Stature from fragmentary bones:* Muller (1935), Steele and McKern (1969) and Steele (1970) carried out studies to calculate total length of humerus, radius and ulna bone by measuring the distance between various landmarks of a particular bone and calculating proportion to the total bone length.

v. Stature from vertebral column and metacarpal lengths have also been used to calculate stature of an individual with some success.

SKELETAL REMAINS BELONG TO HOW MANY INDIVIDUALS?

In wars and mass disasters there may be number of individuals buried together. Hence the forensic expert may be called into match skeletal remains. Bones are arranged in their anatomical position, any duplicate bone or bones from different sex, race, stature and age help the expert to decide that the skeletal remains belong to how many individuals.

Other Features Helpful in Individualization of Bones

Skeletal remains sometimes show some characteristic findings which help in identification.

1. **Skeletal injuries:** Skeletal injuries, loss of bone due to amputation, malunited fracture and bones showing various stages of healing may be of importance in matching the skeletal remains with some missing individual with history of skeletal trauma.

2. **Congenital abnormalities:** Many congenital abnormalities of the human skeleton may help in identification of an individual from the skeletal remains like kyphosis, dwarfism or scoliosis.

3. **Bone diseases:** Some of the bone diseases like osteomyelitis, tumors, gigantism, rickets or poliomyelitis may help in identification of an individual from skeletal remains.

Burnt Bones

In some cases bones subjected to heat are forwarded to forensic experts. Burnt bones show various changes in colour, shrinkage in size, texture and weight. Depending upon the temperature and duration of exposure to heat the colour may change from yellowish brown initially with low intensity heat, then to grayish black or blue with moderate heat and finally with intense heat there is complete calcinations and the bones are recovered as lightweight, fragmentary white pieces and ashes.

Shrinkage and distortion of the burnt bones may pose a problem to forensic experts in providing proper information regarding identification of the skeletal remains.

20 | Torture and Medical Ethics

United nations convention against torture and other cruel, inhuman or degrading treatment or punishment of 10th December 1984 defined torture as follows.

"Any act by which severe pain or suffering whether physical or mental is intentionally inflicted on a person for such purposes as obtaining from him or third person information or confession, punishing him for an act he or third person has committed or is suspected of having committed or intimidating or coercing him or third person, or for any reason based on discrimination of any kind, when such pain or suffering is inflicted by or at the instigation of or with the consent or acquiescence of a public official or other person acting in an official capacity. It does not include any pain or suffering arising only from inherent in or incidental to lawful sanctions."

United Nations Universal Declaration of Human Rights (1948) emphasized on freedom from torture.

"No one shall be subjected to torture, cruel, inhuman or degrading treatment or punishment."

In medical profession ethics and code of conduct is practiced with high level of integrity. *Charak* (700 BC) devised a rigid code of conduct for physicians. *Hippocratic oath* (5th century BC) primarily centered on the principle of "Primus non nocere" meaning above all, do no harm.

World Medical Association as per *declaration of geneva* (1948, 1968 and 1983) emphasized that a "physician should consecrate his life to the service of humanity" and "health of the patient will be his first consideration". It also stressed to "maintain the honour and traditions of medical profession and respect human life from the beginning, even under threat."

International code of medical ethics (1949, 1968 and 1983) expected that a physician is required to "maintain the highest standard of professional conduct and act only in the patient's interest". He will "always bear in mind the obligation of preserving human life".

The declaration of Tokyo (1975) framed guidelines by the World Medical Assembly expressing that "doctors shall not condone or participate in the practice of torture or other forms of cruel, inhuman or degrading procedure, in all situations. Doctor shall not provide any premises, instruments, substances or knowledge to facilitate the practice of torture. A doctor shall not be present during such procedures". They also assured the doctors that world medical association will support doctors in face of threat or reprisals resulting from refusal.

World Psychiatrists Association in declaration of Hawaii (1977 and 1983) has provided detailed guidelines on the role of a psychiatrist in torture procedures. Similarly *International Council of Nurses* (1978) projected guidelines on the role of nurses in care of detainees and prisoners".

United Nations (1948) in *universal declaration of human rights*, article 5, stipulates that "No one shall be subjected to torture, cruel, inhumane or degrading treatment or punishment. Principles of medical ethics (1982) enumerated six principles of medical ethics relevant to the role of health professionals in protection of prisoners and detainees against torture. Even *United nations declaration against torture* (1975) came out with a detailed document on protection of all persons from torture and other cruel, inhuman or degrading treatment.

In India *article 21 of the constitution* guarantees that no person shall be deprived of his life and personal liberty except according to the procedure established by law. Under *IPC section 330* any person in authority, for resorting to torture of a person in custody for extortion of information, is liable for penal action.

Government of India enacted *human rights act* (1993) and established national human rights commission to act as a watch dog.

Code of medical ethics advocated by Indian medical council specifically mentions that medical personal shall not use medical knowledge contrary to the laws of humanity and the health of the patient will be the first consideration.

Unfortunately medical professionals as a group, despite all above provisions, have failed to react appropriately to minimize this abuse.

REASONS FOR TORTURE

a. *Political or governmental:* Government agencies may suspect someone as enemy of the state; to force compliance or force them to leave their lands.

b. *War time torture:* Usually done against prisoners of war; suspected spies or traitors; any person suspected of harboring enemies or civilians in the occupied territories to subjugate them.

c. *Police:* So as to extract information or confession; disobedient prisoner or person trying to escape.

d. *Organized crime:* So as to establish an aura of fear; to extort money; to avenge or torture of witnesses to prevent reporting of crime.

e. *Others:* This group includes torture on religious maters; torture on land disputes; as a revenge for any reason or family violence.

METHODS OF TORTURE

Torture may be inflicted in many ways on a victim:

a. *Physical torture:* Most common physical form of torture is severe beating. A person may be beaten by hands, feet, shoes or weapons like rods, wooden lathis, rifle butts, whips or belts. Some of these weapons produce typical patterned injuries. When a person is given severe beating on the soles it is called **"Falanga"**. Hitting a person on the ears with hands so as to impair his hearing is known as **"Telephono"**. Finger torture may be done by pressing fingers after placing sticks in between the fingers.

A person may be tied up or put up in abnormal posture for prolonged period of time. Other forms of physical torture may include suspension by legs, use of blinding lights, dragging, pulled from hair, pulling out nails, infliction of injuries with a sharp pointed weapon or exposure to extremes of temperature.

b. *Asphyxia:* Repeated submersion of head under water or even sewage so as to partially asphyxiate a victim, this is called **"wet submarino"**. In some cases a plastic bag may be put on the head so as to cause disorientation as well as partial suffocation.

c. *Electrical torture:* High voltage low amperage current is used to inflict pain to a victim. Use of 240 volts domestic current may induce arrhythmias and death in some cases apart from local burns.

d. *Burn injuries:* Burn injuries are commonly seen on the torture victims. Burns may be produced by smoldering end of the cigarettes, putting tyre around the neck and setting that to fire or by heated rods.

e. *Psychological torture:* A victim may be subjected to psychological torture by means of humiliation, isolation, sleep deprivation, hygienic deprivation and use of communication techniques.

f. *Sexual torture:* This type of torture is entirely carried out by men. Female torture victims are subjected to verbal sexual humiliation, forced to undress in front of others and paraded naked, forced to masturbate in front of others, sexual violence by instruments and rape.

SIGNS AND SYMPTOMS

Torture survivors are a special category of patients because they have been subjected to different forms of physical and mental tortures. Signs and symptoms vary from one survivor to another due to degree, intensity and duration of torture suffered. However, the most frequent complaints of torture victims relate to general stress rather than exposure to specific torture methods.

a. *Neurological:* Headache is the most common complaint which improves with psychotherapy. Other complaints like impaired memory, impaired concentration, cognitive difficulties and disorientation are not necessarily caused by the lesions or abnormalities in the brain. Other symptoms may include vertigo, confusion, convulsions, postconcussion syndrome and paresthesia of hand or fingers because of tight rope or electric torture.

b. *Psychiatric:* Sleep disturbance, nightmares, hallucinations, anxiety, depression, suicidal tendencies, lack of control over emotions and aggressive behavior are some of the psychiatric symptoms. Some of these symptoms are grouped under **"Post-traumatic Stress Syndrome"** and the person may constantly recall the experiences with low response to outside world.

c. *Musculoskeletal:* Person may complain of pain and swelling in the muscles and joints, back pain, restrictive movements, pain in the thighs or soles of the feet (Falanga).

d. *Cardiopulmonary:* Includes chest pain, palpitations, fracture of ribs, hemothorax and wet submarino leading to dyspnea, cough, expectoration and even pulmonary infections.

e. *Gastrointestinal:* Intra-abdominal lesions like vomiting, hematemesis or epigastric discomfort and lower abdominal pain are usually the result of severe beating of the abdominal wall.

f. *Urogenital:* Common complaints are hematuria, dysuria and local trauma due to electric torture or insertion of foreign object in vagina, atrophy of testes from injury in that area. Local genital injuries may be seen as a result of rape with associated injuries to the breast.

g. *Dermatological:* May be seen as a result of torture forms as beating, burning and electric damage, in the form of bruises, abrasions, burns or electric burn injuries.

h. *Miscellaneous injuries:* These may include impaired hearing (associated with telephono), nasal bleeding, broken teeth or painful teeth.

MANAGEMENT OF TORTURE VICTIMS

Most of the torture victims are so scared that they do not come forward on their own; hence they require psychological guidance and reassurance. Proper detailed history, along with clinical examination and investigations must be carried out to diagnose cases of torture. Apart from treating the injuries, psychiatric help is of immense importance. Other family members may also require psychological support in such situations.

CUSTODIAL DEATHS

National Human Rights Commission (NHRC) has directed that all custodial deaths occurring while a person is being detained or under arrest or in prison, must be reported within 24 hours. They have further instructed that the postmortem examination on all such cases be recorded by means of videography and still photography for future reference and review.

CAUSES OF CUSTODIAL DEATHS

a. *To overpower resistance:* In some cases the victim may offer resistance while the police are trying to arrest or detain him. Such a person may sustain injuries, especially head injuries from baton, sticks or rifle butts or from fall on the ground. He may be drunk and pickup fight with the authorities during which he may sustain injuries. Neck hold to restrain a person may lead to vagal inhibition of heart along with asphyxia. In Police encounters the victim may die in the exchange of fire.

b. *Torture during interrogation:* Various forms of torture as described earlier may be applied so as to extract information or to accept commission of crime.

c. *Use of drugs:* Invariably addictive drugs like charas, ganja, opium, heroine, amphetamines, cocaine or LSD, are made available to the prisoner by illicit means, which may cause death due to overdose or hypersensitivity in some cases.

d. *Suicides:* Few cases of suicide either by consumption of drugs or asphyxia may take place in custody. Mostly partial hanging is deployed to commit suicide. Any available ligature material like belts, cloth pieces rolled into a rope, electric wires even shoelaces may be used to commit suicide.

e. *Natural diseases:* Emotional and physical distress during detention may cause increase in the blood pressure and may precipitate heart attack especially in elderly person. In some cases pre-existing diseases like diabetes, hypertension, epilepsy or asthma may cause death, which may be evident on postmortem examination by the history of the case and ruling out other causes of unnatural deaths.

POSTMORTEM FEATURES

In some cases victim may succumb to the torture injuries and bodies may be recovered as abandoned. Therefore, autopsy surgeon must be vigilant and try to find features of torture in such cases.

Normally there are features of physical trauma like scars, bruises, lacerations and multiple fractures which have not been medically treated. Hemorrhages are seen in the soft tissues of the soles, ankles and thigh muscles. There may be fracture of bones of the feet with aseptic necrosis in "Falanga". Ruptured or scarred tympanic membrane along with injuries to external ear is seen in "Telephono". In operation table trauma where the upper part of the body is not supported there are bruises on the abdomen and back with rupture of internal abdominal organs.

Where the person is suspended there are bruises on the wrist or ankles at the site of binding. In wet submarino there may be debris in the mouth larynx and trachea with froth and petechial hemorrhages. Signs of asphyxia in dry submarino may be seen.

Sexual abuse injuries to the genitalia and breast may be observed. On prolonged standing dependent parts normally show edema with petechial hemorrhages. Scrotal injuries or perineal hematoma may be seen when victim is forced to straddle a bar.

Electric burn marks depending on the age of the injury, e.g. circular reddish or grayish macular scar may be seen. Burn area may depend upon the object causing burns.

Internal examination may reveal soft tissue hemorrhages, bony injuries or visceral damage in some cases.

In all torture deaths viscera, blood and urine must be preserved to rule out poisoning, swabs from mouth, anal area and vagina should be preserved in sexual assault cases along with nail scrapings.

21 | Criminal Interrogation Techniques

In courts the prosecution mainly depends upon the evidence provided by the police, most important being the confession of the accused. Majority of time the confession is obtained by putting pressure and it becomes difficult to differentiate the innocent victim breaking down during such interrogations and implicating himself by giving a false admission to the crime. Briefly the police interrogation methods can be categorized under following groups.

TRADITIONAL THIRD DEGREE METHODS

Most of the times police rely on third degree methods by depriving food, water or sleep, intimidation, threats, physical discomfort or beating (using various techniques as described under torture). Gradually these methods are being discouraged world over.

REID TECHNIQUE

This is extensively used in the United States for interrogation. It is primarily based on the observation of the accused body language due to anxiety from answering control questions where answers are known. However there are certain objections raised by many as normal person may be stressed under such a situation and on the other hand a professional liar may not exhibit any signs of anxiety.

THE GOOD COP AND BAD COP METHOD

It is normally observed that an accused under stress may open up to the person offering compassion with a belief that such a person will continue to protect him in future also.

THE PEACE METHOD

This method being used in united kingdom is thought to be an effective method to discover truth. The peace (preparation or planning, engage or explain, account closure and evaluate) method is based on the facts that a liar will gradually build up a series of false explanations leading to more inconsistencies in his explanations. These inconsistencies will eventually help the investigators to trap him.

KINESIC INTERVIEW METHOD

Two step approach is adopted in this method, the "Practical kinesic analysis phase" and the "Practical kinesic interrogation phase". In the initial stage behaviour of the accused is observed and based on the information obtained; the interrogation process is devised in such a manner so as to break the cycle of deception.

MODERN MEDICAL TECHNIQUES

In the present day scenario help is being taken in such cases, from newer techniques for finding the truth, when the above mentioned methods fail to yield desired results.

Polygraph

Polygraph or popularly known as lie detector test is based on the changes noted in the measurements in physiological indices like *pulse, blood pressure, respiration and skin conductivity*. It is believed that any false or deceptive answer can be deciphered by the associated physiological changes which are not present in case of a correct answer. Credit for inventing this technique goes to a medical student John Agustus Larson along with a police officer, at the university of california in 1921. This technique is also known as psycho-physiological detection of deception (PDD) examination. Polygraph test is conducted in three stage interview:

a. A *pretest interview* in which the examiner prepares a set of questions based on the information provided by the investigation team like earlier statements made by the accused, facts of the case and criminal charges. A base line is established by questioning the accused and his responses to these questions.

b. *Chart recording* is done by the examiner by mixing questions from the earlier interview and relevant questions (RQ) about the case.

c. *Inference* of the examiner in such a case is based on the responses to relevant questions recorded on the polygraph machine and any deviation from the base line, established earlier, is taken as a false answer. However, this technique is more effective to investigate specific event in comparison to screen an accused.

Though apart from using control question test (CQT) technique as interrogation method, it is also used for selection or screening of candidates for sensitive posts in the government or public sector in some countries.

Reliability of this technique: Accuracy of this technique is debatable. Experts in favour of this technique claim an accuracy of 90%; however, the highest court in United States have concluded that there is no consensus in the scientific community that evidence adduced through polygraph is reliable.

Admissibility in courts: This technique is primarily used as collaborative evidence in the courts.

Narcoanalysis or Truth Serum

When the accused is uncooperative or unwilling to provide information narcoanalysis can be of great help. Narcoanalysis test involves administration of short acting barbiturates or other drugs to induce sleep like state so as to lower his inhibitions for freely sharing of information.

Sedatives and hypnotics like alcohol, scopolamine, benzodiazepines, sodium thiopental or sodium amytal (amobarbital) are commonly used. A team of qualified anesthetist, psychologist, psychiatrist and videographer conduct this test jointly. Normally this test is done by administering slowly 3 gm of sodium thiopental in 3 litres of distilled water in an adult. The dose may vary depending upon the age, sex and built of that person. Normally a person tells lies by using his imagination which is not available for him during narcoanalysis; hence it becomes difficult for him to tell lies. Though during the test a person is not in position to speak on his own but can answer simple questions put to him.

P-300 or Brain Mapping Test

This method also known as *"Brain wave finger-printing"* was developed by a neurologist Dr Lawrence A. Farwell in 1955. Dr Farwell found that a Memory and Encoding Related Multi-faceted Electroencephalographic Response (MERMER) is initiated in the accused when the brain recognizes information pertaining to the crime. The accused is initially interviewed to find out his knowledge about that case, after which sensors are attached to his head and the individual is made to see some pictures on a computer monitor or is made to hear some sounds related to that case. Sensors attached to his head record electric activities in his brain in the form of P-300 waves. These waves are generated only if the accused find any relationship with any stimulus he was shown.

Thus brain mapping matches any information stored in the brain with the stimulus provided to him related to the crime scene. There is no verbal response elicited from the accused during the recording of the EEG in this method. Only drawback of this technique is that the investigator requires detailed information regarding the crime. Experts handling brain mapping are reporting a very high accuracy of this method.

India's only forensic science laboratory that conducts brain-mapping or brain-wave fingerprinting test is located in Bengaluru, where tests were performed on *fake stamp paper case accused* **Telgi** or *gangster* **Abu Salem.**

Courts in United States have started using this technique to convict criminals.

Legal issues: Subjecting accused to undergo these tests is considered to be a violation of the article 20(3) of the Indian constitution, which states that "No person accused of any offence shall be compelled to be a witness against himself". It also is as per legal dictum of *"Nemo Tenetur se lpsum Accusare"* which means that "No man not even the accused himself can be compelled to answer any question which may prove him guilty of a crime". However Mumbai High court in 2004 in fake stamp paper case ruled that narco-analysis of the accused does not violate self-incrimination under article 20(3). Even though the evidence is not admissible in court of law but recoveries made from such interrogation is admissible as collaborating evidence.

Right to remain silent is also given under section 161(2) CrPC which states that every person is bound to answer truthfully all questions put to him by a police officer, other than questions the answer to which would have a tendency to expose that person to a criminal charge, penalty or forfeiture.

Section 45 IEA states that when the court has to form an opinion upon appoint of foreign law or of science or art or as to identity of handwriting or fingerprints the opinion upon that point or persons especially skilled in such foreign law or of science or art or as to identity of handwriting or finger impressions are relevant. However, experts in the field of Narcoanalysis or brain mapping are not included but are gradually finding acceptance by the courts.

22 | Blood and Other Body Fluid Stains

Stains are normally encountered at the scene of crime. Forensic expert is required to preserve those stains and determine the nature, species of origin and identify the individual by blood grouping and DNA analysis.

BLOODSTAINS

Bloodstains may be present on the body parts, clothing or other articles present at the crime scene. Amount of bloodstains and their distribution may provide valuable information about the manner and cause of death. Large amount of blood at the scene indicate injury to a major blood vessel. In case an artery is damaged spurting of blood is seen on the walls and floor. Fall of blood drop from few centimeters produces around stain but as the distance increase there are projections or rays coming out from the spot. Spurting on the walls may produce stain in an exclamation sign indicating the direction from which the blood has come.

Collection of Bloodstains

(i) In case the blood has not dried it can be collected on a white filter paper by putting it on the stain so that the blood gets soaked by the filter paper. Filter paper is then dried at the room temperature before dispatching it to the forensic laboratory; (ii) If a dry stain is present on a smooth surface like metal, glass, plastic or polished stone it is scrapped and

preserved in a glass vial; (iii) Stain present on porous material can be preserved as such along with some unstained portion; (iv) Stains present on the clothing are preserved as such. Clothing belonging to the victim should be examined for any damage corresponding to the injuries present on the body along with the position of the stains before sending them to the forensic laboratory; (v) Bloodstains present on the body surface should be lifted with a moist cotton swab (with distilled water or weak solution of ammonia).

Screening Tests for Blood

A number of chemical tests are available for screening of bloodstains. These tests are based on the presence of peroxidase enzyme in the blood. These are screening tests only as pus; sputum; rust or earth may also give positive results.

i. *Benzidine test:* To the stain extract in a test tube two drops of benzidine solution (10% solution of benzidine in glacial acetic acid) and two drops of hydrogen peroxide gives blue colour. Same test can be done with a moist filter paper pressed on the stain and to which one drop of benzidine solution and a drop of hydrogen peroxide gives blue colour in presence of blood. This test is not favoured these days due to the carcinogenic nature of the ingredients.

ii. *Phenolphthalein test (Kastle meyer test):* The test is performed in the similar manner in which benzidine test is performed, however in place of benzidine solution reduced alkaline phenolphthalein solution (2 gm of phenolphthalein is added to 100 ml of 20% potassium hydroxide solution which is then reduced by boiling with zinc granules) is used which gives pink colouration on addition of hydrogen peroxide. Test is highly sensitive and can detect blood in dilution of one part in five millions.

iii. *Orthotolidine test:* To the stain extract 4% Orthotolidine solution is added followed by hydrogen peroxide. Blue discoloration is produced in presence of blood.

iv. *Leucomalachite test:* To the stain extract few drops of leucomalachite solution (1 gram of leucomalachite is mixed with 100 ml of glacial acetic acid and 150 ml of distilled water is added) along with hydrogen peroxide which gives bright green colour in presence of blood.

Confirmatory Test

To confirm the presence of blood following tests are performed on the stains:

i. *Microscopic examination:* Microscopic examination can confirm the presence of blood in fresh stains as morphology of the blood cells may be properly recognized under microscope. Stain extract is placed on a glass slide and covered with a cover slip which is examined under microscope for intact red cells. Red cell morphology can also help in detecting the species of origin. Human RBCs are biconcave, 7μ in diameter, non-nucleated and circular whereas the mammalian cells are also same except in camel, which are convex. Amphibians, fishes and avian have nucleated, oval and biconvex cells. A dried film of the stain extract can be stained with Leishman stain and blood cells are examined. Presence of davidson bodies in the polymorphs may even help in diagnosing the sex of the individual.

ii. *Spectroscopic examination:* The test is based on the absorption pattern of the substance when the sunlight is passed through a thin film of that material. The sunlight is then passed through a prism to observe the absorption pattern in the light spectrum as black bands. Oxyhemoglobin produces two bands between D and E lines of the spectrum. Reduced hemoglobin produces a broad band between D and E lines.

iii. *Chemical tests (crystal tests):*

a. Haemin crystal test (Teichmann's test): Small quantities of stain extract are dried over a slide and few crystals of pure sodium chloride are added which is then covered with a cover slip and glacial acetic acid is added from the sides. The slide is warmed slightly. The dark brown, rhombic crystals are confirmatory for blood (Fig. 22.1).

b. Haemochromogen test (Takayama test): Small quantities of stain extract are dried over a slide, which is covered with a cover slip and Takayama reagent (3 gm of pyridin, 3 ml of 10% sodium hydroxide, 3 ml of saturated solution of glucose are mixed with 7 ml of distilled water and allowed to mature for two days) is added from the side. The slide is warmed slightly.

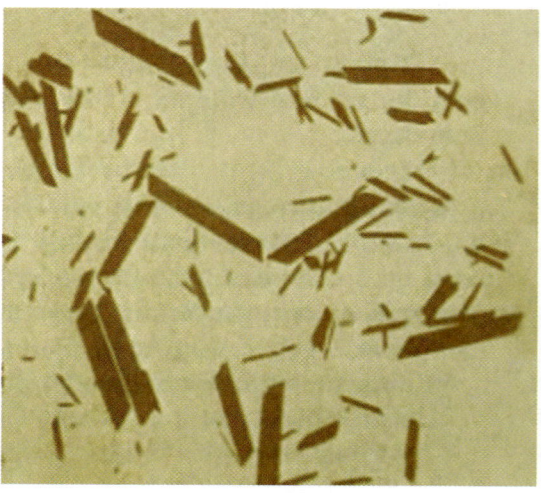

Fig. 22.1: Haemin crystals

Pink feathery crystals of hemochromogen are confirmatory of presence of blood (Fig. 22.2).

Age of the Stains

A rough estimate about the age of the blood-stain can be made out by morphological examination.

1. **Colour of the stain:** Bloodstains normally takes about one hour to dry completely except in humid conditions. The stain remains reddish for a day (fresh stain) and then gradually becomes dark brown or even black (old stain).
2. **Solubility:** Solubility of the stain reduces with increase in the time interval.
3. **Spectroscopic examination:** (Kind, 1972) It was observed that with time hemoglobin in the stain due to slow oxidation gets converted to methemoglobin which can be detected on spectroscopic examination of the blood extract. Methemoglobin produces four bands one band between C and D lines, two bands between D and E and the fourth band is seen between E and F lines of the spectrum.
4. **Photoelectric reflectance colorimetry:** Studies have been carried out to know the age of the stain by photoelectric reflectance colorimetry.

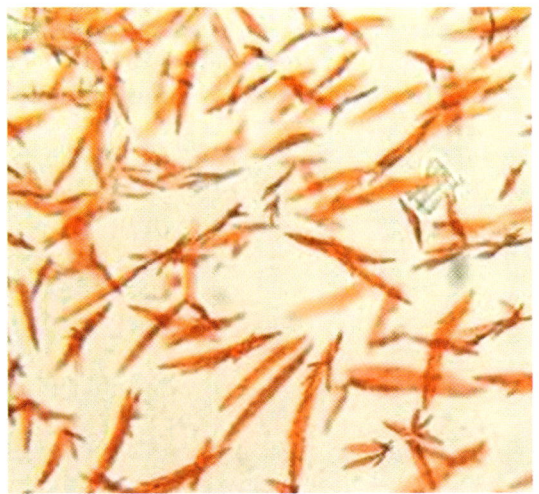

Fig. 22.2: Takayama crystals

5. **Fluorescence reduction:** With age blood stains show reduction in the fluorescence seen with ultraviolet rays.

Species Identification

1. **Precipitin test (Ring test):** Precipitin test is performed with about two drops of the stain extract taken in a precipitin tube or a capillary and antiserum is added carefully along the side of the tube. A precipitin ring is formed at the junction of two fluids. The test show positive reaction even with 1 in 1000 dilution of the stain extract.
2. **Antiglobulin consumption test:** The test is based on the consumption of anti-globulin reagent by the globulin contained in the stain extract. Any reduction in the strength of the antiglobulin is tested for agglutination of Rh positive red cells sensitized with incomplete anti-D. The test is highly sensitive and can detect globulin in 1 to 50,000 dilutions. For other species the test requires red cells coated with globulin from animal species to be tested.
3. **Gel diffusion test:** The test is performed by punching a central well surrounded by six wells in an agar gel on a slide or plate. This test is useful when stain extract material is limited, which is placed in the central well and tested against various species specific antisera placed in the surrounding wells. Precipitin band will develop between the corresponding antigen and species specific antiserum.
4. **Precipitation electrophoresis:** Wells are punched out in the agar on electrophoresis plate. Stain extract is placed in cathodic well and antisera in the anodic well. After electrophoresis a band appears between the corresponding sera and antisera of the same species.
5. **Latex particle agglutination test:** Latex particles are used as a carrier of anti-globulins. These particles when mixed with the stain extract containing globulins of the corresponding species exhibits agglutination. This again is a very sensitive test and

can detect globulin concentration up to 1 µg per ml. Cross reactivity may be seen in some closely related primate cases, however in higher dilutions this problem is not observed.

6. **Passive hemagglutination test:** The test is done with modified red cells treated with tannic acid or other chemicals, which are used to adsorve antigens on their surface. These cells agglutinate in the presence of specific antisera of a species.

Source of Blood

After determination that stain is of human blood, it is equally important in some cases to know the source of blood. Blood loss during life can be removed in flakes due to presence of fibrin. Bloodshed after death tends to breakup in powder on drying.

 i. Menstrual blood has to be differentiated from vaginal bleeding in sexual assault. Finding endometrial cells in the blood is indicative of menstrual bleeding. Fibrinolysin content in the menstrual blood does not allow it to clot. Hence higher proportion of fibrinolysin and fibrin products helps in the detection of menstrual blood. Menstrual blood is acidic in nature. Electrophoresis of lactate dehydrogenase enzyme in the stain extract shows low levels of LDH-1 and LDH-2 whereas LDH-4 and LDH-5 levels are higher. However this is possible only in the fresh stains.

 ii. Hemoptysis blood is bright red in colour and is frothy as it is coming from the lungs.

 iii. Hematemesis blood is dark in colour because of formation of acid hematin and is acidic.

Sex of the Individual

Sex can be determined from the fresh blood-stains by demonstrating Davidson's body in the leucocytes. Y chromosome fluorescence has also been used to demonstrate male blood. However, in majority of cases much reliance cannot be placed on sex determination.

Blood Grouping

Detection of blood groups from the dried bloodstains is of immense value in medico-legal practice. A number of blood group systems have been described based on the specific antigens. However, from medicolegal point of view, the important blood groups are ABO, MNSs and Rh. Results of Rh blood grouping are rather disappointing and N antigen of MNSs blood group disappear rapidly in dried bloodstains. ABO system besides being of importance in disputed paternity cases is of immense value in grouping of stains because of strong antigenic character.

1. **Detection of ABO agglutinins:** Lattes (1932) devised glass slide technique for detection of ABO agglutinins from dried blood crust by adding diluted suspension of standard A and B blood group cells separately and observing agglutination. This method can only be used when the blood crust is fairly fresh and sufficient crust material is available. The above method was modified to increase the sensitivity by test tube technique of kind; cavity slide technique of outteridge and fluorescent antibody technique of Hesbe (1962). In a tropical country like India where humidity and temperature remains high the above mentioned test cannot be relied upon. Presence of earth, dust, secretions and excretions interfere with the test.

2. **Detection of ABO agglutinogens:** Blood agglutination tests as used for blood transfusion are not possible from dried stains as the red blood cells are damaged by drying. Detection of agglutinogens in the bloodstains rests on the demonstration of the specific absorption of the antibodies and is grouped under indirect or direct techniques.

 a. *Indirect methods:* "Absorption-inhibition" method was introduced by Holzer (1931) in this the specific absorption of the anti-sera was allowed by placing antigenic material in contact with its homologous antisera along with a control. Reduced titer of these sera was compared with that of original sera. This method was further modified by kind, capillary technique of pansold (1934) and technique of hausbrant (1938). "Absorption detection" technique was a modification suggested by Grewal and Roychowdhary (1946). The method becomes inapplicable when the material is not sufficient or there is presence of interfering substances like earth, dust, detergents or bacterial contamination. Contamination by *E. Coli* and similar organisms produce antigens like antigen B and to some extent antigen A, which interfere in the blood group detection.

b. *Direct methods:*

i. *Absorption elution technique:* In this method for ABO grouping by Kind (1960,) the bloodstained material was immersed in specific blood antisera and allowed absorption of antisera to the optimum. After which the antisera was discarded and the material was washed free of uncombined antibodies, homologous red blood cells were added and heated together. Thus, the absorbed antibodies get dissociated from the bloodstain and agglutinate indicator cells. He advocated that the test material to be fixed in McIlvaine's buffer before testing them in the reaction chambers formed by applying beeswax to glass slides. Separate anti-A and anti-B serum along with group O serum was used. Advantage of this technique was that the results could be observed with naked eyes. He also applied this technique to stained fabrics. The method of kind was modified by outteridge for use in the common laboratory; he used cavity slides as used for bacteriology. An extraction technique was devised and the stain material was transferred to cotton threads. Clear results were obtained with 10 microgram of dried blood. He further modified the technique and named it as "Micro absorption Elution technique" by using a synthetic resin to stick the bloodstained fibers. This technique has since been modified by various scientists for routine use in the Forensic laboratories.

ii. *Mixed agglutination technique:* Method proposed by coombs and dodd was based on the similar method used in bacteriology. They pretreated the fibers with dilute acetic acid for fixation. Specific absorption of the homologous antibodies was allowed to take place and then the test material was washed free of the uncombined antibodies. On application of homologous indicator red cells the positive result were observed under a microscope, as indicator cells adhering to the fibrils. Fiori (1963) modified the test by using methyl alcohol as fixative and antibody absorption was done at 4°C and not at room temperature. Mitra and Ganguli, Outtridge, Weiner and other forensic experts suggested other modifications.

iii. *Hemagglutination on a smear:* Ogata's (1960) method of hemagglutination on a smear was performed on a thin smear made on a slide, dried and fixed with methyl alcohol. The smear was covered with homologous antisera, incubated, excessive antisera washed out and 2% indicator cells spread over the smear. Slides were again incubated and washed. Microscopic examination showed specific and clear cut results.

iv. *Fluorescent antibody technique:* Kind and cleevely (1970) tried fluorescent antibody technique to detect ABO blood group from stains. Advantage if this technique were that no indicator cells were required and subgroups of blood group A could be distinguished.

Presence of A and B Antigen in Other Body Fluids and Tissues

Blood group antigens of ABO blood group are not confined to red blood cells but are found in most of the body secretions and tissues of the body. However only 75 to 80% of the population secrete their corresponding blood group antigens in their body fluids and are known as secretors. A, B and H antigens are secreted in high concentration in seminal fluid, saliva gastric juices and vaginal secretions. These antigens are present in low concentration in tears sweat and urine whereas in cerebrospinal fluid no antigen can be demonstrated. ABO antigens are predominantly glycolipids and partly glycoproteins, which is water soluble. In nonsecretors A and B antigens are found only in glycolipid fraction.

Normal hemoglobin: Hemoglobin is the respiratory pigment present in the blood. Oxygen in lungs gets attached to the iron ion in haem component to be carried by blood to the tissues for utilization in metabolism. Any abnormality in the hemoglobin can be used for identification as well as in the paternity testing. All individuals have three types of normal hemoglobins.

i. *Hemoglobin A:* This is the normal adult hemoglobin and each molecule has four polypeptide chains two similar chains are called "alpha" chains and two other identical chains are labeled as "beta" chains.

ii. *Hemoglobin A2:* This type of hemoglobin is also present in adult individual in low levels of about 2%. This type of hemoglobin has two alpha chains and two delta chains.

iii. *Hemoglobin F:* During early life a child has different type of hemoglobin which goes on reducing with age and by 2 years it disappears or the level goes below 2%. This hemoglobin has two alpha chains and two gamma chains.

Abnormal hemoglobins: Abnormal hemoglobins are divided in 3 main groups.

i. Abnormally conjugated chains: This may give rise to a situation when all the four chains are similar. When all the chains are gamma chains it is called hemoglobin Bart's and when all the chains are beta then it is known as hemoglobin H.

ii. Substitution in the polypeptide chain: A different amino acid is substituted in alpha or beta polypeptide chain. Beta chain substitutions are known as hemoglobin S, C, D Punjab or E.

iii. Addition or deletion of amino acids: In some rare cases amino acid is either deleted or added in the polypeptide chains or the chains are fused together like in Lepore hemoglobins.

STAINS OF OTHER BODY FLUIDS

Saliva Stains

1. Saliva stains can be detected by examining the stain for amylase which is present in high concentration (350000 units). Disappearance of blue colour given by iodine on starch is used as an indicator of amylase activity. Amylase preset in plants can be differentiated from salivary amylase as it uses chloride ion as an activator and optimum pH is 6.6 to 6.8. Plant amylase requires low pH of 4.4 to 4.5 and does not require chloride ion.

2. On microscopic examination of the stain extract may reveal buccal squamous cells.

3. Presence of thiocyanates, nitrites and phosphates may also indicate presence of salivary stains.

Seminal Stains

Seminal stains are white or yellowish white in colour and feel stiff to touch.

1. The stain when examined under ultraviolet light gives bluish white fluorescence. Similar fluorescence is also given by albuminous materials like mucous and vaginal discharge.

2. Acid phosphatase test can be used as a screening test to exclude nonseminal stains. Seminal fluids contain about 400 to 8000 units per ml which is 20 times or more than in other body fluids. The test is conducted

by using alpha nephthyl phosphatase and black K dye which gives characteristic pink-purple colour.

3. Microscopic examination is confirmative for seminal fluid in case a single intact sperm is seen. However, intact sperms may not be seen in dried seminal stains. Evidence may only be accepted from expert hands provided multiple distinct sperm heads are seen in the slide made from the seminal stain extract.

4. Creatinine phosphokinase concentration which is almost double than any other body fluid can help in detecting seminal stains. Levels above 400 units per ml could be taken as positive result. This enzyme is relatively quite stable and can give positive results in few months old stains.

5. Ammonium molybdate test is primarily used as a screening test.

6. Immunological methods to detect seminal stains have been developed by using anti human sperm serum.

7. *Chemical tests:* (a) Florence test is performed on a drop of stain extract obtained with 10% hydrochloric acid on a slide and a cover slip is placed over it. A drop of florence solution (iodine, potassium iodide and water) is placed near the edge of the cover slip. Brown rhombic crystals of choline iodide are seen under a microscope. Choline is secreted by the seminal vesicles (Fig. 22.3). (b) Barberio test: when picric acid is added to the stain extract yellowish needle shaped spermine picrate crystals are formed. Spermine is part of the prostatic secretions (Fig. 22.4).

Vaginal Stains

Mainly shows vaginal epithelial cells on microscopic examination of the stain extract. Gel electrophoresis technique has been used to differentiate between seminal and vaginal phosphatases. This technique can also be used for the presence of seminal fluid in the vaginal swabs especially in sexual assault by a sterile person or a person who has undergone vasectomy operation.

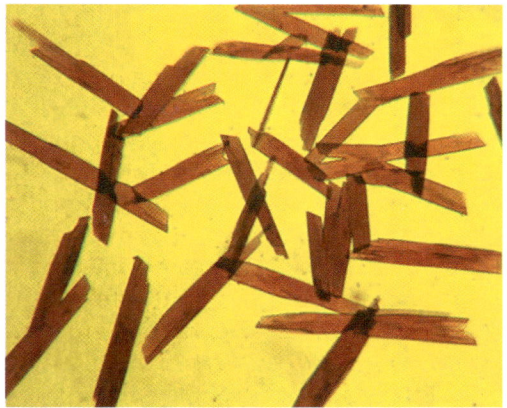

Fig. 22.3: Florence test

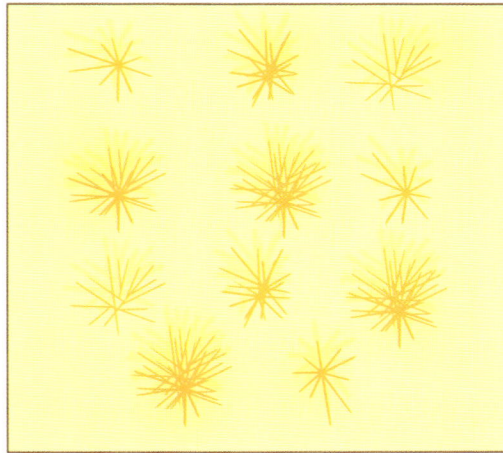

Fig. 22.4: Spermine picrate crystals

Urinary Stains

These stains normally give characteristic odor of urine; (i) urease tablets are used to detect urine stains; (ii) presence of creatinine also helps in deciding whether the stain is of urine or not.

PATERNITY DETERMINATION

The question of disputed paternity comes up in many situations like the husband denies being the father of that child; a lady accusing of a man to be the father of the child or a fictitious child is produced by feigning pregnancy and delivery to claim the property.

Blood groups apart from the identification are very frequently used to solve paternity dispute problems. Genes controlling blood groups are inherited according to the **Mendelian law** of inheritance. Hence, a blood group antigen cannot appear in a child unless it is present in one of the parents and if a parent is homologous (having two similar genes) for a blood group factor that gene must appear in all his children. These blood group antigens inherited from parents are permanent and remain same throughout the life. Position of the gene DNA sequence present on the chromosome is "Locus" and the alternative forms of genes present at the same place are known as "Alleles".

Blood group systems used for paternity testing:

Blood groups and some of the other polymorphism are used in paternity testing.

Red Cell Antigens

Quite a good number of red cell antigens are used for exclusion studies in paternity testing. Main blood groups which are helpful in such studies are ABO, MNSs, Rh, Kell Duffy and Kidd. However some laboratories use other red cell antigens also.

a. *ABO blood group:* Landsteiner (1901) depending upon the presence of A, B, both AB and none of the antigens (agglutinogens) on the surface of red blood cells, divided human beings into four distinct groups. There is no O antigen but group O individual react with anti-H serum hence identified as H group. A and B antigens are equally dominant. Therefore, possible genotypes are AA, AO, BB, BO, AB and OO. Along with the antigen these groups also have opposite antibodies (Agglutinins) like A group has Anti-B, B group has Anti-A, O group has both Anti-A and Anti-B agglutinins, but AB group has none of the agglutinins, therefore, it is known as universal recipient group. Many variants of A and B agglutinogens have been observed but except for A1 and A2 other variants are rare and weak, therefore, has limited utility in the medicolegal application. ABO

blood group alone may be able to exclude paternity in about 17 to 18 % cases.

b. *MNSs blood groups:* This blood group is based on the presence of M, N and closely allied S antigens. Many satellite antigens of MNSs system have been worked out with corresponding antibodies. This blood group system has the potential to exclude paternity in about 32% of cases.

c. *Rh blood groups:* Landsteiner and Wiener (1940) discovered this important blood grouping system. This factor is present in about 80% of the individuals, which are called Rh positive. There are main six antigens, D, d, C, c, E and e apart from many allelic antigens. Actually there is no d antigen and absence of D antigen is donated as presence of d. Combination of main antigens of Rh system can generate 36 genotypes.

d. *Other blood groups:* Besides three main blood groups a number of different blood groups have been discovered. Most of them are antigenic weak as compared to main blood group antigens hence of limited practical use. Some of them are P (P1 and P2 antigens), Lutheran (having Lua and Lub antigens), Kell, Duffy (Having Fya and Fyb antigens), Kidd (having Jka and Jkb antigens), Diego, Yt, Auberger, Dombrock, Colton, sid and scianna. There are number of private blood group antigens which are found in a particular individual or families.

e. *Sex linked blood groups:* The above mentioned blood group antigens are carried by autosomal genes, however there are number of blood group antigens which are controlled by genes present on the X chromosome, out of them earliest detected was Xg system.

Serum Groups

Some antigenic factors are also inherited in Serum.

a. *Haptoglobulins (Hp):* Haptoglobulin is a protein produced by liver and it attaches to free hemoglobin released from the erythrocytes in the blood. Two allelic genes are responsible for Hp1 and Hp2 types of haptoglobulins in the plasma. Combination of these divides the population into three groups like Group-1 (homozygous Hp1 and Hp1), Group-2 (homozygous Hp2 and Hp2) and Group-3 (heterozygous Hp1 and Hp2). These haptoglobulins can be differentiated on electrophoresis and is used in paternity testing. This test alone has an exclusion rate of about 17–18% in paternity disputes.

b. *Gm system:* Gamma factor is also helpful in paternity disputes. Many antigens have been observed in this system, which are inherited from parents as per mendelian law.

c. *Gc system:* This system is based on presence of two allelic genes inherited from each parent. Similar to heptoglobulins this system divide individuals into three groups. This system can help to exclude about 14–15% of disputed paternity cases. Immunoelectrophoresis is used to detect various fractions of Gc system.

Red Cell Enzymes

Red cell enzymes like phosphoglucomutase (PGM), erythrocyte acid phosphatase (EAP), glutamate-pyruvate transaminase (GPT), esterase D (Es D), 6 phosphogluconate dehydrogenase (6-PGD), adenylate kinase (ADK) and adenosine deaminase (ADA) are of some help in paternity disputes. In majority of cases first three red cell enzymes are commonly employed.

Expected rate of exclusion from red cell antigens, serum groups and red cell enzymes together is about 90 to 92 %.

HLA Typing

HLA antigens are surface glycoproteins found on many tissues including leucocytes, platelets, fibroblasts, placental tissues, kidney, liver and epidermal cells. Lymphocytotoxic test is the most commonly used method for determining HLA specificity by incubating target cells with antiserum and rabbit complement. Other techniques include leucoagglutination, complement fixation, fluorochomasia and variation of lymphocytotoxicity tests. Most of the individuals do not have antibodies in their serum. Antibodies against HLA antigens are seen in the sera of those individuals who have received multiple transfusions or as a result of organ or tissue transplantation. Most of the HLA antigens are determined by two autosomal genes known as LA and four loci with extreme polymorphism. HLA antigens are placed in three groups with HLA, W and no prefix. HLA system is primarily used for tissue matching in transplantation along with paternity tests. Exclusion rate in combination with red cell antigens, red cell enzymes and serum groups is up to 98% of disputed paternity cases.

DNA Profile

Absolute determination of paternity is possible by matching DNA profiles of the father, mother and the child in question. Discussed in detail in chapter on identification.

DOUBTFUL MATERNITY

There are cases when maternity of the child is in question, like cases of feigned pregnancy and delivery to claim property or to implicate certain individual so as to marry him. There may be exchange of babies in the hospital or the baby is kidnapped from the legal guardianship and claiming it to be their offspring by another couple. In all such cases the blood of all the parents and the infants is tested for blood grouping which in most of the cases is able to resolve this problem and in rare cases HLA and DNA profile may be required.

23 | Blood Transfusion Mishap

Blood transfusion can be life-saving and provides great clinical benefit to many patients but it is not without risks.

ACUTE COMPLICATIONS OF TRANSFUSION

Early complications of transfusion are rare, occurring in less than 1 in 1,000 transfusions, but tend to be more severe.

a. **Acute hemolytic transfusion reaction (AHTR):** ABO incompatible transfused red cells react with the patient's own anti-A or anti-B antibodies leading to hemolytic reaction. Non-ABO red cell antibody hemolytic reactions tend to be less severe but the Kidd and Duffy antigens also activate complement and can cause severe intravascular hemolysis. Most AHTRs occur within one to two hours of the transfusion but may occur within 24 hours of the offending transfusion. Transfusion of as little as 10–15 ml of incompatible blood may trigger an AHTR, but more severe reactions usually occur after transfusion of more than 200 ml. Laboratory findings suggestive of AHTR include hemoglobinemia, hemoglobinuria, decreased hematocrit values, decreased haptoglobin and increased LDH and bilirubin.

b. **Infective shock:** Bacterial contamination of a blood component, even when the organisms are nonpathogenic or dead, is very rare but severe and sometimes fatal cause of transfusion reactions. This may be seen as acute onset of shock with sudden drop in blood pressure; rigors and feeling of sever pressure on the chest.

c. **Transfusion-related acute lung injury (TRALI):** TRALI is a form of acute respiratory distress due to donor plasma containing antibodies against the patient's leukocytes. Within 6 hours of transfusion there is development of prominent non-productive cough, breathlessness, hypoxia and frothy sputum along with fever and rigors. In such cases donors are usually multiparous women, who have become alloimmunised.

d. **Fluid overload:** This occurs when too much fluid is transfused or too quickly before a transfusion is administered, leading to pulmonary edema and acute respiratory failure.

e. **Nonhemolytic febrile reactions to transfusion of platelets and red cells:** Fever and rigors may develop during red cell or platelet transfusion due to patient's antibodies reacting with transfused white cells. This type of reaction may be seen in 1–2% of patients. Usually symptoms develop towards the end of a transfusion or in the subsequent 1 to 2 hours. Most febrile reactions can be managed by slowing or stopping the transfusion and giving paracetamol.

f. **Anaphylaxis:** Anaphylaxis occurs where an individual has previously been sensitized to an allergen present in the blood and on re-exposure, releases immunoglobulin E (IgE), or IgG, antibodies. Patients with anaphylaxis become acutely dyspneic due to bronchospasm and laryngeal edema and may complain of chest pain, abdominal pain and nausea. Urticaria and itching are common within minutes of starting a transfusion.

g. **Miscellaneous effects:** Other adverse reactions may include hypothermia, especially in infants undergoing replacement transfusion.

Citrate toxicity may develop in those with liver dysfunction or neonates with immature liver function having rapid large volume transfusion. Citrate is the anticoagulant used in blood products. It is usually rapidly metabolized by the liver. Rapid administration of large quantities of stored blood may cause hypocalcemia and hypomagnesemia.

Hyperkalemia can occur during rapid, large volume transfusion of older red cell units in small infants and children.

Presentation

Patients should be observed closely at the start of each blood unit transfused. The recipient may complain of nausea, flushing, chills, pain abdomen, breathing problem and myalgia in some cases. On examination there may be fever, hypotension, tachycardia, respiratory distress, stained urine suggestive of hemoglobinuria.

Investigations

Where a serious acute transfusion reaction has taken place or is suspected, stop the transfusion and keep intravenous transfusion set, sample of post-transfusion blood of the recipient, pretransfusion sample of the recipient if available along with transfused blood in safe custody. Post-transfusion blood is examined for microscopic analysis (agglutinates may be seen), centrifuged plasma for pink-red discolouration, clotting, repeat type and cross match, antibody screen and direct antiglobulin (Coombs') test. An elution and antibody identification should also be performed even if the DAT is negative. Urine specimen from the transfusion recipient is also collected for detection of urinary hemoglobinuria.

Where an anaphylactic reaction is suspected, usual investigations include serum Ig levels, HLA antibody investigations and mast cell tryptase.

Where bacterial contamination is suspected, send blood cultures from patient and remnants of blood in the bag.

DELAYED COMPLICATIONS OF TRANSFUSION

a. **Delayed hemolysis of transfused red cells:** It happens in those who have previously been immunized to a red cell antigen during pregnancy or by transfusion. However, after transfusion of red cells bearing that antigen, a rapid, secondary immune response raises the antibody level drastically leading to the rapid destruction of transfused cells. It is normally seen after 5–10 days post-transfusion, patients present with fever, falling hemoglobin, jaundice and hemoglobinuria.

b. **Development of antibodies to red cells in patient's plasma:** Transfusion of red cells of a different phenotype to the recipient like in RhD-negative patients, who have received RhD-positive cells, will cause alloimmunisation. In case the patient later receives a red cell transfusion, it may cause hemolytic disease.

c. **Development of antibodies that react with antigens of white cells or platelets:** Transfusing red cells of a different phenotype to the patients can also cause the development of leukocyte or platelet antibodies. This can cause nonhemolytic febrile transfusion reactions in the future.

d. **Post-transfusion purpura:** This is a serious complication caused by platelet-specific allo-antibodies, more often seen in female transfusion recipients.

e. **Graft versus host disease (GvHD):** Even though it is a rare complication of transfusion, transfusion-associated GvHD, caused by T-lymphocytes, is almost always fatal. Immunodeficient patients, especially allogenic bone marrow recipients are at greater risk. There is high fever and diffuse erythematous skin rash, diarrhea and abnormal liver function.

f. **Iron overload:** Every unit of blood contains about 250 mg of iron; patients receiving red cells over a long period may develop iron accumulation in cardiac and liver tissues. This is mostly seen in thalassemia patients.

g. **Infection:** The risk of HIV, hepatitis B or hepatitis C from transfusion is extremely rare as blood is screened before transfusion.

Postmortem Examination

Before starting postmortem examination history of the case must be examined for risk factors and necessity of blood transfusion. History of previous transfusions and allergic reactions must be enquired from the near relatives. All clinical records must also be examined including request form, cross matching, label on the transfusion bottle that the blood bank issued it for the same patient and the notes by the physician on the case sheet. Intravenous drip set, sample of post-transfusion blood, pretransfusion sample of the recipient if available along with transfused blood bag must be handed over to police for laboratory testing including microbiological studies.

External Examination

Body should be thoroughly examined for any erythema, cyanosis, jaundice, frothing at the mouth and injection marks.

Internal Examination

Larynx must be examined for laryngeal edema. Bladder for bloodstained urine. Kidneys are examined for acute renal failure in the form of casts and myoglobin. In bacterial contamination there may be sub-endocardial hemorrhages on the interventricular septum. Other body organs must be examined and tissue samples taken from each. Blood, bile and vitreous samples must be collected.

24 | Medicolegal Autopsy

Autopsy is the postmortem examination of a dead body. Medicolegal autopsy is required in all cases of unnatural, sudden and suspicious deaths. In such cases the investigating agencies like Police or Magistrate forward the body for postmortem examination under section 174 Cr PC or 176 Cr PC respectively.

AIMS AND OBJECTIVES

Medicolegal postmortem are done with following objectives.

1. **To find out cause of death:** Primary aim of postmortem is to determine the cause of death like in a case death occurs from shock as a result of hemorrhage from injury to a specific blood vessel or heart. In rare cases the cause of death may not be apparent from postmortem examination alone, hence biochemical, histopathological or toxicological investigations are conducted so as to reach the final conclusion regarding cause of death.

2. **To find out manner of death:** It is imperative on the forensic expert to provide the information to the investigating agency regarding the manner of death, i.e. whether the death is homicidal suicidal or accidental.

3. **To find out time since death:** In most of the criminal cases it is very important to know the time of death so as to corroborate evidence. It may not be possible for a forensic expert to give exact time of death, however

from various changes occurring after death fairly accurate estimation can be done.

4. **To help in identification:** In cases of unidentified persons, mass disasters, advanced putrefaction, mutilated or skeletonised remains it is important to provide all possible help to the investigating agency to identify dead bodies.

5. **To help in proper recovery and preservation of evidence:** While conducting autopsy care is taken to recover and preserve all the trace evidences present on the body of the deceased. These may help the investigating agency to catch the perpetrator of that crime.

6. **To find out whether the newly born was born alive, stillborn or dead born:** From the dead body of a newly born baby, the forensic expert has to find out the period of gestation and whether the baby was born alive, stillborn or dead born.

Medical Officer Authorized to Conduct Autopsy

Investigating officer forward the body under section 174 or 176 of Cr PC to the nearest civil surgeon or other qualified registered medical officer appointed by the state government. In majority of cases the autopsy centers are located in government hospitals or medical colleges. In medical colleges the responsibility to conduct autopsy is normally with the department of forensic medicine. Medical officer conducting autopsy has no powers to waive off the autopsy in a medicolegal case. This can be done by the area magistrate or assistant commissioner of police having judicial powers, on the request of the relatives, provided he does not find any foul play and is satisfied with the documentary evidence produced before him. Medical officer may have an advisory role in such cases.

Documents Required at the Time of Autopsy

A written request, in duplicate, to conduct autopsy is submitted by the investigation police officer not below the rank of an assistant subinspector in all routine cases except murders, death of a woman within seven years of marriage and custody deaths. One copy is retained for departmental records. In a case of murder the request for postmortem is submitted by the police officer of the rank of inspector and in cases of death of a newly married woman, custody death or death in police firing the inquest is done by the magistrate so empowered and submits requests for the postmortem. Without written request postmortem examination should not be conducted.

Along with the request other inquest papers are also submitted. Police form 25/35 A, B or C as per need, is required in all cases. Statements of panchas (witnesses to inquest procedure) and relatives should be a part of inquest papers. Death summary or death certificate in case of hospital deaths, photographs, crime scene report by CSI or homicidal team of the police and seizure memo mentioning any item recovered from the crime scene may also be enclosed with the inquest papers, if possible. In important cases copies of all the inquest papers submitted may be retained.

Transportation of Dead Body to Autopsy Center

The dead body is normally transported from the scene of crime by the police officer investigating the case. It is always preferred to transport the body in a plastic bag which should be opened in the presence of forensic expert in the mortuary otherwise plastic bags may be tied over the head and hands to prevent loss of vital trace evidences like fingernail scrapings.

Rules for Conducting Autopsy

Whenever a dead body along with inquest papers is received for postmortem examination; (i) the authorized medical officer must read all the documents submitted so that important aspects of the case are clear to him; (ii) before starting autopsy the body must be identified by the police officer and the relatives mentioned in the inquest; (iii) in case of unidentified body as many as possible identification marks should be recorded along with the fingerprints and photographs; (iv) autopsy should be conducted as far as possible in a properly equipped and manned mortuary with adequate lighting, availability of water and drainage; (v) no unauthorized person should be present at the time of postmortem examination, presence of police officer may be allowed in certain cases to explain certain facts or findings; (vi) autopsy is normally done during the day time so that colour changes of injuries could be appreciated, however it can be done at anytime of the day provided proper white light and the manpower is made available by the administration; (vii) autopsy must be complete and through. All body cavities must be opened and all the visceral organs examined even in those cases with evident cause of death; (viii) if possible, cases showing advanced putrefaction, mutilation or skeletonisation should be conducted in a separate designated autopsy room; and (ix) removal of clothing and cleaning of the body must be done in presence of the medical officer conducting the autopsy.

Postmortem Examination

Medicolegal autopsy must be done with open, unbiased mind without any fear and favour.

Postmortem examination is started after the body is identified by the police investigating officer along with relatives or identification points are recorded in unidentified case. The body is photographed in presence of a doctor, in the same state in which it was brought for postmortem. After recording the preliminary information in the postmortem report like name, age, sex, address, etc. time, date and place of examination is recorded. Brief history must also be mentioned in the report. The body should be searched for any trace evidence as hair, fibers or stains over the body or clothing.

Examination of the Clothing

Articles of clothing are air dried in case they are wet before examination. They are examined for any cut, tear, loss of buttons or any other damage. In case the clothing are cut to facilitate removal, precaution is taken to avoid those areas having cuts, tears or stains corresponding to the injuries present on the body. Bloodstains are described in detail especially whether they are present prominently on the inner surface or not. Tyre mark impression or presence of grease marks in case of runover accident may be seen on the clothing. It is advisable to examine clothing by the forensic pathologist before sending them to the forensic laboratory. Forensic science expert in the forensic laboratories may make some cuts in the clothing for their testing which may cause confusion at a later date. Wet clothing should be air dried before packing and sealing them.

Collection of Specimen

Any specimen required by the police or thought to be relevant by the forensic expert conducting the autopsy are collected before proper autopsy is started so as to avoid contamination. Hair should be plucked from the roots in the scalp or pubic regions. Swabs can also be collected depending on the case requirements, from vagina, anus or mouth. Fingernail clipping should be collected at this stage. The above mentioned specimen are properly labelled and sealed before handing them to the police investigation officer for forensic analysis.

External Examination

Build, height, weight, age and sex of the dead person is recorded in the postmortem report. The body is examined for the changes occurring after death so as to ascertain time since death like distribution of postmortem lividity, stage of rigor mortis and putrefaction changes, if any. Any finding to suggest change in the position or tempering with the body should be observed. Any evidence of disease like jaundice should also be recorded. Rectal temperature should ideally be taken before putting the body in cold storage along with room temperature reading.

In unidentified bodies, marks of identification like scars, moles, tattoo marks, deformities, dental charting, any congenital abnormality, colour of the eyes, distribution and colour of hair and belongings must be recorded.

Body must be thoroughly examined from head to toes. Though examiner can device his own method of examining the complete body, but normally the sequence of examination include head, face, neck, front of the chest and abdomen, genital area, back of the chest and abdomen, right leg, left leg, right arm and left arm.

Scalp should be examined for contusions and lacerations, as it may be difficult to find them in thick growth of hair and are normally seen after the scalp is reflected. Eyes must be examined for injuries, petechial hemorrhages, periorbital extravasation and other abnormalities. Ear, nose and mouth are examined for any injury, bleeding, damage to teeth and associated injuries. Neck must be examined for abrasions, bruises or ligature marks. If required, photographs of the injuries or ligature marks may be taken or sketches may be prepared. Thorax, abdomen, legs and arms are examined from front and back side for any injury or deformity suggesting underneath fracture.

External injuries whether minor or major must be measured and presence of any age related changes are recorded. Their location in relation to any bony prominence, direction of infliction if possible and any peculiarity or pattern of injury must be noted. Body should be examined for any abnormal mobility of a part indicating underneath fracture. Body orifices should be thoroughly examined for injuries in attempted sexual assault.

Special attention is given to the external appearance of a firearm injury to know the range from which the gun was fired like muzzle impression, cruciate splitting of entrance wound, presence of singeing, blackening, tattooing, abrasion collar and spreading of pellets in shotguns. Corresponding exit wound if present should be noted.

Similarly stab wounds are also described in detail. Their margins, angles must be examined to know whether caused by single edged or double edged weapon, direction of infliction, any tailing and presence of hilt mark if present should be recorded.

Internal Examination

Internal examination of the body is done in a comprehensive manner so as to perform complete autopsy. There is no provision of performing partial autopsy under Indian laws.

a. *Scalp, skull and brain:* An incision is made starting from behind one ear passing through top of the head preferably behind the hairline ending behind the other ear. The scalp is reflected, separating it and exposing skull from supraorbital ridges to occiput. The scalp may reveal bruises, petechial hemorrhages or edema. Skull is examined for any fracture. In case fracture is not visible, skull is tapped with any metallic instrument to note cracking sound which may reveal presence of hairline fractures of the skull. Skull is opened by cutting it with a saw avoiding damage to the meninges and brain. Location, thick-

ness and volume of the extradural hemorrhage if present are noted. Sagittal sinus is then opened to note presence of any antemortem thrombus. Meninges are then cut along the cuts in the skull or parallel to the sagittal suture and note any subdural or subarachnoid hemorrhages. Any midline shift in the brain or any depression on the brain surface is also noted. A cut is made in the fox cerebri and the frontal lobes of the brain are lifted to expose pituitary stalk which is cut along with other cranial nerves. Temporal lobes are gently lifted and tentorium cerebri is cut from the anterior margins on both sides. The medulla is divided near the foramen magnum and the entire brain is lifted out of the skull. Dura is then stripped off the base of the skull for detecting presence of any fractures.

Base of the brain is examined for the vessels especially of the circle of Willis. Major vessels are opened with fine scissors to find any aneurism or thrombus. A cut is made in the midbrain to separate cerebellum. Parallel incisions are given in pons, medulla and cerebellum to observe any pathology. Both cerebral lobes are separated and medial surface examined for any abnormality. Uncus area on both the sides are examined for any signs of herniation. Cerebral lobes are then divided by giving parallel incisions and each surface is examined for presence of any disease or injury. Lateral ventricles should be examined for presence of blood. For better visibility each surface should be examined under slow stream of water. If required the pituitary gland, middle ear, posterior part of the orbits and air sinuses are examined by removing the bone covering over that area with a chisel or bone forceps.

b. *Other body organs:* Other body organs are examined by making any of the following incisions (i) I-shaped incision: This is the most commonly employed incision and is made from the base of the chin to pubic symphysis vertically going by the side of the umbilicus; (ii) Y-shaped incision: the incision starts from behind each ear and joining together at upper boarder of the manubrium sterni and then running vertically downwards till the pubic symphysis going by the side of the umbilicus; (iii) modified Y-shaped incision: the incision starts from the acromian process on both sides, going along the mammary line and joining together at xiphoid process and then running vertically downwards till the pubic symphysis going by the side of the umbilicus. This incision is employed when the face and neck is required to be exposed for viewing (Fig. 24.1).

EVISCERATION TECHNIQUES

Various techniques are used in forensic practice to remove visceral organs for their examinations.

i. *Letulle's technique:* In this method all organs of the body are removed en-block. The organs are then dissected and examined in detail. This method is best suited to study organs in their anatomical position outside the body cavities.

ii. *Ghon's technique:* In this method organs are removed in separate blocks from body cavities. Organs are the separated, dissected and examined.

iii. *Virchow's technique:* In this method all organ are removed individually. Spinal cord is also examined by dissection on the back if required. Major disadvantage of this method is that anatomical relationship between various organs is lost.

iv. *Rokitansky's technique:* In this method *in situ* dissection of the internal organs is done. However there are certain limitations in the examination of organs. This method may be used to prevent spread of certain diseases like AIDS or hepatitis.

In routine practice after giving I-shaped or Y-shaped incision the skin is reflected from the front of the neck up to the jaw bone. Neck structures are examined for presence of any bruises or appearance of ligature mark base. Skin is also reflected from the front of the

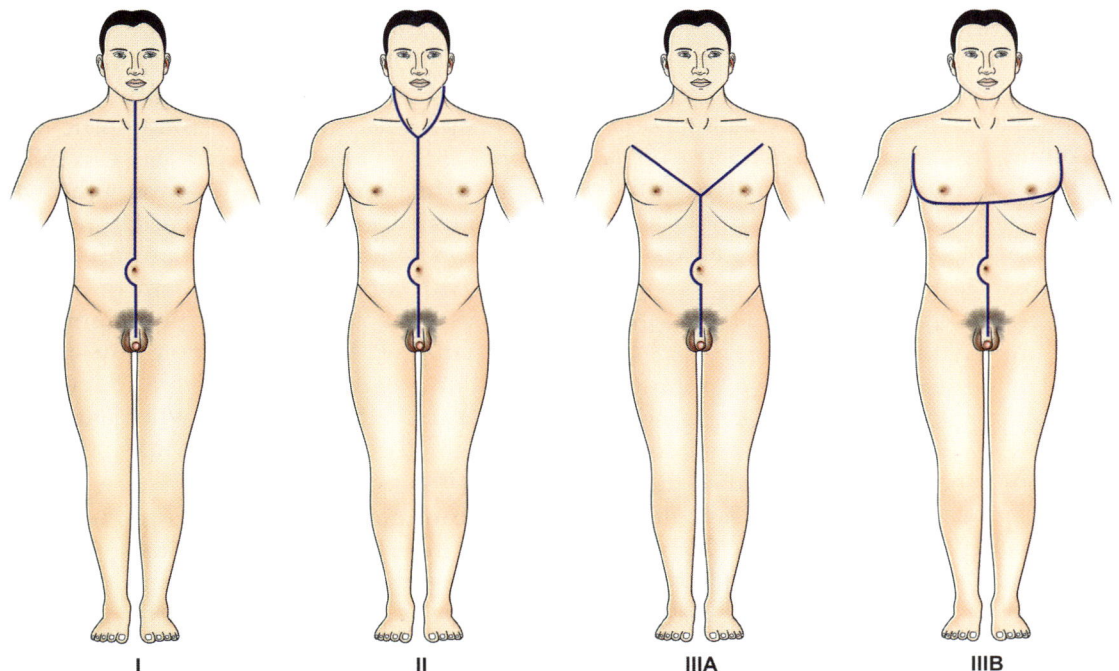

| I | II | IIIA | IIIB |

Fig. 24.1: Postmortem incisions

chest exposing costal cartilages. Presence of pneumothorax can be checked by putting water in the skin pouch on the chest wall, made from the reflected skin and making a cut with a knife in intercostal space. In case of pneumothorax air in the form of bubbles will escape on pressing the chest. Remove water before releasing pressure so that water does not enter the chest cavity. Medial ends of both clavicles are separated from the manubrium by dividing sternoclavicular joints. Costal cartilages are the cut and sternum is removed. Pleural cavities are examined for pleural effusion, hemothorax or pyothorax.

Soft tissues and muscular attachment along the jaw bone are cut with a knife and tongue is pulled in front below the jaw exposing oral cavity and pharynx which are examined at this stage. Carotid arteries and soft tissues are then divided from the base of the skull. By holding the tongue soft tissues are dissected from the front of the vertebrae and chest cavity to separate neck structures, lungs and heart. Esophagus and aorta are divided above the diaphragm after putting double ligatures. Neck structures and the chest organs are then taken out in a block. Esophagus and trachea is divided from the posterior surface to look for presence of any foreign material, blood or blackening from soot particles apart from any pathological changes. Carotid arteries near the bifurcation are examined for any blockage. Hyoid bone, laryngeal cartilages and thyroid gland are examined in detail.

Heart, lungs and major vessels of the thorax are examined in detail. Major vessels are opened up with scissors to note any abnormality like thrombus, aneurism or presence of any growth. Lungs are examined for any pneumonic consolidation, fibrosis, tumors, cavities, pulmonary embolism, unilateral or bilateral collapse and mediastinal shift. Lungs bronchi and bronchioles are dissected starting from the hilar region and proceeding towards periphery. Any foreign material or froth, if present, is recorded. Pulmonary vessels are also dissected for the presence of emboli or atheromatous changes. Lungs are sliced with a brain knife and each lobe parenchyma is examined for any pathology.

Heart pericardium is examined for any injury. Pericardial sac is explored for presence of blood. Heart surface is examined for any change in shape due to aneurism and colour changes like grayish or pale, mottled and hemorrhagic areas suggestive of old or recent infarct. After dividing appendages, coronary arteries are examined by dividing them transversally at half a centimeter distance to observe any narrowing due to atherosis or hemorrhage in atheromatous plaque and calcification in the walls giving a gritty sensation while cutting the artery. In coronary artery occlusion the percentage of narrowing is mentioned.

Heart chambers are opened along the flow of the blood or slicing the heart 3–4 cm from the tip of the ventricles and cutting through various valves to open all the chambers along with aorta and pulmonary artery. Before opening of the chambers valves are examined, circumference measured and any vegetation or calcification on the valves or any abnormality is noted. Circumference of the mitral valve is 8 to 10.5 cm admitting two fingers; tricuspid valve measures from 10 to 12.5 cm; aortic valve from 6 to 8 cm and pulmonary valve from 7 to 9 cm. After opening the chambers the wall thickness is noted, in case the left ventricle thickness is more than 1.5 cm or right ventricular wall is more than 0.5 cm thick, it is indicative of ventricular hypertrophy. The ventricular wall is sliced to note any signs of recent or past infarction. Weight of the heart is measured after dissection, whereas, in case of other body organs weight is taken just after separating the organ.

Abdominal viscera are examined after cutting the mesentery and dividing the small intestines at duodenojejunal junction. Large intestine is separated from the posterior abdominal wall. Renal arteries are examined for any abnormality. Abdominal organs are then removed en-block after dividing the diaphragm from the peripheral attachments leaving behind pelvic structures.

Gallbladder is examined for any dilatation or any bile stones. Adrenals are examined before the renal sheath is removed to expose kidneys. Weight and measurements of the liver, spleen, kidneys and pancreas are taken after separation. They are then examined for any injuries or pathology. Parallel cuts are given with a brain knife to examine parenchyma of each organ for any pathology. Urinary bladder is opened carefully so as to prevent any contamination. Pelvic organs are removed en-block or examined after removing them separately. Uterus and cervix is examined carefully for any signs of pregnancy, attempted abortion, perforation or tears. Bladder is examined and opened carefully to take urine sample with a syringe for preservation, if required.

Spine and spinal cord are examined when indicated with posterior approach, a midline incision is given and muscles and soft tissues are reflected to the sides. Spines and arches of the vertebrae are examined for any damage or injuries. The laminae of the vertebrae are then divided with a saw. Spines and the arches are removed to expose spinal cord. Dura matter covering is opened with a midline cut and the entire spinal cord is removed and examined.

Pelvis, ribs and limb bones are examined for any fracture or damage. X-ray examination must be done in cases of firearms and suspected fractures.

Details about penetrating or perforating firearm or stab injuries are mentioned in details, correlating entrance wound and exit wound along with the track through the body. Projectiles recovered from the body are collected and preserved.

Preservation of Viscera: In all cases of suspected poisoning or when requested by the investigative officer or absence of definitive cause of death, viscera is collected, preserved and handed over to the police. In routine cases following viscera is collected in clean containers:

i. *Stomach and stomach contents:* Stomach is opened and the entire contents along with the stomach wall after it is examined is preserved in 1st bottle.

ii. *Small intestines and contents:* Small intestine piece about 30 to 100 cm, along with contents are preserved in second bottle. Mostly these are preserved along with stomach and its contents in a single bottle.

iii. *Liver spleen and kidneys:* Piece of liver about 500 gm, half of spleen and half of each kidney are placed in third bottle.

iv. *Blood:* Minimum of 30 ml of blood is collected from peripheral sites and placed in the 4th bottle.

v. *Sample of preservative:* Preservative used is added in the 5th bottle.

Preservatives used: For preservation of viscera saturated solution of common salt (which is cheap and easily available) is preferred even though rectified spirit is the ideal preservative. Hand full of salt is added to the contents in each viscera bottle, which draws water from the viscera and make a saturated solution around it. Spirit is not used in alcohol, kerosene, ether, chloroform, phosphorus and related poisons, moreover it is expensive and chances of pilferage are there. Blood sample is commonly preserved without any preservative, but in alcohol and cyanide poisoning potassium fluoride and potassium oxalate are used 10 mg and 3 mg per ml of blood respectively. In carbon monoxide poisoning a layer of liquid paraffin is added over blood or the container is filled up to the brim. **Formalin should never be used as preservative for toxicological analysis.**

In special cases total volume of urine sample is collected in a separate bottle. Urine is preserved by adding few crystals of thymol or phenyl mercuric nitrate. Hair sample from the head and pubic area are collected by plucking them from the roots. Skin sample preferably of 2 cm radius around the injection site should be incised and preserved. A 10 cm long bone piece from the shaft of the femur is preserved if required.

Histopathology: In case some pathology is suspected, small pieces of the liver, spleen, kidney, lung or heart myocardium is preserved along with normal tissue in 10% formalin.

Bacteriological or viral studies: Blood may be collected from various organs in sterile syringe after searing the surface of the organ with hot spatula. Glycerin can be used as preservative for virology studies.

Obscure and Negative Autopsy

The term obscure autopsy is used when on postmortem examination no definite cause of death could be found. Usually there are minimal or nonconclusive findings leading to confusion. In most of these cases, cause of death could be made out by detailed examination, laboratory, histopathological, bacteriological, viral investigations and medical history of the case. Causes of obscure autopsy are mentioned below.

i. *Natural diseases:* Some of the natural diseases like epilepsy, fibrillation, arrhythmias or sudden cardiac arrest.
ii. *Concealed trauma:* Blunt injury to heart, severe concussion, vagal inhibition of heart and fracture dislocation of cervical vertebrae.
iii. *Poisoning:* In cases of narcotic poisoning, anesthetic drugs and neurotoxic poisoning.
iv. *Endocrine disturbance:* Diabetes and adrenal or thyroid over activity.
v. *Metabolic disturbances:* Hyperkalemia or uremia.
vi. *Allergic reactions:* Drug idiosyncrasy.

In few cases of obscure autopsy the cause of death still remains undermined even though all investigations are conducted and such cases are labelled as "negative autopsy". Major reason of negative autopsy is inexperience of the autopsy surgeon. Other reason may include inadequate history, inadequate postmortem examination, when very minimal findings are there, certain poisons not detected on toxicological examina-

tion or histopathology by inexperienced pathologist.

Second Autopsy

In rare cases second autopsy is conducted on the order of magistrate or senior police officer by a board of doctors either from same institution or from different institutions. The doctor who conducted the first autopsy, if possible, should be available to explain any discrepancy noted during second autopsy.

Virtual Autopsy

When instead of conducting proper autopsy, the body is subjected to noninvasive investigative techniques like CT scan or MRI, is known as virtual autopsy. Three dimensional image obtained may be of great help in finding out the cause of death. In cases of head injuries; pneumothorax or aspiration as a cause of death can be ascertained by means of virtual autopsy.

Exhumation

It is the lawful digging out of a buried body from the grave for postmortem examination. There is no time limit for exhumation in India whereas in France it is up to 10 years and in Germany it is up to 30 years. In criminal cases exhumation is conducted in suspected homicide or cases of criminal abortion. In civil cases it may be conducted for identification of the deceased for insurance, disputed identity, burial of wrong body or inheritance, etc.

Authorisation: Body can only be exhumed on the written directive by first class magistrate (judicial or executive).

Procedure: Exhumation is done during the daylight; hence it should be started during the morning hours so that it could be completed before the sunsets. The exhumation is done under the supervision of a doctor, police officer, and magistrate. The grave is identified by the relatives and grave-maker or from the headstone so that wrong body is not exhumed. The area should be cordoned off from the onlookers. As soon as the coffin is exposed soil samples from all sides must be taken and preserved separately. Doctor normally should stand on the side from which wind is blowing. Disinfectants and pesticides should not be sprinkled on the body as it may interfere with toxicological examination. The body is then examined inside the coffin or grave and photographs are taken from all angles. The body is then lifted on a wooden plank or plastic sheet. Body should normally be transferred to a mortuary for detailed postmortem examination. In advanced putrefaction the body is searched for any foreign material like projectiles of a firearm or fractures. In all cases the viscera should be preserved for toxicological analysis. Detailed notes are prepared mentioning the exhumation order, persons present, location diagrams, name of the person identifying the grave, condition in which body recovered, position of limbs, state of putrefaction, photographs and detailed postmortem examination report.

Postmortem Artefacts

Postmortem artefacts are those changes seen in a dead body, which are introduced at the time of death or after death and may mislead the forensic pathologist while conducting the autopsy. Misinterpretation of such findings may lead to wrong conclusions regarding cause and manner of death.

Artefacts are produced in a body due to; (i) agonal changes at the time of death; (ii) due to postmortem changes or (iii) changes introduced while conducting the autopsy procedure by an inexperienced person.

Perimortem Artefacts

These changes normally take place at the time of death due to resuscitation or agonal changes.

Resuscitation artefacts: These artefacts are very commonly seen in hospital deaths. So as to revive a person artificial respiration and external cardiac massage is practically given to most of the patients dying in the hospital. Forceful cardiac massage may lead to fractures of the ribs and some times of the sternum. These changes may be interpreted in the form of blunt force injuries to the front of the chest; however there is very minimum bruising of the intercostal muscles in such cases.

Intracardiac injections may cause bruising in the cardiac muscles. Hence it is important to go through the clinical records of the patient to find out the treatment provided. Patches of hyperemia over the chest may be due to the application of defibrillator, which may be confused with bruising.

Rarely a hole for putting a drainage tube in the chest may be confused with a bullet injury.

Agonal changes: Some agonal changes like regurgitation leading to aspiration of gastric contents may take place in few cases. In such cases finding other asphyxial findings are most important before the case is labelled as death from aspiration.

Artefacts Produced After Death

These artefacts are mainly due to postmortem changes or changes produced by insects and animals. Handling of the body while embalming or burial may produce certain changes which may lead to misinterpretation while conducting autopsy.

Artefacts seen due to postmortem changes: Putrefaction of the body produces certain changes which may be misinterpreted for injuries or pathological changes.

Bloodstained fluid coming out of mouth and nostrils may indicate falsely of hemorrhage from lungs or stomach. Production of skin slippage may give impression of an abrasion but mostly the base is pale and no age related changes are observed. Patches of postmortem lividity may be interpreted as bruises especially when such patches are present on the front of upper part of the chest and can be easily differentiated by giving a cut in the area and observing no extravasation of blood. Blebs formed after deaths may be confused with scalds but these blebs apart from having fluids contain gases. Presence of gases in the heart chambers may suggest air embolism but can be differentiated by analysis of the gases as oxygen is present in air embolism cases.

Cherry red discolouration of the hypostasis normally observed in carbon monoxide poisoning may be observed in case the body is put in a cold chamber or is exposed to extremely cold atmosphere. Hypostasis in the internal organs may be confused with visceral hemorrhage. Death from sunstroke may show high temperature after death and may interfere in determination of time since death.

Toxicological artefacts: Putrefaction of tissues after death produces some amount of alcohol. Some studies have reported production of alcohol in body tissues with bacterial action seen in advanced putrefaction, up to 100 mg% normaly but few authors have reported up 200 mg% of alchol; however addition of sodium fluoride as a preservative prevents production of alcohol in preserved tissues for toxicological analysis. In cases showing advanced putrefaction, estimation of alcohol from vitreous humor may give accurate results. EDTA should not be used as preservative in such cases.

Changes produced by insects or animals: Maggots may alter the shape of injuries or even make hole in the body which may look like gunshot injuries. Rodent bites are sometime seen in the stored bodies and are differentiated by presence of teeth marks and absence of antemortem features.

Changes due to mishandling of the body: Sometimes the rigor mortis is broken so as to transport the body conveniently which may interfere in the time since death calculations. Body may be dragged which may produce postmortem abrasions on the bony prominences.

Artefacts due to embalming or burial: In case the autopsy has to be conducted on an embalmed body or after exhumation, autopsy surgeon has to be careful so that he may not take a hole caused by a trocar for embalming process as a gunshot injury. Sometimes head falling back from embalming table may result in cervical fractures at C-6 or C-7 level known as *"Undertaker's fracture"*. Presence of fungal growth in buried bodies may interfere in the interpretation of injuries.

Misinterpretation of Certain Findings or Production of Artefacts During Autopsy

Sometimes due to inexperience of the autopsy surgeon he may either produce certain artefacts or misinterpret certain findings.

Production of artifacts on autopsy: In certain cases when the neck structures are opened first and left as such for some time the blood from the vessels may stain the neck structures and may give impression of throttling. Even mishandling of neck structures may produce postmortem fracture of hyoid bone. When the viscera is being removed from chest or abdomen the blood may be seen in the body cavities which may escape from the major blood vessels or air may enter blood vessels giving impression of air embolism. Fracture of skull bones or extension of existing fracture line may be seen after the skull is opened with chisel and hammer.

Misinterpretation of findings: A groove may be seen on the uncus gyrus which may be interpreted as edema of the brain. Uncal herniation usually produces a groove which may show minute hemorrhages. Liver may show staining on the under surface in contact with colon may be taken as bruising or hypostasis in the loops of intestines may be recorded wrongly as infarcted areas.

25 | AIDS and Medicolegal Aspects of AIDS

Acquired immune deficiency syndrome (AIDS) is caused by human immunodeficiency virus (HIV) infection. Infection with HIV gradually lowers the immune defence of the person against infections and diseases. The human immunodeficiency virus, a type of retrovirus, destroy T-helper cells (Type of white blood cells) also known as CD4 cells. HIV is also known as human T-lymphotropic virus type-III or lymph-adenopathy associated virus. There are many strains of the HIV; however this virus is divided into two types; HIV-1 and HIV-2. HIV-1 is common variant infecting people across the world, whereas, HIV-2 is mainly seen in western Africa. In an infected person virus can be detected in semen, blood, breast milk and vaginal fluids. Therefore, most common way of transmission of this infection is by having sex or anal sex. Condoms provide sufficient protection against HIV. Infection can also spread through infected needles especially in drug addicts or mother to child during pregnancy. In case no treatment is provided to an infected person, AIDS develop in about 10 to 15 years. However with early diagnosis and antiretroviral treatment, infected person can live healthy life.

Acquired immune deficiency syndrome (AIDS) is advanced stage of HIV infection. CD4 count in the blood is a good indicator of AIDS and CD4 count in such cases goes below 200 per ml of blood. There is wide range of opportunistic infections like bacterial pneumonia, thrush, tuberculosis, toxoplasmosis, cytomegalovirus and fungal infections. There are chances of developing cancers like Kaposi's sarcoma or lymphoma of the brain.

However there is no pathological lesion by which AIDS can be diagnosed properly. Patient may present with low grade fever, generalized lymphadenopathy, weight loss and diarrhea.

MEDICOLEGAL ASPECTS OF AIDS

Apart from the ethical obligations of the medical profession, legal rights of the AIDS patient must be respected. Some of the questions which are raised during handling HIV infected person are confidentiality, consent for testing or mandatory testing, employment of HIV infected person, blood donations, etc.

Consent

Even though code of medical ethics of Indian Medical Council does not mention that one has to take consent before taking a blood test for HIV but National Aids Control Organization (NACO) recommends that blood testing for HIV must be done on voluntary basis and rules out mandatory testing for HIV. Therefore, blood testing for HIV requires informed consent. NACO encourages pre and post-testing counseling. A person may refuse giving sample for blood testing because of the attached stigma. Results must be kept confidential.

Even in the United States of America it is mandatory to obtain consent to test for HIV. In case of minors the consent of parents is taken.

Confidentiality

Confidential information entrusted by a patient or any information a physician comes to know while treating should never be disclosed unless required by the law or in interest of the society. Code of medical ethics directs that in order to protect a healthy individual from a communicable disease a physician should act as he would act towards one of his own family member in similar circumstances.

Supreme court of India has ruled on the issue of right to confidentiality of the subject with HIV infection and breach of confidentiality in order to protect third party. The opinion of the court is that the right to privacy and confidentiality is not absolute. The right may be lawfully restricted in situations where third party is at risk.

NACO encourages motivation of the HIV positive persons to disclose their status to sex partners.

Blood Donation

Prior testing for HIV is not done before any volunteer comes to donate blood. However, all the units of collected blood are tested both for HIV-1 and HIV-2. Only after those units which are found negative after HIV testing are declared fit for use as such or used for preparations of blood components. Blood unit found positive are destroyed preferably by incineration.

Blood donor of HIV positive blood is not informed about his positive status as per the policy of the Government of India. In case the donor wants to know his HIV status, he is referred to the nearby HIV testing center for testing along with pre and post-test counselling.

Marriage

There is no bar on the marriage of a HIV positive person. However, it is mandated that an informed consent is obtained from the marriage partner before marriage. Person getting married without informing other partner can be punished under **section 269 IPC** for negligent act likely to spread infection of disease dangerous to life and is punishable with imprisonment of either description for a term which may extend to six months or with fine or with both. Such a person can also be punished under **section 270 IPC** for malignant act likely to spread infection of disease dangerous to life with imprisonment of either description for a term which may extend to two years or with fine or with both.

Women and HIV

Women are more vulnerable to HIV infections, especially commercial sex workers (CSW). Even when such CSW are willing for the safe sex practices, measures to prevent the spread are likely to fail, unless the clients are educated properly. In Thailand and in red light areas of Kolkata and Mumbai such interventions have yielded excellent results in reducing infection rate.

HIV positive woman is provided with proper counselling; however decision to avoid pregnancy sterilization or abortion when pregnant is left to the woman to decide. As breast mild is having high load of HIV, they are advised to avoid breastfeeding their child.

Right to Treatment

Right to treatment or medical care is fundamental right of the person and state is duty bound to provide facilities for such treatment. All cases brought before doctors in government service are required to treat such cases and if required admission in the hospital may be provided. Even in private setup it is unethical not to provide treatment. However doctors in private practice may decide depending upon the facilities available with them to treat such cases or refer them to appropriate center for treatment. However, in emergency or when HIV positive status is detected during treatment the doctor must continue to provide proper treatment.

Clinical Trials

During conduct of any study or vaccine trials on HIV positive individuals' informed consent is required. A registered medical practitioner shall not publish photographs or case reports of his/her patients without their permission, in any medical or other journal in a manner in which their identity could be made out.

Employment

HIV status of an individual does not affect his right to employment. Even employer cannot subject an individual before employing or after employing to undergo mandatory testing for HIV. Person infected with HIV does not pose any threat to his co-workers. Such persons are permitted to work till they are able to perform their job responsibilities.

Partner Notification

Global Programme on AIDS (GPA) of WHO passed a resolution for avoidance of discrimination of HIV infected persons or individuals with AIDS and laid norms regarding partner notifications like; (i) respecting the human rights of such an individual; (ii) infected person and his partner should have access to treatment facilities independently of their willingness for partner notification on voluntary basis; (iii) confidentiality in maintaining all the records including locating information of the partners; and (iv) counselling and testing facilities on voluntary basis and assured heath facilities to be regularly monitored.

There are two approaches adopted in partner notifications; (i) contact tracing is based on voluntary disclosure of the names of partners; however it requires full confidentiality of details; and (ii) duty to warn approach is adopted when the contact partner

is known like wife of the infected person. Such a contact is informed about the risks without the consent of the infected person. Supreme court has approved such an approach.

PRECAUTIONS FOR HEALTH CARE WORKERS

Doctors especially in the casualty must take proper universal precautions while handling suspected cases like homosexuals or drug addicts. Invasive procedures in HIV infected cases must be done with full barrier protection like gloves, masks plastic aprons, eye protection and gum boots to prevent contact with blood of the patient. Needle prick injuries or other injuries by sharp instruments are to be prevented like avoiding recapping of needles or cleaning sharp instruments with care.

PRECAUTIONS DURING CONDUCT OF POST-MORTEMS

Conduct of postmortem on a known case of HIV infected person requires all precautions so that mortuary staff is well protected. Such a body must be properly labelled by the hospital or mortuary staff. Some of the measures taken during such an autopsy are mentioned below:

a. Double gloves must be used while conducting autopsy. If available, wire mesh protected gloves must be used.
b. High quality face mask to cover mouth and nostrils of the person conducting autopsy.
c. Goggles to cover eyes so that any blood splash could not enter eyes.
d. Plastic apron to cover the front.
e. Gum boots so as to avoid contact with spilled blood on the floor.
f. Avoid pricks from needles, sharp instruments or bone fragments.
g. Use bleaching powder to cover blood spills.
h. Stitch and cover the body properly so that there is no leakage of blood, if possible put some bleaching powder in body cavities.
i. Instruct relatives to handle and cremate the body properly.

26 | Starvation

Starvation is deprivation of food leading to severe deficiency of energy required for maintaining body functions, and in extreme cases resulting in death. Even use of unsuitable food articles may lead to starvation. As per WHO statics, malnutrition is the main reason for mortality in children. Depending upon the consumption of food articles starvation can be divided into two categories:

1. **Acute starvation:** When the food is completely withdrawn like a person trapped in mines or pits.
2. **Chronic starvation:** Chronic starvation occurs when the food supply is deficient or unsuitable food articles are consumed like in famine when sufficient food is not available, neglect of a child by guardian, excessive fasting when food is wilfully refused, certain medical conditions when the patient is incapacitated to consume required quantities of food or in case of poverty when the person is not able to buy required amount of food articles.

ENERGY GENERATION IN FASTING

The energy requirements of a person depend on the physical work. Caloric requirements varies from 2000 calories to 3000 calories per day depending upon whether an adult person is doing sedentary work or engaged in heavy physical work. Features of starvation start appearing when the daily caloric intake from food falls below critical level, i.e. minimum required for the body.

In normal conditions glucose is stored in body as glycogen. In fasting energy requirements of the body is initially met from the glycogen stores of the body through glycogenolysis with the help of glucagon. Gradually body fats are utilised for providing energy by formation of ketones. Acetone which is one of ketone bodies imparts typical smell to the breath. Muscle protein is also used by body for energy production after removing amino group from amino acids. Amino acids are converted to urea and excreted through kidneys.

Features of Starvation

Manifestations depends upon whether the food withdrawal is acute or chronic.

Acute Starvation

There is craving for food for a day or two and then gradually the feeling of hunger is lost. There is pain in epigastric region which can be relieved by pressure. However, feeling of thirst remains. The person feels fatigued and listless. There is gradual loss of weight due to loss of subcutaneous fat. Skin is dry and wrinkled. There is gradual loss of muscles mass. Person finds it difficult to move or to do some activity due to muscular atrophy. Eyes are sunken, cheeks are hollow and lips are dry and cracked. Bones become prominent. Body emits offensive odor. Blood pressure is low and pulse is feeble and slow but on slight exertion may show increase in the pulse rate. Gallbladder is found distended. There is constipation but during terminal stages there is diarrhea. Mind is clear till end; however, in some cases there may be confusion and delirium. Loss of more than 40% of body weight is usually fatal.

When both water and food is deprived the person may survive for 7 to 10 days, but in case only food is withheld the person may survive for 50 to 75 days. There are instances where the person has survived fasting for 25 weeks. Shaheed Bhagat Singh and Batukeshwar Dutt fasted up to 116 days before British agreed to their demands.

Survival period depends on the state of health, amount of body fat, atmospheric temperature, age and sex of the person. Healthy individual can survive for more time than a diseased person. Young and old persons suffer more from fasting, whereas, females can tolerate fasting for longer periods.

Chronic Starvation

Chronic starvation features which are seen due to deficient food supply or consumption of unsuitable food material often lead to vitamin deficiency like beriberi, pellagra and scurvy apart from anemia. There are hunger pains, person feel lethargic, body temperature is below normal (hypothermia) with loss of body weight. There is edema of the feet, which may gradually involve rest of the body. The individual may suffer from diarrhea, dysentery and opportunistic infections. Fungus growth in esophagus may make it difficult to swallow even small quantities of available food.

Death is from brown atrophy of the heart leading to circulatory failure or concomitant infections.

Treatment

Cautious approach is required to treat a case of fasting, initially sips of water mixed with glucose is given at frequent intervals.

Intravenous fluids may be required in serious cases. Fruit juice is also administered to the patient. Gradually semisolid food is given in small quantities before sold food articles are added. Chronic starvation requires additional vitamins and proteins.

Postmortem Features

External Findings

The body is emaciated, skin is dry, pigmented and cracked. There is loss of body fat, except female breasts. Eyes are sunken, bones are prominent. Edema may be seen around ankles or lower legs. Abdomen is concave however in chronic starvation there is ascites. Hairs are dry, brittle and lusterless.

Internal Findings

Subcutaneous fat is completely lost in chronic starvation but in acute starvation some amount may be present. Fat is also lost from mesentery and internal organs which is characteristic of starvation. In chronic starvation especially in children features of malnutrition like rickets, bony deformities, beriberi and pellagra are seen. Muscles show atrophy and are darker in colour due to lipochrome increase. Organs of the body are reduced in size and weight except brain. Stomach and intestine show atrophy and become thin. **Gallbladder is distended and is full of bile**. There are signs of dehydration and urinary bladder is empty in majority of cases. Heart is small in size with features of brown atrophy.

MEDICOLEGAL ISSUES

a. *Conditions simulating starvation:* Starvation deaths have to be differentiated from emaciating diseases like malignancies, diabetes, Addison's disease, tuberculosis or chronic diarrhea. In such cases the cause of death must be pronounced after excluding such conditions.

b. *Accidental starvation:* Accidental starvation may take place in person trapped in pits or mines, person stranded in shipwrecks and famine. In certain conditions the person may not be in a position to ingest food, e.g. person may not be in a position to take medical help or medical support in esophageal strictures or malignancies.

c. *Homicidal starvation:* This is mostly seen in infants or small children who are deprived of the proper food leading to chronic starvation. Such situation is most common in unwanted children or mentally diseased individuals.

d. *Suicidal starvation:* Some individuals voluntarily fast and unless they are forced to feed, death may occur due to acute starvation. Force feeding is permitted under law as under article 21 of the constitution of India right to life does not include right to die, more over doctors under medical ethics has obligation to preserve life, hence person on fast is medically supervised and is advised force feeding when there is loss of weight and acidosis.

27 | Role of Forensic Pathologist at Scene of Crime

Criminal investigations into the cause and manner of sudden and unexpected deaths are required to establish the facts beyond reasonable doubts to the satisfaction of the court so as to penalize the offender. It is pertinent to mention that most of the vital clues are recovered from the scene of crime. Therefore, an immediate, thorough and methodical investigation by investigating agency is a must to bring the culprit to justice. Collection of evidence, including physical findings, biological and trace elements is primary responsibility of the investigating team. Unfortunately in Indian scenario the information which a medical professional can help in collecting from the scene of crime is missing in majority of times. Author in his long experience in the field of forensic medicine can hardly recall very few cases when his services were required on the scene of crime in the city of New Delhi. Interpretation from photographs may not be easy at a later date. Under ideal conditions the investigating office of the police should include a forensic pathologist in his team when visiting the scene of crime.

DUTIES OF A DOCTOR AT THE SCENE OF CRIME

Whenever a doctor is requested to visit a scene of crime, he should be prompt in responding and should arrive as soon as possible so that he is in a position to observe the scene before it is disturbed by other members of the team. He should make a sketch of the scene; any disturbance in the surrounding articles; note the clothing; any sign of struggle; posture of the body; injuries present; presence of trace elements; weapon of offence and their relative position to the body. He must allow the photographic record to be completed before observing condition of the body. If required he can advise the photographer for taking some pictures to record some significant findings. It is advisable not to change the position of the body or touch anything at the scene of crime before taking permission of the investigating officer. Help the investigating team in collecting trace evidence from the scene. After completing your examination inform the investigating office about your interpretation of the findings. In case the doctor himself has to conduct the autopsy, the final conclusion should be offered after Post-mortem examination.

ADVANTAGES OF PRESENCE OF A DOCTOR AT SCENE OF CRIME

Apart from certifying death, a doctor is required to provide information regarding time since death and probable cause and manner of death. Some of the advantages are mentioned below:

a. *Certification of death:* Foremost duty of a doctor on reaching the scene of crime is to examine the person whether he is alive or dead. In case the person is alive it is the duty of the doctor to provide resuscitative measures and to shift that person to a nearest medical center for necessary treatment.

b. *Collection and preservation of evidence:* Collection of the evidence from the scene of crime and their preservation is highly important in the courts to prove that they are connected with the crime. Hence, these are properly labelled and proper chain of custody is maintained. For collection of evidence the scene of crime is searched thoroughly by the investigating team. A Forensic expert could be helpful in collection of trace elements. Following are some of the methods employed to search crime scene:

   i. *Line search:* The scene is search by the team by searching in straight line to cover the entire area.

   ii. *Spiral search:* The examination is done starting from the center and going over the entire area in a spiral.

   iii. *Zone method:* The entire scene is divided into various zones and each zone is searched separately.

   iv. *Grid method:* the scene is searched by going in a radial direction from the center and covering the entire area.

c. *Identification:* In a case when body is not of a known person, it is responsibility of the doctor to provide any helpful information to the inquiry officer like tattoo marks, deformities, age related changes or presence of any document on the body helpful in identification, etc.

d. *Position and location of body:* Position and location of body must be recorded. Body recovered from a locked room from inside may suggest suicide.

e. *Clothing:* Cloths worn by the victim must be carefully examined for any signs of struggle; presence of bloodstains on the inner aspect; tears or cuts and presence of

firearm discharge from a close range may be of help in interpretation of injuries and cause of death.

f. *Postmortem changes:* Changes after death especially the postmortem staining, rigor mortis and changes of putrefaction are recorded.

g. *Time since death:* Body inner core temperature is recorded along with ambient temperature of the surroundings. In case the body is present outdoor, then the climatic conditions like rain and humidity levels are also noted. Mention statement of a witness regarding the time of incident which may help in determination of the time since death.

h. *Any change in the body position:* This is normally inference by the present of fixation of hypostasis on presently non-dependent parts or rigor mortis not consistent with the position of the body.

i. *Cause and manner of death:* Changes in the body like presence of cadaveric spasm may be helpful in interpretation of the manner of death. Presence of drugs or empty wrappers can be interpreted better by a doctor to provide clues to the investigating police officer. Presence of vomitus may suggest poisoning and collection of the same for toxicological analysis, as it may contain the maximum amount of the ingested poison. Presence of stab injuries, defence wounds or distant range firearm injuries are mostly suggestive of homicidal nature of the death.

j. *Injuries:* All the injuries along with their location and dimensions are recorded as far as possible.

k. *Avoiding misinterpretation due to artifacts:* When postmortem is conducted at a later stage; due to passage of time or mishandling of the body during transportation, postmortem artifacts may be produced. These can easily be differentiated when the body is examined at the scene of crime.

l. *Better understanding of requirements at the time of postmortem examination:* Most of the time detailed information about the circumstances and observations at the scene of crime are not provided to a doctor conducting autopsy. Therefore, visit to the scene of crime may help a doctor regarding the requirements of the case.

CRIME SCENE EXAMINATION KIT

A doctor proceeding to the scene of crime must carry with him a standard kit having following articles:

a. A pair of surgical gloves
b. Containers for collecting trace evidence like plastic and glass bottles with tight fitting lids
c. Cotton swabs, slides, self-sealing envelops and labels
d. Rectal thermometers
e. Hand lens
f. Measuring tape
g. Digital camera and flash light
h. Surgical blades, forceps, probes and a pair of scissors
i. Stethoscope and ultraviolet lamp
j. Note pad and pen.

DIFFICULTIES IN VISITING SCENE OF CRIME BY A DOCTOR

Though presence of a forensic pathologist is of great importance in interpretation of various findings at the scene of crime, but presently there are many difficulties which are faced in such situations.

a. *Reluctance of medical persons to visit a scene of crime:* Medical officers working in government service are overworked and do not show any interest in visiting a scene of crime.

b. *Lack of training:* Routine medical persons are not properly trained in this field as there is no motivation or incentives available for doing such services.

c. *Interference in police work:* Most of the police officers take it as interference in their work. Moreover they find it difficult to request a doctor for scene visit as no doctor is designated for this work by the health department except for doctors working in forensic field.

28 | Sexual Offences

Sexual offences are acts of obtaining sexual gratification by means of sexual intercourse or otherwise with a person or an animal against the provision of the law. These can be classified into following groups:

    i. **Natural sexual offences:** Include rape, incest and adultery.

    ii. **Unnatural sexual offences:** These include sodomy, lesbianism or tribadism, buccal coitus and bestiality.

    iii. **Sexual perversions:** Perversions include sadism, masochism, fetishism, transvestism, voyeurism, exhibitionism, undinism and froutterism.

    iv. **Miscellaneous:** These include indecent assault and prostitution.

NATURAL SEXUAL OFFENCES

Rape

The need for a new law on sexual assault was felt as the law at that time did not define and reflect the various kinds of sexual assault that women are subjected to in our country. Hence changes were introduced by means of criminal law amendment act 2006 and criminal law amendment act 2013. This act extends to the whole of India except the state of Jammu and Kashmir.

A man is said to commit "rape" if he (**section 375 IPC**);

a. Penetrates his penis, to any extent, into the vagina, mouth, urethra or anus of a woman or makes her to do so with him or any other person; or

b. Inserts, to any extent, any object or a part of the body, not being the penis, into the vagina, the urethra or anus of a woman or makes her to do so with him or any other person; or

c. Manipulates any part of the body of a woman so as to cause penetration into the vagina, urethra, anus or any of body of such woman or makes her to do so with him or any other person; or

d. Applies his mouth to the vagina, anus and urethra of a woman or makes her to do so with him or any other person.

Under the Circumstances Falling Under Any of the Following Seven Descriptions:

Firstly: Against her will.

Secondly: Without her consent.

Thirdly: With her consent, when her consent has been obtained by putting her or any person in whom she is interested, in fear of death or of hurt.

Fourthly: With her consent, when the man knows that he is not her husband and that her consent is given because she believes that he is another man to whom she is or believes herself to be lawfully married.

Fifthly: With her consent when, at the time of giving such consent, by reason of unsoundness of mind or intoxication or the administration by him personally or through another of any stupefying or unwholesome substance, she is unable to understand the nature and consequences of that to which she gives consent.

Sixthly: With or without her consent, when she is under eighteen years of age.

Seventhly: When she is unable to communicate consent.

Explanation 1: For the purposes of this section, "vagina" shall also include labia majora.

Explanation 2: Consent means an unequivocal voluntary agreement when the woman by words, gestures or any form of verbal or nonverbal communication, communicates willingness to participate in the specific sexual act.

Provided that a woman who does not physically resist to the act of penetration shall not by the reason only of that fact, be regarded as consenting to the sexual activity.

There are following exceptions under section 375 IPC.

Exception 1: A medical procedure or intervention shall not constitute rape.

Exception 2: Sexual intercourse or sexual acts by a man with his own wife, the wife not being under fifteen years of age, is not rape' (not being under 13 years in the union territory of Manipur).

Consent and Will

Willingness of a person differs from the consent given for the act. A girl may be willing but may not give consent because of the fear of society or in some cases the consent is invalid when she is intoxicated or below the age of giving consent. The consent must be obtained prior to the sexual act, therefore, consent obtained after the act is not a valid consent. Presence of struggle marks due to resistance offered by the victim is taken as proof of absence of consent, however as per the explanation 2 of the Section 375 it has been clarified that absence of physical resistance to

penetration should not regarded as consent for the act.

Punishment for Rape (Section 376 IPC)

1. Whoever, except in the cases provided for in subsection (2), commits rape shall be punished with rigorous imprisonment of either description for a term which shall not be less than seven years, but which may extend to imprisonment for life, and shall also be liable to fine.

2. Whoever:

   a. Being a police officer, commits rape:
      i. Within the limits of the police station to which such police officer is appointed.
      ii. In the premises of any station house.
      iii. On a woman in such police officer's custody or in the custody of a police officer subordinate to such police officer.

   b. Being a public servant, commits rape on a woman in such public servant's custody or in the custody of a public servant subordinate to such public servant; or

   c. Being a member of the armed forces deployed in an area by the central or a state government commits rape in such area; or

   d. Being on the management or on the staff of a jail, remand home or other place of custody established by or under any law for the time being in force or of a women's or children's institution, commits rape on any inmate of such jail, remand home, place or institution; or

   e. Being on the management or on the staff of a hospital, commits rape on a woman in that hospital; or

   f. Being a relative, guardian or teacher of, or a person in a position of trust or authority towards the woman, commits rape on such woman; or

   g. Commits rape during communal or sectarian violence; or

   h. Commits rape on a woman knowing her to be pregnant; or

i. Commits rape on a woman when she is under sixteen years of age; or

j. Commits rape, on a woman incapable of giving consent; or

k. Being in a position of control or dominance over a woman, commits rape on such woman; or

l. Commits rape on a woman suffering from mental or physical disability; or

m. While committing rape causes grievous bodily harm or maims or disfigures or endangers the life of a woman; or

n. Commits rape repeatedly on the same woman, shall be punished with rigorous imprisonment for a term which shall not be less than ten years, but which may extend to imprisonment for life, which shall mean imprisonment for the remainder of that person's natural life, and shall also be liable to fine.

Explanation: For the purposes of this subsection:

i. "Armed forces" means the naval, military and air forces and includes any member of the armed forces constituted under any jaw for the time being in force, including the paramilitary forces and any auxiliary forces that are under the control of the central government!, or the state government.

ii. "Hospital" means the precincts of the hospital and includes the precincts of any institution for the reception and treatment of persons during convalescence or of persons requiring medical attention or rehabilitation.

iii. "Police officer" shall have the same meaning as assigned to the expression "police" under the police act, 1861.

iv. "Women's or children's institution" means an institution, whether called an orphanage or a home for neglected women or children or a widow's home or an institution called by any other name, which is established and maintained for the reception and care of women or children.

Punishment for Causing Death or Resulting in Persistent Vegetative State of Victim

Section 376-A IPC: Whoever, commits an offence punishable under subsection (1) or subsection (2) of section 376 and in the course of such commission inflicts an injury which causes the death of the woman or causes the woman to be in a persistent vegetative state, shall be punished with rigorous imprisonment for a term which shall not be less than twenty years, but which may extend to imprisonment for life, which shall mean imprisonment for the remainder of that person's natural life, or with death.

Sexual Intercourse by Husband Upon his Wife During Separation

Section 376-B IPC: Whoever has sexual intercourse with his own wife, who is living separately, whether under a decree of separation or otherwise, without her consent, shall be punished with imprisonment of either description for a term which shall not be less than two years but which may extend to seven years, and shall also be liable to fine.

Sexual Intercourse by Person in Authority

Section 376-C IPC: Whoever, being;

a. In a position of authority or in a fiduciary relationship; or

b. A public servant; or

c. Superintendent or manager of a jail, remand home or other place of custody established by or under any law for the time being in force, or a women's or children's institution; or

d. On the management of a hospital or being on the staff of a hospital, abuses such position or fiduciary relationship to induce or seduce any woman either in his custody or under his charge or present in the premises to have sexual intercourse with him, such sexual intercourse not amounting to the offence of rape, shall be punished with rigorous imprisonment of either description for a term which shall not be less than five years, but which may extend to ten years, and shall also be liable to fine.

Explanation 1: In this section, "sexual intercourse" shall mean any of the acts mentioned in clauses (a) to (d) of section 375.

Explanation 2: For the purposes of this section, Explanation I to section 375 shall also be applicable.

Explanation 3: "Superintendent", in relation to a jail, remand home or other place of custody or a women's or children's institution, includes a person holding any other office in such jail, remand home, place or institution by virtue of which such person can exercise any authority or control over its inmates.

Explanation 4: The expressions "hospital" and "women's or children's institution" shall respectively have the same meaning as in Explanation to subsection (2) of section 376.

Gang Rape

Section 376-D IPC: Where a woman is raped by one or more persons constituting a group or acting in furtherance of a common intention, each of those persons shall be deemed to have committed the offence of rape and shall be punished with rigorous imprisonment for a term which shall not be less than twenty years, but which may extend to life which shall mean imprisonment for the remainder of that person's natural life, and with fine:

Provided that such fine shall be just and reasonable to meet the medical expenses and rehabilitation of the victim:

Provided further that any fine imposed under this section shall be paid to the victim.

Punishment for Repeat Offenders

Section 376-E IPC: Whoever has been previously convicted of an offence punishable under section 376 or section 376A and is subsequently convicted of an offence punishable under any of the said sections shall be punished with imprisonment for life which shall mean imprisonment for the remainder of that person's natural life, or with death.

Absence of Consent or Quality of Consent in Prosecution for Rape

Section 114-A of the Indian evidence act: In a prosecution for rape under section 376 of the Indian penal code, where sexual intercourse by the accused is proved and the question is whether it was without the consent of the woman alleged to have been raped and such woman states in her evidence before the court, that she did not consent, the court shall presume that she did not consent.

Section 146 of the Indian evidence act: Provided that in a prosecution for an offence under section 376, section 376A, section 376B, section 376C, section 376D or section 376E of the Indian penal code or for attempt to commit any such offence, where the question of consent is an issue, it shall not be permissible to adduce evidence or to put questions in the cross-examination of the victim as to the general immoral character or previous sexual experience of such victim with any person for proving such consent or the quality of consent."

Section 53-A of the Indian evidence act: In a prosecution for an offence under section 354 or section 376 of the Indian penal code or for attempt to commit any such offence, where the question of consent is in issue, evidence of the character of the victim or of such person's previous sexual experience with any person shall not be relevant on the issue of such consent or the quality of consent.

Public Servant Disobeying Direction Under Law

Section 166-A IPC subsection (c): Whoever, being a public servant, fails to record any information given to him under subsection (I) of section 154 of the Code of Criminal Procedure, 1973, in relation to cognisable offence punishable under section 326A, section 326B, section 354, section 354B, section 370, section 370A, section 376, section 376A, section 376B, section 376C, section 376D, section 376E or section 509, shall be punished with rigorous imprisonment for a term which shall not be less than six months but which may extend to two years, and shall also be liable to fine.

Punishment for nontreatment of Victim

(Section 166-B IPC): Whoever, being incharge of a hospital, public or private, whether run by the central government, the state government, local bodies or any other person, contravenes the provisions of section 357C of the code of criminal procedure shall be punished with imprisonment for a term which may extend to one year or with fine or with both.

Recording of Statement

Section 161 of the code of criminal procedure, subsection (3): It has been included that the statement of a woman against whom an offence under section 354, section 376 or section 509 of the Indian penal code is alleged to have been committed or attempted shall be recorded, by a woman police officer or any woman officer.

Disclosure of Identity of the Victim of Certain Offences

Section 228-A of the code of criminal procedure: Whoever prints or publishes the name or any matter which may make known the identity of any person against whom an offence under section 376, section 376A, section 376B, section 376C or section 376D shall be punished with imprisonment of either description for a term which may extend to two years and shall also be liable to fine.

MEDICAL EXAMINATION OF VICTIM OF SEXUAL ASSAULT

Sexual assault on women and children are some of the most heinous crimes. Delhi high court vide order dated 23-4-2009 recommended guidelines as suggested by *"Delhi commission of women"* to effectively tackle sexual assault cases. Sexual assault, like any other form of violence, results in physical and psychological consequences. Thus, health care providers have a dual responsibility vis-à-vis victims of sexual assault. The first is to provide the victim/patient with the required medical and psychological treatment care, while the second is to assist the victims in their medico-legal proceedings by collecting evidence and performing good quality and thorough forensic medical examination and documentation.

Section 164-A criminal procedure code which deals with medical examination of the victim of rape says that medical examination shall be conducted by a registered medical practitioner employed in a hospital run by the government or a local authority and in the absence of such a practitioner, by any other registered medical practitioner, with the consent of such woman or of a person competent to give such consent on her behalf.

General Information and Consent

1. Enter the OPD number/IPD number or other registration number of the victim. Also mention the MLC number in the place provided.
2. Enter the full name of the patient/victim.
3. Enter the age and sex of the patient. Also enter the marital status of the patient, i.e. whether single, married, divorced, etc.
4. Enter the patients' address with contact number if any.
5. Enter the date and time of arrival of the patient or victim at the hospital.
6. Brought by: If the patient is accompanied by a police or law enforcement officer, enter the officer's name, identification number (if applicable) and police station with letter number and date, wherever such information is available.

   If the patient comes on her own accompanied by another person then enter the name of that person with relation (if any).
7. Consent: The doctor is required to give the patient an explanation of what the examination comprises and how the various procedures will be carried out in the language which the patient can understand. Consent is most important as no one can force victim of sexual assault to undergo examination. Obtain informed consent on consent form.

Consent must be taken from the guardian/parent if the survivor is under the age of 12 years or if the survivor is unable to give her consent due to mental disability or mental illness or intoxication. If female patient is to be examined by a male doctor then such examination shall be made in presence of a female, i.e. nurse/attendant, etc. with the consent of the patient.

8. Two identification marks must be recorded in the report.

History/Details of Alleged Sexual Assault

As far as possible history shall be obtained from the victim in her own words. If it is not possible to collect the history from the victim because of medical reasons then history is taken from the accompanying person. One must be very sensitive and compassionate while eliciting the history. While taking history, no third person or police is allowed. Any history of sexually transmitted diseases or infections prior to assault must be asked. Activities undertaken by the survivor after the assault like bathing, urinating, douching, or defecating are recorded. History of any drug including alcohol being given to the victim before or during the assault is also important.

Medical, Obstetrical and Surgical History

Enter the relevant details regarding menarche or menopause and menstrual status at the time of examination. Record the date of last menstrual period. Enter the obstetric details of the patient about pregnancies, deliveries, live births, abortions and deaths. If the victim is pregnant at the time of assault, then details like length of gestation must be recorded. Details about past medical and surgical history must be recorded.

General Physical Examination

a. General mental conditions including orientation as regards to time, place and person. Record whether she is agitated, restless, numb, anxious and able to respond to questions.

b. Record blood pressure, pulse and respiration rate.

c. Signs of intoxication by alcohol or drugs like gamma hydroxibutyric acid, ketamine and benzodiazepines; which are the most commonly used as date rape drugs.

d. Collection of foreign material and examination of clothes worn at the time of assault: Patient is made to undress over a large sheet of paper to collect any foreign material falling onto the paper. Cloths are examined for evidence of tears, loss of parts, stains, loss of buttons, and other damage sustained as a result of the assault, foreign materials including fibers, twigs, hair, grass, soil or material from the suspect or the crime scene like blood or seminal stains, etc.

e. *Stains/foreign materials on body:* Any soiled area must be swabbed with plain cotton swabs, moistened with sterile water. Skin may be examined by an ultraviolet light for areas of fluorescence.

f. *Fingernails examination:* Nails are examined for presence of ragged or broken ends, any chipping of nail varnish and any foreign material under nails.

g. *Gait of victim:* The gait of the victim should be carefully observed, with emphasis for pain in any specific posture.

Injury Examination

Injuries on Body (if Any)

Body charts may be used for recording the injuries. If there is history of buccal or anal penetration and presence of bite marks, appropriate swabs should be taken as indicated. While describing the injury always note the type of injury, site, dimensions, margins, color, associated tenderness, directions and evidence of any foreign body in the injured area.

Local Examination of Genitals, Anus and Oral Cavity

A careful observation of the perineum is made for evidence of injuries, seminal stains and stray pubic hairs. If the patient is menstruating at the time of examination then the process of examination and sample collection of other areas be done. The patient can be requested to come back for re-examination immediately after the period is over. A swab of the external genitalia should be taken before any digital exploration or speculum examination is attempted.

a. *Pubic hairs:* Examined for matting, any loose hairs, and foreign material. If the hairs are matted together, a portion must be cut off and preserved. Combing the pubic hair for specimens of free foreign hair and clippings of a few of the patient's pubic hairs for comparison may be done at this point of examination.

b. *Labia majora, labia minora, clitoris, fourchette and introitus/vagina:* Look for bruises, abrasion, redness, bleeding, and tears, which may even extend into the perineum, especially in the case of girl child. A gentle stretch at the posterior fourchette area may reveal abrasions that are otherwise difficult to see, particularly if they are hidden within slight swelling or within the folds of the mucosal tissue. Asking the patient to bear down may assist the visualizing of the introitus. In case injuries are not visible but suspected; 1% Toluidine blue dye test may be done. If there is vaginal discharge, comment on the colour, texture and odor.

Finger test of sexual assault victims: The procedure is degrading and medically and scientifically irrelevant. **This procedure should not be performed in cases of sexual assault.**

c. *Hymen:* Evidence of disruption of the hymenal ring, such as reddening, laceration or tear, bleeding, edema, position of tears and its age should be noted.

d. *Perineal tear if any:* Examine for swelling, bleeding and degree of tear.

e. *Urethra:* Look for redness, swelling, discharge, injuries, bleeding, etc. Swabs from these sites should be collected.

f. *Per-speculum examination:* Findings relevant to the assault should be noted.

g. *Anus:* Record any bleeding, swelling, injuries, discharge, stains and warts around the anus. Examine the anal sphincter and document the findings. Per-rectal examination to detect injuries, stains, fissures or hemorrhoids in the anal canal must be carried out and relevant swabs from these sites should be collected.

h. *Oral cavity:* It should be inspected carefully, checking for bruising, abrasions and lacerations of buccal mucosa, petechial hemorrhages on the hard/soft palate, torn frenulum and broken teeth. Collect an oral swab, if indicated.

i. *Any other findings:* Look for various signs suggestive of sexually transmitted infections like HIV, syphilis or gonorrhea.

Examination to Determine the Age of the Victim

If the victim appears to be below the age of consenting the age of the girl is determined by general physical, dental and radiological examination.

Sample collection for hospital/clinical laboratory

As per the order of the Delhi high court *"Sexual assault forensic examination"* (**SAFE**) kit must be available at all centers comprising of following articles: (a) detailed instructions for the examiner; (b) forms for documentation; (c) tube for blood sample; (d) urine sample container; (e) paper bag for cloths; (f) large sheet of paper for patient to undress; (g) cotton swabs for biological evidence collection; (h) sterile water; (i) glass slides; (j) unwaxed dental floss; (k) wooden sticks for fingernail scrapings; (l) envelops for evidence samples; (m) wood's lamp; (n) toluidine blue dye; (o) patients gown; (p) needle syringes, speculum, colonoscope, microscope; (q) camera; and (r) required medicine.

Laboratory tests: Where appropriate laboratory facilities exist, tests for sexually transmitted infections (STI) should be done. Cultures for neisseria gonorrhea, trichomonas vaginalis and chlamydia trachomatis; wet mount microscopy slides and blood samples for syphilis, HIV, and hepatitis B must be collected and tested.

Various Samples to be Preserved

1. Debris with collection paper (on which the victim has undressed).
2. *Clothing:* Each garment should be properly labelled and placed separately in paper bag after drying.
3. Any sanitary napkins, panty liner, diapers or tampons (worn by the patient for the period of up to 24 hours after the assault)
4. Swabs from suspected or alleged bite marks and from the places that have been licked and kissed along with control sample.
5. *Semen-like stains on body:* Collect and specify site from where the swab was collected.
6. *Combing of the patient's head hair:* For collection of loose hairs and to compare with the reference sample of hairs of the victim.
7. High vaginal/cervical swab (sterile cotton) for microscopy and culture in plain sterile test tube.

   After the speculum is in place remove any mucus with cotton or gauze. Insert the swab and collect the specimen with a gentle side-to-side motion. Allow a few seconds for the organism to adsorb onto the swab surface. Sample any cervical discharge if present.
8. Urethral swab (sterile cotton) for micros- copy and culture in plain sterile test tube.
9. Swab (sterile cotton) from vaginal dis- charge for microscopy and culture in plain sterile test tube.
10. Blood for serology (for syphilis, HIV and hepatitis B) in plain sterile tube, blood grouping and DNA profile.
11. Urine (midstream) for microscopy and culture in plain sterile bottle.
12. Swab (sterile cotton) from rectum for microscopy and culture in plain sterile tube may be taken in required cases. Insert the swab 4–5 cm into the anal canal and gently move it from side to side to sample the anal crypts.
13. Fingernail scrapings of both hands sepa- rately.

Specific Examinations

Examination of seminal fluid and stains: Seminal fluid is a viscid mucilaginous fluid with faint yellow colour and characteristic odor. It is a suspension of spermatozoa in seminal plasma and contains about 50,000 to 350000 spermatozoa per ml. Seminal stains commonly show a slight degree of viscosity and they are readily visible, because they exhibit a stiff, starchy and crusty appearance. A seminal stain allows the fluorescence to be generated under ultraviolet light. The fluore- scence from semen stains can be significantly enhanced using appropriate interference filters. Handling of articles bearing stains should be done very carefully to avoid damage to spermatozoa. Vaginal, anal and penile swabs should be collected along with their smears on slides.

Ultraviolet (UV) light exam of clothes and skin: The seminal, blood and salivary stains (dried or moist), fluorescent fibers and subtle injuries, exhibits characteristic appearance when subjected to visual examination by using long wave UV light. These lights are used to scan the body for evidence such as: dried or moist secretions.

Microscopic examination: Sperm may be detected in the vagina, rectum or mouth. Preservation of sperm in the mouth is usually not as good as in the vagina, since salivation, drinking and expectoration tend to cleanse the oral cavity. Defecation may get rid of sperm and seminal fluid from the rectum. The spermatozoa is produced in the testis by the process of spermatogenesis. The total length of spermatozoa is about 50 microns. The head is flat; oval shaped of 4.6 × 2.6 × 1.6 microns size and is covered with microsomal cap. The tail portion is responsible for the movement of sperm. (Fig. 28.1)

Detection of sperms in seminal stains: Inspection of the *wet mount slide* of the vaginal swab or *stained slide* prepared from the vaginal swabs is undertaken to determine the presence or absence of motile or nonmotile human spermatozoa in the vagina of the patient. In recent specimens, motile spermatozoa may be found and to identify them absolutely, it is necessary to find complete sperm with head and tail. Finding of single spermatozoa is confirmatory of recent sexual act. However, this is not always feasible, since spermatozoa are extremely fragile when dry and easily disintegrate. Furthermore, sexual crimes may involve males with oligospermia who have an abnormally low sperm count or may involve individuals who have no spermatozoa at all in their seminal fluid (aspermia). Presence of spermatozoa in the vaginal cavity also provides important information regarding the time of sexual activity. Which can be obtained from the knowledge that motile sperms may generally survive up to four to six hours in the vaginal cavity of a living person, however, intact sperm (sperm with tails) are not normally found 18–24 hours after intercourse, but in some rare cases they have been reported to be found as late as 72 hours after intercourse.

Chemical and Other Tests for the Detection of Seminal Fluid

1. **Florence test:** A few drops of the stain extract is taken on a slide and a drop of florence reagent (solution of iodine and potassium iodide) is added and allowed to mix slowly under a cover slip. Dark brown, needle shaped crystals of choline per-iodide are formed with in a few minutes. However, false negative results are often observed. Choline is secreted by seminal vesicles.

2. **Barberio's test:** A few drops of Barberio's reagent (saturated solution of picric acid) when added to spermatic fluid produces needle shaped, rhombic and yellow coloured crystals of spermine picrate. Spermine is secreted by prostate.

3. **Acid phosphatase test:** Acid phosphatase is an enzyme that is secreted by the prostate gland into seminal fluid and it is present in all portions of the ejaculate. Its concentrations in seminal fluid are up to 400 times greater than those found in any other body fluid. The fluid extract obtained from a small stained cloth piece is placed in a cavity on a porcelain tile and two drops each of citrate buffer and 1% aqueous solution of disodium phenyl phosphate are added. After 10 minutes, addition of 2 drops of phenol reagent and 2 drops of 20% solution of sodium carbonate, presence of blue colour indicates presence of acid

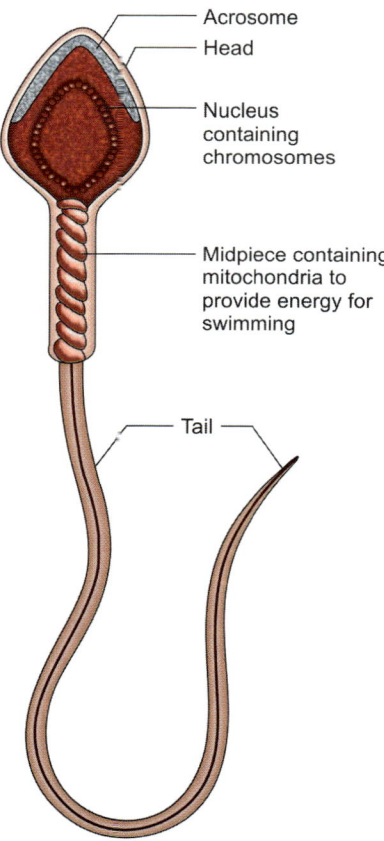

Acrosome
Head
Nucleus containing chromosomes
Midpiece containing mitochondria to provide energy for swimming
Tail

Fig. 28.1: Morphology of sperm

phosphatase. Negative test is normally used for ruling out seminal stains.

4. **LDH isoenzyme method:** Equal quantities (0.25 ml) of clear extract of seminal stain and 40% of sucrose solution are mixed. 0.1 ml of this mixture is subjected to vertical polyacryl amide gel electrophoresis. electrophoresis is carried out in refrigerator for 150 minutes using a current of 5 mA. Isoenzyme bands are revealed by staining. This method gives a specific biochemical detection of spermatozoa in semen in the presence of vaginal fluid, blood, nasal secretion, saliva and urine.

5. **Acid phosphatase isoenzyme method:** Seminal stains are extracted with water and are used in polyacryl amide gel electrophoresis method followed by staining with methyl belliferyl. Phosphate reagent enables the seminal acid phosphatase to be distinguished from that of other substance like vaginal secretions. The method is sufficiently specific and applicable to semen derived from normal, oligospermic, azoospermic and vasectomised individuals.

6. **Creatinine phosphokinase:** Creatinine phosphokinase concentration is almost double in seminal fluid in comparison with other body fluids. Normal seminal fluid concentration of creatinine phosphokinase is 385–14000 units/ml. It is diagnostic if the levels are found to be more than 400 units of CPK/ml. Major advantage of this enzyme is that it stable and can be demonstrated in old stains up to six months duration.

7. **Thin layer chromatographic technique for the detection of choline and spermine:** Thin layer chromatographic technique has been used for the detection of both choline and spermine in seminal stains.

8. **Protein p30 test:** Protein p30 is unique to seminal plasma and it is measured with a crossed electrophoresis technique. This protein is a useful semen marker particularly in cases of azoospermia.

9. **Monoclonal antibodies against human seminal plasma:** Monoclonal antibodies are also used for detection of human semen.

10. **Prostate specific antigen:** Prostate specific antigen (PSA) has been found to be present in high concentrations in semen. Simple, sensitive and reproducible methods have been developed for analysis of the presence of PSA, including the tandem-E PSA Immunoenzymetric Assay. This method can be used to identify the presence of PSA that is of seminal origin in a biological stain in forensically significant specimens.

11. **FISH test:** Since not all cases of sexual assault result in the deposit of semen, recent research with "fluorescence *in situ* hybridization" (FISH) has been found to be a very sensitive and specific method for detection of the Y chromosome from male cells in the absence of semen. This method demonstrates the presence of epithelial cells of male origin in the postcoital vaginal tract for extended amounts of time after sexual assault, using a commercially available probe. This can occur during penetration, ejaculation or from the saliva of the assailant. Y chromosome may be identified in intact epithelial cells up to 4th postcoital day. Additionally, Y chromosome positive epithelial cells may be identified in vaginal swabs obtained following intercourse with no ejaculation.

12. **Semenogelin test:** It is a protein originating in the seminal vesicles, it is a substrate for prostate specific antigen (PSA) and it is a useful marker for the identification of semen.

Toluidine Blue Dye Test

Toluidine blue dye is used to assist in the identification of recent genital and perianal injuries especially when injuries are not appreciated by naked eye examination. After the initial examination of the posterior fourchette and fossa navicularis and the collection of vaginal samples and swabs, apply 1% aqueous solution of toluidine blue dye to the posterior fourchette and fossa navicularis. After allowing a minute for the dye uptake, remove the excess with lubricant, such as K-Y jelly or 10% acetic acid. Dye uptake is considered positive and affirms injury when there is residual blue colouring of the laceration or its border after the excess dye has been removed.

Anoscopy: Anoscopic examination should only be done in cases of anal bleeding or severe anal pain or injury suspected or if the presence of a foreign body in the rectum is suspected.

Colposcopic examination: Colposcopic examination is required to be done when injuries are not appreciated by naked eye examination and collection of photographic evidence required. Minor skin and/or mucosal surface trauma such as abrasions, lacerations, petechiae, focal edema, hymenal tears, and anal fissures are more easily seen with magnification, and photographs can be taken for documentation. Camera can be attached to colposcope to record images.

Pregnancy test: Possibility of pregnancy resulting from the assault should be discussed and female patients should be assessed for the possibility of pregnancy. When available, pregnancy testing kits can be offered. However, most of the testing kits will not detect a pregnancy before expected menses. Patient should be advised to return for pregnancy testing if she misses her next period. Parent or guardian may come to know about the sexual assault when the victim becomes pregnant. In such circumstances, proper assessment of gestational age of fetus may become important from therapeutic and legal point of view. If pregnancy test is positive, then advise USG for confirmation and to calculate gestational age of fetus.

Labelling and sealing evidence containers or envelopes: All items of evidence must be clearly labelled to enable the person who collected the evidence to identify it in court later and to ensure that the chain of custody is maintained.

Label the envelopes or containers with the following information: Sample number, full name of patient, date of collection, MLC No, name of the sample and signature of the doctor.

Proper sealing of containers: Proper sealing of containers ensures that contents cannot escape and that nothing can be added or altered. Doctor must sign over the sealing tape with name, age of the victim; reference number and date of examination.

Treatment Guidelines

a. Injuries are treated immediately.

b. If clinical signs are suggestive of STD, collect relevant swabs and start post-exposure prophylaxis. If there are no clinical signs, wait for lab results. For non-pregnant women, the preferred choice is azithromycin 1 gm stat or doxycycline for 7 days, with metronidazole for 7 days with antacid.

c. For pregnant women, amoxycillin/azithromycin with metronidazole is preferred. Metronidazole should not to be given in the 1st trimester of pregnancy.

d. Draw a sample of blood for HBsAg and administer 0.06 ml/kg hepatitis B immune globulin immediately (anytime up to 72 hours after sexual act).

e. Pregnancy prophylaxis (emergency contraception) the preferred choice of treatment is 2 tablets of levonorgestrel within 72 hours. If vomiting occurs, repeat within 3 hours. OR Mala D2 tablets stat repeated 12 hours within 72 hours of sexual act.

f. Pregnancy assessment must be done on follow-up and the victim must be advised to get tested for pregnancy in case she misses her next period.

g. Tetanus toxoid in case of injuries.

h. Postexposure prophylaxis (PEP) for HIV should be given if a survivor reports within 72 hours of the assault. Before PEP is prescribed, HIV risk should be assessed.

i. *Follow-up:* It is ideal to call the survivor for re-examination 2 days after the assault to note the development of bruises and other injuries; thereafter at 3 and 6 weeks.

EXAMINATION OF THE ACCUSED IN SEXUAL ASSAULT

Examination of the accused in a sexual assault case is done on the same lines as has been described for the victim in sexual assault. General information, history, general physical examination and examination of the injuries are undertaken in the similar manner.

Consent

Consent is normally obtained from the accused, however, on the request of the police officer under section 53 CrPC a registered medical practitioner can examine the accused person even using force reasonably necessary.

Examination of the Genitalia

a. Pubic hair are examined for any foreign pubic hair or matting of pubic hair. These are collected and preserved for detection of seminal fluid and blood grouping and if required for DNA profile.
b. The penis is examined for any malformation and presence of **smegma** in case prepuce is present and not retracted (indicative of no sexual intercourse in last 24 hours).
c. A swab is taken from the glance penis to detect vaginal epithelium (moist blotting paper is rubbed around the glance and exposed to iodine vapours, which turns brown indicating presence of vaginal epithelium as they are rich in glycogen) and monilia by microscopic examination.
d. Any tear in the frenulum should be noted.
e. Any injuries or nail marks in the pubic area must be recorded.

Material for Preservation

Almost same material is preserved in a case of accused as is done in a case of victim except in place of vaginal smears, swab from the glance is preserved.

INCEST

The english word incest is derived from the Latin *incestus*, which has a general meaning of "impure, unchaste". It is sexual relationship between close or blood relations belonging to the socially prohibited group like between father and daughter, brother and sister, mother and son or father and step daughter. Incest is not a crime in India unless it falls under the category of rape or adultery. Some of the predisposing factors include low mental development, psychiatric problems, drugs or alcohol abuse or close living conditions.

ADULTERY

The term comes from the words "ad" (towards) and "alter"(other). At the time of its origin, it referred exclusively to sex between a married woman and a man other than her spouse. The definition of the term 'adultery' and its consequences vary between religions, cultures, and legal jurisdictions, but the concept is similar in Judaism, Christianity, Hinduism and Islam.

Section 497 of IPC deals with Adultery "Whoever has sexual intercourse with a person who is and whom he knows or has reason to believe to be the wife of another man, without the consent or connivance of that man, such sexual intercourse not amounting to the offence of rape, is guilty of the offence of adultery, and shall be punished with imprisonment of either description for a term which may extend to five years, or with fine, or with both. In such case the wife shall not be punishable as an abettor".

UNNATURAL SEXUAL OFFENCES

Section 377 of IPC defines unnatural sexual offences as carnal (sexual) intercourse against the order of nature with any man, woman or animal. It is punished with imprisonment for life, or with imprisonment of either description for a term which may extend to ten years, and shall also be liable to fine.

Explanation: Penetration is sufficient to constitute the carnal intercourse necessary to the offence described in this section. When offence is done without the consent of passive agent, only active agent is guilty.

Supreme court of India dismissed a review petition on 11th Dec. 2013 thereby holding homosexuality under section 377 IPC to be an offence and set aside the Delhi high court order of 2009 to hold that consensual sex between two adults of the same gender is not a criminal offence. However, recently on 2nd February 2016 Supreme Court has referred this matter to a constitutional bench of 5 Judges.

Sodomy: Also known as Greek Love or Buggery. It was named sodomy as it used to be practised in the town of Sodom. It is defined as anal intercourse between 2 males (homosexual sodomy), or male and female (heterosexual sodomy) which is *included under rape as per The Criminal Law (Amendment) Bill, 2013*. It is called **Pederasty** when passive agent is a young boy and the passive boy is called **Catamite**. If the passive agent is elderly; it is called **Gerontophilia**. Active agent is one who performs act and passive agent is one on whom act is performed. Habitual passive agents are called *fairies, gays* or *queen* in west. In India some of them are known as "**Zananas**" and "**Hinjras**". Zananas are actually males dressed up like females but their male genitals are intact, whereas Hinjras are castrated males dressed up in female attires. Homosexual offence is frequent among sailors, prisoners, hostellers' and persons in military barracks who are sex starved. Hermaphrodites may also act as passive agents.

Examination of the passive agent: Examination of the passive agent is done on the same manner in which a rape victim is examined. In a nonhabitual passive agent there is pain and swelling around the anal region, loss of tone on digital examination, linear abrasions, tears or fissures are seen, seminal stains around that area along with other physical injuries due to resistance. Presence of foreign hair, bloodstains along with anal swabs are also collected and preserved. In a habitual passive agent there is no pain or tenderness. On examination, shaving of the anal area may be present, funnel shaped depression towards the anus, there is relaxation of the anal sphincters on touching the perianal region,

anal fissures or old scars or venereal warts may be seen.

Examination of the active agent: the examination is done on the same lines as is performed on the accused in a rape case.

Buccal coitus, Sin of Gomorrah or Fellatio or Cunnilingus

Means the oral stimulation or manipulation of the genitals either by male or female. "*Fellatio*" means the oral stimulation or manipulation of the penis either by male or female which is *included under rape as per the Criminal law (Amendment) bill, 2013*. "*Cunnilingus*" means the oral stimulation of the female genitals. Buccal coitus is also called "*Sin of Gomorrah*" because it was prevalent in a Biblical town of that name. When a male organ is introduced into mouth, buccal swabs of victim teeth within few hours of act will reveal seminal traces, provided there was no cleaning of teeth or consumption of food or drinks. Rarely, faint teeth marks and abrasions on penis of assailant may be seen. Death during the act is very rare but may take place from aspiration of semen or impaction of penis in oropharynx. On postmortem examination semen may be detected in respiratory tract or stomach.

Tribadism or Lesbian Love or Lesbianism

It is also known as female homosexuality. In Greek mythology, the female population of the isle of Lesbos practised this perversion and hence the name. It is gratification of sexual desire of a woman by another woman. The instrument of passion is usually the clitoris which may be enlarged. Tribadism is a form of mental aberration and is indulged by women who have repulsion for men or who suffer from "*nymphomania*" (Perverted uncontrollable sexual desire). As there is no penetration, the condition is not covered under section 377 IPC, hence is of little medicolegal interest and the medical examination is of no value in deciding whether the offence has taken place or not.

Bestiality

It means sexual intercourse by a human being with a lower animal, either through the anus or the vagina. The offence is punishable under Section 377 IPC. Any animal, either domesticated farm animals or pets – calves, sheep, ducks, geese, donkeys, and dogs may be used. Generally sheep are used by the males, dogs and cats by the females. On most occasions, the animal manipulates the genitalia by mouth and actual coitus is not common. The accused may be a young person employed to look after the animals, sex- starved lonely individual, or one suffering from some mental aberration. The superstitious belief that STDs are cured by sexual intercourse with a lower animal may also lead to bestiality.

SEXUAL PERVERSIONS

Sexual perversions are habitual acts to obtain sexual gratification without indulging in sexual intercourse. This is also described by the term paraphilia (Greek para: beside, philos: loving) meaning recurrent, intense sexual urges, fantasies, or behaviors that involve unusual objects, activities, or situations and cause clinically significant distress or impairment in social, occupational or other important areas of functioning.

Sadism or Algolagnia

Obtaining sexual gratification by means of beating, biting, whipping or inflicting injuries on the other individual. The name sadism is derived from the French writer Marquis de Sade (1740–1814), who wrote books in which characters enjoyed being cruel.

"Necrophagia" is an extreme form of sadistic practice. After death of the female he may tear out the genitalia or other organs and may suck or lick the wounds or eat the flesh of the victim to derive sexual pleasure.

"Lust murder" is the consequences of extreme sadistic practice which starts with torturing the victim and getting sexual gratification by killing the sexual partner. These sadists have sexual obsession with their victims, and organised lust murderers may stalk their victims for months or weeks before the actual killing. This type of act is seen in mentally aberrated individuals.

Masochism or Passive Algolagnia

This is opposite of sadism where a person gets sexual gratification by being bodily tortured or abused by the sexual partner and is more common in males. The term is derived from the 19th century author Leopard Von Sacher Masoch, an Austrian novelist who portrayed characters suffering from this perversion. As a stimulus to write, he liked to be whipped by his wife. This is found in all age groups and among all socioeconomic strata. These acts of cruelty may completely substitute the sexual intercourse. Sadism and Masochism are mostly seen together in an individual in a combined form known as *"sadomasochism"* with one type dominant over the other. Masochistic asphyxial death (sexual asphyxia) may occur due to accidental hanging or strangulation in a masochist due to failure of safety mechanism. In sexual asphyxia, sexual gratification is obtained by partial reduction of blood supply to brain.

Fetishism: This type of perversion is mainly seen in males. Fetishism is a perversion in which sexual gratification is associated with contact and sight of certain parts of the female body or even clothing or other articles known as fetish objects. Any article like clothing, shoes or particularly the undergarments like panties or bra of a female acts as stimulus. He would like to have these articles for sexual gratification and may masturbate in them. He may develop an irresistible habit to steal these objects. Alfred Binet, the French psychologist coined this term meaning mystical qualities to inanimate objects.

Exhibitionism: This is a desire to the expose genitalia in public places in presence of others mostly in front of females so as to obtain sexual pleasure. This act may be accompanied by with or without masturbatory acts. Rarely females may expose themselves in public. This perversion is more in males and such persons are called "flashers". Most of them are psychopathic or suffer from compulsive neurosis. Exhibitionism is an obscene act punishable under section 294 IPC with imprisonment up to 3 months and or fine.

Transvestism or Eonism: In this condition sexual gratification is obtained by wearing cloths of the opposite sex. The clothes worn are usually underclothes, brassier, knickers, etc. of an expersive and alluring type. The perversion is also seen in females who dress themselves in male attire. Zananas who wear female cloths are not true transvestites.

Voyeurism or Scoptophilia: In this the pervert has morbid desire to secretly observe people undress, taking bath, see the genitalia or watch sex performance of others to get erotic excitement and sexual gratification. Voyeurs (French voir: to see, observer) frequently peep into the bedrooms of others and are therefore called "Peeping Toms". This act may be accompanied by exhibitionism or masturbation.

Frotteurism: This is a perversion mostly seen in males; in which the pervert try to rub the genitalia against a female's body in crowded place or bus to get sexual gratification and even orgasm. This is an offence and punishable under section 290 IPC (fine up to ₹ 200) and section 291 IPC (imprisonment for 6 months and/or fine).

Urolagnia or urophilia or undinism: The pervert gets sexual gratification by the sight or odor of urine and by urination. The word is derived from Greek (ouron: urine, lagneia: lust) and these types of perverts may enjoy urinating on another person or being urinated upon.

Coprophilia: It is a morbid attraction and sexual gratification obtained from feces (liking, smell, taste or feel). The term has originated from Greek language (kopros: excrement, filia fondness).

Troilism: Such a person gets sexual gratification by observing his wife having sexual intercourse with another man.

There are many other forms of perversions like **Autagonistophilia** getting pleasure by having sex in front of others, **Formicophilia** is finding pleasure in having ants, spiders, etc. crawl on their body or bite them, **Hematolagnia** is finding sexual gratification through blood and bleeding, etc.

MISCELLANEOUS SEXUAL OFFENCES

Prostitution

Prostitution has been defined under section 2 of immoral trafficking prevention Act 1956 as the sexual exploitation or abuse of persons for commercial purposes. Prostitution is punishable with rigorous imprisonment up to 7 years but not less than 3 years with fine up to ₹ 2000 which can be extended on second offence from 7 to 14 years. Person visiting prostitutes are also liable for imprisonment for 3 months with fine or fine up to 2000 but on second visit imprisonment can be for six months with fine up to ₹ 50,000.

Indecent Assault

Any offence committed on a female with the intention or knowledge to outrage her modesty is punishable under **section 354 IPC** with imprisonment for a term which may extend to five years but not less than one year and shall also be liable to fine. This can mean anything, from an unproven rape to merely touching the buttocks in a crowded bus, fondling the breast, thighs, perineum, kissing a woman forcefully, or putting up a hand in woman's skirt constitute indecent assault.

Section 354-A IPC deals with the definition of **"sexual harassment"** which is very broadly defined and criminalizes acts like forcibly showing pornography, physical contact and advances involving unwelcome and explicit sexual remarks, demanding or requesting sexual favours, any other unwelcome physical, verbal or nonverbal conduct of sexual nature. This section further deals with the punishment to be awarded for the offence depending upon the act in question. While demanding or requesting sexual favours and physical contact or advances which involve unwelcome and explicit sexual remarks are punishable with rigorous imprisonment of a term which may extend to five years or with fine or with both, for making sexually coloured remarks a lesser term which may extend to one year or fine or both can be awarded.

Section 354-B IPC deals with offence where criminal force or assault is used on a woman with the intention of disrobing her or compelling her to be naked in public. Such a person can be penalized with an imprisonment term which shall not be less than three years but may extend to seven years and also liable to fine.

Section 354-C IPC also deals with the specific act of either watching or capturing the images of a woman engaging in a private act where she expects privacy and observation by the perpetrator or any other person at the behest of the perpetrator or disseminates such image attracts an imprisonment term which shall not be less than one year but may extend to three years and fine. But on a subsequent conviction the minimum imprisonment term shall be that of three years extendable to seven years and also fine.

Section 354-D IPC criminalizes the act of illegally stalking a woman which interferes with the mental peace of a person or causes distress, fear of violence or alarm. The same is punishable with a minimum imprisonment term of one year which may extend to three years and also liable with fine on subsequent conviction the term may be extended to five years.

SEXUAL HARASSMENT OF WOMEN AT WORK PLACE

To prevent harassment of women at their place of work "**Sexual harassment of women at work place (prevention, prohibition and redressal) act of 2013**" was promulgated by the Government of India. Internal or local complaints committee to be constituted at all places; employing 10 or more workers, for the redressal of various complaints received from aggrieved women workers. The committee can summon and examine a person on oath and shall complete the inquiry within 90 days. The committee can recommend action as per service rules and can also award compensation to the aggrieved women. In case the complaint is proved to be false or malicious the action against the woman is to be recommended as per service rules for misconduct.

TRAFFICKING OF PERSON: (Section 370 IPC)

Whoever, for the purpose of exploitation (physical or any form of sexual exploitation): (a) recruits; (b) transports; (c) harbours; (d) transfers; or (e) receives, a person or persons, by use of force, by abduction, by fraud, by threats, by use of power or by inducement shall be punished with rigorous imprisonment for a term which shall not be less than seven years, but which may extend to ten years, and shall also be liable to fine. Where the offence involves the trafficking of more than one person or a minor, it shall be punishable with rigorous imprisonment for a term which shall not be less than ten years but which may extend to imprisonment for life, and shall also be liable to fine.

If a person is convicted of the offence of trafficking of minor on more than one occasion or when a public servant or a police officer is involved in the trafficking, then such person shall be punished with imprisonment for life, which shall mean imprisonment for the remainder of that person's natural life, and shall also be liable to fine.

Exploitation of a Trafficked Person
(Section 370A IPC)

Trafficking of a Minor

Whoever, knowingly or having reason to believe that a minor has been trafficked, engages such *minor* for sexual exploitation in any manner, shall be punished with rigorous imprisonment for a term which shall not be less than five years, but which may extend to seven years, and shall also be liable to fine.

Trafficking of an Adult

Whoever, knowingly by or having reason to believe that a person has been trafficked, engages such person for sexual exploitation in any manner, shall be punished with rigorous imprisonment for a term which shall not be less than three years, but which may extend to five years, and shall also be liable to fine.

THE PROTECTION OF CHILDREN FROM SEXUAL OFFENCES ACT (POCSO ACT) 2012

The protection of children from sexual offences act (POCSO act) 2012 was enacted by the Indian parliament in order to effectively address sexual abuse and sexual exploitation of children. Even though there are some acts under IPC to deal with sexual offences but they are not much effective against sexual harassment of the children especially males below the age of 18 years.

The act defines a child as any person below eighteen years of age. It defines different forms of sexual abuse, including penetrative and nonpenetrative assault, as well as sexual harassment and pornography. The protection of children from sexual offences (POCSO) act 2012 is applicable to the whole of India.

Offences under the act have been grouped under various categories like: (a) penetrative and aggravated penetrative sexual assault; (b) sexual and aggravated sexual assault; (c) sexual harassment; and (d) using a child for pornographic purposes. Offence under this act is treated as **aggravated** when the abused child is mentally ill or when the abuse is committed by a person in a position of trust or authority like a family member, police officer, teacher, or doctor.

A child's statement can be recorded even at the child's residence or a place of his choice and should be preferably done by a female police officer not below the rank of sub-inspector.

As per this act, the investigating office has the discretion to get the child's medical examination conducted even prior to registration of an FIR. The investigating police officer has to get the child medically examined in a government hospital or local hospital within 24 hours of receiving information about the offence. This is done with the consent of the child or parent or a competent person whom the child trusts and in their presence. Following are some of the child-friendly measures included under the POCSO act:

   i. At night no child to be detained in the police station.
  ii. The statement of the child to be recorded as spoken by the child.
 iii. Frequent breaks for the child during trial.
  iv. Child not to be called repeatedly to testify.

Above all, the act stipulates that a case of child sexual abuse must be disposed of within one year from the date the offence is reported.

Punishments

a. Punishment for penetrative sexual assault is imprisonment for minimum of 7 years or more which may extend up to life imprisonment and fine. For aggravated penetrative sexual assault the imprisonment may be for minimum of 10 years which may be extended up to life imprisonment and fine.

b. Punishment for sexual assault is imprisonment for minimum for 3 years extendable up to 5 years and fine. In case of aggravated sexual assault imprisonment may be minimum of 5 years extendable up to 7 years and fine.

c. Punishment for sexual harassment is imprisonment up to 3 years and fine.

d. Punishment for using a child for pornographic purposes is imprisonment for 5 years and fine.

e. The punishment for the attempt to commit is up to half the punishment prescribed for the commission of that offence.

f. The act also provides for mandatory reporting of sexual offences. This casts a legal duty upon a person who has knowledge that a child has been sexually abused to report the offence; if he fails to do so, he may be punished with six months' imprisonment and/or a fine.

g. The media has been barred from disclosing the identity of the child without the permission of the special court. The punishment for breaching this provision by media is imprisonment from six months to one year.

For offences under this act the burden of proof is shifted on the accused, keeping in view the vulnerability and innocence of children. To prevent misuse of the law, punishment has been provided for false complaints or false information with malicious intent.

29 | Impotency and Sterility

Impotency is the inability of a person to perform sexual intercourse. **Erectile dysfunction** (ED) commonly used in medical practice means that a male cannot get or maintain an erection. In some cases the penis becomes partly erect but not hard enough to have sex properly, whereas *"frigidity"* (absence of desire for sexual intercourse) and *"vaginismus"* (spasm of pelvic muscles preventing sexual intercourse) are the terms used to describe female impotency.

Sterility is inability to procreate, i.e. a male is unable to impregnate a female or a female is unable to conceive a child. An impotent person may or may not be sterile and vice versa a sterile person may or may not be impotent. The question of impotency, sometimes sterility, may arise in many civil as well as criminal cases.

Civil cases: Impotency is a ground for divorce and also of importance in cases of legitimacy, adultery, nullity of marriage, adoption, disputed paternity and cases of compensation for causing impotency.

Criminal cases: The question may arise in adultery, rape, unnatural sexual offences or injuries resulting in impotency.

CAUSES OF MALE IMPOTENCE OR ERECTILE DYSFUNCTION

There are several causes of male impotency which can be grouped into those that are mainly (i) physical and those that are mainly due to (ii) psychological reasons.

Physical Causes

Majority of impotency cases are due to physical causes:

a. **Age:** At extremes of age, a male is considered to be impotent. A male becomes potent at the age of puberty. As the age advances the potency decreases. However there is no definite age prescribed for the same.

b. **Malformations and local diseases:** Congenital malformations like epispadias, hypospadias, or scrotal adhesions may render a person impotent but not necessarily sterile. Local diseases like scrotal elephantiasis, scrotal herniation, phimosis, malignancy, tuberculosis or infections may result in impotency which can be correct by surgical or medical intervention.

c. **Reduced blood flow to the penis:** This is, by far, the most common cause of impotency in men over the age of 40. Like in other parts of the body, arteries which take blood to the penis can become narrowed. Blood flow may then not be enough to cause an erection.

d. **Diseases which affect the nerves going to the penis:** Neurological conditions like multiple sclerosis, stroke or parkinson's disease may result in impotency.

e. **Diabetes:** This is one of the most common causes of impotency in males. Diabetes can affect blood vessels and nerves.

f. **Hormonal causes:** Lack of testosterone, which is not very commonly seen, could be one of the causes. A head injury can sometimes affect the function of the pituitary gland in the brain. The pituitary gland makes a hormone that stimulates the testes to make testosterone. Other symptoms of a low testosterone level include a reduced sex drive (libido) and changes in mood.

g. **Injury to the nerves going to the penis:** Spinal injury, following surgery to nearby structures like prostate, fractured pelvis or radiotherapy to the genital area may lead to impotency due to injury to nerves going to penis.

h. **Side-effect of certain medicines:** The most common are antidepressants, beta-blockers such as propranolol, atenolol; some diuretics or cimetidine.

i. **Alcohol and drug abuse:** Chronic abuse of alcohol and other addicting drugs may lead to impotency.

j. **Long distance cycling:** Temporary impotency after long-distance cycling may be observed, probably due to pressure on the nerves going to the penis, from sitting on the saddle for long periods.

k. **Excessive outflow of blood from the penis:** Blood outflow from the penis take place through the veins (venous leak). This is rare but can be caused by various conditions of the penis.

In most cases due to physical causes (apart from injury or after surgery), the erectile dysfunction tends to develop slowly.

Psychological Causes

1. In some cases the impotency may result from psychological reasons like fear, anxiety or worry, stress, depression and sense of guilt especially from excessive masturbation.

2. Quoad: A male may be selectively impotent with a particular woman and such a situation is known as "**Impotence quoad hoc**".

EXAMINATION OF A MALE FOR IMPOTENCY

Examination is done on the request of law enforcing agency like court or police officer investigating a case.

1. **Preliminary information:** The examination include recording of preliminary information about the person to be examined.

2. **Consent:** The examination is carried out after taking proper consent except when examining an accused on the request of a police officer under section 53 Cr PC.

3. **History:** History about the incident as well as the medical history and treatment taken for the same.

4. **General examination:** Complete physical examination is done including central nervous system.

5. **Psychological evaluation:** Psychological evaluation by using a standard questionnaire.

6. **Local examination:** Any abnormality, malformations or venereal infections are recorded which may make a person impotent.

7. **Laboratory tests and potency tests:** Individual is subjected to many tests which are directed to ascertain potency of that person.

   a. *Blood test:* This is done to know whether the person is suffering from diabetes or kidney related disorders which may affect his potency.

   b. *Nocturnal penile tumescence or rigiscan monitoring:* This test involves measuring the number of spontaneous erections that occur at night. Two self-calibrating loops are attached to the penis, one near the tip and other at the base. The machine is strapped to the thigh. The equipment measures the blood flow in the organ, the size and hardness during erection. This is done to check whether the person gets 5 to 6 nocturnal erection during sleep as a physiological response and is thus capable of getting spontaneous erection. It also tests morning erection. Even psychologically impotent person also have two or more erections during the night. Absence may indicate defect in the nerve functioning.

c. *Serum testosterone level:* Testosterone plays a very small role in letting a man get an erection. By this test, testosterone level is measured biochemically in a laboratory.

d. *Penile doppler scan:* This test shows how much and how well blood flows in and out of the penis to detect any atherosclerotic changes.

e. *Visual erection examination:* During the visual examination, the doctor examines the penis in both states, i.e. aroused and flaccid. Intracorporeal injection of about 80 mg of papaverine hydrochloride is done to observe real time measurement of erection. This is done to check for any sort of dysfunction or damage.

f. *Penile biothesiometry:* Electromagnetic vibrations are used to test the nerve functions and sensitivity in the glance and penile shaft.

Opinion

In case where malformations or local conditions are present rendering a person impotent, opinion is given citing the reason for impotency. However when there is no physical condition causing impotency, opinion is expressed in double negative form *"on physical examination of the male, there is nothing to suggest that person is incapable of performing sexual intercourse".* This type of opinion is given as psychological impotency cannot be ruled out.

These days after testing a person thoroughly for impotency by *urologists* after performing above mentioned tests a positive or negative opinion is normally forwarded to the courts in majority of cases.

Opinion regarding sterility is primarily based on the clinical and laboratory findings in a case, i.e. production of normal sperms in required quantities and intact delivery system in males.

CAUSES OF IMPOTENCY AND STERILITY IN FEMALES

Even though the female is a passive partner in sexual intercourse, still there are many causes which may render a female impotent or sterile.

1. **Age:** Age has no direct effect on impotency in a female however a female is normally taken as sterile before menarche and after menopause. There are reported cases where a female may become pregnant after menopause or before menarche.

2. **Malformations:** Occlusion of vagina, strictures, adhesions, imperforate hymen may result in impotence in females; however, these conditions are correctable by surgery.

3. **Local diseases:** Painful infective conditions prolapsed of uterus, inflamed Bartholin cyst, chancre of vulval region, rectovaginal fistula, strictures as a result of perineal tears or local surgery may result in impotence. Strictures in fallopian tubes, big fibroids in uterus, endometriosis and peritoneal adhesions may cause sterility.

4. **General diseases:** General dilapidating conditions from chronic illness may result in sterility.

5. **Chronic poisoning:** Chronic heavy metal poisoning especially lead may cause sterility. Lead causes blastophoric action on the ovum. Radiation injuries also cause sterility.

6. **Drug abuse:** Drug addiction may cause sterility in some cases.

7. **Psychological:** Fear, prior traumatic sexual experience, apprehension may sometimes result in spasm of the levator ani and adductor femoris muscles causing spasm of the lower part of the vagina preventing penetration by male organ and is known as **Vaginismus.** Sometimes there is no desire for the sexual intercourse and female may not allow the male partner to have sexual intercourse is known as **Frigidity.**

EXAMINATION OF A FEMALE

1. **Preliminary information:** The examination include recording of preliminary information about the person to be examined.
2. The examination is carried out after taking proper consent and should normally be done by a female doctor. In case female doctor is not available then it can be done by a male doctor after taking consent for the same and is always done in presence of a female attendant.
3. **History:** History about the incident as well as the medical history and treatment taken for the same must be asked.
4. **General examination:** Complete physical examination is done including central nervous system.
5. **Psychological evaluation:** Psychological evaluation by using a standard questionnaire along with previous sexual experiences.
6. **Gynecological examination:** Local examination is carried out to find any painful condition or presence of any venereal diseases. Swab should be collected from vagina and cervix for venereal diseases. Position of the uterus, presence of fibroids, size of the uterus or tenderness can be observed by bimanual examination.
7. **Laboratory tests:** Apart from routine tests, estrogen levels, ultrasonography, CT scan or even MRI may be undertaken if required.

Opinion

Based on the clinical and laboratory findings opinion is expressed whether a female is capable of participating in sexual intercourse *(Aptavira)* or not *(Nonaptavira)*.

Opinion regarding sterility is primarily based on the clinical and laboratory findings in a case, i.e. production of ovum, patent fallopian tubes and normal uterus for implantation of fertilised ovum.

30 | Virginity, Pregnancy and Delivery

The word *virgin* comes from the latin word *"virgo"* literally meaning "maiden". **Virginity** is the state of a female who has never engaged in sexual intercourse (virgo intacta). Loss of virginity in a female is known as defloration. There are cultural and religious traditions which place special value and significance on this state, especially in the case of unmarried females.

The traditional view is that virginity is only lost through vaginal penetration by the penis, consensual or nonconsensual, and that acts of oral sex, anal sex, masturbation or other forms of nonpenetrative sex do not result in loss of virginity.

SIGNS OF VIRGINITY

Breasts

Breasts in a young adult female are firm and hemispherical. Areola is pink or slightly darker and nipples are small. Breasts normally become large and pendulous after pregnancy or with frequent handling. Few acts of intercourse will not result in any change in the breast.

Genitals

a. **Mons-veneris:** The mons-veneris, Latin for "hill of Venus" is the pad of fatty tissue that covers the pubic bone below the abdomen but above the labia. It is covered with pubic hair in adult females.

b. **Labia majora:** The labia majora are the outer lips of the vulva, pads of fatty tissue that wrap around the vulva from the mons-veneris to the perineum. These labia are usually covered with pubic hair, and contain numerous sweat and oil glands.

c. **Labia minora:** The labia minora are the inner lips of the vulva, thin stretches of tissue within the labia majora that fold and protect the vagina, urethra, and clitoris. The appearance of labia minora can vary widely, from tiny lips that hide between the labia majora to large lips that protrude.

d. **Clitoris:** The clitoris is a small body of spongy tissue. Only the tip or glans of the clitoris shows externally, but the organ itself is elongated and branched into two forks, the crura, which extend downward along the rim of the vaginal opening toward the perineum. The clitoral glans or external tip of the clitoris is protected by the prepuce, or clitoral hood, a covering of tissue similar to the foreskin of the male penis.

e. **Hymen:** *Hymen* is a fold of mucous membrane about 1 mm thick that partially covers the vaginal opening. It is usually elastic but rarely hymen may be rigid and fibrous. Hymen is the traditional "symbol" of virginity, although being a very thin membrane; it can be torn by surgical manipulations or the insertion of a tampon.

Some common types of hymen are annular, septate, cribriform, imperforate, parous introitus, fimbriate, semilunar or carunculae myrtiformes (Fig. 30.1). Imperforate hymen that completely closes the vagina may require surgical intervention to provide for a normal flow of blood once menstruation begins. In fimbriate hymen the notches are symmetrical, located anteriorly and do not reach the vaginal wall, by which it can be differentiated from hymen rupture.

Presence of intact hymen is not an absolute proof of virginity. In some cases the hymen is so elastic and fleshy that it can admit male organ without its being ruptured. In case other features are indicative of defloration but the hymen is intact the female is known as *"False Virgin"*.

Causes of Rupture of Hymen

1. *Sexual intercourse:* It is the most common cause of the rupture of the hymen. In such cases the rupture is mostly seen at the lower back portion on the either side of the midline.
2. *Gynecological examination or surgeries:* Hymen may get ruptured during examination or surgical operation being performed in that area. Hymen does not rupture with jumping, riding or vigorous exercises.
3. *Use of tampons:* Use of sanitary tampons may lead to rupture of the hymen.
4. *Insertion of foreign material:* Sometimes foreign material like sola pith is introduced in the vagina, which swells up by absorbing water, so as to render a female fit for sexual activity.

f. **Vagina:** The vagina extends from the vaginal opening to the cervix, the opening to the uterus. The vagina serves as receptacle for the penis during sexual intercourse and as birth canal through which the baby passes during labour. The average vaginal canal is three inches long, possibly four in women who have given birth. This may seem short in relation to the penis, but during sexual arousal the cervix will lift upwards and the fornix may extend upwards into the body as long as necessary to receive the penis. After intercourse, the contraction of the vagina will allow the cervix to rest inside the fornix, which in its relaxed state is a bowl-shaped fitting perfect for the pooling of semen.

Medicolegal Importance

Question of virginity arises in cases of nullity of marriage, in divorce, defamation and rape.

a. *Nullity of marriage:* Marriage can be annulled in case it has not been consummated owing to husband being impotent. On examination the female will be virgin. When there is question of impotency of the husband then he is also examined. Other reasons for nullity of marriage under section 12 of the Hindu Marriage Act, 1955 are: (i) Either party below the age of marriage; (ii) Either party was already

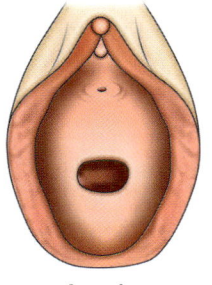 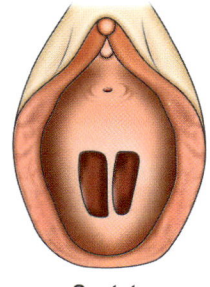 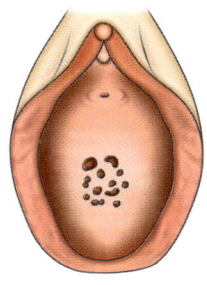 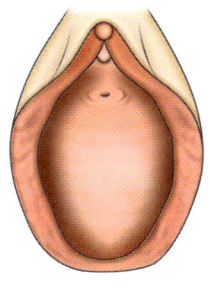 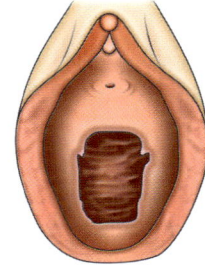

| **Annular** | **Septate** | **Cribriform** | **Imperforate** | **Parous introitous** |

Fig. 30.1: Hymen shapes

married at the time of marriage; (iii) Female was at the time of the marriage pregnant by some person other than the petitioner; or (iv) Either party is incapable of giving a valid consent to it in consequence of unsoundness of mind; or though capable of giving a valid consent, has been suffering from mental disorder of such a kind or to such an extent as to be unfit for marriage and the procreation of children.

b. *Divorce:* Marriage can be dissolved by a decree of divorce on the ground that the other party has; (i) after the solemnisation of the marriage; had voluntary sexual intercourse with any person other than his or her spouse; or (ii) has, after the solemnisation of the marriage, treated the petitioner with cruelty; or (iii) has deserted the petitioner for a continues period of not less than two years immediately preceding the presentation of the petition; (iv) the passing of a decree for restitution of conjugal rights in a proceeding to which they were parties; (v) A wife may also present a petition for the dissolution of her marriage by a decree of divorce on the ground; that the husband has, since the solemnisation of the marriage, been guilty of rape, sodomy or bestiality; and (vi) divorce can also be obtained on mutual consent, on the ground that they are living separately for the last one year.

c. *Rape:* When a rape is reported to police the victim is brought before a medical officer for examination to provide evidence of sexual assault.

Defloration

Following features are observed in a case when a woman has experienced sexual intercourse. All these features may not be present in a woman who has not experienced frequent sexual acts. Normally intact hymen is taken as a proof of virginity.

a. Hymen showing a rupture on the posterior lower side on either side of midline at 5 or 7 o'clock position. Margins are red and swollen and bleed on touching when rupture is recent. Margins heal in about 5 to 7 days and gradually they shrink and appear as granular tags. Hymen is seen as small tags along the hymnal ring with frequent sexual acts or with child birth, known as *"Crunculae myrituformis or hymenalis"*.

b. Labia majora are less fleshy and do not oppose each other and may reveal vaginal opening.

c. Labia minora get enlarged and pigmented.

d. Vagina loose rugae and become roomy.

e. Fossa navicularis may not be observed.

f. Fourchette may show scars for old tears.

g. Vestibule is wide and spacious.

h. Clitoris may be enlarged.

i. Posterior commissure may show tears in few cases.

j. breasts are large and pendulous. Areola also gets enlarged and pigmented.

There are cases of women with damaged hymens undergoing *"hymenorrhaphy"* or *"hymenoplasty"* to repair or replace their hymens, known as **born-again virgins,** and cause vaginal bleeding on the next intercourse as proof of virginity. Some authors consider the practice to be virginity fraud.

Medical virginity tests are practiced in many regions of the world, but are condemned these days as a form of abuse of women. According to the World Health Organization (WHO); sexual violence compasses a wide range of acts including *"obligatory inspections for virginity"*. Two finger test earlier recommended for testing virginity is not permitted these days.

PREGNANCY

A female is pregnant when she carries a fertilised ovum in her uterus.

Features of pregnancy in living can be divided into; (i) presumptive signs; (ii) probable signs; and (iii) definite or confirmatory signs.

Presumptive Signs

1. **Amenorrhea:** Cessation of menstruation is an important sign of pregnancy. However amenorrhea may occur in a female due to ill health or fear of pregnancy.

2. **Changes in breast:** There is increase in the size of the breast, nipples get dark pigmentation and are more erectile, areola also becomes dark-brown with "*Montgomery*" tubercles due to enlarged sebaceous glands by third month and striae lines are seen due to overstretching of skin after sixth month of pregnancy. Breast signs are diagnostic only in primigravida. In multigravida, it may be due to the previous pregnancies.

3. **Morning sickness:** may be present during the middle of the first trimester till the end of third month. There is nausea and vomiting during the early hours of the morning.

4. **Quickening:** Fetal movements are normally felt by the mother from 16th week onwards. It may be slightly delayed, i.e. from 18th week onwards in primigravida.

5. **Pigmentation of skin:** Skin around axilla, vulva and abdomen gets pigmentation. Linea nigra are dark lines over abdomen from pubis to umbilicus seen from 20th week onwards.

6. **Changes in vagina:** As a result of venous stagnation the vaginal colour changes from pink to violet or blue from 8th week of pregnancy onwards known as *Chadwick's or Jacquemier's sign.*

7. **Urinary disturbances:** From pressure of the uterus there is increased frequency which is seen between 6 to 12th weeks of pregnancy.

8. **Sympathetic disturbances:** Perverted appetite with craving for certain types of food like pickles or ice creams or aversion to certain food. Some pregnant ladies have irritable temper and salivation.

9. **Fatigue:** The pregnant woman normally complains of fatigue frequently.

10. **Backache:** It is common to experience a dull backache throughout pregnancy.

Probable Signs

1. **Fundal height or McDonald's rule:** It is a measure of the size of the uterus used to assess fetal growth and development during pregnancy. It is measured from the top of the mother's uterus to the top of the mother's pubic bone in centimeters. Fundal height roughly corresponds to gestational age in weeks between 16 and 36 weeks. The fundus is at the level of pubic symphysis by 12th week; reaches umbilicus by 24th week; near xiphoid process by 36–38th week and comes down slightly by 40th week (Fig. 30.2). According to McDonald's rule fundal height in cm divided by 3.5 gives gestation period in months.

2. **Hegar's sign:** This sign is demonstrated by placing two fingers in the vagina and other handover the abdomen. Isthmus of the uterus is felt as soft and compressible area between firm and hard cervix and elastic uterus. This sign is observed between 6 and to 10th weeks of pregnancy.

3. **Softening of cervix or goodell's sign:** Softening of the cervix which is hard as tip of the nose in nonpregnant woman, starts

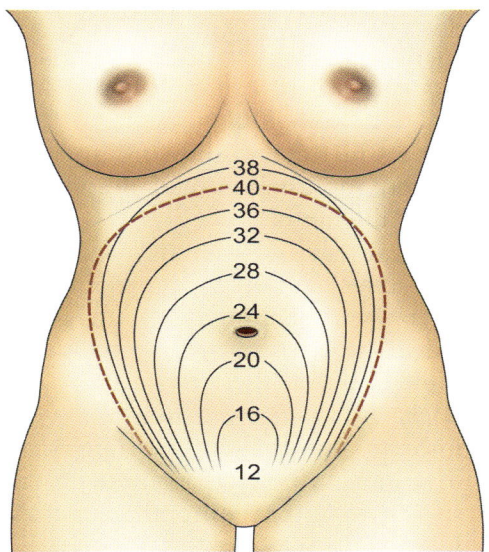

Fig. 30.2: Fundal height during pregnancy

from 2nd month onwards and is completely soft like lips by 4th month. The opening of the cervix become circular and may admit tip of the little finger easily.

4. **Uterine contractions or braxton hick's sign:** These are intermittent uterine contractions observed after 3rd or 4th month onwards. Contraction lasts for a minute and there is relaxation period of 2 to 3 minutes between these contractions. These contractions may be observed even when the fetus has died inside the uterus.

5. **Palmer's sign:** Uterine contractions felt during bimanual examination as early as 2nd month of pregnancy.

6. **Ballottement:** Ballottement refers to bouncing of fetus like a ball in the uterus. This sign is observed during 4th and 5th month of pregnancy.
   a. *Internal ballottement:* When two fingers are placed in the anterior fornix and the uterus is pushed up the fetus moves up and then fall back which can be felt by the fingertips.
   b. *External ballottement:* When the side of the abdomen is given a push the fetus moves to the other side and then rebounds back.

7. **Palpation of fetal parts:** Fetal parts can be felt on palpation through the abdominal wall, after 5th month.

8. **Uterine soufflé:** Soft blowing murmur is heard on auscultation matching with the pulse of the mother.

9. **Biological tests:** Test animals are injected with serum or urine of the pregnant woman to test presence of human chorionic gonadotropins. These tests are replaced with immunological tests these days.
   a. *Aschheim zondek test:* Immature white mice are injected with morning sample of urine and positive result is observed in the form of hemorrhagic corpus luteum.
   b. *Rapid rat test:* Immature albino rats are tested with morning sample of urine and

positive result is observed in the form of hemorrhagic ovaries.
   c. *Friedman's test:* Adult female rabbits are used and positive result is observed in the form of hemorrhagic follicles in ovaries.
   d. *Hogben test:* African toads are injected with morning sample of urine and ovulation is observed.
   e. *Gallimainini test:* Male frogs are injected with morning sample of urine and presence of sperms in the urine of the frog is observed.

Immunological Tests

a. Based on human chorionic gonadotropins:
   i. *Agglutination test:* Latex particles or sheep erythrocyte coated with anti-HCG are incubated with urine sample and observe agglutination.
   ii. *Agglutination inhibition tests:* The urine sample is mixed with anti HCG serum. In a pregnant woman anti HCG will neutralise the HCG present in the urine and will not be able to agglutinate sheep erythrocyte coated with anti-HCG.
   iii. *Rapid dip stick test:* It is used to test HCG in urine. The stick is dipped in urine for 10 seconds to get the result.
   iv. Rapid and simple tests based on enzyme-labelled monoclonal antibodies assay can detect low level of HCG in urine.

Causes of false positive results

1. Proteinuria.
2. Hematuria.
3. At time of ovulation (cross reaction with LH).
4. HCG injection for infertility treatment within the previous 30 days.
5. Thyrotoxicosis (high TSH).
6. Premature menopause (high LH and FSH).
7. Early days after delivery or abortion.
8. Trophoblastic diseases.
9. HCG secreting tumors.

Causes of false negative results

1. Missed abortion.
2. Ectopic pregnancy.
3. Too early pregnancy.
4. Urine stored too long in room temperature.
5. Interfering medications.

b. Serum pregnancy tests
  1. Radioimmunoassay of b-subunit of HCG.
  2. Radioreceptor assay.

c. Enzyme-linked immunosorbent assay (ELISA).
  Can be used for urine and serum.

The pregnancy test becomes negative in about:

a. One week after delivery
b. 2 weeks after abortion
c. 4 weeks after evacuation of vesicular mole.

Positive or Confirmative Signs

1. **Fetal movements:** Fetal movements can be felt on palpation of the abdomen by 4th month onwards.
2. **Fetal heart sounds:** Fetal heart sounds can be heard by a stethoscope after 5th month.
3. **X-ray diagnosis:** Fetal shadow can be made out by 4th month on radiological examination. Small dots in linear arrangement are seen for vertebral column, annular shadows for skull bones curved lines for ribs and linear lines for limbs are observed on X-ray examination.
4. **Ultrasonography examination:** Gestational sac can be detected after 4–5 weeks of amenorrhea. Fetal heart pulsation can be detected as early as 7 weeks.

Signs of Pregnancy in Dead

When pregnancy is suspected in a dead, examination of the pelvic organs on autopsy is important.

a. *Uterine changes:* Enlarged uterus may be observed when the pregnancy is advanced, however internal examination of uterine wall may show attachment of the placenta after 2nd month onwards.

b. *Presence of ovum or fetus in the uterus:* Presence of product of conception confirms that female was pregnant.

c. *Corpus luteum:* Corpus luteum continues to develop during pregnancy and maximum size may be observed during 4th and 5th month.

Medicolegal Significance

Under several circumstances the question of pregnancy is disputed and a medical practitioner may be required to determine whether the woman is pregnant or not.

  i. *Attendance in the court:* Absence from appearing in the court may be granted in advanced pregnancy or complications due to pregnancy.

  ii. *Execution:* Capital punishment awarded to a woman may be postponed or convert into life imprisonment in case the woman is quick with the child.

  iii. *Defrauding regarding rightful heir of a property:* a Woman may contest a will after the death of the husband by posing to be pregnant.

  iv. *Marriage contract:* Marriage is declared null and void in case a female is pregnant at the time of marriage by some person other than the petition.

  v. *Forcing a person into marriage contract:* She may pose to be pregnant after marriage promise by that person.

  vi. *Blackmailing a person:* A female may be blackmailing on grounds of pregnancy by that person.

  vii. *Defamation:* A widow or an unmarried girl may be defamed alleging her to be pregnant.

  viii. *Secure greater compensation:* In order to secure greater compensation from some person through whose culpable neglect her husband has died.

  ix. *Pseudocyesis:* It is a psychosomatic state in a woman when she believe that she is pregnant but actually there is no conception and is marked by some of the physical symptoms as cessation of menses, enlargement of the abdomen, and apparent fetal movements and changes in hormonal balance of pregnancy.

It is normally seen in women badly desirous of having a child. Medical examination including investigations like ultrasonography may clear her doubts.

x. *Superfecundation:* In this condition two ova released from the same ovulatory cycle in a female are fertilised by two separate acts of coitus. It is possible that two different males may father these twins known as "Heteropaternal superfecundation". Such babies may show different features and doubt of adultery or infidelity may arise.

Superfecundation most commonly happens within hours or days of the first instance of fertilization with other ova released during the same cycle. The time window when eggs are able to be fertilised is small. Sperm cells can live inside a female's body for four to five days. Once ovulation occurs, the egg remains viable for 12–48 hours before it begins to disintegrate. Thus, the fertile period can span five to seven days.

Normal twins are either monozygotic, i.e. from single ovum or bizygotic from two ova but are fertilized at the same time by single act of coitus. Sometimes one fetus grows at the cost of another and the second fetus is under developed or rarely it may die and even get mummified known as "Fetus compressus" or "Fetus pypyraceus".

xi. *Superfetation:* Fertilisation of two ova from different ovulatory cycles by two acts of coitus. Fertilisation of second ovum is possible within first three months of the fertilisation of the first ovum in an already pregnant woman. In such a case the babies born are of different ages or maturation stages. Superfetation is claimed to be common in some animal species but is rare in humans.

xii. *Normal period of pregnancy:* The period from conception to delivery is normally taken in medicolegal practice as 10 lunar months or in obstetrics as 9 calendar months plus one week or about 280 days.

xiii. *Maximum period of pregnancy:* Some courts in order to establish legitimacy has taken 350 days as the maximum period of pregnancy. Whenever, the period is more than the normal period of pregnancy the fetus must show signs of maturation as per the extended period of pregnancy.

xiv. *Illegitimate child:* A child born out of the wedlock or within the specified time after cessation of the relationship between husband and wife or when conception by her husband is not possible, such a child is known as illegitimate child or bastard child.

DELIVERY

Delivery is normal culmination of pregnancy with expulsion of fetus. A medical practitioner may be asked whether a woman has delivered or not. Findings in a woman may suggest of the following:

1. **Recent delivery:** When the delivery has taken place within two weeks.
2. **Remote delivery:** When the delivery has taken place beyond more than two weeks.

Signs of Recent Delivery

a. *General disposition:* Fatigue and general indisposition is present for 3 to 4 days. There may be "after pains" due to uterine contractions.

b. *Breasts:* Breasts are full, firm and enlarged. Colostrum is seen in first 24 hours. Nipple is enlarged and areola becomes well marked with montgomery's tubercles.

c. *Abdomen:* Lax abdomen with linea albicantes, which are pink in the beginning. Linea nigra are also present over lower abdominal wall.

d. *Uterus:* Uterus is felt as flabby mass 4 to 5 cm below the umbilicus, just after delivery. Gradually it becomes hard and felt as hard ball felt up to mid-point between pubic symphysis and umbilicus. After two weeks it goes behind the pubic symphysis.

e. *Vagina:* Vagina is dilated and may show tears or lacerations which normally heal in a week. Deep lacerations, if present, may take more time to heal.

f. *Labia majora and labia minora:* These are congested and tender to touch.

g. *Cervix:* Cervix is soft and show transverse laceration. It admits two fingers for few days and only one finger after a week. The opening is closed after two weeks.

h. *Lochia:* This is a watery discharge with disagreeable smell from the uterus. Normally lochia is present up to two weeks after delivery.

    i. Lochia rubra: Reddish stained fluid containing traces of blood and shreds of fetal membranes for 4 to 5 days.

    ii. Lochia serosa: Pale watery fluid is discharged for next 4 to 5 days.

    iii. Lochia alba: It is whitish and thick discharge and disappears after next 4 to 5 days.

i. *Biological tests:* These tests remain positive after few days to a week after delivery.

Signs of Recent Delivery in Dead

On postmortem examination a forensic pathologist usually examine breast and genital tract for various signs.

1. *Breast:* They are full, enlarged and firm to feel.
2. *Uterus:* Size of the uterus depends on the period after delivery the woman has died.
3. Tears are seen in cervix and vagina.
4. Lochia may be seen.
5. Corpus luteum is present in one of the ovaries.
6. Uterus walls show pink raw area for placental attachment site.

Signs of Remote Delivery in Living or Dead

1. **Breasts:** Breasts are enlarged and pendulous. Nipples are enlarged and areola is dark with Montgomery tubercles.
2. **Abdomen:** Abdomen is lax with linea albicantes.
3. **Uterus:** Uterus is seen bulky and enlarged (Table 30.1).
4. **Vagina:** Vagina is dilated with healed tears.
5. **Cervix:** Cervix show transverse cleft.

It is possible to calculate time of delivery up to 2 months; after this period exact time cannot be properly calculated.

Medicolegal Importance

a. Delivery may be feigned for inheritance purposes.
b. To claim maintenance from the husband a child is produced in affiliation cases.
c. Abandoning a child.
d. Concealing birth of a child.
e. Disputed maternity cases.

Table 30.1: Differences between Nulliparous and Multiparous uterus		
Feature	Multiparous	Nulliparous
Size	Large (10 × 6 × 2.5 cm)	Small (7 × 5 × 2 cm)
Cervical length	It is half of the body length	Body and cervix are equal
Shape of cervix	It is cylindrical in shape	It is conical in shape
weight	More (80–100 gram)	Less (40–50 gram)
Uterine cavity	Spacious with concave walls	Small with convex walls
External os	Small rounded opening	Transverse opening
Internal os	circular	Wrinkled margins
Fundus height	Above the broad ligament	At the level of broad ligament
Placental attachment	Scar may be observed	No such scar is present

31 | Abortion

In legal terms abortion means "expulsion of products of conception at any time before confinement, i.e. full term. However, depending on the trimester in which this expulsion of products of conception takes place, medically they are called abortion (occurring during first trimester), miscarriage (which occurs during second trimester) and premature labour (when it takes place during third trimester till full term).

Abortion can be classified into mainly two types:

a. *Natural:* This can be spontaneous or accidental.

b. *Artificial or induced:* These are either therapeutic or criminal abortions.

Depending on the medical status of abortion they are also known as threatened; inevitable; incomplete; complete or septic abortions.

NATURAL ABORTIONS

Natural abortions are most common, about 80% during the first trimester of the pregnancy. Majority of these take place before the woman is even aware about her pregnancy.

Causes of Natural Abortions

Causes of natural abortions could be because of maternal, fetal and miscellaneous reasons.

Maternal

a. *Systemic diseases:* These include syphilis, anemia, diabetes, high fever like in malaria, viral infections like rubella or variola, AIDS and bacterial infections.

b. *Trauma:* Local trauma in the abdominal region may cause separation of the placenta. even fear or shock may result in abortion.

c. *Local diseases or deformities:* Fibroid, malformation of uterus or inflammatory conditions may result in abortions.

d. *Endocrinal disturbances:* Low progesterone levels may result in abortion.

e. *Heavy metal poisoning:* Especially in cases of chronic lead poisoning.

f. *Low implantation of zygote.*

Fetal

a. *Chromosomal abnormalities:* Almost 50% of spontaneous abortions are due to chromosomal abnormalities like autosomal trisomy.

b. *Hydatid mole.*

c. *Placental or decidual diseases.*

d. *Rh Blood group incompatibility.*

Miscellaneous

a. *In about 30 to 40% of cases there is no evident cause.*

b. *Smoking and drug abuse.*

c. *Exposure to X-rays or anticancer drugs.*

Artificial Abortions

These are either therapeutic or criminal abortions.

THERAPEUTIC OR LEGAL ABORTIONS

During the last fifty years many countries including India have liberalised their abortion laws. Today only 8% of the world's population lives in countries where the law prevents abortion. In India, Shantilal Shah Committee (formed in 1964) recommended liberalisation of abortion law in 1966 to reduce maternal morbidity and mortality associated with illegal abortions. On these recommendations, in 1969 Medical termination of pregnancy bill was introduced in Rajya Sabha and Lok Sabha, which was passed by Indian Parliament in August, 1971. Medical Termination of Pregnancy Act, 1971 (MTP Act) was implemented from April, 1972 and was amended in 1975 and 2002.

THE MEDICAL TERMINATION OF PREGNANCY ACT, 1971

An act to provide for the termination of certain pregnancies by registered medical practitioners.

Reason for Termination by a Registered Medical Practitioner

1. **Therapeutic:** The continuance of the pregnancy would involve a risk to the life of the pregnant woman or of grave injury to her physical or mental health.

   Some of the reasons under this clause may include severe eclampsia, hypertensive crisis, malignancy, cardiovascular conditions, nephrotic syndrome or severe uncontrolled diabetes, etc.

   The MTP act also include grave injury to the mental health of the pregnant woman under following explanations:

   a. *Explanation 1:* Where any pregnancy is alleged by the pregnant woman to have been caused by **rape**, the anguish caused by such pregnancy shall be presumed to constitute a grave injury to the mental health of the pregnant woman.

   b. *Explanation 2:* Where any pregnancy occurs as a result of **failure of any device or method** used by any *married woman* *or her husband* for the purpose of limiting the number of children, the anguish caused by such unwanted pregnancy may be resumed to constitute a grave injury to the mental health of the pregnant woman.

   In determining whether the continuance of a pregnancy would involve such risk of injury to the health account may be taken of the pregnant women actual or reasonable foreseeable environment.

2. **Eugenic:** There is a substantial risk that if the child were born, it would suffer from such physical or mental abnormalities to be seriously handicapped.

   Such conditions include infections by rubella or mumps in pregnant woman, exposure of pregnant woman to radiations or administration of certain teratogenic drugs.

Period of Gestation for Termination of Pregnancy

a. Where the length of the pregnancy does not exceed twelve weeks by a single doctor.

b. Where the length of the pregnancy exceeds twelve weeks but does not exceed twenty weeks, than two registered medical practitioner are, of opinion, formed in good faith, that termination is required then anyone of them can terminate the pregnancy.

Consent

No pregnancy shall be terminated except with the consent of the pregnant woman, who has attained the age of eighteen years. However, no pregnancy in a female who has not attained the age of eighteen years, or, who is mentally ill, shall be terminated except with the consent in writing of her guardian. As per MTP ACT, consent of the husband is not required if the women fulfills the conditions and wants to end her pregnancy. However, in case of **Samar Ghosh and Jaya Ghosh**, supreme court of India held that unilateral decision of sterilization, **abortion,** and refusing to have intercourse for considerable period may also amount to mental cruelty.

Place where pregnancy may be terminated (MTP rules, 1975 and 2003): Termination of pregnancy shall be made in accordance with this act at either of the following places.

    i. A hospital established or maintained by government.

    ii. A place for the time being approved for the purpose of this act by government.

Emergency Situations

The length of the pregnancy and the opinion of not less than two registered medical practitioners, shall not apply to the termination of a pregnancy by a registered medical practitioner in a case where he is of opinion, formed in good faith, that the termination of such pregnancy is immediately necessary to *save the life of the pregnant woman.*

    Experience and training required for termination (MTP rules, 1975 and 2003): For the purpose of medical termination, a registered medical practitioner shall have one or more of the following experience or training in gynecology and obstetrics:

a. In the case of a medical practitioner, who was registered in a state medical register before the commencement of the act; experience in the practice of gynecology and obstetrics for a period of not less than three years.

b. In the case of other medical practitioner, who is registered in a state medical register after 1971.

    i. If he has completed six months of house surgeonship in gynecology and obstetrics.

    ii. If he had experience at any hospital for a period of not less than one year in the practice of obstetrics and gynecology.

    iii. If he has assisted a registered medical practitioner in the performance of twenty-five cases of medical termination of pregnancy of which at least five have been performed independently, in a hospital established or maintained or a training institute approved for this purpose by the government. However, this training would enable the registered medical practitioner (RMP) to do only 1st Trimester terminations.

    iv. Registered medical practitioner, who holds a postgraduate degree or diploma in gynecology and obstetrics.

Maintenance of records (MTP rules, 1975 and 2003): All forms and records filled for the procedure for the conduct of termination of pregnancy must be kept confidential.

Penalties

Termination of pregnancy by a person who is not a registered medical practitioner shall be an offence punishable with rigorous imprisonment for a term which shall not be less than two years but which may extend to seven years.

    Whoever terminates any pregnancy in a place other than approved places shall be punishable with rigorous imprisonment for a term which shall not be less than two years but which may extend to seven years.

    Any person being owner of a place (who is the administrative head or otherwise responsible for the working or maintenance of a hospital) which is not approved under clause (b) of section 4 shall be punishable with rigorous imprisonment for a term which shall not be less than two years but which may extend to seven years.

    Protection of action taken in good faith (Section-8): No suit or legal proceedings shall lie against any registered medical practitioner for any damage caused or likely to be caused by anything, which is in good faith done or intended to be done under this act.

ILLEGAL OR CRIMINAL ABORTIONS

When pregnancy is terminated contravening the provisions of the MTP act 1971 is known as illegal or criminal abortion. Mostly there is no therapeutic indication for abortion in such cases. Mostly such terminations are done in widows; unmarried girls or for female feticides. In such cases termination of pregnancy is undertaken mostly during first trimester especially in 2nd or 3rd month. Majority of such cases go unnoticed. Only when the condition of the woman become serious or they die due to complications only then these cases are brought to the notice of the police or hospitals. Such abortions may be under taken by a qualified doctor, a midwife or nurse who is semiskilled, untrained quacks or the pregnant woman by self-medication.

To prove that the complications or death has taken place due to abortion, following things are to be established:

a. The woman was pregnant.
b. An act was done for the termination of pregnancy.
c. Abortion was as a result of that action.
d. The act was unlawful (not as per MTP act 1971).

All cases of criminal abortions need to be made medicolegal, investigated and police informed.

Methods of Criminal Abortions

Criminal abortion can be undertaken by means of:

Use of Drugs or Chemicals

1. Acting directly on the uterus:
   a. *Ecbolics:* These drugs increase uterine contractions like ergometrine or ergot alkaloids, quinine, potassium permanganate and posterior pituitary extract (oxytocin).
   b. *Emmenogogues:* These drugs increase menstrual blood flow. These drugs when given in large doses may induce abortion like savin oil or leaves, borax and prostaglandins.
2. Acting on the uterus through gastrointestinal tract:
   a. *Emetics:* Strong emetics like tartar emetic can reflexly result in abortion.
   b. *Purgatives:* Croton oil, aloe or castor oil can result in abortion.
3. Acting of the uterus through genitourinary system: Oil of turpentine, oil of pennyroyal or tancy and cantharides act as abortifacient through genitourinary system.
4. Drugs having generalised poisonous effects:
   a. *Vegetable poisons:* Like unripe papaya fruit and seeds, unripe pineapple fruit, madar juice and lal chitra.
   b. *Metallic poisons:* Especially lead having effect on trophoblastic epithelium resulting in abortion.

Mechanical violence

1. General violence:
   a. Pressure over abdomen by tight belts or by jumping.
   b. *Violent exercises:* Riding, cycling, lifting heavy weights or swimming.
   c. *Cupping:* By lighting a wick over abdomen and placing an inverted glass, cup or "Lota" over it. When it becomes adherent to abdominal wall, due to vacuum, pulling the same with a jerk is known as cupping.
   d. Application of leaches over thighs or perineum.
   e. Alternate hot and cold hip baths.
2. Local violence:
   a. *Dilatation of cervix:* It is normally done along with rupture of membranes with uterine sound, hair pin or a glass rod. *Laminaria tent* bark of slippery elm may be placed in cervix, which swells up causing dilatation. *Abortion stick* which is about 5 to 6 inches long, one end wrapped with cotton wool with application of irritant substances like marking nut juice, calotropis, or red lead is used for dilatation of cervix and causing abortion. Dilatation and curettage is done for medical termination of pregnancy.
   b. *Syringing:* Irritant substances like soap water, lysol in hot water is injected with *Higginson's* syringe into uterus.

c. *Passage of electric current:* Electric current is passed by placing positive pole over sacrum and negative pole in cervix to cause contraction of the uterus.

d. *Air insufflations:* Air is pumped into vagina or cervix with a pump or syringe.

e. Vacuum extractor for abortion is normally used by medical practitioners.

Causes of Death in Criminal Abortion

a. Immediate causes:

i. *Reflex shock:* Vagal inhibition of heart may take place during abortion.

ii. *Hemorrhage:* Hemorrhage from vaginal or uterine injuries may cause death. Sometimes incomplete separation of the placenta may lead to massive hemorrhage.

iii. *Pulmonary air embolism:* Injecting soap water with bubbles can cause air embolism resulting in death of a female. About 100 cc of air can cause fatal air embolism.

iv. *Amniotic fluid embolism:* Rarely amniotic fluid may result in pulmonary embolism.

b. Delayed causes:

i. *Infections:* Use of un-sterilized instruments may cause infection. Tetanus also has been reported in few cases.

ii. Rupture of uterus may lead to peritonitis.

iii. Necrosis of cervix may cause death in few cases.

c. Remote causes: Bacterial endocarditis, renal failure, meningitis, pneumonia, delayed pulmonary embolism, chronic poisoning effects may be responsible for deaths in few cases.

Medicolegal Conditions in which a Female is Examined for Signs of Abortion

1. A woman is alleging abortion after a blow on the abdomen.
2. A woman alleging that abortion is as a result of some abortifacient drugs administered to her.
3. A woman trying to conceal abortion after being charged with it.

Signs of Abortion

Living Person

Signs of abortion mainly depend on the stage of pregnancy and time elapsed after abortion. Discharge of colostrum may be seen. Undergarments may show bloodstaining. Signs of injury to the vagina with blood clots, dilatation of cervix, enlarged uterus and rise in temperature due to presence of infection are mostly observed. Urine may be positive for HCG up to 2 weeks.

Dead Person

Signs of recent delivery with enlarged uterus and signs of local trauma to the labia majora, vagina, cervix or uterus. In air embolism cases pelvic veins may show air bubbles. Undergarments stained with blood, presence of abortifacient drugs or instruments for abortion and products of conception may be present on the scene of crime.

Punishment for Criminal Abortion

Section 312 IPC: Causing miscarriage: Whoever voluntarily causes a woman with child to miscarry, shall, if such miscarriage be not caused in good faith for the purpose of saving the life of the woman, be punished with imprisonment of either description for a term which may extend to three years, or with fine, or with both; and, if the woman be quick with child, shall be punished with imprisonment of either description for a term which may extend to seven years, and shall also be liable to fine. A woman, who causes herself to miscarry, is within the meaning of this section.

Section 313 IPC: Causing miscarriage without woman's consent: Whoever commits the offence defined in the last preceding section without the consent of the woman, whether the woman is quick with child or not, shall be punished with imprisonment for life or with imprisonment of either description for a term which may extend to ten years, and shall also be liable to fine.

Section 314 IPC: Death caused by act done with intent to cause miscarriage: Whoever, with intent to cause the miscarriage of a woman with child, does any act which causes the death of such woman, shall be punished with imprisonment of either description for a term which may extend to ten years, and shall also be liable to fine; if the act is done without the consent of the woman, shall be punished either with imprisonment for life or with the punishment above mentioned.

Explanation: It is not essential to this offence that the offender should know that the act is likely to cause death.

Section 315 IPC: Act done with intent to prevent child being born alive or to cause it to die after birth: Whoever before the birth of any child does any act with the intention of thereby preventing that child from being born alive or causing it to die after its birth, and does by such act prevent that child from being born alive, or causes it to die after its birth, shall, if such act be not caused in good faith for the purpose of saving the life of the mother, be punished with imprisonment of either description for a term which may extend to ten years, or with fine, or with both.

Section 316 IPC: Causing death of quick unborn child by act amounting to culpable homicide: Whoever does any act under such circumstances, that if he thereby caused death he would be guilty of culpable homicide, and does by such act cause the death of a quick unborn child, shall be punished with imprisonment of either description for a term which may extend to ten years, and shall also be liable to fine.

PRECONCEPTION AND PRENATAL DIAGNOSTIC TECHNIQUES (PROHIBITION OF SEX SELECTION) ACT, 1994 (PCPNDT ACT)

An act to provide for the regulation of the use of preconception and prenatal diagnostic techniques for the purpose of detecting genetic or metabolic disorders or chromosomal abnormalities or certain congenital malformations or sex-linked disorders and for the prevention of the misuse of such techniques for the purpose of prenatal sex determination leading to female feticides.

Only genetic counselling centre, genetic laboratory or genetic clinic registered under this act, shall conduct or help in, conducting activities relating to prenatal diagnostic techniques by employing persons who possess the prescribed qualifications. No person shall conduct any prenatal diagnostic techniques at a place other than a place registered under this act. Supreme Court of India in 2001 gave a verdict to include ultrasound clinics under the act.

Regulation of Genetic Counselling Centers, Genetic Laboratories and Genetic Clinics

1. No genetic counselling centre, genetic laboratory or genetic clinic unless registered under this act, shall conduct or associate with, or help in, conducting activities relating to prenatal diagnostic techniques.
2. No genetic counselling centre or genetic laboratory or genetic clinic shall employ or cause to be employed or take services of any person, whether on honorary basis or on payment who does not possess qualifications.
3. No medical geneticist, gynecologist, pediatrician, registered medical practitioner or any other person shall conduct or cause to be conducted or aid in conducting by himself or through any other person, any prenatal diagnostic techniques at a place other than a place registered under this act.

Prohibition of Sex-Selection

No person, including a specialist or a team of specialists in the field of infertility, shall conduct or cause to be conducted or aid in conducting by himself or by any other person, sex selection on a woman or a man or on both or on any tissue, embryo, conceptus, fluid or gametes derived from either or both of them.

Prohibition on sale of ultrasound machines, etc. to persons, laboratories, clinics, etc. not registered under the act: No person shall sell any ultrasound machine or imaging machine or scanner or any other equipment capable of detecting sex of fetus to any genetic counselling centre, genetic laboratory, genetic clinic or any other person not registered under the act.

Regulation of Prenatal Diagnostic Techniques

Clause 1: No place including a registered genetic counselling centre or genetic laboratory or genetic clinic shall be used or caused to be used by any person for conducting prenatal diagnostic techniques except for the purposes specified in clause (2) and after satisfying any of the conditions specified in clause (3).

Clause 2: No prenatal diagnostic techniques shall be conducted except for the purposes of detection of any of the following abnormalities, namely:

  i. Chromosomal abnormalities
  ii. Genetic metabolic diseases
  iii. Hemoglobinopathies
  iv. Sex-linked genetic diseases
  v. Congenital anomalies
  vi. Any other abnormalities or diseases as may be specified by the central supervisory board.

Clause 3: No prenatal diagnostic techniques shall be used or conducted unless the person qualified to do so is satisfied for reasons to be recorded in writing that any of the following conditions are fulfilled, namely:

  i. Age of the pregnant woman is above thirty-five years.
  ii. The pregnant woman has undergone two or more spontaneous abortions or fetal loss.
  iii. The pregnant woman had been exposed to potentially teratogenic agents such as drugs, radiation, infection or chemicals.
  iv. The pregnant woman or her spouse has a family history of mental retardation or physical deformities such as, spasticity or any other genetic disease.
  v. Any other condition as may be specified by the central supervisory board.

Written consent of pregnant woman required and prohibition of communicating the sex of fetus:

1. Prenatal diagnostic test should not be undertaken unless:
   a. The doctor has explained all known side and after effects of such procedures to the pregnant woman concerned before such procedures.
   b. The doctor has obtained in the prescribed form her written consent to undergo such procedures in the language which she understands.
   c. A copy of her written consent obtained under clause (b) is given to the pregnant woman.
2. Person conducting the prenatal diagnostic procedure should not communicate to the woman or her relatives by any means the sex of the fetus and also give a declaration to that effect on the report of that patient.
3. Woman before undergoing prenatal diagnostic test should also declare that she does not want to know the sex of her fetus.

Determination of Sex Prohibited

a. No genetic counselling centre or genetic laboratory or genetic clinic shall conduct or cause to be conducted in its centre, laboratory or clinic, prenatal diagnostic techniques including ultrasonography, for the purpose of determining the sex of a fetus.
b. No person shall conduct or cause to be conducted any prenatal diagnostic techniques including ultrasonography for the purpose of determining the sex of a fetus.
c. No person shall, by whatever means, cause or allow to be caused selection of sex before or after conception.

Registration of genetic counselling centers, genetic laboratories or genetic clinics: No person shall open any genetic counselling centre, genetic laboratory or genetic clinic, including clinic, laboratory or centre having ultrasound or imaging machine or scanner or any other technology capable of undertaking determination of sex of fetus and sex selection, or render services to any of them, after the commencement of the prenatal diagnostic techniques (regulation and prevention of misuse) amendment act, 2002 unless such centre, laboratory or clinic is duly registered under the act.

Advertisements Prohibited

No person or organisation including genetic counselling centre, genetic laboratory or genetic clinic shall issue, publish, distribute, communicate or cause to be issued, published, distributed or communicated any advertisement in any manner regarding prenatal determination or preconception selection of sex by any means whatsoever, scientific or otherwise.

Any person who contravenes the provisions shall be punishable with imprisonment for a term which may extend to three years and with fine which may extend to ten thousand rupees.

Maintenance and Preservation of Records

1. All registered centers should maintain a register showing details of all cases examined.
2. In all cases related records, consent forms, laboratory slides, sonographic pictures and observations should be preserved for at least 2 years or till the final disposal in a legal case.
3. A printed copy of computer based records duly authenticated by the concerned person must be preserved.

Offences and Penalties

1. Any medical geneticist, gynecologist, registered medical practitioner or any person who owns a genetic counselling centre, a genetic laboratory or a genetic clinic or is employed in such a centre, laboratory or clinic and renders his professional or technical services to or at such a centre, laboratory or clinic, whether on an honorary basis or otherwise, and who contravenes any of the provisions of this act or rules made thereunder shall be punishable with imprisonment for a term which may extend to three years and with fine which may extend to ten thousand rupees and on any subsequent conviction, with imprisonment which may extend to five years and with fine which may extend to fifty thousand rupees.
2. The name of the registered medical practitioner shall be reported by the appropriate authority to the state medical council concerned for taking necessary action including suspension of the registration if the charges are framed by the court and till the case is disposed of and on conviction for removal of his name from the register of the council for a period of five years for the first offence and permanently for the subsequent offence.
3. Any person who seeks the aid of a genetic counselling centre, genetic laboratory, genetic clinic or ultrasound clinic or imaging clinic or of a medical geneticist, gynecologist, sonologist or imaging specialist or registered medical practitioner or any other person for sex selection or for conducting prenatal diagnostic techniques on any pregnant women for the purposes other than those specified, he shall, be punishable with imprisonment for a term which may extend to three years and with fine which may extend to fifty thousand rupees for the first offence and for any subsequent offence with imprisonment which may extend to five years and with fine which may extend to one lakh rupees.
4. All offences under the act are considered as cognizable, non-bailable and non-compoundable.

32 | Fetal and Infant Deaths

Dead body of a fetus, newly born or an infant poses a complex problem before a forensic expert to decide whether the death is natural, accidental or homicidal in nature. Some of the terms associated with fetal and infant deaths are mentioned below:

Feticide: It is killing of fetus anytime before childbirth.

Filicide (from latin filius: Son): It is killing of child by its parents.

Neonaticide: It is killing of neonate within 24 hours of its birth.

INFANTICIDE

It is defined as "unlawful destruction of a child any time from birth up to one year of age".

According to infanticide act (1938) section I, of England, "where a woman by any willful act or omission causes the death of her child under the age of twelve months but at the time the balance of her mind was disturbed by not having fully recovered from the effects of giving birth to the child or by reason of the effects of lactation, she shall be guilty of infanticide". A lesser punishment is awarded to the mother in such a case.

Infanticide in India

According to Indian Law, killing of all infants either by mother or by any other individual is equated with murder. Infanticide does not include death of fetus during labour when it is destroyed by craniotomy or decapitation. Hence, according to Indian law, killing of an infant before it is live born is not homicide. But destruction of an infant after any part of a child, showing signs of life, has been brought forth external to the mother, even though it is not completely born constitutes homicide.

Infanticide is usually committed by young unmarried women or widow with the intention of concealing the birth. In every case of infanticide, legal presumption is that the child is born dead and the onus of proving that the child was born alive and died from criminal violence rests on the prosecution.

In case of death of a child, following factors are required to establish infanticide:

i. That the child was capable of being born alive, e.g. child is not a monster.
ii. The pregnancy must have reached 28th weeks or above to prove that the child was viable.
iii. It must be proved that a willful act was done to cause its death.
iv. The above act resulted in the death of the child.

Killing a child in the act of birth and before it is fully born is not infanticide, but if injuries are inflicted before birth which result in death after birth, it is homicide.

Autopsy in Suspicious Death of Newborn Infant

Whenever a dead body of an infant is brought for postmortem examination by investigating police officer, proper identification by parents or relatives must be undertaken. Hospital labels, identification tags can also be used for this purpose. Clothing worn by infant and any other clothes in which body is wrapped should be preserved for identification. A detailed history as alleged by police officer is important in such cases. If possible, detailed photography of the body should be done and injuries should be recorded. In suspected cases of physical abuse of the child, radiological examination is of importance before proceeding for autopsy.

Autopsy is carried out to find, whether the infant is stillborn, dead born or live born, the age of the fetus or infant and cause and manner of death.

WHETHER THE CHILD WAS STILLBORN, DEAD BORN OR LIVE BORN?

Dead Born Fetus

It means death of the fetus *in utero,* irrespective of the duration of pregnancy and on being born manifests signs indicating death of the fetus prior to the complete expulsion or extraction from its mother of a product of human conception except in case of an induced termination of pregnancy.

Signs of Dead Born Fetus

1. Maceration (Macerare = soften by soaking): Maceration is aseptic autolysis resulting in changes which occur in a fetus retained in uterus after its death. This is also known as *Mors fetus intrauterine* meaning fetal demise during pregnancy, usually showing maceration. Presence of liquor amnii facilitates maceration process.

In case female retains dead fetus for some time, she may suffer from DIC, a fatal condition.

Stages of Maceration

Stage 0: Parboiled, reddened skin.
Stage 1: Skin slippage and peeling.
Stage 2: Extensive skin peeling, red serous effusions in chest and abdomen.
Stage 3: Yellow-brown liver, turbid effusion and even mummification in some cases.

General Features of Child Having Undergone Intrauterine Maceration

Body of fetus is flaccid and flattened; body emits sweetish disagreeable smell and the umbilical cord is seen straight and flaccid. Detailed changes are mentioned below:

i. *Skin:* The earliest sign of macerations are seen in the skin in about 12 to 24 hours after intrauterine death. Initially epidermis separates from the dermis on applying a pressure **(skin slipping)**. Large blebs appear with collection of fluid beneath the epidermis. The desquamation regularly progresses in time to extensive skin separation on the face, neck, abdomen, limbs and external genitalia exposing red and moist dermal surface.

ii. *Head:* Collapse of the skull with overlapping cranial bones (*Spalding sign*). Gradually cranial bones become separated from the dura and periosteum. Widely open mouth and eyes are frequent with progressive maceration.

iii. *Internal organs:* Uniform reddish discolouration, due to progressive hemolysis, yellow-brown discolouration occurs. With retention of fetus for several weeks, dystrophic calcification is possible. Organs most severely affected by autolysis are those from abdominal cavity (liver, spleen, adrenals) and brain which is very soft or semiliquid in severe maceration. There is softening of all organs and connective tissues, laxity of joints, exudation of fluid and hemolysed blood into pleural, pericardial and peritoneal cavities. The fetus may look edematous **(hydrops fetalis)**.

2. **Rigor mortis:** Rigor mortis is the usual change after death and suggests death *in utero* at least 2–3 hours before birth.
3. **Mummification:** In later stages, progressive loss of fluid results in mummification.
4. **Adipocere:** When sufficient liquor amnii is there, adipocere formation may be seen in rare cases.

Examination of Placenta

Placenta remains viable after fetal death *in utero*. Placenta should be thoroughly examined for placental abnormalities such as infarction, retroplacental hemorrhage and cord accidents.

Radiological Signs of Dead Born Fetus

1. **Robert's sign:** An earliest sign; Air in aorta, pulmonary vessels and abdomen appears 12 hours after death.
2. **Spalding's sign:** When overridding cranial bones of fetal skull are observed in an X-ray taken of the mother before the fetus is delivered is known as **spalding sign**. This sign becomes positive after 2 to 4 days or more after the death of the fetus inside uterus (Table 32.1).
3. Hyperflexion of the spine along with crowding of the ribs.

Stillbirth

Stillbirth is a baby who after 28 weeks (In English law, the age is 24 weeks) of gestation, did not at any time after being completely expelled from its mother, breathe or show any other signs of life. The child dies during the process of labour and do not show any sign of dead born fetus. This is also known as *mors fetus intrapartum* which means death occurs during delivery. Such a fetus mostly weighs 900 gm or more.

Causes of Stillbirth

Following are some of the causes of stillbirth:
  i. Anoxia
 ii. Birth trauma
iii. Prolonged labour
 iv. Congenital abnormalities
  v. Rh incompatibility in fetus
 vi. Premature fetus
vii. Toxemia of pregnancy.

Features of Stillborn Fetus

Signs of prolonged labour like subscalpel hemorrhage, caput succedaneum, severe molding of head are mostly observed. There are no features of a dead born fetus. Other specific features are mentioned below:
  i. On microscopic examination of the lungs, the air sacs retain a gland like appearance, which indicates that the child has not breathed and therefore was stillborn.
 ii. Lungs are flooded with liquor amnii.
iii. Evidence of phagocytosis of meconium by cells lining air sacs.
 iv. Bronchial epithelial desquamation.
  v. Distension of lower intestine with meconium.

Live Birth

Live birth is defined as "the complete expulsion or extraction from its mother of a product of human conception, irrespective of the duration of pregnancy, which, after such expulsion or extraction, breathes, or shows

Table 32.1: Differences between macerated fetus and decomposed fetus		
Findings	*Macerated fetus*	*Decomposed fetus*
Appearance	Brownish-pink	Greenish
Surface	Slimy, blistered, jelly-like	Fluid filled blisters with brownish-black fluid
Joints	Loose	Not so
Cranial plates	Detached, overriding	No detachment
Spalding sign	Characteristic	Not so

any other evidence of life such as beating of the heart, pulsation of the umbilical cord, or definite movement of voluntary muscles, whether or not the umbilical cord has been cut or the placenta is attached".

In india live birth is defined as "*if any part of a living child has been brought forth external to the mother, though the child may not have breathed or completely born*". To constitute live birth, the child must have been alive when at least one part of its body was entirely outside the maternal passages and it must have had an independent circulation, though this does not imply the severance of the umbilical cord.

According to Indian laws a newly born child found dead is held to be born dead until it has been shown to have been born alive, whereas, in United Kingdom, baby is presumed to be alive after birth.

Signs Suggestive of Live Birth

In civil cases any sign of life after complete birth of child is accepted as a proof of live birth.
1. **Subjective signs:** Signs which are suggestive of live birth
   i. *Cry of baby:* Baby's cry and respiration is an important sign of live birth. Baby can inhale air and cry inside the uterus (vagitus uterinus) or inside the vagina (vagitus vaginalis) and may even die.
   ii. Muscle twitching/limb movements.
   iii. Sneezing and yawning.
2. **Objective signs:** In criminal cases demonstrable signs are relied upon to demonstrate live birth. Some of these signs provide strong indications towards live birth.

Signs of Live Birth Prior to Respiration

Under normal circumstances it is difficult to give opinion regarding live birth before a child has respired after birth, however, in some cases following observations may suggest live birth:
1. Injuries are found on the body consistent with having been inflicted during birth, and are associated with such hemorrhage as could only have occurred while the blood was circulating.

2. Fractures of the skull from accidental falls (precipitate labour) are as a rule stellate, and are situated on the vertex or in the parietal protuberance. The fractures from violence are more extensive, usually depressed, and accompanied by laceration of the scalp.

Signs of Live Birth After Respiration

Most of the reliable signs are seen in the chest and lungs during postmortem examination of the child. Shape of the chest becomes rounded or drum shaped, the diaphragm dome corresponds to sixth or seventh rib and the lung consistency becomes spongy and crepitant with rounded margins and increase in weight as well as volume of the lungs are seen after the child has respired. Differentiating features between respired lung and non-respired lung are mentioned in Table 32.2.

Some of the test performed to confirm live birth are primarily based on the weight or volume of the respired lungs.

a. **Hydrostatic test (Raygat's test):** Once the child has respired, the weight and volume of lungs tend to increase due to inflow of blood and air respectively, however the specific gravity of the lungs decreases from 1.04–1.05 to 0.94–0.95.
   i. This test originally consisted of placing the lungs along with the heart, in water, and noticing whether they sink or float. A piece of liver serves as control. If liver floats in water, which can float due to putrefaction, then test is of no value.
   ii. The test is now modified and done in four steps. (Step-I) Placing the lungs along with the heart, in water and noticing whether they sink or float. In case they float (Step-II) the bronchus are tied and lungs severed above the ligature and each lung is placed in water one by one. If individual lung float (Step-III) cut the lung into 15 to 20 pieces and these pieces are placed in water to observe floatation of these pieces. When these

Table 32.2: Differences in chest and lungs before and after respiration

Findings	Before Respiration	After respiration
Shape of chest	Flat, circumference 1–2 cm less than that of abdomen	Expanded, drum shaped
Shape and position of diaphragm	More arched, higher (at level of 5th–6th rib)	Less arched, lower (at level of 6–7th rib)
Lungs:	a. Surface smooth	a. Surface uneven
	b. Situated in the back of the thorax	b. Expand closely surround the heart and thymus gland
	c. Do not fill thoracic cavity.	c. Occupy the whole thorax
	d. They are of a dark, red-brown colour	d. The portions containing air are of a light brick-red colour.
	e. Consistency is of liver, dense, firm, non-crepitant	e. Soft spongy and crepitate.
	f. Lungs are without mottling	f. Lungs are mottled from the presence of islands of aerated tissue.
Blood within lungs	Less	more
Weight of lungs (Fodere's test)	35 gm	70 gm (double)
Ploucquet's test (Ratio of weight of lungs to that of body)	1 : 70	1 : 35
Specific gravity	1.04–1.05	0.94–0.95
Hydrostatic test	Negative, sinks	Positive, floats
On dissection, oozing of blood	Little blood, no froth oozes out on pressure	Abundant frothy blood oozes out
Medicolegal importance	Suggestive of stillborn or dead born fetus	Suggestive of live born fetus

pieces float (Step-IV) lung pieces are squeezed between two hard surfaces like cardboard pieces to expel tidal air but the residual air is still present in the respired alveoli. If these pieces float, it indicates that respiration has taken place. A piece of liver is used as control.

Hydrostatic test is not necessary when:
1. Fetus is born before the age of viability.
2. Fetus is dead born, showing signs of maceration, mummification or putrefaction.
3. Stomach and duodenum contains curdled milk.
4. Umbilical cord separated showing signs of healing.
5. Monster fetus.

False positive results are seen when there is presence of putrefaction or forceful artificial respiration has taken place.

False negative results in hydrostatic test may be observed in atelectasis, presence of alveolar duct membrane, pulmonary edema or pneumonia.

b. **Weight of lungs (Fodere's test):** With establishment of circulation and expansion of lungs with air the weight of the lungs almost doubles. Before respiration lungs weigh 35 gm, whereas, after respiration it increases to 70 gm.

c. **Ploucquet's test:** This test is based on the ratio of weight of lungs to that of body. The ratio before respiration is 1:70, whereas, after respiration it is 1:35.

d. Microscopic examination of lungs: After opening the thoracic cage, thoracic block to be removed intact by cutting with a scalpel, the parts being controlled by holding the tongue or larynx with the forceps. The block is fixed for 48 hours and later on samples for microscopic examination are taken of whole lung in cross-section. This technique is called 'No touch technique' by Osborn. Unrespired lung of a fetus, alveoli has hallowed gland like appearance with thick walled ductules, lined by cubicle or columnar epithelial cells. Cellular changes in the alveoli (cells becoming flat/thin) take some time after respiration has been established.

e. Other findings suggestive of live birth:

i. *Blood:* By 24 hours, nucleated RBCs disappear and by 3rd month of life fetal hemoglobin (normal 70–80%) is reduced to 7–8% and disappears completely by 6th month. Fall of reticulocyte count (2%) in the peripheral blood occur by 10 days after birth.

ii. *Presence of meconium:* Meconium is a green viscid substance consisting of thickened bile and mucous. It is completely expelled from the intestinal tract within 24–48 hours of birth. The large intestines in stillborn children are filled with meconium while in those born alive they are usually empty. In anoxia and breech presentation, it is completely excreted before birth.

iii. *Caput succedaneum:* Caput is an area of soft swelling that forms between the layers of the scalp over presenting part of head in vertex presentation that disappears in 1–7 days. It commonly seen in prolonged labour, difficult deliveries, forceps delivery or vacuum extraction.

iv. *Cephalhematoma:* Cephalhematoma is localised accumulation of blood deep to scalp between periosteum and bone surface that occurs in less than 1% of the newborn infants. It is a hemorrhage that is limited by attachment of the pericranium to the fibrous tissue between the sutures. It never crosses suture line and is commonly limited to periosteal sheath of single bone usually right parietal bone. This swelling of 1–5 cm size increases during the first two days after birth due to accumulation of more blood. However, it gradually decreases during the next weeks due to absorption of blood.

v. *Skin changes:* The skin is in a condition of exfoliation soon after birth. Skin of the abdomen exfoliates for the first three days after birth. After birth, the skin is bright red in colour but is darker and brick red by 2–3 days. It changes to yellow and is normal by 7th day. Vernix caseosa persists for 1–2 days and covers the skin in the axilla, inguinal region and neck folds. It may be absent at birth and can be removed by washing.

vi. *Findings in the gastrointestinal tract:* The stomach may contain milk, recognized by the microscope and by Trommer's test for sugar. The air travels in the GIT at the same speed in full term infants as in premature infants. The air reaches the stomach after 15 minutes, small intestine after 1–2 hours, colon after 5–6 hours and rectum after 12 hours. The attempts at resuscitation and bacterial gas formation may result in false interpretation.

Breslau's second life (Stomach-bowel) test: During respiration, air is engulfed in stomach and intestine making them buoyant.

Stomach and bowel are removed after tying double ligature at each end and put in water. If the stomach and duodenum contain air and consequently float in water, the chances are that the child did not die immediately after birth; this is known as Breslau's second life test, and the lower the air in the intestinal canal, the greater is the probability that the child survived birth.

False positive results may be seen in; (1) resuscitative efforts; (2) decomposition and (3) in stillborn fetus while clearing air passages by suction, stomach and bowel tend to engulf air.

vii. *The urinary bladder* is generally emptied soon after birth

viii. *Changes in umbilical cord:* The umbilical cord in a newborn child is fresh, firm, round, and bluish in colour; blood is contained in its vessels. The cord may be ruptured by the child falling from the maternal parts in a precipitate labour, and the ruptured parts present ragged ends. It is seldom that a child bleeds to death from an untied or cut umbilical cord, and the chances in a torn cord are still more remote. The changes in the cord are as follows:

2 hours	Blood clots at cut end.
12–24 hours	Cord shrinks and dries.
36–48 hours	Inflammatory ring forms at the base (stage of inflammation)
2–3rd day	Reddish brown, shrivels and mummifies (stage of desiccation and mummification).
5–6th day	Cord falls off leaving a raw area (stage of cicatrisation).
10–12 day	Heals and leaves the scar (Stage of healing).

ix. *Changes in fetal circulation:* Fetal circulation undergoes various changes seen in umbilical artery, umbilical vein, ductus arteriosis, ductus venosus and foramen ovale after birth. Extent to which these changes have advanced will give an idea of how long the child has survived after birth. Features in detail are mentioned in Table 32.3.

x. *Changes in middle ear (Wreden's Test):* During embryonic life, middle ear contains gelatinous tissue. With respiratory efforts sphincter at pharyngeal end of eustachian tube relaxes and some air enters middle ear.

After removing skull cap submerge base of skull in water and opening petrous temporal bone, if air bubbles escape out suggestive of air in middle ear, child has respired and born alive.

xi. *Other miscellaneous features:*
- Unequivocal neonatal line in the enamel of unerupted teeth is suggestive of separate existence (Gustafson 1966).
- Development of incremental lines (Stack 1960) begins after birth.
- Presence of extraneous material; material which could enter only when infant is completely born, present either in the respiratory tract in secondary bronchi or beyond or in the digestive tract may suggest live birth e.g. presence of milk in infant's stomach and duodenum.

Determination of Intrauterine Age

Intrauterine age is the period starting from time of conception till delivery. The various medical terms used for describing products

Table 32.3: Changes in the fetal circulation		
Vessels	*Closure commences*	*Complete closure*
Umbilical artery	10 hours	3rd day
Umbilical vein (right)	6–7 months IUL	
Umbilical vein (left)	3rd day	4–5th day
Ductus venosus		5th day
Ductus arteriosus		10th day
Foramen ovale	Few seconds of birth	3rd month/rarely unobliterated in adults

of conception are: (i) *Ovum:* from fertilization till second week of gestation; (ii) *embryo:* from second week of gestation till third month of intrauterine life; (iii) *fetus:* from third month of gestation till full term.

Intrauterine age of the fetus for medico-legal purposes is calculated in lunar months, i.e. a month of 4 weeks and the full term is 10 lunar months. Whereas for obstetrical examination it is calculated in calendar months and a normal full term fetus is 9 months and one week.

Hasse's Rule: Intrauterine period can be calculated from the crown heel length using the Hasse's rule.

i. According to this rule the age of the fetus is calculated by the square root of the crown heel length in centimeters for first five months. For example, if the crown heel length is 16 cm, the age of the fetus is about 4 months of intrauterine life.

ii. After 5 months of intrauterine life, crown heel length of the fetus in centimeters, divided by five gives the age in months, e.g. if the length is 40 cm, the age is 8 months. This part of the rule is also known as *Morrison's Rule.*

Determination of the age of a fetus: Various features which help in determination of the age of a fetus at the end of each month are mentioned below:

a. *One month:* length is 1 cm and weight is 2.5 gm.

b. *Second month:* Length is 4 cm; weight is 10 gm; placenta is formed; eyes can be recognised; hands and feet are webbed; and anus is seen as a dark spot.

c. *Third month:* Length is about 9 cm; weight is 30 gm; limbs well developed; neck is formed and pupillary membrane appears.

d. *Fourth month:* Length is 16 cm; weight is about 120 gm; sex can be recognised; lanugo hair visible; pupillary membrane visible and meconium is seen in upper part of the small intestines.

e. *Fifth month:* Length is 25 cm; weight is about 400 gm; **ossification center at calcaneum**; thin light hair over scalp; meconium at the beginning of large intestines and vernix caseosa over the body.

f. *Sixth month:* Length is 30 cm; weight is 700 gm; eyebrows and eyelashes appear and meconium in transverse colon.

g. *Seventh month* (viable fetus): Length is 35 cm; weight is about 900 gm; **Ossification center for talus appears**; pupillary membrane disappears: eyelids are open; meconium is entire large intestines; nails are thick; testis at external inguinal ring and placenta is 350 to 400 gm in weight.

h. *Eighth month:* Length is 40 cm; weight is about 1.2 to 1.5 kg; scalp hair are thick; nails reach to the ends of fingertips; skin is not wrinkled due to subcutaneous fat; left testes has descended in the scrotum and skin covered with lanugo hair.

i. *Ninth month:* Length is 45 cm; weight is about 2.5 kg; scrotum contains both testes; scalp hair about 4 cm long; **ossification center appears at lower end of femur** and posterior fontanel is closed.

j. *Tenth month (full term):* Length is 50 cm; weight is about 3 to 5 kg; **ossification center at upper end of tibia and cuboid bone**; nails grow beyond the fingertips; umbilicus located between pubis and xiphoid.

Autopsy Examination

While conducting autopsy on a newly born infant for age estimation following observations are recorded:

a. Body weight, body length, crown-rump or crown–heel length and head circumference to assess gestational age to be noted.

b. The placenta and umbilical cord must be studied in detail while conducting autopsy in infant or child.

c. In infants the whole chest cavity can be opened under water in order to demonstrate a pneumothorax. In infants and fetuses,

Letulle's technique of *en masse* removal is the preferred technique in most cases so that certain rare malformations can be properly preserved for example, pulmonary venous connections. Histological sections should be taken from lungs, liver, kidney, brain, thymus, placenta, umbilical cord and the free margin of falciform ligament. Fetal circulation changes are recorded.

d. Demonstration of ossification centers:

 i. *Ossification centers of lower end of femur and upper end of tibia:* A transverse incision is made into the joint after flexing the knee joint. The incisions are given in a parallel fashion in the lower end of femur until the largest part of ossification center is reached. The center is identified by its brownish red appearance surrounded by bluish white cartilage. The serial incisions may continue till the diaphyseal center. At 37–38 weeks of intrauterine life, diameter of center is 2–5 mm, whereas it is 6–8 mm at full term.

 ii. *Centers of foot:* The ossification centers of foot that is talus, calcaneum and cuboid are shown by making an incision between the web of third and fourth toes, when the foot is grasped from the ankle. The incision is extended backwards through the sole of foot and middle of the heel.

 iii. *Sternum:* The sternum is divided along its long-axis to demonstrate various ossification centers in sternum.

e. Examination of skull and brain: In this age group, the skull is often difficult to separate from the dura as in adults. *"Beneke's technique"* by making para sagittal cuts with scissor and making parietal flaps, is used to open the skull when the sutures are not closed and the skull bones are soft.

f. Decomposition changes: Bodies of newborn child is normally sterile and when they respire and swallow, microorganisms tend to enter into the body, in live borne infant, putrefaction occurs from within to outwards whereas in a stillborn baby, putrefaction sets in from outside to inwards.

Decomposition and maceration are completely different entities and need to be differentiated.

g. Vernix caseosa over body of child: If vernix caseosa is absent it is suggestive of washing the baby and its survival for some time after birth.

h. Placenta: Placenta should be properly weighed and measured. Normal placenta weighs 1.2 kg at term; it is about 22 cm in diameter and 1.5 cm thick. It should be examined for any abnormality.

i. Umbilical cord: Umbilical cord should be examined that whether its ends are sharp clean-cut or torn and whether it is tied or not. Look for vital reactions at the ends. Look for any abnormal twists, knots and whether infected or not.

j. All the injuries and other findings such as presence of caput succedaneum to be noted.

Whether the Child has Attained Viability

Viability means the stage of maturity at which a fetus with normal intrauterine development is able to maintain a separate existence after birth. In India, a child is viable after 28 weeks or seven months of intrauterine life, Youngest premature baby known to have survived was Amillia Taylar born just after 21 weeks and 6 days of pregnancy. With advanced and well-equipped hospitals in western countries premature babies above 24 weeks may survive.

In law, a fetus which has not attained completion of 7th month of intrauterine life is said to be incapable of maintaining a separate existence and therefore nonviable. Where it can be shown that the child was premature, there is a strong presumption of stillbirth or death from prematurity shortly after live birth.

General Features Suggestive of Viable Fetus

1. *General condition:* General condition of fetus when it is plump or fat and there is lack of any apparent disease or malformation.

2. *Weight of the fetus:* In multiple births, the weight of each of the infants is appreciably less than that of a single birth at the same stage of gestation. The female fetus is 100 gm less in weight than the male foetus.

3. *Crown-heel length of the fetus:* It has been established that there is a close relationship between age and height of the fetus. To calculate age from height, crown-heel length is the best criteria.

4. At 28 weeks, on histopathological examination, respiratory bronchioles proliferate and end in alveolar ducts and sacs. Pulmonary surfactant appears in alveoli of lungs. The surfactant decreases surface tension of alveoli and thus alveoli develop ability to inflate. Due to deficiency of pulmonary surfactant, infant respiratory distress syndrome can occur.

5. Ossification center at Talus is observed at the end of 7th month of intrauterine life.

6. Pupillary membrane disappears, nails are thick but may not reach up to the tips of the fingers and meconium is present in the entire large intestine.

WHETHER DEATH WAS DUE TO NATURAL CAUSES OR DUE TO ANY ACT OF OMISSION OR COMMISSION

Natural Causes of Death

Natural causes in the mother: Death of a child may take place from natural causes in the mother like (i) infectious diseases in the mother, e.g. syphilis, smallpox; (ii) pre-eclamptic toxemia; (iii) placenta previa; and (iv) abnormal gestation (ectopic pregnancy).

Natural causes in newborn: Some of the causes related to new born deaths are; (i) anoxia; (ii) immaturity; (iii) debility; (iv) congenital diseases of heart and lungs; (v) malformations; (vi) hemorrhage from umbilical cord; (vii) prematurity; (viii) neonatal infections; (ix) cerebral trauma; (x) erythroblastosis fetalis or hemolytic disease of the newborn which may manifest in following forms; (a) congenital hydrops fetalis; (b) icterus gravis neonatorum or (c) anemia of the newborn.

Accidental Causes

1. During birth:

a. *Prolonged labour:* Intracranial hemorrhage and death with or without linear fracture of parietal bones of skull may result when the head is severely compressed against the contracted or deformed pelvis. Subdural hemorrhages are present on both sides. Rarely extradural hemorrhage may occur. The cause of hemorrhage is rupture of bridging veins and internal or great cerebral veins and rarely tears of falx cerebri. The finding of moulding and caput succedaneum are usually seen. In addition fracture dislocations of clavicles and limb bones may be present.

b. *Prolapse or pressure on the cord:* In breech presentations when the cord gets compressed by head of fetus, resultant anoxic damage may result in death of the fetus. On autopsy blood, meconium, liquor amnii, vernix caseosa is found in bronchial tubes.

c. *Intravaginal or intrauterine strangulation:* The twisting of the cord and knots in the cord can cause death by strangulating the fetus. The cord gets compressed and there are normally no findings of abrasions or ecchymosis in the cord.

d. *Injury to the mother:* When the mother's abdomen is hit by heavy blows or kicks or fall from height, there may be fracture of skull or rupture of blood vessels and signs of concussion of brain.

e. *Death of the mother:* The child may die with death of the mother and can only be saved when delivered within 5–10 minutes of her death.

2. After birth:

a. *Asphyxia due to suffocation:* The child may die when the fetal membranes cover the head during birth; face gets pressed accidently onto the clothes or when the fetus is submerged in the blood, liquor amnii or meconium discharge, it may die of suffocation. There are chances that the fetus may survive when covered by membranes only for 20–30 minutes.

b. *Suffocation by falling into the lavatory pan:* If birth occurs in the toilet bowel, the infant may inhale the liquid, blood, meconium and vaginal mucus that may be found in the air passages. On microscopic examination of the lungs on the slide under low magnification, the foreign particles can be seen in the drowning fluid. Examination of the cord may reveal torn ends of the cord.

c. *Head injury and fracture of skull:* In accidental fall usually bilateral subdural hemorrhage is present. The average length of the cord is 50 cm that is sufficient to protect the child from falling on the ground. It can withstand the weight of the infant. In these cases, caput succedaneum is not formed. Fissured fracture of skull is present limited to the parietal bone and may extend to frontal or squamous part of the temporal bone. Hemorrhage occurs usually from a fall from 75 cm height but it can also occur in some cases in a fall from a height of 45 cm.

d. *Hemorrhage from the torn ends of the cord:* Though it is not frequently seen.

e. *Precipitate labour:* In precipitate labour all three stages of labour are merged into one. The disproportionately shorter time is taken than an average either by a primipara or multipara. There is expulsion of fetus within less than three hour of commencement of contractions. All the stages of labour are merged into one and woman may deliver unconsciously because the contractile power of uterus is independent of volition. Fetus is normal or premature. It usually occurs in multiparous woman with large, roomy pelvis.

Risk factors: (1) multipara; (2) abruptioplacentae; (3) large, roomy pelvis; (4) small premature baby, mother cannot distinguish between sense of fullness due to descent of child from bulky evacuation.

Postmortem findings: Fractures of the skull from precipitate labour are as a rule stellate, and are situated on the vertex or in the parietal protuberance. The fractures from violence are more extensive, usually depressed, and accompanied by laceration of the scalp.

Medicolegal aspects: Mother or her relative may be accused of infanticide, whilst the death of the fetus may be due to injuries or asphyxia. Differences in detail are mentioned in Table 32.4.

Conditions when delivery can occur without knowledge of mother: Anesthesia, apoplexy, coma, drunkenness, delirium, hypnosis, eclamptic seizures, epileptic fits, influence of narcotics or other intoxicants may be responsible.

Table 32.4: Head injury due to precipitate labour or blunt force trauma		
Findings	*Head injury due to precipitate labour*	*Head injury due to blunt force trauma*
Manner	Accidental	Homicidal
Mechanism	Sudden fall of infant from pelvis to floor	Intention trauma to head
Bruises	On vertex, area in contact with floor	Anywhere on scalp
Scalp lacerations	Absent usually	Present
Fractures	Stellate or linear fracture of parietal bones,	Extensive comminuted, depressed
Brain	Usually no injuries	Injuries present: Hemorrhages, contusions, lacerations

Legal provisions for concealment of birth or abandonment of a child:

Section 318 IPC (concealment of birth by secret disposal of dead body): Law makes it an offence for every person who has tried to intentionally conceal the birth of the child by burying or otherwise disposing of its dead body, whether the child dies during or after its birth, with imprisonment up to 2 years. If the person is charged with murder of the child and later acquitted, he may still be convicted under concealment of birth, depending upon the evidence. There is no need to prove live birth. It is sufficient that there has been a birth and that the child was dead at the time of concealment.

Section 317 I.P.C. (Exposure and abandonment of a child under 12 years by parent or person having care of it): If the mother or father of a child under the age of twelve years, or anyone having care of such child, leaves such child in any place with the intention of abandoning the child, shall be punished with imprisonment up to seven years with/or fine. Average length and weight of Indian infants are mentioned in Table 32.5.

CHILD ABUSE

In 1999, the WHO consultation on child abuse prevention compared definitions of abuse from 58 countries and drafted the following definition:

"Child abuse or maltreatment constitutes all forms of physical and/or emotional ill-treatment, sexual abuse, neglect or negligent treatment or commercial or other exploitation, resulting in actual or potential harm to the child's health, survival, development or dignity in the context of a relationship of responsibility, trust or power".

Brandel's university (Massachusetts) definition of child abuse is "Nonaccidental physical attack or physical injury including minimal as well as fatal injury, inflicted upon children by persons caring for them".

Types of Child Abuse

Physical Abuse

Physical abuse is any nonaccidental injury to a child under the age of 18 by a parent or caretaker. These injuries may include beatings, shaking, burns, human bites, strangulation, or immersion in scalding water or others, with resulting bruises, fractures, scars, burns, internal injuries or other injuries.

a. **Battered baby syndrome:**

Definition: The term battered baby syndrome was coined by "**Henry Kempe**". It is also known as the "**Cafey's syndrome**", "**child abuse syndrome**" or the "**child maltreatment syndrome**". This term was coined to characterise the clinical manifestations of serious physical abuse in young children. This term is generally applied to children showing intentional, repeated and devastating injuries to the skin, skeletal system or nervous system.

Classical features of the syndrome are obscure illness or unexplained injury in infants of six or eight weeks up to four or five years, due to repeated abuse, physical hurt over a period of weeks or months by either or both parents, guardian or baby sitter, who fail to report or delay reporting

Age	Boys		Girls	
	Weight (Kg)	Length (cm)	Weight (Kg)	Length (cm)
At birth	3.3	61.1	3.2	49.9
3 months	6	61.1	5.4	60.2
6 months	7.8	67.8	7.2	66.6
9 months	9.2	72.3	8.6	71.1
1 year	10.2	76.1	9.5	75.0

Table 32.5: Determination of extrauterine age

Average height and weight of Indian infants as per aarogya.com

the incidents, and, who, when they do mislead, indeed deliberately deceive, the nurse or the doctor over the cause.

Predisposing factors:

a. Incidences are more common between the ages of one to three years. The mean age is fourteen months.

b. Incidence is more common in boys.

c. Usually there is only one child in the family.

d. The child is often unwanted or may be born before marriage due to failure of contraception and is usually an illegitimate child.

e. The child may be interfering with the freedom of movements or earning capacity.

f. The incidences are higher in low socio-economic families living in areas of high density.

g. The age of the parents is in early twenties having marital discords and the family is usually isolated.

h. The battering parents were themselves battered children.

i. In the family of battered children, if one child is battered other will be battered too.

j. Adult caregivers may suffer greater stress and social difficulties and have lack of control over stressful situations.

k. Parents are usually of low intelligence and may lack education.

l. Alcoholism or other drug addictions in parents.

Triggering factors: The act of the child like crying, refusal to be quiet and persistent soiling of napkins or acts of "disobedience" precipitates the violence of the parents.

Nature of injuries: The injuries are non-instrumental, but sometimes objects that are handy or in nearby vicinity such as feeding bottles, may be used for hitting. Injuries over the body of child may be observed in the form of:

1. *Injuries to the skin and soft tissue:* Bruises abrasions and lacerations are commonly produced. Soft tissue injuries are almost universal with an incidence of 80–100%. The areas' most commonly affected are head, face and neck. Approximately 50% of physically abused patients have head or facial injuries. Bruises are in various stages of healing and they can be linear or unusual shaped bruises. Multiple bruises matching the shape of a hand, fist or belt are seen. Punching/slapping of face produces characteristic bruises. Bruising of scalp and forehead and underlying skull and brain injuries are produced that may be visible on autopsy. Bruising of external ear, cheeks and the lips especially the upper lip associated with tears or laceration of frenulum of upper lip is characteristic finding. Fingertip pressure marks and grip marks in the form of bruises are seen on neck and sides of the chest formed while gripping the child firmly and violently shaking while stopping him from crying. Encircled bruise around wrists or ankles (indicating twisting) are seen. There are multiple fractures of the posterior parts of the ribs. Bruising of the abdomen is most common after head injuries. The rupture of abdominal viscera may occur. The limbs show bilateral multiple bruising of the forearms, arms and legs.

2. *Human bite marks:* The bites are very commonly produced by the mother that is to be differentiated from the bites by other children. Bites strongly suggest abuse and are easily overlooked.

3. *Head, facial, oral injuries:* Head is a common area of injury in a battered child.

4. *Abusive burn patterns:* Cigarette butt marks in the form of punctuate burns, Scalds due to immersion into hot liquid and splash Burns may be seen. Electric radiator burn marks from child being made to sit upon a stove or electric radiator.

5. *Eye injuries:* The injuries to the eye that are found in battered baby syndrome are black eyes, retinal separation, lens displacement, subconjunctival and retinal hemorrhages.

6. *Visceral injuries:* Rupture of internal organs such as liver, intestine and mesentery account for most of the fatalities due to blows over front of abdomen. The visceral injuries are the most common cause of death.

7. Miscellaneous findings:
   a. Loss of tuft of hair as a result of pulling the child by holding his hair.
   b. In most cases history of fall is given by the parents, which according to them has resulted in injuries. If a child is reported to have had a fall but has severe injuries of different durations; this inconsistency of the history with the injuries indicates child abuse.

8. *Radiological examination:* Whole body X-ray before autopsy is important in such cases. Other imaging techniques, such as MRI or scans, may confirm or reveal other internal injuries. Fractures of skull and ribs (beading effect) along with spiral fracture of long bones resulting from twisting are indicative of child battering. The characteristic finding is of multiple fractures in different stages of healing. Callous formation is important in identifying and approximately dating old healing fractures. Epiphyseal separation is seen around elbow and knee joint when limb is involved. Another characteristic finding is subperiosteal calcification in periosteal hemorrhages due to shearing and elevation.

b. **Shaken baby syndrome:** Shaking is a prevalent form of abuse seen in very young children (less than 1 year). Most perpetrators of such abuse are males. Intracranial hemorrhages, retinal hemorrhages and chip fractures of the child's extremities can result from very rapid shaking of an infant.

c. **Corporal punishment of children:** Corporal punishment in the form of hitting, punching, kicking or beating is socially and legally accepted in some countries. In many, it is a significant phenomenon in schools and other institutions and in penal systems for young offenders.

Sexual Abuse

Child sexual abuse is the exploitation of a child or adolescent for the sexual gratification of another person.

Emotional Abuse

Emotional abuse includes the failure of a caregiver to provide an appropriate and supportive environment, and includes acts that have an adverse effect on the emotional health and development of a child.

Such acts include restricting a child's movements, denigration, ridicule, threats and intimidation, discrimination, rejection and other nonphysical forms of hostile treatment.

Neglect

Neglect refers to the failure of a parent to provide for the development of the child, where the parent is in a position to do so, in one or more of the following areas; health, education, emotional development, nutrition, shelter and safe living conditions.

Neglect is thus distinguished from circumstances of poverty in that neglect can occur only in cases where reasonable resources are available to the family or caregiver.

SUDDEN INFANT DEATH SYNDROME

Sudden infant death syndrome (SIDS) is the sudden unexplained natural death of a child less than one year of age that remains unexplained even after a thorough autopsy, detailed death scene investigation and review of clinical and social history. SIDS usually occurs during sleep. SIDS is also known as "**crib death** or **cot death**" because many babies who die of SIDS are found in their cribs/cots.

It is not a recognised cause of death in India due to much higher level of infant mortality as the increased rate of death from causes like infections and malnourishment overshadows cot deaths.

Predisposing Factors

a. *Age of the infant:* SIDS is the leading cause of death in children between one month and one year old. Most SIDS deaths occur when babies are between two months and four months old.
b. *Sex incidence:* More common in male babies.
c. *Season:* In temperate countries mostly seen in winter months. It may coincide with infection prone period.
d. *Prematurity:* Premature babies with low birth weight have a higher risk of SIDS.
e. *Time of death:* Mostly at home between 6 PM in the evening to 10 AM in the morning.
f. *Socioeconomic status:* More frequent in low socioeconomic group living in areas of high density population.

Mode of Death

Suggest a rapid terminal event. The baby dies silently in sleep.

Classic presentation of SIDS begins with an infant who is put to bed, typically after breastfeeding or bottle-feeding. Checks of the baby at varying intervals are unremarkable, but the baby is found dead, usually in the position in which he or she had been placed at bedtime or naptime. Most of infants are apparently healthy except in some cases where upper respiratory tract infections may be present.

Examination of Scene of Death

No disturbance is seen at the scene of death. Efforts must be made to distinguish death from various forms of suffocation (as in abuse). At the scene of death examine for signs of environmental factors that may have contributed to the death.

The forensic pathologist's diagnosis of SIDS is one of exclusion. To confirm the diagnosis of SIDS, a complete forensic autopsy needs to be performed, using information gathered from the scene investigation, interview of caregivers and review of medical and social history. It is more accurate to use **"Sudden unexpected infant death" (SUID)** if there is no external evidence of injury to the infant and no scene information to suggest another cause of death.

In very few cases some histopathological changes are observed like upper respiratory infection, intraalveolar mononuclear cells with explosive desquamation of bronchial epithelial cells, mild diffuse alveolar distension with some amount of pulmonary edema. Few cases may even show petechial hemorrhages. Cardiac conduction system may show hemorrhage and degeneration of cardiac ganglia. Few cases may show colloid depletion of thyroid follicles. Area of fibrinoid necrosis on the vocal cords may suggest fatal laryngospasm.

Causes of SIDS

Even though no definite cause is known, some of the following theories have been suggested for deaths from SIDS:

1. The morphological differences in the brainstem of infants who have died from SIDS indicate that such cases may represent immature development of centers responsible for arousal, cardiovascular, and respiratory functions. When the cardiorespiratory system becomes compromised due to noxious environmental conditions (hypoxia, hypercarbia) during sleep, such infants may not become aroused to defend against these conditions, resulting in sudden death.
2. Suffocation is suspected in many cases but not proved. Hypoxia resulting from face pressing against a pillow especially in obligatory mouth breathers. Laryngospasm also has been postulated as one of the reason. *Sleep apnea* is one of the most accepted theories for causation of SIDS. Prone sleep position, maternal smoking and accidental suffocation such as during bed sharing with another adult/child may also play a role.
3. Hypersensitivity to cow's milk or to viral infections has been advocated as the child is mostly bottle-fed, there is high level of milk antibodies and milk has been seen in the lungs in few cases.

4. Ammonia poisoning resulting when the baby is fully covered and ammonia gas is liberated from nappies loaded with urine and feces.

5. Other probable causes include infections (viral or bacterial), genetic disorders, conduction disorders in heart, adrenal and parathyroid abnormality and subclinical amino acid disorder.

Even when a thorough investigation is conducted, it may be difficult to separate SIDS from other types of sudden unexplained infant deaths (SUIDs), especially unintentional suffocation in an adult bed. After a thorough case investigation, some of these SUIDs may be explained.

MUNCHAUSEN SYNDROME BY PROXY

Munchausen by proxy syndrome was described using that term in 1977 by Roy Meadow in cases involving caregivers who fake symptoms by causing injury to someone else, often a child, and then want to be with that person in a hospital or similar medical setting. Since mothers continue to be the primary caregivers in many societies, the mother is often the individual identified as having Munchausen syndrome by proxy, but anyone in the role of parent or caregiver may develop this condition.

Symptoms

The mother can do extreme things to fake symptoms of illness in her child. For example, she may:

1. Add blood to the child's urine or stool.
2. Withhold food so the child looks like they cannot gain weight.
3. Heat up thermometers so it looks like the child has a fever.
4. Make up lab results.
5. Give the child drugs to make the child throw up or have diarrhea.
6. Infect an intravenous line to make the child sick.

These mothers are really involved with their children. They seem devoted to the child. This makes it hard for health professionals to see a diagnosis of Munchausen syndrome by proxy.

The mother makes frequent visits to different doctors and hospitals. The child may undergoes various tests, surgeries or other procedures but without any improvement. The symptoms of the child do not match the test results. The child's symptoms are reported by the mother, but are never seen by health care professionals. Even the blood samples do not match the child's blood type. However, drugs or chemicals may be found in the child's urine, blood, or stool.

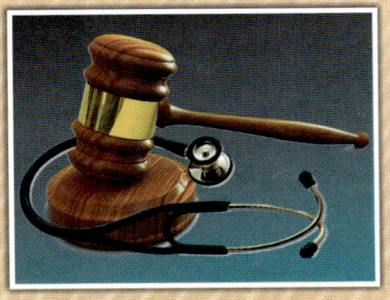

Medical Jurisprudence

33 | Medical Jurisprudence

Medical Jurisprudence (Juris = law, Prudence = knowledge): It deals with legal aspects of the practice of medicine like responsibilities of a medical professional, medical negligence, ethics, duties, etiquette and laws governing medical practice.

Medical ethics is a system of moral principles or code of conduct derived by the governing professional bodies that apply values and judgements to the practice of **medicine**. As a scholarly discipline, **medical ethics** encompasses its practical application in clinical settings as well as work on its history, philosophy, theology, and sociology.

A common framework used in the analysis of medical ethics recognises four basic moral principles, which are to be judged and weighed against each other, with attention given to the scope of their application. The four principles are as follows:

i. *Respect for autonomy:* The patient has the right to refuse or choose his or her treatment. This is rooted in society's respect for individuals' ability to make informed decisions about personal matters.

ii. *Beneficence:* A practitioner should act in the best interest of the patient.

iii. *Nonmaleficence:* The concept of nonmaleficence is embodied by the phrase "first, do no harm". Many consider that should be the main or primary consideration, that it is more important not to harm your patient, than to do them good.

iv. *Justice (fairness and equality):* Concerns the distribution of scarce health resources, and the decision of who gets what treatment.

When moral values are in conflict, the result may be an ethical dilemma or crisis, for example the principles of autonomy and beneficence clash when patients refuse blood transfusions or when a patient does not want a treatment because of cultural or religious beliefs.

Double effect: Double effect refers to two types of consequences that may be produced by a single action and in medical ethics it is usually regarded as the **combined effect of beneficence and nonmaleficence.** A commonly cited example of this phenomenon is the **use of morphine or other analgesic in the dying patient**. Such use of morphine can have the beneficial effect of easing the pain and suffering of the patient while simultaneously having the maleficent effect of shortening the life of the patient through suppression of the respiratory system.

THE INDIAN MEDICAL DEGREES ACT, 1916

An act to regulate the grant of titles implying qualification in western medical science and the assumption and use by unqualified persons of such title is punishable under the act.

MEDICAL COUNCIL OF INDIA (MCI)

Medical Council of India (MCI) is a statutory body with the responsibility of establishing and maintaining high standards of medical education and recognition of medical qualifications in India. It registers doctors to practice in India, in order to protect and promote the health and safety of the public by ensuring proper standards in the practice of medicine.

The medical council of India was established in 1934 under the Indian medical council act, 1933, now repealed, with the main function of establishing uniform standards of higher qualifications in medicine and recognition of medical qualifications in India and abroad. The number of medical colleges had increased steadily after independence. It was felt that the provisions of Indian medical council act were not adequate to meet with the challenges posed by the very fast development and the progress of medical education in the country. As a result, in 1956, the old act was repealed and a new one was enacted. This was further modified in 1964, 1993 and 2001.

The Objectives and Functions of the Indian Medical Council (MCI)

1. **Medical education:** It is responsible for the maintenance of uniform standards of medical education throughout the country for both undergraduate and postgraduate courses. Prior approval of the MCI is required to start any undergraduate or postgraduate course. Medical inspectors appointed by the MCI visit the medical college for verification of the staff; infrastructure and clinical load required for starting a course, increase in the seats or renewal of recognition and submit their report. MCI based on the inspection report sends its recommendations to the health ministry, Government of India for grant of approval or to withdraw recognition.

2. **Maintenance of medical register:** MCI maintain a register of doctors with recognised medical qualifications. State medical councils send the name of medical practioner registered with them to the MCI to be entered in the medical register. Similarly, if the name of any medical practitioner has been removed for medical negligence or unethical conduct by the state medical council the same is also intimated to the MCI.

3. **Recognition of foreign medical qualifications:** Such foreign degrees which are mentioned under part-II of the third schedule are recognised by the MCI. In a case where a degree is not mentioned in the part-II of the third schedule the medical council may negotiate with a foreign country and on the basis of reciprocity, mutual recognition of medical qualifications may be undertaken.

4. **Appeal against disciplinary action:** Any medical practitioner aggrieved by the action of the state medical council may appeal to the central ministry of health within 60 days, which refers the case to MCI for examination. Ethics committee of the MCI after thorough examination recommends their decision which is binding on the state medical council.

5. **Warning notice**: In case any medical practitioner fails to abide by the code of ethics and professional conduct prescribed by the MCI, a warning notice is issued to him.

Constitution of Medical Council

Following members are appointed for a period of 5 years:

i. One member from each university elected amongst the medical faculty by the university court or senate.

ii. One member to be elected from the registered medical practioners enrolled in a state medical council register.

iii. One member from each state to be nominated by the central government in consultation with state governments.

iv. Seven members to be elected from the enrolled members in any state medical register possessing qualifications included in part-I of the third schedule.

v. Eight members to be nominated by the central government.

President and vice president are elected amongst the members. The council members also constitute an executive committee and other committees as per the constitution of the MCI. Secretary is appointed by the members to look after routine work of the council.

THE INDIAN MEDICAL COUNCIL ACT, 1956

(As amended by the Indian medical council amendment acts, 1964, 1993 and 2001): An act to provide for the reconstitution of the medical council of India and the maintenance of a medical register for India and for matters connected therewith.

1. **The first schedule of IMC act:** List of colleges and courses as per the first schedule of IMC act, i.e. UG and PG degrees recognised in India.
2. **The second schedule:** Recognised medical qualifications granted by medical institutions outside India.
3. **The third schedule (Part I):** Recognised medical qualifications granted by medical institutions not included in the first schedule.

Formation of national medical commission is under active consideration of the Government of India. A draft National Medical Commission Bill 2016 has been circulated by the Niti Aayog so as to create a world class medical education system and to repeal Indian Medical Council Act 1956.

STATE MEDICAL COUNCILS (SMCs)

These are bodies instituted by state governments for registration and to regulate conduct of the medical practitioners working in that state. The state medical council is constituted by members of the medical profession from (i) elected members from the medical teachers from various universities/medical colleges in the state; (ii) elected members from the registered medical practitioners in that state; (iii) nominated members by the state government; and (iv) some exofficio members.

All these members elect a president and a vice president and other bodies like executive body, disciplinary body and financial body for executing the work assigned to the state medical council.

Duties and Responsibilities of SMC

State medical council has primarily two responsibilities:

i. *Maintenance of medical register:* On payment of prescribed fee the names of the medical practioners working in the jurisdiction of the state medical council are entered in a medical register. This registration may be provisional as granted to medical students after clearing final MBBS examination, during internship training or permanent registration after completing internship training. Every person whose name is entered in the register is given a certificate in the prescribed form. Such certificate may remain valid for a specified period as mentioned on them and after that period they have to be renewed.

ii. *Disciplinary control:* All registered medical practitioners of that state are under the disciplinary control of that particular state medical council. Any professional misconduct brought to the notice of the state medical council by any law enforcing agency, any public person including patients and their relatives or body and conviction by a court on account of any criminal act are enquired. The registrar of the state medical council on receipt of a complaint brings it to the knowledge of the president of the state medical council. The complaint is then handed over to the disciplinary committee for conduct of disciplinary enquiry. If required the disciplinary committee may co-opt any expert from the concerned field to help the committee. Complainant as well as the doctor concerned is called for providing evidence to prove charges or to defend himself respectively. In case a doctor is found guilty of professional misconduct the disciplinary committee recommends to reprimand a practitioner by issuing a warning; removal of the name from the register altogether or for a specified period of time. These recommendations are placed before the general body of the state medical council for approval. Decision on the complaint is taken within six months by the state medical council. Appeal against the verdict of state medical council is done within 60 days to the central health ministry (representations are received by MCI as per MCI regulations). Indian medical council review such cases as per MCI regulations and recommendations are forwarded to the central health ministry.

INDIAN MEDICAL COUNCIL (PROFESSIONAL CONDUCT, ETIQUETTE AND ETHICS) REGULATIONS, 2002 (AS AMENDED UP TO 2016)

The Medical Council of India, with the approval of the central government, made regulations relating to the general duties and responsibilities, duties towards their patients, duties in consultation, etiquette, unethical acts, professional misconduct, and punishment and disciplinary action for professional misconduct of registered medical practitioners.

Chapter 1: Code of Medical Ethics

A. Declaration

Each applicant, at the time of making an application for registration under the provisions of the act, shall be provided a copy of the declaration and shall submit a duly signed declaration. The applicant shall also certify that he/she had read and agreed to abide by the same.

B. Duties and Responsibilities of the Physician in General

1.1. Character of physician: Doctors with qualification of MBBS or MBBS with postgraduate degree/diploma or with equivalent qualification in any medical discipline:

1.1.1. A physician shall uphold the dignity and honour of his profession.

1.1.2. The prime object of the medical profession is to render service to humanity; reward or financial gain is a subordinate consideration. A physician should be an upright man, instructed in the art of healings. He shall keep himself pure in character and be diligent in caring for the sick; he should be modest, sober, patient, prompt in discharging his duty without anxiety; conducting himself with propriety in his profession and in all the actions of his life.

1.1.3. No person other than a doctor having qualification recognised by medical council of India and registered with medical council of India/State medical council (s) is allowed to practice modern system of medicine or surgery.

1.2. Maintaining good medical practice:

1.2.1. The principal objective of the medical profession is to render service to humanity with full respect for the dignity of profession and man. Physicians should merit the confidence of patients entrusted to their care, rendering to each a full measure of service and devotion. Physicians should try continuously to improve medical knowledge and skills and should make available to their patients and colleagues the benefits of their professional attainments. The physician should practice methods of healing founded on scientific basis and should not associate professionally with anyone who violates this principle. The honoured ideals of the medical profession imply that the responsibilities of the physician extend not only to individuals but also to society.

1.2.2. Membership in medical society: For the advancement of his profession, a physician should affiliate with associations and societies of allopathic medical professions and involve actively in the functioning of such bodies.

1.2.3. A physician should participate in professional meetings as part of continuing medical education programmes, for at least 30 hours every five years, organized by reputed professional academic bodies or any other authorized organisations. The compliance of this requirement shall be informed regularly to medical council of India or the state medical councils as the case may be.

1.3. Maintenance of medical records:

1.3.1. Every physician shall maintain the medical records pertaining to his/her **indoor patients for a period of 3 years** from the date of commencement of the treatment in a standard proforma laid down by the medical council of India.

1.3.2. If any request is made for medical records either by the patients/authorised attendant or legal authorities involved, the same may be duly acknowledged and documents shall be issued within the period of 72 hours.

1.3.3. A registered medical practitioner shall maintain a register of medical certificates giving full details of certificates issued. When issuing a medical certificate he/she shall always enter the identification marks of the patient and keep a copy of the certificate. He/she shall not omit to record the signature and/or thumb mark, address and at least one identification mark of the patient on the medical certificates or report.

1.3.4. Efforts shall be made to computerize medical records for quick retrieval.

1.4. Display of registration numbers:

1.4.1. Every physician shall display the registration number accorded to him by the state medical council/medical council of India in his clinic and in all his prescriptions, certificates, money receipts given to his patients.

1.4.2. Physicians shall display as suffix to their names only recognized medical degrees or such certificates/diplomas and memberships/honours which confer professional knowledge or recognizes any exemplary qualification/achievements.

1.5. Use of generic names of drugs: Every physician shall prescribe drugs with generic names legibly and preferably in capital letters and he/she shall ensure that there is a rational prescription and use of drugs.

1.6. Highest quality assurance in patient care: Every physician should aid in safeguarding the profession against admission to it of those who are deficient in moral character or education. Physician shall not employ in connection with his professional practice any attendant who is neither registered nor enlisted under the Medical Acts in force and shall not permit such persons to attend, treat or perform operations upon patients wherever professional discretion or skill is required.

1.7. Exposure of unethical conduct: A physician should expose, without fear or favour, incompetent or corrupt, dishonest or unethical conduct on the part of members of the profession.

1.8. Payment of professional services: The physician, engaged in the practice of medicine shall give priority to the interests of patients. The personal financial interests of a physician should not conflict with the medical interests of patients. A physician should announce his fees before rendering service and not after the operation or treatment is under way. Remuneration received for such services should be in the form and amount specifically announced to the patient at the time the service is rendered. It is unethical to enter into a contract of "no cure no payment". Physician rendering service on behalf of the state shall refrain from anticipating or accepting any consideration.

1.9. Evasion of legal restrictions: The physician shall observe the laws of the country in regulating the practice of medicine and shall also not assist others to evade such laws. He should be cooperative in observance and enforcement of sanitary laws and regulations in the interest of public health. A physician should observe the provisions of the acts, rules, regulations made by the central/state governments or local administrative bodies or any other relevant act relating to the protection and promotion of public health.

Chapter 2: Duties of Physicians to their Patients

2.1. Obligations to the sick

2.1.1. Though a physician is not bound to treat each and every person asking his services, he should not only be ever ready to respond to the calls of the sick and the injured, but should be mindful of the high character of his mission and the responsibility he discharges in the course of his professional duties. In his treatment, he should never forget that the health and the lives of those entrusted to his care depend on his skill and attention. A physician should endeavour to add to the comfort of the sick by making his visits at the hour indicated to the patients. A physician advising a patient to seek service of another physician is acceptable; however, in case of emergency a physician must treat the patient. No physician shall arbitrarily refuse treatment to a patient. However for good reason, when a patient is suffering from an ailment which is not within the range of experience of the treating physician, the physician may refuse treatment and refer the patient to another physician.

Medical practitioner having any incapacity detrimental to the patient or which can affect his performance vis-à-vis the patient is not permitted to practice his profession.

2.2. Patience, delicacy and secrecy: Patience and delicacy should characterize the physician. Confidences concerning individual or domestic life entrusted by patients to a physician and defects in the disposition or character of patients observed during medical attendance should never be revealed unless their revelation is required by the laws of the State. Sometimes, however, a physician must determine whether his duty to society requires him to employ knowledge, obtained through confidence as a physician, to protect a healthy person against a communicable disease to which he is about to be exposed. In such instance, the physician should act as he would wish another to act toward one of his own family in like circumstances.

2.3. Prognosis: The physician should neither exaggerate nor minimize the gravity of a patient's condition. He should ensure himself that the patient, his relatives or his responsible friends have such knowledge of the patient's condition as will serve the best interests of the patient and the family.

2.4. The patient must not be neglected: A physician is free to choose whom he will serve. He should, however, respond to any request for his assistance in an emergency. Once having undertaken a case, the physician should not neglect the patient, nor should he withdraw from the case without giving adequate notice to the patient and his family. Provisionally or fully registered medical practitioner shall not wilfully commit an act of negligence that may deprive his patient or patients from necessary medical care.

2.5. Engagement for an obstetric case: When a physician who has been engaged to attend an obstetric case is absent and another is sent for and delivery accomplished, the acting physician is entitled to his professional fees, but should secure the patient's consent to resign on the arrival of the physician engaged.

Chapter 3: Duties of Physician in Consultation

3.1. Unnecessary consultations should be avoided:

3.1.1. However in case of serious illness and in doubtful or difficult conditions, the physician should request consultation, but under any circumstances such consultation should be justifiable and in the interest of the patient only and not for any other consideration.

3.1.2. Consulting pathologists/radiologists asking for any other diagnostic lab investigation should be done judiciously and not in a routine manner.

3.2. Consultation for patient's benefit: In every consultation, the benefit to the patient is of foremost importance. All physicians engaged in the case should be frank with the patient and his attendants.

3.3. Punctuality in consultation: Utmost punctuality should be observed by a physician in making themselves available for consultations.

3.4. Statement to patient after consultation:

3.4.1. All statements to the patient or his representatives should take place in the presence of the consulting physicians, except as otherwise agreed. The disclosure of the opinion to the patient or his relatives or friends shall rest with the medical attendant.

3.4.2. Differences of opinion should not be divulged unnecessarily but when there is irreconcilable difference of opinion the circumstances should be frankly and impartially explained to the patient or his relatives or friends. It would be opened to them to seek further advice as they so desire.

3.5. Treatment after consultation: No decision should restrain the attending physician from making such subsequent variations in the treatment if any unexpected change occurs, but at the next consultation, reasons for the variations should be discussed/explained. The same privilege, with its obligations, belongs to the consultant when sent for in an emergency during the absence of attending physician. The attending physician may prescribe medicine at any time for the patient, whereas the consultant may prescribe only in case of emergency or as an expert when called for.

3.6. Patients referred to specialists: When a patient is referred to a specialist by the attending physician, a case summary of the patient should be given to the specialist, who should communicate his opinion in writing to the attending physician.

3.7. Fees and other charges:

3.7.1. A physician shall clearly display his fees and other charges on the board of his chamber and/or the hospitals he is visiting. Prescription should also make clear if the physician himself dispensed any medicine.

3.7.2. A physician shall write his name and designation in full along with registration particulars in his prescription letter head.

Note: In government hospital where the patient–load is heavy, the name of the prescribing doctor must be written below his/her signature.

Chapter 4: Responsibilities of Physicians to Each Other

4.1. A physician should consider it as a pleasure and privilege to render gratuitous service to all physicians and their immediate family dependents.

4.2. Conduct in consultation: In consultations, no insincerity, rivalry or envy should be indulged in. All due respect should be observed towards the physician incharge of the case and no statement or remark be made, which would impair the confidence reposed in him. For this purpose no discussion should be carried on in the presence of the patient or his representatives.

4.3. Consultant not to take charge of the case: When a physician has been called for consultation, the consultant should normally not take charge of the case, especially on the solicitation of the patient or friends. The consultant shall not criticize the referring physician. He/she shall discuss the diagnosis and treatment plan with the referring physician.

4.4. Appointment of substitute: Whenever a physician requests another physician to attend his patients during his temporary absence from his practice, professional courtesy requires the acceptance of such appointment only when he has the capacity to discharge the additional responsibility along with his/her other duties. The physician acting under such an appointment should give the utmost consideration to the interests and reputation of the absent physician and all such patients should be restored to the care of the latter upon his/her return.

4.5. Visiting another physician's case: When it becomes the duty of a physician occupying an official position to see and report upon an illness or injury, he should communicate to the physician in attendance so as to give him an option of being present. The medical officer/physician occupying an official position should avoid remarks upon the diagnosis or the treatment that has been adopted.

Chapter 5: Duties of Physician to the Public and to the Paramedical Profession

5.1. Physicians as citizens: Physicians, as good citizens, possessed of special training should disseminate advice on public health issues. They should play their part in enforcing the laws of the community and in sustaining the institutions that advance the interests of humanity. They should particularly co-operate with the authorities in the administration of sanitary/public health laws and regulations.

5.2. Public and community health: Physicians, especially those engaged in public health work, should enlighten the public concerning quarantine regulations and measures for the prevention of epidemic and communicable diseases. At all times the physician should notify the constituted public health authorities of every case of communicable disease under his care, in accordance with the laws, rules and regulations of the health authorities. When an epidemic occurs a physician should not abandon his duty for fear of contracting the disease himself.

5.3. Pharmacists/Nurses: Physicians should recognize and promote the practice of different paramedical services such as, pharmacy and nursing as professions and should seek their cooperation wherever required.

Chapter 6: Unethical Acts

A physician shall not aid or abet or commit any of the following acts which shall be construed as unethical.

6.1. Advertising

6.1.1. Soliciting of patients directly or indirectly, by a physician, by a group of physicians or by institutions or organisations is unethical. A physician shall not make use of him/her (or his/her name) as subject of any form or manner of advertising or publicity through any mode either alone or in conjunction with others which is of such a character as to invite attention to him or to his professional position, skill, qualification, achievements, attainments, specialities, appointments, associations, affiliations or honours and/or of such character as would ordinarily result in his self-aggrandizement. A physician shall not give to any person, whether for compensation or otherwise, any approval, recommendation, endorsement, certificate, report or statement with respect of any drug, medicine, nostrum remedy, surgical, or therapeutic article, apparatus or appliance or any commercial product or article with respect of any property, quality or use thereof or any test, demonstration or trial thereof, for use in connection with his name, signature, or photograph in any form or manner of advertising through any mode nor shall he boast of cases, operations, cures or remedies or permit the publication of report thereof through any mode. A medical practitioner is however permitted to make a formal announcement in press regarding the following:

1. On starting practice.
2. On change of type of practice.
3. On changing address.
4. On temporary absence from duty.
5. On resumption of another practice.
6. On succeeding to another practice.
7. Public declaration of charges.

6.1.2. Printing of self-photograph or any such material of publicity in the letter head or on sign board of the consulting room or any such clinical establishment shall be regarded as acts of self-advertisement and unethical conduct on the part of the physician. However, printing of sketches, diagrams, picture of human system shall not be treated as unethical.

6.2. Patent and copyrights: A physician may patent surgical instruments, appliances and medicine or copyright applications, methods and procedures. However, it shall be unethical if the benefits of such patents or copyrights are not made available in situations where the interest of large population is involved.

6.3. Running an open shop (dispensing of drugs and appliances by Physicians): A physician should not run an open shop for sale of medicine for dispensing prescriptions prescribed by doctors other than himself or for sale of medical or surgical appliances. It is not unethical for a physician to prescribe or supply drugs,

remedies or appliances as long as there is no exploitation of the patient. Drugs prescribed by a physician or brought from the market for a patient should explicitly state the proprietary formulae as well as generic name of the drug.

6.4. Rebates and commission:

6.4.1. A physician shall not give, solicit, or receive nor shall he offer to give solicit or receive, any gift, gratuity, commission or bonus in consideration of or return for the referring, recommending or procuring of any patient for medical, surgical or other treatment. A physician shall not directly or indirectly, participate in or be a party to act of division, transference, assignment, subordination, rebating, splitting or refunding of any fee for medical, surgical or other treatment.

6.4.2. Provisions of para 6.4.1 shall apply with equal force to the referring, recommending or procuring by a physician or any person, specimen or material for diagnostic purposes or other study/work. Nothing in this section, however, shall prohibit payment of salaries by a qualified physician to other duly qualified person rendering medical care under his supervision.

6.5. Secret remedies: The prescribing or dispensing by a physician of secret remedial agents of which he does not know the composition, or the manufacture or promotion of their use is unethical and as such prohibited. All the drugs prescribed by a physician should always carry a proprietary formula and clear name.

6.6. Human rights: The physician shall not aid or abet torture nor shall he be a party to either infliction of mental or physical trauma or concealment of torture inflicted by some other person or agency in clear violation of human rights.

6.7. Euthanasia: Practicing euthanasia shall constitute unethical conduct. However on specific occasion, the question of withdrawing supporting devices to sustain cardiopulmonary function even after brain death, shall be decided only by a team of doctors and not merely by the treating physician alone. A team of doctors shall declare withdrawal of support system. Such team shall consist of the doctor incharge of the patient, chief medical officer/medical officer incharge of the hospital and a doctor nominated by the incharge of the hospital from the hospital staff or in accordance with the provisions of the transplantation of human organ act, 1994.

6.8. Code of conduct for doctors in their relationship with pharmaceutical and allied health sector industry.

6.8.1. In dealing with pharmaceutical and allied health sector industry, a medical practitioner shall follow and adhere to the stipulations given below:

a. *Gifts:* A medical practitioner shall not receive any gift from any pharmaceutical or allied health care industry and their sales people or representatives. Gifts more than ₹ 1,000/- up to ₹ 5,000/-: Censure. Gifts more than ₹ 5,000/- up to ₹ 10,000/-: Removal from Indian Medical Register or State Medical Register for 3 (three) months. Gifts more than ₹ 10,000/- to ₹ 50,000/-: Removal from Indian Medical Register or State Medical Register for 6 (six) months. Gifts more than ₹ 50,000/- to ₹ 1,00,000/-: Removal from Indian Medical Register or State Medical Register for 1 (one) year. Gifts more than ₹ 1,00,000/-: Removal for a period of more than 1 (one) year from Indian Medical Register or State Medical Register.

b. *Travel facilities:* A medical practitioner shall not accept any travel facility inside the country or outside, including rail, road, air, ship, cruise tickets, paid vacations, etc. from any pharmaceutical or allied healthcare industry or their representatives for self and family members for vacation or for attending conferences, seminars, workshops, CME programme, etc. as a delegate. Expenses for travel facilities more than ₹ 1,000/- up to ₹ 5,000/-: Censure. Expenses for travel facilities more than ₹ 5,000/- up to ₹ 10,000/-: Removal from Indian Medical Register or State Medical Register for 3 (three) months. Expenses for travel facilities more than ₹ 10,000/- to ₹ 50,000/-: Removal from Indian Medical Register or State medical Register for 6 (six) months. Expenses for travel facilities more than more than ₹ 50,000/- to ₹ 1,00,000/-: Removal from Indian Medical Register or State Medical Register for 1 (one) year. Expenses for travel facilities more than ₹ 1,00,000/-: Removal for a period of more than 1 (one) year from Indian Medical Register or State Medical Register.

c. *Hospitality:* A medical practitioner shall not accept individually any hospitality like hotel accommodation for self and family members under any pretext. Expenses for Hospitality more than ₹ 1,000/- up to ₹ 5,000 -: Censure Expenses for Hospitality more than ₹ 5,000/- up to ₹ 10,000/-: Removal from Indian Medical Register or State Medical Register for 3 (three) months. Expenses for Hospitality more than ₹ 10,000/- to ₹ 50,000/-: Removal from Indian Medical Register or State medical Register for 6 (six) months. Expenses for Hospitality more than ₹ 50,000/- to ₹ 1,00,000/: Removal from Indian Medical Register or State Medical Register for 1 (one) year. Expenses for Hospitality more than ₹ 1,00,000/-: Removal for a period of more 11 than

1 (one) year from Indian Medical Register or State Medical Register.

d. *Cash or monetary grants:* A medical practitioner shall not receive any cash or monetary grants from any pharmaceutical and allied healthcare industry for individual purpose in individual capacity under any pretext. Funding for medical research, study, etc. can only be received through approved institutions by modalities laid down by law/rules/guidelines adopted by such approved institutions, in a transparent manner. It shall always be fully disclosed. Cash or monetary grants more than ₹ 1,000/- up to ₹ 5,000/-: Censure Cash or monetary grants more than ₹ 5,000/- up to ₹ 10,000/-: Removal from Indian Medical Register or State Medical Register for 3 (three) months. Cash or monetary grants more than ₹ 10,000/- to ₹ 50,000/-: Removal from Indian Medical Register or State Medical Register for 6 (six) months. Cash or monetary grants more than ₹ 50,000/- to ₹ 1,00,000/-: Removal from Indian Medical Register or State Medical Register for 1 (one) year. Cash or monetary grants more than ₹ 1,00,000/-: Removal for a period of more than 1 (one) year from Indian Medical Register or State Medical Register.

e. *Medical Research:* A medical practitioner may carry-out, participate in, work in research projects funded by pharmaceutical and allied healthcare industries. A medical practitioner is obliged to know that the fulfillment of the following items (i) to (vii) will be an imperative for undertaking any research assignment/project funded by industry – for being proper and ethical. Thus, in accepting such a position a medical practitioner shall:- (i) ensure that the particular research proposal(s) has the due permission from the competent concerned authorities. (ii) ensure that such a research project(s) has the clearance of national/state/institutional ethics committees/bodies. (iii) ensure that it fulfils all the legal requirements prescribed for medical research. (iv) ensure that the source and amount of funding is publicly disclosed at the beginning itself. (v) ensure that proper care and facilities are provided to human volunteers, if they are necessary for the research project(s). First time censure, and thereafter removal of name from Indian Medical Register or State Medical Register for a period depending upon the violation of the clause. (vi) ensure that undue animal experimentations are not done and when these are necessary they are done in a scientific and a humane way. (vii) ensure that while accepting such an assignment a medical practitioner shall have the freedom to publish the results of the research in the greater interest of the society by inserting such a clause in the MoU or any other documents/agreement for any such assignment.

f. *Maintaining Professional Autonomy:* In dealing with pharmaceutical and allied healthcare industry a medical practitioner shall always ensure that there shall never be any compromise either with his/her own professional autonomy and/or with the autonomy and freedom of the medical institution. First time censure, and thereafter removal of name from Indian Medical Register or State Medical Register.

g. *Affiliation:* A medical practitioner may work for pharmaceutical and allied healthcare industries in advisory capacities, as consultants, as researchers, as treating doctors or in any other professional capacity. In doing so, a medical practitioner shall always: (i) ensure that his professional integrity and freedom are maintained. (ii) ensure that patients' interests are not compromised in any way. (iii) ensure that such affiliations are within the law. (iv) ensure that such affiliations/employments are fully transparent and disclosed. First time censure, and thereafter removal of name from Indian Medical Register or State Medical Register for a period depending upon the violaton of the clause.

h. *Endorsement:* A medical practitioner shall not endorse any drug or product of the industry publically. Any study conducted on the efficacy or otherwise of such products shall be presented to and/or through appropriate scientific bodies or published in appropriate scientific journals in a proper way. First time censure, and thereafter removal of name from Indian Medical Register or State Medical Register.

6.8.2: **Travel Facilities:** A medical practitioner shall not accept any travel facility inside the country or outside, including rail, road, air, ship, cruise tickets, paid vacation, etc. from any pharmaceutical or allied healthcare industry or their representatives for self and family members for vacation or for attending conferences, seminars, workshops, CME Programme, etc. as a delegate.

Chapter 7: Misconduct

The following acts of commission or omission on the part of a physician shall constitute *professional misconduct* rendering him/her liable for disciplinary action:

7.1. **Violation of the regulations**: If he/she commits any violation of these regulations.

7.2. If he/she does not maintain the medical records of his/her indoor patients for a period of three years as per regulation 1.3 and refuses to provide the same within 72 hours when the patient or his/her authorised representative makes a request for it as per the regulation 1.3.2.

7.3. If he/she does not display the registration number accorded to him/her by the state medical council or the medical council of India in his clinic, prescriptions and certificates, etc. issued by him or violates the provisions of regulation 1.4.2.

7.4. **Adultery or improper conduct:** Abuse of professional position by committing adultery or improper conduct with a patient or by maintaining an improper association with a patient will render a physician liable for disciplinary action as provided under the Indian medical council act, 1956 or the concerned State medical council act.

7.5. **Conviction by court of law:** Conviction by a court of law for offences involving moral turpitude/criminal acts.

7.6. **Sex determination tests:** On no account sex determination test shall be undertaken with the intent to terminate the life of a female fetus developing in her mother's womb, unless there are other absolute indications for termination of pregnancy as specified in the medical termination of pregnancy act, 1971. Any act of termination of pregnancy of normal female fetus amounting to female feticide shall be regarded as professional misconduct on the part of the physician leading to penal erasure besides rendering him liable to criminal proceedings as per the provisions of this act.

7.7. **Signing professional certificates, reports and other documents:** Registered medical practitioners are in certain cases bound by law to give, or may from time to time be called upon or requested to give certificates, notification, reports and other documents of similar character signed by them in their professional capacity for subsequent use in the courts or for administrative purposes, etc. Such documents, among others, include the ones given at Appendix–4. Any registered practitioner who is shown to have signed or given under his name and authority any such certificate, notification, report or document of a similar character which is untrue, misleading or improper, is liable to have his name deleted from the register.

7.8. A registered medical practitioner shall not contravene the provisions of the drugs and cosmetics act and regulations made thereunder. Accordingly; (1) prescribing steroids/psychotropic drugs when there is no absolute medical indication; (2) selling schedule 'H' and 'L' drugs and poisons to the public except to his patient; in contravention of the above provisions shall constitute gross professional misconduct on the part of the physician.

7.9. Performing or enabling unqualified person to perform an abortion or any illegal operation for which there is no medical, surgical or psychological indication.

7.10. A registered medical practitioner shall not issue certificates of efficiency in modern medicine to unqualified or non-medical person. (Note: The foregoing does not restrict the proper training and instruction of bonafide students, midwives, dispensers, surgical attendants, or skilled mechanical and technical assistants and therapy assistants under the personal supervision of physicians.)

7.11. A physician should not contribute to the lay press articles and give interviews regarding diseases and treatments which may have the effect of advertising himself or soliciting practices; but is open to write to the lay press under his own name on matters of public health, hygienic living or to deliver public lectures, give talks on the radio/TV/internet chat for the same purpose and send announcement of the same to lay press.

7.12. An institution run by a physician for a particular purpose such as a maternity home, nursing home, private hospital, rehabilitation center or any type of training institution, etc. may be advertised in the lay press, but such advertisements should not contain anything more than the name of the institution, type of patients admitted, type of training and other facilities offered and the fees.

7.13. It is improper for a physician to use an unusually large sign board and write on it anything other than his name, qualifications obtained from a university or a statutory body, titles and name of his specialty, registration number including the name of the State Medical Council under which registered. The same should be the contents of his prescription papers. It is improper to affix a signboard on a chemist's shop or in places where he does not reside or work.

7.14. The registered medical practitioner shall not disclose the secrets of a patient that have been learnt in the exercise of his/her profession except in a court of law under orders of the presiding judge:

  i. In circumstances where there is a serious and identified risk to a specific person and/or community.

  ii. Notifiable diseases.
  In case of communicable/notifiable diseases, concerned public health authorities should be informed immediately.

7.15. The registered medical practitioner shall not refuse on religious grounds alone to give assistance in or conduct of sterility, birth control, circumcision and medical termination of pregnancy when there is medical indication, unless the medical practitioner feels himself/herself incompetent to do so.

7.16. Before performing an operation the physician should obtain in writing the consent from the husband or wife, parent or guardian in the case of minor, or the patient himself as the case may be. In an operation which may result in sterility the consent of both husband and wife is needed.

7.17. A registered medical practitioner shall not publish photographs or case reports of his/her patients without their permission, in any medical or other journal in a manner by which their identity could be made out. If the identity is not to be disclosed, the consent is not needed.

7.18. In the case of running of a nursing home by a physician and employing assistants to help him/her, the ultimate responsibility rests on the physician.

7.19. A physician shall not use touts or agents for procuring patients.

7.20. A physician shall not claim to be specialist unless he has a special qualification in that branch.

7.21. No act of *in vitro* fertilization or artificial insemination shall be undertaken without the informed consent of the female patient and her spouse as well as the donor. Such consent shall be obtained in writing only after the patient is provided, at her own level of comprehension, with sufficient information about the purpose, methods, risks, inconveniences, disappointments of the procedure and possible risks and hazards.

7.22. Research: Clinical drug trials or other research involving patients or volunteers as per the guidelines of ICMR can be undertaken, provided ethical considerations are borne in mind. Violation of existing ICMR guidelines in this regard shall constitute misconduct. Consent taken from the patient for trial of drug or therapy which is not as per the guidelines shall also be construed as misconduct.

Chapter 8: Punishment and Disciplinary Action

8.1. It must be clearly understood that the instances of offences and of professional misconduct which are given above do not constitute and are not intended to constitute a complete list of the infamous acts which calls for disciplinary action, and that by issuing this notice the medical council of India and or state medical councils are in no way precluded from considering and dealing with any other form of professional misconduct on the part of a registered practitioner. Circumstances may and do arise from time to time in relation to which there may occur questions of professional misconduct which do not come within any of these categories. Every care should be taken that the code is not violated in letter or spirit. In such instances as in all others, the medical council of India and/or state medical councils have to consider and decide upon the facts brought before the medical council of India and/or state medical councils.

8.2. It is made clear that any complaint with regard to professional misconduct can be brought before the appropriate medical council for disciplinary action. Upon receipt of any complaint of professional misconduct, the appropriate medical council would hold an enquiry and give opportunity to the registered medical practitioner to be heard in person or by pleader. If the medical practitioner is found to be guilty of committing professional misconduct, the appropriate medical council may award such punishment as deemed necessary or may direct the removal altogether or for a specified period, from the register of the name of the delinquent registered practitioner. deletion from the register shall be widely publicized in local press as well as in the publications of different medical associations/societies/bodies.

8.3. In case the punishment of removal from the register is for a limited period, the appropriate council may also direct that the name so removed shall be restored in the register after the expiry of the period for which the name was ordered to be removed.

8.4. Decision on complaint against delinquent physician shall be taken within a time limit of 6 months.

8.5. During the pendency of the complaint the appropriate council may restrain the physician from performing the procedure or practice which is under scrutiny.

8.6. Professional incompetence shall be judged by peer group as per guidelines prescribed by medical council of India.

8.7. Where either on a request or otherwise the medical council of India is informed that any complaint against a delinquent physician has not been decided by a state medical council within a period of six months from the date of receipt of complaint by it and further the MCI has reason to believe that there is no justified reason for not deciding the complaint within the said prescribed period, the Medical Council of India may: (i) impress upon the concerned state medical council to conclude and decide the complaint within a time bound schedule; (ii) may decide to withdraw the said complaint pending with the concerned state medical council straightaway or after the expiry of the period which had been stipulated by the MCI in accordance with para (i) above, to itself and refer the same to the ethical committee of the council for its expeditious disposal in a period of not more than six months from the receipt of the complaint in the office of the medical council of India.

8.8. Any person aggrieved by the decision of the state medical council on any complaint against a delinquent physician, shall have the right to file an appeal to the MCI within a period of 60 days from the date of receipt of the order passed by the said medical council: Provided that the MCI may, if it is satisfied that the appellant was prevented by sufficient cause from presenting the appeal within the aforesaid period of 60 days, allow it to be presented within a further period of 60 days.

DECLARATION

At the time of registration, each applicant shall be given a copy of the following declaration by the registrar concerned and the applicant shall read and agree to abide by the same:

a. I solemnly pledge myself to consecrate my life to service of humanity.

b. Even under threat, I will not use my medical knowledge contrary to the laws of humanity.

c. I will maintain the utmost respect for human life from the time of conception.

d. I will not permit considerations of religion, nationality, race, party politics or social standing to intervene between my duty and my patient.

e. I will practice my profession with conscience and dignity.

f. The health of my patient will be my first consideration.

g. I will respect the secrets which are confined in me.

h. I will give to my teachers the respect and gratitude which is their due.

i. I will maintain by all means in my power, the honour and noble traditions of medical profession.

j. I will treat my colleagues with all respect and dignity.

k. I shall abide by the code of medical ethics as enunciated in the Indian medical council (Professional conduct, etiquette and ethics) regulations 2002.

I. Make these promises solemnly, freely and upon my honour.

MEDICAL MALPRACTICE (MEDICAL MALPRAXIS)

This term is used to denote failure on the part of the medical practitioner to conduct himself according to the rules framed by the medical council of India or laws of the land in relation to his obligations towards his patients. Hence medical malpractice can be divided into two types:

1. **Professional misconduct:** This is also called as ethical malpractice when the medical practitioner is found wanting in his professional behavior as envisaged by the MCI in **Indian medical council (professional conduct, etiquette and ethics) regulations, 2002 (Chapter 6, 7 and 8)**.

2. **Medical negligence:** Medical negligence or professional negligence is defined as "want of reasonable care and skill by act or omission by a health care provider in which the treatment provided falls below the accepted standard of practice in the medical community and causes injury or death to the patient". (Fig. 33.1)

Justice Baron Alderson (1856) defined negligence as "omission to do something which a reasonable person would do or doing something which a reasonable and prudent person would not do".

Medical negligence happens when the medical practitioner fails to provide the care (*acts of omission*) which is expected in such a case or doing something (*acts of commission*) which a reasonable medical practitioner under the circumstance would not do. This can be any tort or breach of contract of health care or professional services rendered by a health care provider to a patient. The standard of skill and care required of every health care provider in rendering professional services or health care to a patient shall be that degree of skill and care ordinarily employed in the same or similar field of medicine as defendant.

In medical negligence cases it is the duty of the patient or his/her relatives to establish that:

1. *Doctor–patient relationship:* There should be an establishment of patient–doctor relationship.
2. *Duty owed:* Due to establishment of patient–doctor relationship, there was a duty of care which the medical practitioner owed to the patient.
3. *Dereliction of duty:* By acts of omission or commission on the part of the medical practitioner, there was a breach of that duty.
4. *Damage to the patient:* The breach of duty resulted in injury or death of the patient.
5. *Direct causation:* The acts of commission or omission were directly responsible in resultant damage to the patient.
6. *Foreseeability:* Without a particular act of omission or commission the resultant damage in the patient would have not taken place.

Types of Medical Negligence

Depending upon the court in which the Trial of medical negligence takes place it is divided into two types.

1. Civil negligence
2. Criminal negligence

1. **Civil negligence:** When the case is filled in civil courts for compensation in simple absence of care and skill cases and there is normally no violation of the criminal laws of the land. Under the civil law, victims of negligence can get relief in the form of compensation from a civil court or the consumer forum. Here, the applicant only needs to prove that an act took place that was wanting in due care and caution, and the victim consequently suffered damage. In some cases when the doctor files a case for recovery of his fee in a civil court, the patient refuses to pay on the ground of negligence. As there is a limiting period of two years to file a case of negligence, doctors suspecting plea of negligence from the patient's side, file such recovery suits only after two years.

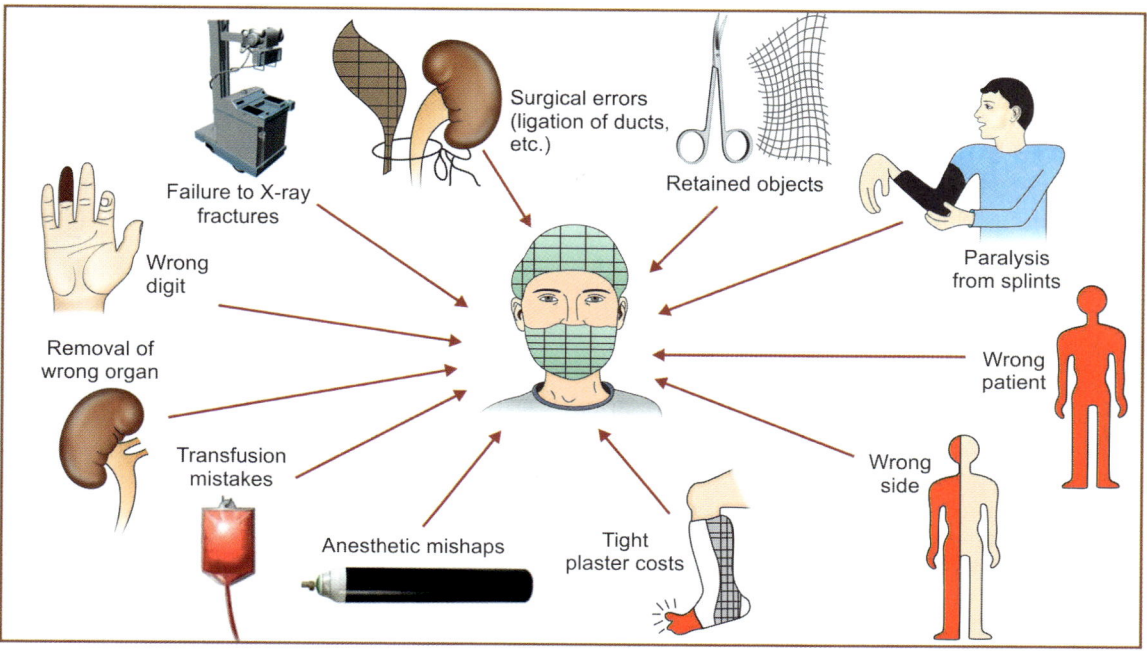

Fig. 33.1: Cases of medical negligence

There is a difference between civil and criminal negligence. However, in certain circumstances, the same negligent act may also be seen as criminal if it constitutes an offence under any law of the land.

2. **Criminal negligence:** According to section 304-A IPC, causing death by doing a rash and negligent act attracts imprisonment for up to two years or a fine or both. The burden to collect evidence of criminal liability is upon the complainant. The accused person will be presumed innocent until proof beyond reasonable doubt is adduced by the prosecution.

The supreme court stated in Dr Jacob Mathew's case that in order to make a doctor criminally responsible for the death of a patient, it must be established that there was negligence or incompetence on the doctor's part which went beyond a mere question of compensation on the basis of civil liability. Criminal liability would arise only if the doctor did something in disregard of the life and safety of the patient.

The main question in the above case was whether different standards could be applied to professionals (medical profession) alone, placing them on a higher pedestal for finding criminal liability for their acts or omissions. The court noted that as citizens become increasingly conscious of their rights, they are filing more cases against doctors in the civil courts, as also under the consumer protection act, 1986, alleging 'deficiency in service'. furthermore, doctors are being prosecuted under section 304-A IPC, section 337 or section 338 IPC.

The court observed that allegations of rashness or negligence are often raised against doctors by persons without adequate medical knowledge, to extract unjust compensation. This results in serious embarrassment and harassment to doctors who are forced to seek bail to escape arrest. If bail is not granted, they will have to suffer incarceration. They may be exonerated of the charges at the end; but in the meantime they would have suffered a loss of reputation; often irreversible. The tendency to initiate such cases has therefore to be curbed.

Since the medical profession renders a noble service, it must be shielded from frivolous or unjust prosecutions. With this perspective in mind the court went into the question as to what is actionable negligence in the case of professionals.

The hon'ble Supreme Court has provided following guidelines:

1. A simple lack of care, an error of judgment or an accident, even fatal, will not constitute culpable medical negligence. If the doctor had followed a practice acceptable to the medical profession at the relevant time, he or she cannot be held liable for negligence merely because a better alternative course or method of treatment was also available, or simply because a more skilled doctor would not have chosen to follow or resort to that practice.

2. Professionals may certainly be held liable for negligence if they did not possess the requisite skill which they claimed, or if they did not exercise with reasonable competence, the skill which they did possess.

3. The word 'gross' has not been used in Section 304-A IPC. However, as far as professionals are concerned, it is to be read into it so as to insist on proof of gross negligence for finding of guilty.

4. The maxim "Res ipsa loquitur" (let the event speak for itself; no other evidence need be insisted) is only a rule of evidence. It might operate in the domain of civil law; but has only a limited application in trial on a charge of criminal negligence.

5. Statutory rules or executive instructions incorporating definite guidelines governing the prosecution of doctors need to be framed and issued by the state and central governments in consultation with the medical council of India (MCI). Until this is done, private complaints must be accompanied by the credible opinion of another competent doctor supporting the charge of rashness or negligence. In the case

of police prosecutions, such an opinion should preferably from a doctor in government service.

6. Doctors accused of rashness or negligence may not be arrested simply because charges have been leveled against them; this may be done only if it is necessary for furthering the investigation, or for collecting evidence, or if the investigating officer fears that the accused will abscond.

The supreme court has not stated, even now, that doctors can never be prosecuted for medical negligence. It has only emphasized the need for care and caution in prosecuting doctors in the interests of society. This immunity is available only in criminal courts and not elsewhere.

Some examples of criminal negligence are as follows:

1. Injecting anesthetic in fatal dosage or in wrong tissues.
2. Amputation of wrong finger, operation on wrong limb or removal of wrong organ.
3. Operation on wrong patient.
4. Leaving instruments or sponges inside the part of body operated upon.
5. Leaving tourniquets too long, resulting in gangrene.
6. Transfusing wrong blood.
7. Applying too tight plaster or splints which may cause gangrene or paralysis.
8. Performing a criminal abortion or violation of statutory provisions of various acts, e.g. sex determination (PCPNDT Act) or transplantation of human organ act.

Doctrine of *Res Ipsa Loquitur*

Res ipsa loquitur (the thing speaks for itself) is a doctrine in tort law that infers negligence from the very nature of an accident or injury. Normally a negligence case is proved in a court of law by the evidence of another doctor. But when the negligence is so evident to apply this doctrine, the patient is not required to prove the case but the doctor has to defend himself. This doctrine is mainly used in civil negligence cases and has limited role in criminal negligence cases.

To establish the doctrine of *res ipsa loquitur* the patient has to satisfy the following criteria:

1. The injury is of the kind that does not ordinarily occur without negligence.
2. The injury is caused by an agency or instrumentality within the exclusive control of the defendant.
3. The injury causing accident is not due to any voluntary action or contribution on the part of the plaintiff (contributory negligence).
4. Defendant's non-negligent explanation does not completely explain plaintiff's injury.

Res ipsa loquitur often arises in the case when a scalpel or a pair of scissors is left behind or there is a failure to remove gauze piece from the abdomen after the surgery.

Res Judicata

Res judicata is a Latin term for "a matter already judged", and is followed in cases, in which there has been a final judgment and the matter cannot be raised again, either in the same court or in a different court on the same grounds and between same parties. A court will use *res judicata* to deny reconsideration of a matter.

The legal concept of *res judicata* arose as a method of preventing injustice to the parties of a case supposedly finished, but perhaps mostly to avoid unnecessary waste of resources in the court system. *Res judicata* does not merely prevent future judgments from contradicting earlier ones, but also prevents litigants from multiplying judgments, and confusion.

Res judicata does not restrict the appeal process, which is considered a linear extension of the same lawsuit. There are limited exceptions to *res judicata* that allow a party to attack the validity of the original judgment, even outside of appeals. These exceptions, usually called collateral attacks, are typically based on procedural or jurisdictional issues.

Vicarious Responsibility

The legal concept of "vicarious liability" and the doctrine of "**Respondent superior**" occur when the servant (employee) commits a tort or civil wrong within the scope of employment and the master (employer) is held liable although the master may have done nothing wrong. It is in a broader sense, the responsibility of any third party that had the "right, ability or duty to control" the activities of a violator. Even when two doctors are working as partners both are liable for the negligent act of anyone of them. This doctrine is based on the principle "that the wrong of the agent is the wrong of his employer" and require following conditions to be satisfied:

1. The wrong doer is having relationship of employee with the employer.
2. The wrongful act is done by the employee while he is on the job.
3. The negligence occurred within the scope of employment.

*To avoid such liability employer must ensure that **all reasonable steps** have been taken by* the employer to reduce this liability.

Borrowed servant doctrine: This doctrine stipulates that the special employer is vicariously held liable for the actions of a borrowed employee which he has taken on loan from some other general employer, though there is no permanent employee and employer relationship but the special employer has control over the work conducted by the borrowed employee.

PREVENTIVE MEDICAL LITIGATION

In view of the patients becoming increasingly conscious of their rights, they are filing cases of medical negligence against doctors in the civil courts, under the consumer protection act, 1986, alleging 'deficiency in service' and criminal courts under section 304-A IPC, section 337 IPC or section 338 IPC.

General Preventive Measures

a. *Proper behavior:* A medical practitioner must always behave in proper and courteous manner with his patients or his relatives. In most of the cases were the patient or his relatives feel offended with the behaviour of the doctor they may drag the doctor into litigations.

b. *No casual remarks:* Casual remarks by the treating doctor may give rise to suspicion in the mind of the patient with regards to the treatment or the outcome of the case.

c. *Proper attention:* Doctor must give proper attention so that the patient or his relatives do not feel neglected.

d. *Avoid professional jealousy:* Never downgrade your colleague by passing casual remarks about the earlier treatment. They may file a case on the earlier treating doctor based on your casual remarks.

e. *No guaranty for cure/days of treatment:* It is advisable that no guarantee should be given to a patient regarding the cure or the days in which the cure will take place.

Specific Preventive Measures

a. *Proper care and skill:* Though in medical negligence cases the court expects competency equated with similarly placed and trained medical practioners, however it is always desired that the doctor must keep himself updated and provide proper care while treating a patient. **Bolam test** is a typical rule for assessing the appropriate standard of reasonable care in negligence cases involving skilled professionals, e.g. doctors. In Bolam v Friern Hospital case the court held that "there is no breach of standard of care if a responsible body, of similar professionals, supports the practice that caused the injury".

b. *Adhere to standard procedures:* While treating a patient a doctor must adhere to standard procedures to be followed as per the routine practice or mentioned in the treatise. In case a new treatment procedure is being adopted proper informed consent and standard guidelines must be followed.

c. *Proper documentation:* All documents related with the treatment must be complete, legible and preserved. In case a patient gives written request for his treatment records, the records must be provided to him within 72 hours.

d. *Proper consent:* Consent is voluntary permission, agreement or compliance. consent has been defined under section 13 of Indian contract act as "Two or more persons are said to consent when they agree upon the same thing in the same sense".

e. *If in doubt, take second opinion:* It is advisable to take a second opinion when there is any doubt in the mind of the treating doctor or when the patient is not responding to the prescribed line of treatment.

f. *Respect rights of the patient:* A doctor has a fiduciary duty of confidentiality towards a patient. This is to encourage disclosure to the doctor of facts which may help in diagnosis or treatment but which may be embarrassing or harmful to the patient if released to others. This **"fiduciary duty"** includes a duty not to disclose any medical information received in connection with treatment. If medical information is disclosed without the client's prior approval, the client may bring a lawsuit against the doctor for breaching their fiduciary duty.

Protective Measures

a. *Indemnity insurance:* Professional indemnity insurance indemnifies the insured against financial loss resulting from a claim brought about due to an error or omission committed while performing a service contracted for. Individual professionals, having an indemnity policy can ensure their personal as well as professional survival should they have to pay a claim. These types of indemnity policies are available for a group of doctors working together or for individual doctor. The indemnity insurance company in case of a medical negligence claim brought against that doctor provides (a) legal help in the form of providing suitable lawyer to defend the case in the court and (b) settling claims including no fault claims.

b. *Redressal forum at the institutional level:* In some bigger institutions they have a redressal forum at the institutional level which provides legal help and settlement of any claim against the doctors working in that institution.

Liability Control Measures

a. *Support from professional bodies*: Professional bodies like Indian Medical Association or State Medical Association support their members in such situations. Apart from providing moral support to the concerned doctor they also provide legal help.

b. *Defending the case in the court:* While defending a case of medical negligence in the court a doctor must observe certain rules like:

i Courteous: A doctor's behaviour in the court must always be courteous.

ii Do not volunteer: Unless some information is required from the doctor, never volunteer any information.

iii. No casual remarks: A doctor should be very careful while defending his case in the court and no casual remarks against the patient should be made.

iv. Show concern for the welfare of the patient: While defending the case always show concern for the welfare of the patient.

Defenses to Malpractice

a. *Denial of liability:* First principle of defense is not to accept liability in medical negligence cases. Inform the court that all possible care and proper skill was utilized while treating the patient. The treatment was provided as per the standard practice as mentioned in the treatise.

b. *Contributory negligence:* Contributory negligence is seen when the plaintiffs/claimants have, through their own negligence, contributed to the harm they suffered due to the negligence of the doctor. Contributory negligence is generally a defense to a claim based on negligence hence it is a defense in civil cases only and has no role in criminal negligence. In these cases the doctor has to prove the negligence on part of the patient. It is the duty of the treating doctor to foresee situations where patient may harm himself and issue instructions in this regard to the patient. Some examples of contributory negligence are failure to follow instructions of the treating doctor in regards to proper drugs, diet, rest and timely review. In India compensation in favour of victim gets reduced in proportion with his negligence.

c. *Assumption of risk:* When the medical procedure or the act not intended and not likely to cause death or grievous hurt done with consent and in good faith or take that risk under Section 87 of IPC or an act not intended to cause death done by consent in good faith for persons' benefit under Section 88 of IPC or an act done in good faith for benefit of child or insane person by consent of the guardian under Section 89 of IPC is not an offence.

d. *Doctrine of calculated risk:* Calculated risk is a hazard or chance of failure whose degree of probability has been previously estimated before some undertaking is entered upon. Such risk of failure, i.e. mortality or morbidity percentage, previously known is always possible in any type of surgery or medical procedure. It is taken as a defense in medical negligence cases.

e. *Emergency:* Under section 92 of IPC when the circumstances are such that it is impossible for a person to give consent and has no guardian, any act done in good faith for the benefit of that person is not an offence.

f. *Res judicata:* This dictum can be used in cases, in which there has been a final judgment so that the matter cannot be raised again, either in the same court or in a different court on the same grounds and between same parties.

g. *Reasonable error of judgment:* Reasonable error of judgment is accepted as a defence in medical negligence cases. Supreme court has held that a doctor cannot straightway be held liable for medical negligence simply because a patient has not favourably responded to treatment or surgery has failed. It was suggested that whenever complaints are received against a doctor or hospital, the consumer forum or criminal court, before issuing notice, should first refer the matter to a competent doctor or a committee of doctors, specialising in the field where negligence was attributed. Only after that committee reports that there is a prima facie case of medical negligence; should notice be issued to the doctor/ hospital concerned.

h. *Medical mal-occurrence and therapeutic misadventure:* Medical mal-occurrence is that bad outcome of a medical procedure which is unrelated to the quality of care provided to the patient. In some cases idiosyncrasy may develop against any drug or a substance used for diagnostic purpose and complications arising unpredictably or which are unavoidable.

i. *Beyond time limit:* In civil cases a limitation period of two years has been prescribed for filling the case in consumer courts. Hence a case filled after this period may be contested.

j. *Novus actus interveniens:* Novus actus interveniens literally means new act intervening. There will be no liability if some new intervening act breaks the chain of causation between a medical negligence and the loss or damage sustained by the claimant. Courts in such cases interpret that the intervening act was the cause of the damage or harm to the patient.

k. *Product liability:* In some cases the doctor takes a plea in medical negligence cases that the damage is as a result of faulty equipment. In this type of liability, manufacturers, distributors, suppliers, retailers, and others who make products available to the public are held responsible for the injuries caused by those products. Product liability is of following types:

a. Manufacturing defects are those that occur in the manufacturing process and usually involve poor-quality materials or shoddy workmanship.

b. Design defects occur where the product design is inherently dangerous or useless, no matter how carefully manufactured.

c. Failure-to-warn defects arise in products that carry inherent nonobvious dangers, regardless of how well the product is manufactured and designed for its intended purpose.

A landmark turn in India's medical negligence law: Anuradha Saha died painfully in May 1998 at the age of 36, her skin sloughed off all over her body, except for her skull. She was diagnosed with toxic epidermal necrolysis and was encased in bandages meant to prevent infections that had already lodged in her system. Her immunity had been compromised after receiving a high dosage of steroids from some of the top doctors in Kolkata. For 15 years, her husband, Dr Kunal Saha pushed Indian courts to hold at least five doctors and the hospital responsible. Though the lower courts rejected his cases, Dr Saha persisted, appealing all the way to the supreme court, which found the doctors and AMRI Hospital (Advanced Medicare and Research Institute Ltd.) in Kolkata guilty of negligence in 2009. It took another four years for the supreme court to award Dr Saha an unprecedented amount in a medical negligence case in India, 60.8 million rupees ($1 million), plus 6 percent annual interest for each of the 15 years that Dr Saha has been fighting his legal battle. The landmark ruling is supposed to remind doctors, hospitals, and nursing homes that they will be dealt with strictly if they do not maintain their standard of care, the supreme court said in its judgment.

"The patients, irrespective of their social, cultural and economic background, are entitled to be treated with dignity, which not only forms their fundamental right but also their human right," wrote Justices Chandramauli KR Prasad and V Gopala Gowda.

CONSENT

In medical practice there are two types of consent:

a. *Implied consent:* When a patient presents himself before a doctor, it is presumed that he is volunteering himself for routine examination. In such situation there is implied consent. However, in case any internal examination like per vaginal or per rectal examination is required expressed consent should be taken.
b. *Expressed consent:* When the patient is required to give consent for specific purpose, it is expressed consent. This consent can be obtained either in oral form or written form.
    i. *Oral consent:* Oral or verbal consent is normally taken for internal examination, minor procedures or withdrawal of blood for therapeutic purposes preferably in presence of a disinterested third party like a nurse.
    ii. *Written consent:* Written consent is always required in major diagnostic procedures or operations. Written legally valid consent is known as informed consent, wherein a patient makes an informed decision regarding his treatment procedure.

Elements of Informed Consent

1. The patient is informed about his illness and prognosis.
2. Provision of the full information in plain language about the procedure to be done.
3. Benefits and risks of the procedure.
4. Alternative procedure available with risks and benefits.
5. Assurance that patient has freedom to decide or take an informed decision to accept or refuse the treatment.

6. Assessment of the capacity of the patient to make a decision.

However there is no defined parameters regarding the information to be provided to the patient but it is desired that reasonable amount of information must always be provided.

Exceptions to Informed Consent

a. *In emergencies:* Under section 92 IPC when the circumstances are such that it is impossible for a person to give consent and has no guardian, any act done in good faith for the benefit of that person is not an offence.
b. *Therapeutic privilege:* In such cases the information is withheld from the patient as disclosure would pose a psychological threat. However, the near relatives are taken into confidence and details are explained to them.
c. *Therapeutic waiver:* In some rare situations a patient may provide prior therapy waiver request, and give up his right to informed consent.
d. *Examination of an accused:* Under Section 53 of CrPC, an accused can be examined without consent, using reasonable force on the written request of the police officer not below the rank of subinspector. However, an accused female must be examined under this section by a female medical practitioner.
e. *Incompetent to give consent:* In certain situations the patient is not able to give consent as he is incompetent to provide valid consent like when the person in unconscious, suffering from psychotic conditions or senility.

Age of Consent

1. Under section 90 of IPC a child under the age of 12 years or a person who is suffering from mental disorders or intoxication, unable to understand nature and consequences of that to which he gives his

consent, or any consent given under fear or misconception is not valid.

2. For routine medical examination the age of consent is more than 12 years. Below 12 years consent of the parents or guardian is required.

3. For any invasive procedure or operations the age of the person should be above 18 years.

CONSUMER PROTECTION ACT, 1986

Introduction

The doctor patient relationship in our country has undergone a sea change in the last decade and a half. The lucky doctors of the past were treated like god and people revered and respected them. We witness today a fast pace of commercialization and as a result, the doctor-patients relationship has deteriorated considerably. Consumer protection act 1986 was introduced to provide faster and in-expensive arbitration. Earlier too, doctors were covered by various laws, i.e. the law of torts, IPC, etc. but since the passing of the consumer protection act in 1986, litigation against doctors is on the increase. **Following consumer rights have been recognised:**

1. **The right to safety:** This means the right to be protected against products, production processes and services which are hazardous to health or life.

2. **The right to be informed:** This means the right to be informed of all the facts needed to make an informed choice or decision. The right to be informed now goes beyond avoiding deception and the protection against misleading advertising, labelling or other practices.

3. **The right to choose:** This means the right to have access to basic goods and services. In medical practice it is the right to select/choose desired line of treatment or surgery.

4. **The right to be heard:** This means the right to be heard and represented in the development of products and services before they are produced or set up; it also implies a representation, not only in

government policies, but also in those of other economic powers.

5. **The right to redress:** This means the right to a fair settlement of just claims and where needed, free legal aid or an accepted form of redress for small claims should be available.

6. **The right to consumer education:** This means the right to acquire the knowledge and the right to consumer education incorporates the right to the knowledge and skills needed for taking action to influence factors which affect consumer decisions.

The consumer rights No. 1 to 6 are also enshrined in our consumer protection act, 1986.

Supreme court ruling: In November,1995 the Supreme Court ruled to bring Health Sector under CPA. Even though the above ruling was contested by various medical professional bodies citing that: (i) that medical profession and services cannot be equated with trade; (ii) this ruling would propagate defensive medicine; (iii) hence this will increase the cost of treatment to the patients; (iv) doctors will avoid complicated cases; (v) rural health care will suffer as doctors will not prefer to go to rural areas in absence of proper investigative facilities; (vi) outcome of the treatment is variable depending upon many factors which are beyond the control of the doctor; and (vii) there is no medical representative in the consumer courts or tribunals.

Supreme court has ruled that health services provided they meet following conditions comes under the preview of CPA:

a. All services in hospitals/nursing homes on payment (even free to some) shall be covered.

b. Third party payments (insurance company or parents of a child) would constitute service under sect. 2(1) (o) of CPA.

c. Services under "contract of employment" shall not be covered. As the services provided by the medical professional to the employer cannot be covered under CPA. However *contract for personal services* are covered.

d. Services provided free of charge to all patients by the medical practitioner are also not covered under CPA.

The act envisages a three-tier quasi-judicial machinery (i) district consumer disputes redressal forum at the district level; (ii) state consumer disputes redressal commission at the state level; and (iii) national consumer disputes redressal commission at the national level. Act has been amended by the consumer protection (amendment) act, 1993.

District Forum

At least one in each district or in certain cases one district forum may cover 2 or more districts. It consists of three members (i) a person who is, or has been, or is qualified to be a district judge, its president; and (ii) two other members shall be persons of ability, integrity and standing and have adequate knowledge or experience or have shown capacity, in dealing with problems relating to economics, law, commerce, accountancy, industry, public affairs or administration, one of whom shall be a woman.

Jurisdiction of the district forum: The district forum shall have jurisdiction to entertain complaints where the value of services and compensation claimed does not exceed ₹ twenty lakhs.

Manner in which complaint shall be made: A complaint may be filed with a district forum by:
a. The consumer to whom such service is provided or is agreed to be provided;
b. Any recognised consumer association, whether the consumer to whom the service is provided or is agreed to be provided is a member of such association or not;
c. One or more consumers, where there are numerous consumers having the same interest, with the permission of the district forum, on behalf of or for the benefit of all consumers so interested; and
d. The central or the state government.

Procedure on receipt of complaint: The district forum shall on receipt of a complaint:

a. Refer a copy of such complaint to the opposite party directing him to give his version of the case within a period of 30 days or such extended period not exceeding 15 days as may be granted by the district forum.
b. Where the opposite party, on receipt of a copy of the complaint, denies or disputes the allegations contained in the complaint, or omits or fails to take any action to represent his case within the time given by the district forum, the district forum shall proceed to settle the consumer dispute:
   i. On the basis of evidence brought to his notice by the complainant and the opposite party, where the opposite denies or disputes the allegations contained in the complaint.
   ii. On the basis of evidence brought to its notice by the complainant where the opposite party omits or fails to take any action to represent his case within the time given by the forum.
   iii. Where the complainant or his authorised agent fails to appear before the district forum on such day, the district forum may in its discretion either dismiss the complaint in default or if a substantial portion of the evidence of the complainant has already been recorded, decide it on merits. Where the opposite party or its authorised agent fails to appear on the day of hearing, the district forum may decide the complaint ex parte.
   iv. Where any party to a complaint to whom time has been granted fails to produce his evidence or to cause the attendance of his witnesses or to perform any other act necessary to the further progress of the complaint, for which time has been allowed, the district forum may notwithstanding such default:
      a. If the parties are present, proceed to decide the complaint forthwith; or
      b. If the parties or any of them is absent, proceed as mentioned above in b. (iii).

v. The district forum may, on such terms as it may think fit at any stage, adjourn the hearing of the complaint but not more than one adjournment shall ordinarily be given and the complaint should be decided within 90 days from the date of notice received by the opposite party where complaint does not require analysis or testing of the goods and within 150 days if it requires analysis or testing of the goods.

Findings of the District Forum

If, after the proceedings, the district forum is satisfied that any of the allegations contained in the complaint about the services are proved, it shall issue an order to the opposite party directing him to do one or more of the following things:

1. To return to the complainant the charges paid.
2. Pay such amount as may be awarded by it as compensation to the consumer for any loss or injury suffered by the consumer due to the negligence of the opposite party.
3. To remove the deficiency in the services in question.
4. To provide for adequate costs to parties.

Appeal Against Orders of the District Forum

Any person aggrieved by an order made by the district forum may appeal against such order to the state commission within a period of 30 days from the date of the order. The state commission may entertain an appeal after 30 days if it is satisfied that there was sufficient cause for not filing it within that period.

State Commission

They shall be located in each state and shall consist of (i) a person who is or has been a Judge of a high court, who shall be its president and (ii) two other members (as for district forum).

Jurisdiction of the State Commission

1. Complaints where the value of services and compensation claimed exceeds ₹ twenty lakhs but does not exceed ₹ one crore;

2. Appeals against the orders of any district forum within the state;
3. Revision petitions against the district forum.

Procedure to be followed by state commission: Same as for district forum.

Procedure for hearing appeals: The state commission may, on such terms as it may think fit and at any stage, adjourn the hearing of appeal, but not more than one adjournment shall ordinarily be given and the appeal should be decided within 90 days from the first date of hearing.

Appeals against orders of state commission: Any person aggrieved by an order made by the state commission may appeal against such order to the national commission within a period of 30 days. The national commission may entertain an appeal after 30 days if it is satisfied that there was sufficient cause for not filing it within that period.

National Commission

Instituted at the national level and consists of (i) a person who is or has been a judge of the supreme court, who shall be its president. (No appointment under this clause shall be made except after consultation with the Chief Justice of India); and (ii) four other members (qualifications: As for district forum/state commission).

The National Commission have Jurisdiction:

a. To entertain
   i. Complaints where the value of services and compensation claimed exceeds ₹ one crore.
   ii. Appeals against the orders of any state commission.
b. To entertain revision petition against the state commission.

Procedure to be Followed by the National Commission

A complaint containing the following particulars shall be presented by the complainant in person or by his agent to the national commission or be sent by registered post, addressed to the national commission (i) the name, description and the address of the complainant; (ii) the name, description and address of the opposite party or parties, as the case may be, so far as they can be ascertained; (iii) the facts relating to the complaint and when and where it arose; (iv) documents in support of the allegations contained in the complaint; and (v) the relief which the complainant claims.

The remaining procedure and the procedure for hearing the appeal are similar to that for state commission.

Appeal against orders of the national commission: Any person, aggrieved by an order made by the national commission, may appeal against such order to the supreme court within a period of 30 days from the date of the order. The supreme court may entertain an appeal after 30 days if it is satisfied that there was sufficient cause for not filing it within that period.

Limitation period: The district forum, the state commission or the national commission shall not admit a complaint unless it is filed within 2 years from the date on which the cause of action has arisen. In case there are sufficient grounds for not filing the complaint within such period, extension may be granted.

Dismissal of frivolous or vexatious complaints: Where a complaint instituted before the district forum, the state commission or the national commission, as the case may be, is found to be frivolous or vexatious, it shall, for reasons to be recorded in writing, dismiss the complaint and make an order that the complainant shall pay to the opposite party such cost, not exceeding 10,000 ₹, as may be specified in the order.

Penalties for failure to comply: Where a person against whom a complaint is made or the complainant fails or omits to comply with any order made by the district forum, the state commission or the national commission, as the case may be, such person or complainant shall be punishable with imprisonment for a term which shall not be less than one month but which may extend to three years, or with fine which shall not be less than 2,000 ₹ but which may extend to 10,000 ₹ or with both. In exceptional circumstances the penalties may be reduced further.

Consumer Protection Councils

The Consumer Protection Act provides for the establishment of councils at state and central levels.

1. **The central consumer protection council** (The central council).
2. **The state consumer protection council** (The state council).

Objectives of the council shall be: To promote and protect the rights of the consumers such as mentioned below:

1. Right to be protected against the marketing of services which are hazardous to life and property.
2. Right to be informed about the quality, quantity, potency, purity, standard and price of services so as to protect the consumer against unfair trade practices.
3. Right to be assured, whenever possible, access to a variety of services at competitive prices.
4. Right to be heard and to be assured that consumer's interests will receive due consideration at appropriate forums.
5. Right to seek redressal against unfair trade practices or restrictive trade practices or unscrupulous exploitation of consumers.
6. Right to consumer education.

The central council shall consist of 150 members. The minister incharge of the consumer affairs in the central government shall be its chairman. The state council shall be chaired by minister incharge of consumer affairs in the state government. The resolution passed by these councils shall be recommendatory in nature.

EUTHANASIA OR MERCY KILLING

The word euthanasia in greek means a good death (Eu = Good; Thanatos = Death) and this practice of intentionally ending a life is undertaken, in order to relieve pain and suffering. The word "euthanasia" was first used in a medical context by **Francis Bacon** in the 17th century, to refer to an easy, painless, happy death, during which it was a physician's responsibility to alleviate the 'physical sufferings' of the body. The definition offered incorporates suffering as a necessary condition, with "the painless killing of a patient suffering from an incurable and painful disease or in an irreversible coma".

Request for premature ending of life has contributed to the debate about the role of such practices in contemporary health care. This debate cuts across complex and dynamic aspects such as, legal, ethical, human rights, health, religious, economic, spiritual, social and cultural aspects of the civilized society.

In India abetment of suicide is criminal offence. In 1994, constitutional validity of Indian penal code (IPC) section 309 (attempt to suicide) was challenged in the supreme court. The supreme court declared that IPC Sec. 309 is unconstitutional, and clearly stated that "a person attempts suicide in a depression, and hence he needs help, rather than punishment". The supreme court recommended to parliament to consider the feasibility of deleting section 309 from the Indian penal code. Union home ministry on 10 December 2014 decided section 309 IPC. However, pending the passage of mental health care bill 2013, section 309 IPC is yet to be repealed.

Euthanasia is categorized into following two types:

a. *Active euthanasia:* When a person directly and deliberately does something which results in the death of patient. Active euthanasia entails the use of lethal substances or forces, such as administering a lethal injection, to kill. Active euthanasia has raised many controversies.

b. *Passive euthanasia:* It involves withholding of medical treatment or withdrawal from life support system required for continuance of life. Hence in passive euthanasia death is brought about by an act of omission.

In India passive euthanasia was deliberated in supreme court in case of Aruna Shanbaug vs Union of India (2011). She was sexually assaulted by a ward boy. He strangulated her with a dog chain. The resultant asphyxiation caused irreversible injury to the brain causing permanent hypoxic damage to her brain and since then, she was in persistent vegetative state. After sometime her family abandoned her, but the nurses at the KEM hospital continued to take care of her. On 17th December 2010, Pinki Virani claiming to be Aruna's friend (a social activist-cum-journalist) made a plea in supreme court for permitting euthanasia on Aruna Shanbaug. On 7th March 2011, the apex court while rejecting Pinki Virani's plea for active euthanasia, the court observed that "the general legal position all over the world seems to be that while active euthanasia is illegal unless there is legislation permitting it, passive euthanasia is legal even without legislation provided certain conditions and safeguards are maintained". Aruna Shanbaug ultimately died in May 2015 after 42 years in coma. Whenever there is a need for passive euthanasia for some patient, permission has to be obtained from the concerned high court before life prolonging measures can be withheld.

Both active and passive euthanasia can be further differentiated into voluntary, involuntary and nonvoluntary.

i. *Voluntary euthanasia*: Euthanasia conducted with the consent of the patient is termed voluntary euthanasia. Active voluntary euthanasia is legal in Belgium, Luxembourg and the Netherlands. Passive voluntary euthanasia is legal throughout the US. Assisted suicide is legal in Switzerland and the US states of Oregon, Washington, Montana and Vermont.

ii. *Nonvoluntary euthanasia:* Euthanasia conducted where the consent of the patient is unavailable is termed nonvoluntary euthanasia.

iii. *Involuntary euthanasia:* Euthanasia conducted against the will of the patient is termed involuntary euthanasia.

Arguments Against Euthanasia

There are some persons who are against euthanasia being adopted legally:

i. *Eliminating the invalid:* Euthanasia opposers argue that if we embrace 'the right to death with dignity', people with incurable and debilitating illnesses will be disposed from our civilized society.

ii. *Constitution of India:* 'Right to life' is a natural right embodied in article 21 but suicide is an unnatural termination or extinction of life and, therefore, incompatible and inconsistent with the concept of 'right to life'. It is the duty of the state to protect life and the physician's duty to provide care and not to harm patients. The supreme court held that the right to life under article 21 of the constitution does not include the right to die.

iii. *Symptom of mental illness:* Attempt to suicide is a psychiatric emergency and it is considered as a desperate call for help or assistance.

iv. *Malafide intention:* In the era of declining morality and justice, there is a possibility of misusing euthanasia by family members or relatives for inheriting the property of the patient.

v. *Emphasis on care:* Earlier majority of them died before they reached the hospital but now science has advanced to the extent that life can be prolonged and some diseases may become curable in near future.

vi. *Commercialisation of health care:* Passive euthanasia occurs in majority of the hospitals across the county, where poor patients and their family members refuse or withdraw treatment because of the huge cost involved in keeping them alive.

Arguments in Favour of Euthanasia

1. *Caregivers burden:* 'Right-to-die' supporters argue that people who have an incurable, degenerative, disabling or debilitating condition should be allowed to die a dignified painless death.

2. *Refusing care:* A patient has right to refuse medical treatment, which is well recognised in law, including medical treatment that sustains or prolongs life.

3. *Right to die:* Many patients in a persistent vegetative state or else in chronic illness do not want to be a burden on their family members.

4. *Encouraging the organ transplantation:* Euthanasia in terminally ill patients provides an opportunity to advocate for organ donation. This in turn will help many patients with organ failure waiting for transplantation.

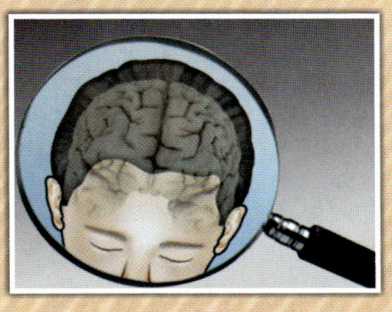

Section 3

Forensic Psychiatry

34 | Forensic Psychiatry

Mental illness is defined as "a state of mind in which the individual loses power to regulate his actions and conduct according to the rules of society or there is conflict between his personality and surroundings".

Mental health care during preindependence period started with Indian lunatic asylum act of 1858. In 1912 Indian lunacy act was passed for treating mentally ill persons. A major step in providing psychiatric help was achieved with mental health act of 1987. Mental health care bill 2013 is being proposed for right of mentally ill person to get proper treatment in mental health establishments.

MENTAL HEALTH ACT 1987

The **mental health act 1987** defines a "mentally ill person" as a person who is in need of treatment by reason of any mental disorder other than mental retardation. The mental health act (MHA) 1987 repeals Indian lunacy act 1912 and lunacy act, 1977 (Jammu and Kashmir) and extends to whole of India. This Act was promulgated primarily to replace offensive terminology to uphold the dignity of mentally ill patients, providing new psychiatric hospitals and establishing licensing authorities.

Psychiatric hospitals and nursing homes can be established or run only after obtaining a license from state or central authorities for mental health services, and are regulated for proper functioning and care of the mentally ill. However, psychiatric services provided from a general hospital or nursing home would not be covered by the licensing and regulating rules (Sec. 3–10 MHA).

Admission in Psychiatric Hospitals

Admission on Voluntary Basis

a. *Admission of a major on voluntary basis:* Any person aged eighteen and above who considers himself to be mentally ill person, can request medical officer incharge of the psychiatric hospital for *voluntarily admission* to get inpatient treatment (section 15 MHA).

b. *Admission of a minor on voluntary basis:* In case of minor (less than 18 years of age) who is mentally ill, can be presented for admission by the guardian as a voluntary patient (section 16 MHA).

Admission of Voluntary Patient

On receipt of a request under Sec.15 or Sec.16 of MHA, the medical officer incharge shall make such inquiry as he may deem fit within a period not exceeding twenty- four hours and if satisfied that the applicant or minor requires treatment as an inpatient, may admit such a person as a voluntary patient. Every voluntary patient admitted to a psychiatric hospital or psychiatric nursing home shall be bound to abide by such regulations as may be made by the medical officer incharge of the psychiatric hospital or psychiatric nursing home.

Discharge of Voluntary Patient

Patients admitted on voluntary basis, if they request for discharge, are obliged to be discharged by the medical officer incharge within 24 hours of receiving the request, unless the medical officer is convinced that the discharge will harm the interest of the voluntary patient. In such case, the medical officer would constitute a board of two medical officers and seek their opinion. If the Board is of the opinion that such voluntary patient needs further treatment in the psychiatric hospital or psychiatric nursing home, the medical officer shall not discharge the voluntary patient but continue his treatment for a period not exceeding 90 days at a time (subsection 3 of section 18 MHA).

Admission to Psychiatric Hospital Under Special Circumstances

Admission can also be made on request of a relative or friend of the patient if the patient is not in a position to express willingness for admission as voluntary patient, provided the medical officer incharge is satisfied that it is in the interest of the patient to do so. This application should be accompanied by two medical certificates (one from a medical officer who is working in government service) stating that the person has such mental illness and it requires inpatient observation and treatment. No person admitted on the request of another person can be kept in the mental hospital for more than 90 days (section 19 MHA).

A mentally ill patient admitted by relative or friend can also apply to the magistrate for discharge (subsection 3 of section 19 MHA).

Admission on Reception Order

Apart from voluntary admission, a mentally ill person can be admitted through reception order. An application for reception order may be made by following:

a. Medical officer incharge of a psychiatric hospital or psychiatric nursing home.

b. Spouse or by any other relative of the mentally ill patient for admission to the magistrate.

The application should be accompanied by two medical certificates from two independent medical practitioners certifying the need for admission for treatment, and that is in the interest, for personal safety of the patient, or that of others. The medical practitioners should have examined the patient within the last ten days prior to the application. The magistrate can pass the reception order or reject the application, after personally reviewing the documents and personally examine the alleged mentally ill person. The consideration of the application should be made in the presence of the applicant, the allegedly mentally ill person, and the person appointed by the allegedly mentally ill to represent him (section 22 MHA). A reception order is valid up to 30 days only or till discharged (section 31 MHA).

Powers and Duties of Police Officers in Respect of Certain mentally ill Persons

Detailed procedures are laid down for being taking into custody by the police, confinement and security of wandering mentally ill persons who are not able to take care of themselves or are dangerous to themselves or others. Such a person has to be produced before the magistrate by the police officer within 24 hours (section 23 MHA).

When such a person is produced before the magistrate, he may examine the person, make necessary inquiries and ask that person to be examined by a medical officer. The magistrate may, from time to time authorize detention of the alleged mentally ill person for ten days at a time, maximum up to 30 days.

The magistrate may pass a reception order authorizing the detention of the said person as an inpatient in a psychiatric hospital or psychiatric nursing home on medical advice or handover that individual under proper care and supervision of a relative or friend with or without sureties as determined by the magistrate (section 25 MHA).

Mentally ill Person Cruelly Treated or not Under Proper Care and Control

Mentally ill person not under proper care and control shall be reported by the police officer incharge of a police station to the area magistrate. The magistrate may cause the mentally ill person to be produced before him, and summon such relative or other person who is, or who ought to be incharge of, such mentally ill person. Magistrate can order the concerned relative to take proper care of the person. Failure to do that shall make such a person liable for fine which may extend to 2000 ₹. In case there is no person legally liable to take care of such mentally ill person the magistrate may order that person to be medically examined and pass a reception order.

Admission After Judicial Inquisition

If any district court holding an inquisition under chapter VI regarding any person who is found to be mentally ill is of opinion that it is necessary in the interest of such person, the court may direct that such person shall be admitted and kept as an inpatient in a psychiatric hospital or psychiatric nursing home.

Admission of Mentally ill Prisoners

Under sec. 330 or sec. 335 of the code of criminal procedure 1973 and various provisions/Acts of armed forces the court/tribunals may direct the reception of a mentally ill prisoner into any psychiatric hospital or psychiatric nursing home to which such person may be lawfully transferred for detention.

Supervision of Psychiatric Hospitals or Psychiatric Nursing Homes

The act provides for regular, thorough supervision of mental hospital and nursing homes by monthly joint inspection of three visitors designated by the central or state authority for health services (section 37 MHA).

DISCHARGE AND LEAVE OF ABSENCE

Any person (other than a prisoner) admitted to a psychiatric hospital who feels he has recovered from his mental illness can apply for discharge to the magistrate, supported by a medical certificate from the medical officer incharge of the hospital (section 43 MHA). Admitted person can be allowed to take leave from the hospital on request of his relatives or friends for a specified period (section 45 MHA).

Detailed procedure of safety in hospital, or during leave or absence or transfer to another hospital has been laid down (sections 45, 46, 47 MHA). Similarly safe custody and protection of property of the patients has been mentioned under sections 50–77 of MHA. Physical or mental cruelty of mentally ill patients is forbidden. Similarly conduct of research on a mental patient is forbidden, unless voluntarily consent is obtained. The human rights of a mentally ill person are protected under section 81 of MHA. Penalties and fines for contravening the provisions of the act have been mentioned under sections 82–87 of MHA.

THE MENTAL HEALTH CARE BILL 2013

The Indian government in 2007 ratified the United Nations Conventions on the Rights of Persons with Disabilities. To that effect, the Mental Health Care Bill, 2013 was first introduced in the Rajya Sabha to repeal the existing Mental Health Act 1987. This bill has been passed by the Rajya Sabha and is likely to be placed in the Lok Sabha.

In this bill the mental illness has been defined as "disorder of mood, thought, perception, orientation and memory which causes significant distress to a person or impairs ability to meet the demands of daily life and include mental conditions associated with abuse of alcohol and other drugs, but does not include mental retardation".

The bill requires any health establishment where PMIs are admitted or kept in for care, treatment, convalescence and rehabilitation to be registered as Mental Health Establishment (MHE), which would then be bound by all the rules framed under the bill by Mental Health Authorities. The provision of "License" under the MHA, 1987 has been replaced by "registration". Within nine months of the bill being passed, state governments will have to establish their own Mental Health Authorities. Main features of the proposed bill are summarized below.

Availability of good quality mental health services: The bill ensures right of every person without discrimination to access affordable and good quality mental health services which are to be made available by the government in sufficient quantity, which is easily accessible.

Human resources requirement of mental health services: Government have to address human resources requirement of mental health services by planning on the internationally accepted guidelines for number of mental health professionals on the basis of population are to be met within a period of ten years.

Access to treatment: Everyone should have access to mental health services which are affordable and easily available and those seeking treatment should not have to travel long distances.

Human rights of the PMI: Unless the persons with mental illness are completely incapable of understanding their illness, they will decide for themselves what kind of treatment they receive.

Decriminalization of Suicide: The act decriminalizes the attempt to suicide, placing it under the ambit of mental illness, instead of punishing the person who attempted suicide.

Imposing ban on unmodified ECT and restrictions on ECT to minors: Unmodified ECT has been prohibited in the bill, i.e. prohibiting ECT without anesthesia and muscle relaxants. Severe restrictions have been placed on the use of ECT to minors in the bill, where prior approval from the Mental Health Review Board has to be obtained.

TERMS COMMONLY USED IN PSYCHIATRIC PRACTICE

Intelligent quotient test (Binet-Simon test): It is used to measure the intellectual level of an individual. IQ of a person is calculated as "mental age (as assessed by his performance on psychological tests)/chronological age X 100". IQ of a person indicates relative brightness of an individual at a particular age.

Delusion

It is a false or erroneous belief in something, which is not a fact and is not in harmony with his educational and social beliefs. This cannot be corrected by any amount of logic, reasoning or arguments. False belief present in normal individuals which can be corrected by logic or reasoning are not delusions. Delusions normally are indicative of psychoses.

Types of Delusions

There are many types of delusions. Some important ones are enumerated below:

a. *Delusion of grandeur:* The person thinks himself to be rich or a big man or a king and behaves like that.

b. *Delusion of persecution:* His thinks that people are trying to kill him.

c. *Delusion of infidelity:* The person thinks that his spouse is not faithful.

d. *Cotard delusions:* Person has false belief that he is dead or does not exist.

e. *Delusion of reference:* He believes that people are talking or discussing about him.

f. *Delusion of jealousy:* He believes that others are jealous of him.

g. *Delusion of influence:* He believes that other peoples are controlling his thought process and actions.

h. *Nihilistic delusions:* He believes that he does not exist or the world does not exist.

i. *Hypochondrial delusions:* That he is suffering from some incurable disease.

J. *Erotomania:* Where an individual believes that a person usually of higher status is in love with him.

Medicolegal Importance

Delusions are important sign of mental illness. Person suffering from delusions may commit crimes under their influence or may commit suicide. In such cases the doctrine of diminished responsibility may be applied and the person may not be held fully responsible for his acts. During medical examination, such a person may be able to hide them hence he has to be observed for a longer duration.

Hallucinations

A false or erroneous sense perception without any external stimulus or object to produce it. Hallucinations of sight or hearing are most common.

Types of Hallucinations

i. *Auditory:* Person may hear some voices or roar of an animal.
ii. *Visual:* Person may visualize some object.
iii. *Olfactory:* He may smell something without any stimulus.
iv. *Tactile:* May feel some insects crawling over or sand grains on his skin.
v. *Psychomotor:* Feeling movement of some part his body.
vi. *Lilliputian:* The person visualizes things much smaller than their actual size.

These hallucinations can be pleasant or unpleasant ones.

Causes of Hallucinations

i. *Drugs:* Cannabis and LSD are few of the hallucinogenic drugs.
ii. *High fever:* Can also induce hallucinations.
iii. *Mental illness:* Presence of hallucination may suggest mental illness.

Illusion

It is false interpretation by a sense of an external object or stimuli, which has real existence, e.g. taking a rope for a snake. A normal person may also have illusions but after close observation he is able to correct himself. However a person suffering from mental illness is not able to correct himself and his actions may result from that false misinterpretation.

Impulse

Sudden and irresistible force compelling a person to the conscious performance of some action without motive or forethought. A normal person can restrain himself realizing the consequences, but a mentally ill person commits the act as soon as an impulse strikes him. Some of the important impulses are mentioned below:

i. *Kleptomania:* Irresistible desire to steal articles of small value.
ii. *Pyromania:* Desire to set fire.
iii. *Dipsomania:* Desire to drink in excess at short intervals.
iv. *Sexual impulses:* These could be nymphomania and satyriasis in females and males respectively.
v. Suicidal or homicidal impulses.

Obsession

Appearance of a persistent and irresistible thought, image, emotion or impulse which cannot be removed from the consciousness inspite of the best efforts of the sufferer to drive it out of his mind like a person checking door bolt again and again at night. This is an important sign of border line mental illness.

Lucid Interval

This is a period between two phases of mental illness when he becomes free of all symptoms of mental illness (or becoming conscious between two periods of unconsciousness in head injury cases). This may be seen in mania, melancholia or depressive psychosis (between manic and depressive phases) and person is held responsible for his actions during this period.

MENTAL DISORDERS

Mental disorders can be divided into two categories:

a. ***Mental deficiency or defectiveness (Amentia, Oligophrenia):*** There is retarded mental development. Depending upon the severity of the incomplete development, such cases are divided into three types as per Indian legal system, i.e.

i. *Idiots or custodial:* These are having IQ levels below 20 and may be associated with other physical abnormalities.

ii. *Imbecile or trainable:* In such cases the IQ levels range from 20 to 50 and can be trained for a specific job.

iii. *Feeble minded or morons (educable):* They have IQ levels from 50 to 75 and have mental development of a child between 6 to 11 years of age and can be educated.

According to international classification these are divided into (a) *borderline:* in such cases the IQ levels are from 70 to 84; (b) *mild:* when the IQ levels are from 55 to 69; (c) *moderate:* in such cases the IQ levels are from 40 to 54; (d) *severe:* in such cases the IQ levels are from 25 to 39; and (e) *profound:* when the IQ level is below 24.

b. *Mental disorders or diseases:* They can be grouped under (a) psychosis; (b) neurosis; (c) personality disorders; (d) sexual perversions; and (e) drug dependence.

The international classification of diseases (ICD) is an international standard diagnostic classification for a wide variety of health conditions. The ICD-10 states that mental disorder is "not an exact term", although generally used to imply the existence of a clinically recognizable set of symptoms or behaviours associated in most cases with distress and with interference with personal functions. Chapter V focuses on "mental and behavioural disorders" and consists of 10 main groups:

i. F0: Organic. including symptomatic, mental disorders

ii. F1: Mental and behavioural disorders due to use of psychoactive substances

iii. F2: Schizophrenia, schizotypal and delusional disorders

iv. F3: Mood [affective] disorders

v. F4: Neurotic, stress-related and somatoform disorders

vi. F5: Behavioural syndromes associated with physiological disturbances and physical factors

vii. F6: Disorders of personality and behaviour in adult persons

viii. F7: Mental retardation

ix. F8: Disorders of psychological development

x. F9: Behavioural and emotional disorders with onset usually occurring in childhood and adolescence.

In addition there is a group of unspecified mental disorders.

Within each group there are more specific subcategories. The ICD includes personality disorders on the same domain as other mental disorders, unlike the DSM.

Diagnostic and Statistical Manual of Mental Disorders, Fifth Edition (DSM-5): American Psychiatric Association in 2013 edition of DSM-5 defines and classify mental disorders in order to improve diagnosis, treatment and research.

Causes of Mental Illness

1. **Hereditary conditions:** Mental illnesses sometimes run in families, suggesting that in case, there is a mental illness in the family other members are likely to be affected. This susceptibility is passed on in families through genes. A family member may be susceptible but may not show any signs of mental illness unless some other factor may precipitate it like stress, illness or head injury.

2. **Environmental factors:** Person who is susceptible to mental illness, any stress may trigger a mental illness. Some of the environmental factors are mentioned below:

   a. Death of a near relative or friend.

   b. Divorce.

   c. Strained family relations.

   d. Loss of job.

   e. Drug abuse.

   f. Low self-esteem, anxiety or anger.

3. **Psychogenic causes:** Psychological factors may also contribute towards development of mental illness in an individual. Some of them are mentioned below:

   a. Psychological trauma from loss of a parent in early age group.

b. Childhood neglect.

c. Physical or sexual abuse suffered during childhood.

4. **Abnormal functioning of nerve pathways:** Neurotransmitters responsible for proper functioning of particular brain pathways are sometimes responsible for certain mental illnesses. Therefore, medication to run these pathways in a proper manner is helpful in treating such cases.

5. **Infections:** Some of the infections are linked with development of mental illnesses. It has been observed that streptococcal infection in children is responsible for obsessive compulsive disorder and some other mental illnesses.

6. **Brain injuries or damage:** It has been observed that anoxic damage during birth may be associated with autism. Even injury to certain area of the brain, occurring during adult age group is responsible for certain group of mental illnesses.

7. **Drugs related causes:** Chronic drug abuse has been linked to depression and paranoia.

Diagnosis of Mental Illness

1. **Family history:** Detailed family history is asked from the patient as well as relatives regarding any family history of mental illness. Loss of any family member in the recent past may also be inquired.

2. **Personal history:** Personal history is very important and the person must be taken into full confidence. History regarding whether the birth was normal or not, milestone of growth, any head injury, performance in the school and college, occupation and interest in the job, sexual indulgence, relation with wife if married and any other medical problems must be asked.

3. **Physical examination:** The patient must be thoroughly examined with especial reference to the nervous system.

4. **Mental status:** The individual must be examined for general appearance, aggressive behaviour, orientation of time and place, whether timid or smart, posture, facial expression, speech, mannerism, prominent thoughts, delusions or hallucinations, presence of any impulse, memory, disturbing intelligence and sleep pattern must be enquired and noted.

5. **Special investigations:** Apart from routine investigations, special investigations, like CT scanning, MRI and EEG may be undertaken if required.

6. **Feigned mental illness:** While diagnosing mental illness, cases of feigned insanity must be excluded. A person may feign insanity for the purposes of evasion, deceit or diversion of suspicion. Such cases can be differentiated by noting motive, habits, symptoms, sleep pattern and eating habits. Detailed differentiating features are mentioned in Table 34.1.

Mental Illness and Responsibility

In law responsibility of a mentally ill person means liability for his acts. Depending upon the type of court involved it can be of two types:

1. Civil responsibilities
2. Criminal responsibilities.

1. **Civil responsibilities:** Question of civil responsibility of a mentally ill person arises in cases like:

   a. *Management of property:* If a person is found mentally ill after judicial inquisition and because of which he is incapable of managing himself and his affairs (like looking after his property), in such cases high court or district court can issue an order for the appointment of a manager to look after his property.

   b. *Contracts:* Under section 12 of the Indian contract act a contract is invalid if one of the parties making it was by the reason of mental illness, incapable of understanding it and making a rational judgment as to its effects upon his interests. However the validity of ordinary contracts entered into by a person of mental illness depends upon the circumstances accompanying the act. A mentally ill

		True mental illness	Feigned mental illness
	Tabe 34.1: Differentiation between True and Feigned Mental illness		
1.	Onset	Gradual, rarely sudden	Always sudden
2.	Motive	Nil	Some motive is there
3.	Symptoms	Can be grouped under one type of mental illness	Bizarre symptoms
4.	Look	Vacant look in advanced cases	Changes from time to time
5.	Exertion	Can stand for days together	Will breakdown after sometime
6.	Habits	Dirty and filthy	Not so
7.	Skin and lips	Dry with furred tongue	Not so
8.	Frequent examinations	Do not mind	Resist
9.	Observed without his knowledge	Symptoms remain	No symptoms
10.	Sleeping	May have insomnia deprivation	Compensate for sleep
11.	Eating habits	Any food available	Only clean food

person is responsible for payment of necessities purchased by him according to his position and status, however in case it is proved that the other person (seller) has taken advantage of his mental illness then there is no liability.

c. *Marriage*: Marriage in law is more than an ordinary contract, it can be declared null and void if it is proved that one of the parties was by reason of mental illness at the time of marriage unable to understand the nature and responsibilities of the contract of marriage. However, mental illness developing subsequently to the marriage was no ground for divorce earlier, but with the amendments in the marriage acts in 1976 this can now be a ground for divorce.

d. *Competency as a witness*: Under section 118 of IEA a mentally ill person is not competent to give evidence in the court of law, if he is prevented by his mental illness to understand a question put to him and giving a rational answer to it.

e. *Consent*: Under section 90 IPC consent by a mentally ill person is invalid, who is unable to understand the nature and consequences of that to which he gives his consent.

f. *Torts and mental illness*: Tort is an infringement of the general rights of the others or failure to respect the general rights of others. A mentally ill person is not liable for the infringement of the rights of others by his actions, because he is incapable of knowing that his act was wrong.

g. *Testamentary capacity*: Testamentary capacity means capacity to make a valid will. Preconditions to make a valid will are as follows:
   i. Testator must be a major.
   ii. Testator must be of sound disposing mind.
   iii. Testator must sign in presence of two disinterested witnesses.

To prove that a person is having sound disposing mind: (a) he must understand the nature of the will; (b) he must have proper knowledge of the property to be distributed; and (c) he must know the persons who have moral claim to his property and their relative strength of claim.

Whenever a medical man is asked to witness a will, he not only signs as a witness but also testifies as to the competency (sound disposing mind) of the testator to make a valid will.

Certain situations associated with testamentary capacity:

i. *Delusions:* Delusions may co-exist with testamentary capacity provided evidence is given that at the time of making a will the testator's mind was not influenced by the delusions.

ii. Underinfluence: A will is held invalid if executed under the influence of any other person or intoxicant.

iii. Lucid interval: A person can make a will during lucid interval. However, in some cases will making may be doubted due to presence of retrograde amnesia in head injury.

iv. Extremes of age: A will made at the point of death in old age is usually doubted.

v. Suicides: The will remains valid even if the testator commits suicide after making a will.

vi. Deaf and dumb: Persons who are deaf or dumb can make a valid will.

vii. Aphasia and will: If a person is able to communicate by writing or indicating by any means, he can make a valid will.

viii. Eccentricity and will: An eccentric person provided he is having sound disposing mind can make a valid will.

2. **Criminal responsibility:** Law presumes that every person is mentally sound until he is proved to be suffering from mental illness to the satisfaction of the court. The plea of mental illness may be raised by way of defense to any criminal charges but because of stigma and admission in a psychiatric hospital, such pleas are mainly confined to the charges of murder in order to escape capital punishment.

The question of mental illness in criminal cases arises at two stages:

a. *At the court of trial:* The person claims that he is unfit to plead the case. The tests applied for this depends upon his inability to; (i) understand the nature of proceedings; (ii) distinguish between pleas of guilty and not guilty; (iii) examine witnesses; (iv) make proper defence; and (v) to follow evidence properly. Opinion of the doctor in such cases must be based on the examination of the accused on the day of trial. Such cases are kept pending till the person concerned becomes fit to stand trial.

b. *At the court of conviction:* When a person takes the plea of mental illness as his defence the court normally applies following rules:

i. *McNaughten's rule:* McNaughten in 1843 shot Mr Drummond the private secretary to Sir Robert Peel, then Prime Minister of England. When he was acquitted on the ground of insanity, the British parliament, due to public uproar, put certain questions to a panel of 14 eminent Judges. McNaughten rule is based on the answers given by the panel of judges.

"That to establish defence on the ground of insanity it must be clearly proved that at the time of committing the act, the party accused was labouring under such a defect of reason, from the disease of mind as not to know the nature and quality of the act he was doing or if he did know it, he did not know that what he was doing was wrong".

This law was incorporated in the Indian laws under section 84 of Indian penal Code which states that "Nothing is offence which is done by a person who at the time of doing it, is by the reason of unsoundness of mind, incapable of knowing the nature of the act or that he is doing is either wrong or contrary to the law".

To establish defence in such a case three things are required to be proved by the accused:

a. Evidence of mental disease or defect.

b. That the mental disease or defect existed at the time of unlawful act.

c. That this mental disease or defect was of such a degree because of which the accused was unable to understand that the act was wrong or contrary to law.

However some criticism has been voiced against the McNaughten's rule. On the grounds that (i) there is no consideration of emotional factors or psychopathic personalities (subnormalities); (ii) diagnosis of insanity is a complex procedure hence should not be trusted to laymen especially to jury; and (iii) There is no provision for disorders affecting reasoning process like in melancholia who may kill a dependent before attempting suicide.

ii. *Diminished responsibility:* In certain mental disorders, e.g. psychopathic personalities, the sufferer strictly from the legal point of view is responsible for his acts but from medical or psychological point of view is not fully responsible. In England under section 2 of the Homicide Act 1957 the principle of diminished responsibility was introduced.

"When a person kills or is a party to the killing of another he shall not be convicted for murder, if he was suffering from such abnormality of mind as to substantially impair his mental responsibility for his act and omissions in doing or being a part to the killing".

iii. *Irresistible impulse rule:* This rule is often expressed in the form of a question.

"If the defendant did know the nature and quality of act and that it was wrong, was he unable, because of mental disease or defect to adhere to the right"?

This is only applicable in those situations where crime is done on sudden impulse. Under section 300 IPC, a homicide is not a murder if it is committed without premeditation in sudden fight.

iv. *Durham's rule:* This rule states that "an accused is not criminally responsible if his unlawful act was the product of mental disease of defect". Interpretation of the word product created confusion in many cases hence now this rule has been dropped by many US courts.

v. *ALI formula:* American Law Institute formulated this rule regarding criminal responsibility.

"A person is not responsible for his criminal conduct if at the time of such conduct as a result of mental disease of defect he lacked substantial capacity to appreciate the criminality of his act or conform his conduct to the requirement of the law".

vi. *Curren's rule:* Judge Briggs modified the ALI formula in Curren case as follows:

"That at the time of committing the act the defendant as a result of mental disease of defect lacked the substantial capacity to conform his conduct to the requirements of the law".

Somnambulism (Sleep Walking)

It is sleep disorder belonging to parasomnia group. The person may walk or perform certain activities in a state of low consciousness like during sleep. Courts have decided that a person is not responsible for the act as he is not aware of the actions and afterwards does not remember anything.

Hypnotism

Normally not taken as defence as the person had willingly consented for hypnotism and even under hypnotism will not do anything against his subconscious desires.

Somnolentia

Also known as sleep drunkenness. This is a condition between sleep and awaking like confused state at sudden awakening from sleep, and the person in confusion may commit some act for which he is not held responsible.

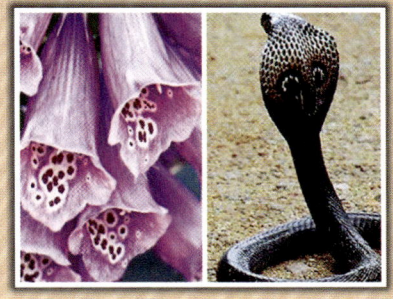

Section 4

Forensic Toxicology

35 | General Toxicology

Toxicology is the science dealing with properties, action, toxicity, fatal dose, detection, estimation and interpretation of the result of toxicological analysis, management and autopsy findings in a case of poisoning.

POISON

A poison is defined as any substance which when administered in living body through any route (inhaled, ingested, absorbed, injected or developed inside the body) will produce symptoms, ill-health or death by its action which is due to its physical, chemical or physiological properties.

Stedman's medical dictionary defines poison as "any substance; either taken internally or applied externally that is injurious to health or dangerous to life".

British toxicologist Alfred Swaine Taylor (1859) wrote that "a poison in small doses is a medicine and a medicine in large doses is a poison".

FORENSIC TOXICOLOGY

Branch of forensic medicine dealing with medical and legal aspects of the harmful effects of poisons, chemicals or toxins on human beings.

Drug

Drug is any substance or product that is used or intended to be used to modify or explore physiological systems or pathological states for the benefit of the recipient. WHO has defined the drug as "any substance that when taken into living organism may modify one or more of its actions".

Clinical Toxicology

Deals with human diseases caused by, or associated with abnormal exposure to chemical substances.

Toxinology

It refers to study of toxins produced by living organism which are dangerous to human like snake venom, fungal and bacterial toxins.

Toxicity Rating

Toxicity rating of a poison depends upon its potency. It is graded from 1 (practically nontoxic) to 6 (highly toxic or supertoxic). Grade 6 supertoxic are those substances where fatal dose is usually less than 5 mg per kg of body weight; Grade 5, i.e. Extremely toxic in which the fatal dose is between 5 to 50 mg per Kg body weight; grade 4 are very toxic and the fatal dose varies from 50 to 500 mg per kilogram of body weight; grade 3 are moderately toxic with fatal dose between 500 mg to 5 gm per kilogram of body weight; grade 2 slightly toxic have fatal dose between 5 to 15 gm per kilogram of body weight and grade -I practically nontoxic are those when the fatal dose is more than 15 gm per Kg body weight.

Fatal Dose

It is the approximate quantity required for fatal consequences in an adult of a particular drug. It varies depending upon age, build, ill-health and many other factors.

NATURE OF POISONING

Intentional Poisoning

Intentional poisoning cases can be further divided into suicidal or homicidal poisoning.

a. *Suicidal poisoning or self-poisoning:* When some poisonous substance is taken by an individual for suicidal purposes. Most common poisons used for this purpose are opium, barbiturates, organophosphorus, KCN, oxalic acid and oleander.

b. *Homicidal poisoning:* When some poison is administered to kill any individual. Common poisons used for this purpose are arsenic, antimony, nux-vomica, madar, powdered glass and aconite.

Accidental Poisoning

Accidental poisoning is very commonly seen in children when they accidentally consume some drugs like paracetamol or kerosene.

Animal poisoning is also common in India to kill animals and the poisons used are strychnine, abrus precatorius, yellow oleander, zinc phosphide, arsenic or aconite.

Presentations of Poisoning

Depending on the dose and frequency of administration the features of poisoning may manifest in following forms:

i. *Fulminant poisoning:* This is seen when a massive dose of a poison is consumed leading to sudden death from shock. Manifesting symptoms of that poisoning may not be observed in such cases.

ii. *Acute poisoning:* This is caused by a large single dose, or several dose of a poison taken over a short interval of time, manifesting symptoms of that poison.

iii. *Subacute poisoning:* In such a case features of both acute and chronic poisoning are present.

iv. *Chronic poisoning:* This is caused by smaller doses over a longer period of time, resulting in gradual manifestation of symptoms of chronic poisoning.

MEDICOLEGAL ASPECTS OF POISONING

Indian law takes cognizance of the intention with which a substance is given to an individual. If it is given to cure then it is medicine but if given with intention to cause bodily harm or death then it is poison.

Sec. 272 IPC: Whoever adulterates food or drink, so as to make the same noxious, intended for sale may be punished with imprisonment of either term extend up to 6 months and/or fine up to 1000 ₹.

Sec. 273 IPC: Whoever sells noxious food or drink may be punished with imprisonment of either description for a period of 6 months and/or fine up to 1000 ₹.

Sec. 274 IPC: Whoever adulterates any drug in any form with any change in its effect knowing that it will be sold and used as unadulterated drug for medicinal purpose, may be punished with imprisonment of either description for a period of 6 months and/or fine which may extend to 1000 ₹.

Sec. 275 IPC: Whoever knowingly sells adulterated drugs with less efficacy or altered action serving it for use as unadulterated may be punished with imprisonment of either description for 6 months and/or fine which may extend to 1000 ₹.

Sec. 276 IPC: For selling a drug as a different drug or preparation may be punished with imprisonment of either description which may extend up to 6 months and or fine which may extend to 1000 ₹.

Sec. 277 IPC: For fouling water of public spring or reservoir may be punished with imprisonment of either description which may extend to a period of 3 months and/or fine which may extend to 500 ₹.

Sec. 278 IPC: For voluntarily making atmosphere noxious to health is punished with fine which may extend up to 500 ₹.

Sec. 284 IPC: Whoever does with respect to poisonous substance any act as to endanger human life is punished with imprisonment of either description which may extend up to 6 months and/or fine which may extend up to 1000 ₹

Sec. 324 IPC: Whoever voluntarily causes hurt by means of any poison or corrosive substance or any substance which is deleterious to the human body to inhale, to swallow or to receive in blood shall be punished with imprisonment of either description for a term which may extend to three years with or without fine.

Sec. 326 IPC: Whoever voluntarily causes grievous hurt by means of any poison or corrosive substance or any substance which is deleterious to the human body to inhale, to swallow or to receive in blood shall be punished with imprisonment of either description for a term which may extend to 10 years or imprisonment for life with or without fine.

Sec. 328 IPC: Whoever causes hurt by means of poison or any stupefying, intoxicating or unwholesome drug or any other thing with the intent to commit an offence shall be punished with imprisonment of either description for a term which may extend to ten years with or without fine.

Sec. 299 IPC (Culpable Homicide) and Sec 300 IPC (Murder): Causing death of a person by an act, with the intention of causing such bodily injury and is likely to cause death, or with the knowledge that he is likely, by such an act to cause death (including poisoning).

LAWS RELATED TO POISONS

a. *The opium act 1857:* This act provided with issue of licenses for cultivation, delivery to the produce to the concerned officers and fixation of the price of opium produced.

b. *The opium act 1858:* This was enacted to regulate possession, transport, import, export and sale of opium in India.

c. *Poison act (1919):* The act was passed to control import of poisons into India, their possession and sale within India.

d. *Dangerous drugs act of 1930:* The act was passed with a view to regulate cultivation, manufacture, import, export, possession, sale and use of drugs derived from opium, Indian hemp and coca leaves causing addiction. This act was in fact passed in accordance with geneva convention and was later amended in 1933, 1938 and 1957.

e. *Drugs act of 1940:* Drug Act was passed to regulate the import, manufacture, distribution and sale of all types of drugs. Main feature of the act was to control the quantity, purity and strength of drugs. The drug act was later amended to include cosmetics and the title was changed to **Drugs and cosmetics act**. In 1955 it was amended to include insecticides disinfectants and contraceptives. The act was further amended in 1962 and also in 1964 to include Unani, Siddha and Ayurvedic drugs.

f. *Drugs and cosmetic rules of 1945:* Drug technical advisory board and central drug laboratory are instituted to advise and help central and state governments. From 1955 the central government has taken over the powers to make rules from state governments related to manufacture, distribution and sale of drugs. These rules regulate the import of drugs, functions of central drug laboratory, appointment of licensing authorities and also have classified the drugs into various schedules:

Important schedules of drugs act are:

C – Biological and special products.

E – List of poisons.

F – Vaccines and sera.

G – Hormones.

H – Drugs and poisons to be sold on prescription of RMP.

J – List of diseases for which drugs should not be advertised.

L – Antibiotics, antihistaminic, chemotherapeutic agents (to be sold on prescription of RMP).

Conditions for dispensing drugs under drugs and cosmetic rules:

1. Must possess a license to stock, sell and distribute drugs.
2. Any prescription by a RMP must be compounded by a qualified pharmacist.
3. Supply of listed drugs must be entered in a register.
4. One prescription must not be dispensed more than once unless specified.
5. Poisons must be kept in separate almirah under lock and key with poison written in red letters.
6. Customers must not have access to these drugs.
7. Schedule H and L drugs must not be sold except on prescription by a RMP.

A prescription must be written, dated and signed by a RMP. It should mention the name and address of the patient and indicate the name of the drugs their doses and amount to be supplied.

g. *The pharmacy act of 1948:* The act made provisions for the regulation of the profession of the pharmacy and to constitute pharmacy council.

h. *Drug control act of 1950:* It controlled supply distribution and sale of drugs. It also gives power to the government to fix maximum price of any drug.

i. *Drugs and magic remedies act of 1954:* Under this act advertisements of magic remedies for miscarriage, contraception, increase sexual potency and treatment of venereal diseases are completely banned.

j. *Insecticide act of 1968 and 1971:* To control the distribution and sale of insecticides all over India.

k. *Narcotic drugs and psychotropic substances act, 1985:* The narcotic drugs and psychotropic substances act, commonly referred to as the NDPS act, came into force on 14 November

1985. Under the NDPS act, it is illegal for a person to produce, manufacture, cultivate, possess, sell, purchase, transport, store, and/or consume any narcotic drug or psychotropic substance. The act has been amended - in 1988, 2001 and 2014. The act extends to the whole of India and it applies also to all Indian citizens outside India and to all persons on ships and aircraft registered in India. The act defines narcotic drugs and psychotropic substances. *Narcotic drugs* include coca leaves, cannabis, opium and related manufactured drugs, whereas psychotropic substances include 76 drugs and their derivatives mentioned in the list.

The *narcotic drugs and psychotropic substances (amendment) act, 2014* (act No. 16 of 2014) amended the NDPS act to relax restrictions placed by the act on essential narcotic drugs (morphine, fentanyl and methadone) making them more accessible for use in pain relief and palliative care.

This act repeals the opium act 1857, the opium act 1878 and dangerous drugs act 1930. Under provisions of the act, the narcotics control bureau was set up with effect from March 1986. The act is designed to fulfil India's treaty obligations under convention on narcotic drugs, convention on psychotropic substances, and united nations convention against illicit trafficking in narcotic drugs and psychotropic substances.

Punishment: Anyone who contravenes the NDPS act will face punishment based on the quantity of the banned substance.

a. Where the contravention involves a *small quantity*, with rigorous imprisonment for a term which may extend to 1 year, or with a fine which may extend to 10000 or both.

b. Where the contravention involves a quantity lesser than *commercial quantity* but greater than a *small quantity*, with rigorous imprisonment for a term which may extend to 10 years and with fine which may extend to 1 lakh.

c. Where the contravention involves a *commercial quantity*, with rigorous imprisonment for a term which shall not be less than 10 years but which may extend to 20 years and also a fine which shall not be less than 1 lakh but which may extend to 2 lakh.

Central government has specified small and commercial quantity of each drug, e.g. for opium small quantity is 25 gm and commercial quantity is 2.5 Kg.

DUTIES OF A MEDICAL PRACTITIONER IN A CASE OF SUSPECTED POISONING

Duties of a medical practitioner are both professional as well as legal.

Professional Duties

Medical treatment should be provided immediately to save the life of an individual hence professional duties have priority over legal responsibilities.

Legal Duties

1. Preliminary information of the patient must be recorded, like name, age, sex, address, occupation, date and time identification marks and brought by whom, etc.
2. A doctor must observe and note the symptoms, signs, presence of any peculiar smell, and any other person similarly affected.
3. In suspected poisoning case the opinion must be expressed with due care.
4. A doctor must preserve vomitus or stomach wash, sample of urine if passed and other material present on the scene like bottle, glass or cup from which the poison was administered. Failing to do so, a doctor can be charged under section 201 IPC for causing disappearance or destruction of evidence.
5. A doctor must safe guard the patient against further administration of poison by either appointing a nurse or shifting the patient to a hospital.
6. A doctor must inform the police in suspected homicidal poisoning case. Noncompliance can be punished under section 176 IPC. However he has the discretion of not informing the police in suicidal poisoning case (not covered under section 39 CrPC). However, for a doctor in government service, he is mostly instructed to inform the police in all poisoning case.
7. If suspected poisoning prove fatal a doctor must not issue a death certificate, rather he should inform the police.

Classification of Poisons

According to mode of action poisons are classified as follows:

Poisons Having Predominantly Local Action

1. **Corrosives:**
   a. *Acids:*
      i. Mineral acids: These are sulfuric acid (car battery fluid), nitric acid (metal cleaners), hydrochloric acid (descalers) and hydrogen fluoride (rust removers).
      ii. Organic acids: These are formic acid, carbolic acids and acetic acid.
   b. *Alkalis:*
      i. Caustics or alkalis, such as hydroxide or carbonates of sodium, potassium or calcium and ammonia when anhydrous or in a concentrated solution.
      ii. Extremely strong bases (super-bases) such as alkoxide, metal amides (e.g. sodium amide) and organometallic bases such as butyllithium.
   c. *Heavy metal salts:* Some of the heavy metal salts also have corrosive properties like calcium oxide , anhydrous zinc chloride, anhydrous aluminum chloride and mercuric chloride (corrosive sublimate).
   d. Miscellaneous substances like formalin, elemental bromine, fluorine, chlorine and iodine, iodine tincture, concentrated hydrogen peroxide, etc.

2. **Irritants:**
   a. *Inorganic metals:* Arsenic, lead, mercury, copper or thallium salts.
   b. *Inorganic nonmetals:* Chlorine, iodine or phosphorus.

c. *Mechanical:* Glass powder, diamond dust or hair

d. *Organic irritants:*

   i. Organic irritant poisons of animal origin like snakes, scorpions, spiders and cantharides.

   ii. Organic irritant poisons of vegetable origin like abrus, castor, croton, capsicum or calotropis, etc.

Poisons Having Remote Action

1. **Neurotoxic:**

   a. *Cerebral poisons:*

      i. Somniferous: Opium and its alkaloids.

      ii. Inebriant (intoxicant): Alcohol, ether, chloroform.

      iii. Hypnotics and sedatives: Barbiturate, chloral hydrate.

      iv. Stimulant: Amphetamine, dextroamphetamine or methamphetamine, etc.

      v. Deliriant: Datura (stupefacient), belladona, hyocyamus, cannabis indica.

      vi. Hallucinogens: LSD, peyote, psilocybin, cannabis.

   b. *Spinal (convulsent) poisons:* Strychnos nux vomica and gelsemium.

   c. Poisons acting on peripheral nerves:

      i. Local anesthetics: cocaine, procaine.

      ii. Relaxants: Curare and conium

2. **Cardiac poisons:** Cyanide, digitalis, aconite, nicotine, quinine, oleander.

3. **Asphyxiants:** Carbon dioxide, CO, hydrogen sulphide

4. **Miscellaneous:** Food poisons, common household poisons, insecticides (organophosphorus, carbamates), herbicides (paraquat, bromoxynil), rodenticides (zinc phosphide, strychnine) and fumigants (aluminum phosphide).

5. Chemical and biological warfare agents.

6. Drugs of abuse and date rape drugs.

Combined Local and Remotes Action

Some poisons have both local and systemic actions like carbolic acid, oxalic acid, phosphorus, etc.

Drugs Having Specific Toxicity

a. *Nephrotoxic:* Oxalic acid, mercury, cantharides, etc.

b. *Hepatotoxic:* Phosphorus, carbon tetrachloride, chloroform, etc.

FACTORS INFLUENCING THE ACTIONS OF A POISON IN THE BODY

1. **Quantity:** Large dose of poison acts quickly and often results in fatal consequences. A small dose may have subclinical effects and causes chronic poisoning on repeated exposure. Very large dose of arsenic may produce death by shock without any irritant symptoms, whereas slightly lower dose causes death by irritation. In copper sulphate a large single dose induces vomiting but small multiple doses result in fatal consequences.

2. **Physical form:** Gaseous or volatile poisons are very quickly absorbed and are thus most rapidly effective. Liquid poisons are more rapid in action than solid poisons which are absorbed slowly. Some poisonous vegetable seeds, in case taken intact, may pass through the intestinal canal without any poisonous effects, when taken crushed, they may result in poisoning.

3. **Chemical form:** Chemical combination of poisons may alter the action of poisons like silver nitrate and hydrochloric acid in combination forms an insoluble compound whereas independently they both are strong poisons. Chemically pure arsenic and mercury are not poisonous because these are insoluble and are not absorbed. But white arsenic trioxide and mercuric chloride are deadly poisonous.

4. **Mechanical combination:** Action of the poison may be altered if combined with some inert substance like alkaloids mixed with active charcoal may be harmless on ingestion.

5. **Concentration (or dilution):** Concentrated form of poison are absorbed more rapidly and are also more fatal like acids but in highly diluted form may not be harmful.

6. **Condition of the stomach:** Presence of food content acts as diluents of the poison and hence protects the stomach wall and also delays absorption of poison. Empty stomach absorbs poison most rapidly. In cases of achlorhydria, KCN and NaCN are ineffective due to lack of hydrochloric acid, which is required for the conversion of KCN and NaCN to HCN before absorption. Absorption of phosphorus is more rapid when taken with fatty foods. Snake venom may be ineffective if taken orally.

7. **Route of administration:** The rapidity of action of poison depends upon the mode in which it is administered. A poison acts more rapidly when inhaled or when given intravenously. Next in rapidity are intramuscular or subcutaneous routes. Oral route is faster than when given per rectum.

8. **Cumulative action of poisons:** Preparations of poisons which are not readily excreted from the body and are retained in different organs of the body for a long time, like lead may not cause any toxic effect when enters the body in low dose, but when consumed over a long period of time, may cause harm due to their cumulative property.

9. **Condition of the body:**
   a. *Age:* Most of the poisons have great effect in extremes of age. However, opium and its alkaloids are tolerated better by elderly subjects but badly by children and infants. Belladonna group of drugs are better tolerated by children than by adults.
   b. *State of body health:* A well-built person with good health can tolerate the action of poison better than a weak person. In certain diseased conditions some drugs are tolerated exceptionally well, e.g. Opium, sedatives and tranquilizers in tetanus or mania and strychnine in paralysis.
   c. *Intoxication and poisoning states:* In certain poisoning cases some drugs are well tolerated, like, in case of strychnine poisoning, barbiturates and sedatives are better tolerated.
   d. *Sleep:* Due to slow metabolic process and depression of other body functions during sleep, usually the absorption and action of the poison is also slow. But depressant drugs may cause, more harm during the state of sleep.
   e. *Exercise:* Action of alcohol on CNS is reduced during exercise because more blood is drawn to the muscles during exercise.
   f. *Tolerance:* Tolerance may develop in certain individuals on long-term exposure to a particular poison and such persons may even tolerate fatal dose of that drug like arsenic.
   g. *Idiosyncrasy:* It is the abnormal response to a drug due to hypersensitivity like penicillin, arsenic, potassium iodide aspirin, etc.

GENERAL PRINCIPLES OF MANAGEMENT

Most important aspect of the management of a poisoning case is that he should be approached in a rational fashion as mentioned below:

a. **Diagnosis:**
   i. Entertain the possibility of poisoning.
   ii. Identify the poison.

b. **Treatment:**
   i. Prevent further absorption.
   ii. Symptomatic and supportive therapy.
   iii. Administration of specific antidotes if possible.
   iv. Hasten excretion of the toxic substance.

c. **Legal and other aspects:**
   i. Preserve physical evidence of poison.
   ii. Anticipate complications.
   iii. Prevent reoccurrence.

Diagnosis of Poisoning

Failure to consider the possibility of poisoning is the most common and often most serious mistake in management. Diagnosis can only be made once the possibility is considered.

Poisoning may not be considered when the manifestation is tetany (fluorides), ataxia (barbiturates), cyanosis (nitrates) or delirium (aconite). In some cases of suicides the patient may even mislead the doctor by giving an alternative explanation. A possibility of double poisoning should also be considered like suicidal attempt with alcohol and barbiturates.

Diagnosis of Poisoning in Living

There is no single symptom or group of symptoms, which are absolutely characteristic of poisoning. Identification of the toxic substance is of importance as specific antidotal therapy can be administered and also help in anticipating and avoiding further complications. However, appropriate symptomatic treatment must not be withheld pending confirmation of the toxic agent.

a. The onset is usually sudden except in chronic poisoning. Poisoning has to be differentiated from diseases which have sudden onset like cholera, gastroenteritis or acute abdomen.

b. Symptoms usually appear immediately or within a short time after consuming some food or drink.

c. Symptoms are uniform in character and rapidly increase in severity.

d. Similar symptom may be seen all the persons consuming the same food or drink.

e. Sometimes characteristic symptoms and smell may indicate the nature of poisoning in some cases.

f. Detection of poison in food, vomit, urine or feces is a strong proof of poisoning hence they must always be preserved. However the results are often received late to be of any use in treating the case.

Diagnosis of Poisoning in Dead

Diagnosis of poisoning is made from the postmortem findings, chemical analysis, animal experimentation and circumstantial evidence.

1. **Postmortem findings:** Before conducting the postmortem examination, inquest papers must be scrutinized for clinical history and circumstantial evidence of the case.

External examination:

a. Clothing must be examined for presence of vomitus.

b. Injection prick marks and other stains should be noted along with their colour.

c. *Colour of the hypostasis:* colour of the hypostasis is bright red in carbon monoxide, brick red in cyanide, chocolate brown in nitrate and yellowish in phosphorus poisonings.

d. Natural orifices specially mouth and nostrils for any sign of poisoning.

e. *Smell:* Some of the poisons can be recognised from their smell like alcohol, opium, cyanides, etc.

Internal examination: A thorough examination should be done.

a. *Mouth and throat:* Examined for any corrosive action.

b. *Stomach:* Contents and the walls of the stomach may suggest the nature of poisoning in some cases specially corrosives or irritant poisoning.

i. Contents are examined for any residue of the poison and characteristic smell.

ii. Stomach wall: may show: (a) hyperemia which is most marked along the greater curvature and the cardiac end. Mostly it is patchy involving the ridges. Colour of the wall may help in finding the type of poisoning like green in ferrous sulphate or copper sulphate, black or charred in sulphuric acid, yellow in nitric acid, grayish white and hardened in carbolic acid and velvety red in potassium cyanide poisoning; (b) softening may result from corrosives or irritant poisons causing damage to superficial layers mainly seen in alkalis. Softening in putrefaction is mainly seen on the dependent portions of the stomach wall; (c) ulceration is mostly seen along the greater curvature. Erosions have thin friable margins surrounded by softened mucosa; (d) perforation may be seen with sulphuric acid poisoning and have ragged and irregular edges.

c. *Liver spleen and kidneys:* These may show congestion.

d. *Heart:* Any subendocardial hemorrhages are noted.

2. **Chemical analysis:** Viscera, blood and other body fluids taken out at the time of postmortem examination are forwarded for chemical analysis. In some cases poison may not be detected in the viscera due to (a) elimination from the body or short life span; (b) destroyed during storage; (c) insufficient material of testing; and (d) some poisons are not tested unless indicated.

3. **Experiments on animals:** Not preferred these days, however domestic animals may be fed on the suspected food material and symptoms noted.

4. **Circumstantial evidence:** Circumstantial evidence in the form of empty containers, prescriptions and through questioning friends, family or co-workers may be of help in finding out the nature of poison consumed and motive of poisoning.

Treatment of Poisoning

Removal of Poison from the Body to Prevent Further Absorption:

1. **Inhaled poison:** Person should be removed to fresh air, provide artificial respiration and keep the air passage clear.

2. **Injected poison:** In case of intramuscular injection, subcutaneous injection or snake bite a bandage is applied over that limb to minimize absorption. Wound is excised and poison is sucked or neutralized by chemicals.

3. **Contact poison:** In such a case the skin is washed with water or neutralized by specific chemical substance.

4. **Ingested poison:**
   i. Gastric lavage is useful within 3 to 4 hours of ingestion of a poison. It is done by Ewald's or Boas tube. In children

Ryle's tube can also be used. Artificial dentures if present should be removed before introducing gastric lavage tube up to 50 cm mark from incisor teeth. To know whether the tube has actually gone into the stomach or in trachea, air is injected into the tube by closing the outer end and compressing the balloon. Auscultation over the epigastrium for escape of air in the stomach confirms its presence in the stomach. Otherwise the free end of the tube can be dipped in water, in case the tube has gone into trachea continuous stream of bubbles will come out. To minimize the danger of aspiration the patient is placed in prone position with head and shoulders lower than the hips and head turned towards one side. About 250 ml of water is passed through the funnel into the stomach and then removed by siphoning action. First sample is preserved for chemical analysis. Depending upon the ingested poison, different chemical antidotes are used to clean the stomach in subsequent washes.

Contraindications of gastric lavage:

a. Absolute contraindications:
   i. Corrosive poisons except carbolic acid.
   ii. Known case of esophageal varices.

b. Relative contraindications:
   i. Convulsent poison
   ii. Comatosed patient
   iii. Volatile poison like kerosene
   iv. Marked hypothermia.

Clinical judgment must be used in deciding whether the advantage of gastric lavage outweigh its dangers. In such cases stomach wash may be attempted only when absolutely required and after taking proper precautions.

ii. *Emetics:* Emesis may occur spontaneously in irritant poisons. Normally emetic are used when there are problems

Solutions for gastric lavage	
Poison	*Specific gastric lavage solution*
Alkaloids	1:5000 potassium permanganate solution
Bleach	5% Sodium thiosulphate
Copper salts	1% pot. ferrocyanide
Fluorides/ Oxalates	5% calcium lactate or milk
Formaldehyde	1% ammonium carbonate
Iodine	Starch solution
Ferrous salts	5–10 gram of desferoxamine in 100 ml of 10% sodium bicarbonate
Salicylates	10% sodium bicarbonate
Silver	5% sodium chloride

in using gastric lavage or lavage tube is not available. Emetics are often ineffective if the poison has antiemetic activity like phenothiazine. Emetics are contraindicated in advanced pregnancy or heart and lung diseases. Emesis can be introduced in following manner:

a. By stimulating pharynx with a finger or a feather in conscious patient.
b. Copious amount of warm water.
c. Table spoon (15 gm) of ground mustard or common salt in 200 ml of water.
d. Zinc sulphate, 1–2 gm in tumbler of water can be repeated after 15 minute
e. Ipecacuanha powder, 1–2 gm or 30 ml of syrup.
f. Ammonium carbonate 1–2 gm.
g. Tartar emetic about 0.1 gm.
h. Apomorphine 60 mg subcutaneously but may result in depression.

Symptomatic and Supportive Therapy

For most of the poisons specific antidotes are not available hence therapy must be directed towards control of symptoms. Even when specific antidotes are available supportive therapy may be required to control hypotension or hypoxia.

1. **Shock:** This requires immediate attention and depending upon the cause of hypotension resulting in shock, treatment should be initiated.
   a. To combat depression of vasomotor centers vasopressor amines are quite effective like methyl amphetamine 15 to 30 mg intramuscularly. Foot end of the bed should also be raised.
   b. Anoxia is commonly overlooked in a patient with shock. Artificial respiration and oxygen inhalation is required to combat anoxia. Without controlling anoxia it is difficult to control blood pressure.
   c. Loss of fluids and blood must be estimated and compensated. Vomiting help in elimination of poison, however in severe cases chlorpromazine 25 to 50 mg may be administered. Patient may be given sips of warm water or tea along with milk of magnesia or aluminum hydroxide.
   d. Autonomic ganglion block, myocardial damage or cardiac arrhythmias must be kept in mind while treating shock.

2. **Hypoxia:** Hypoxia has to be treated urgently which may be due to:
   a. Central respiratory depression may require assisted ventilation in case the cyanosis does not improve with 100% oxygen.
   b. Muscular paralysis and retained secretions can be diagnosed with presence of feeble cough. In such cases even minor airway obstruction may cause respiratory arrest. Secretions must be cleared and if required early tracheostomy should be performed.
   c. Bronchospasm may be as a result of inhalation or aspiration of a toxic substance. Course rhonchi may be diagnostic and steam inhalation and tracheostomy may be required.
   d. Laryngeal spasm or edema may result from inhalation of toxic fumes which may require tracheostomy or endotracheal intubation.

e. Pulmonary edema may be seen in injury to alveoli from toxic gases or overdose of heroin, which can be treated with hyperbaric oxygen, atropine sulphate 0.5 to 1 gm subcutaneously, steroids, aminophylline 0.25 to 0.5 gm or morphine if not contradicted.

f. Defective oxygen transport may be from methemoglobinemia formation or carboxyhemoglobinemia. 100% oxygen or hyperbaric oxygen, assisted ventilation and in methemoglobinemia, 1% methylene blue by slow infusion may be administered.

3. **Pain:** For intestinal colic atropine sulphate 0.5 mg or other antispasmodic should be administered whereas for cutaneous lesions topical anesthetic agents along with aspirin may be given. In severe cases pethidine (50 to 100 mg) or paraldehyde may be used.

4. **Diarrhea:** In case of diarrhea kaolin mixture, activated charcoal 1–2 TSF, bismuth subcarbonate 1 gram or aluminum oxide gel or atropine sulphate may be given. Electrolyte imbalance due to severe diarrhea or vomiting must be properly corrected.

5. **Delirium:** Delirium can be treated by chlorpromazine hydrochloride 50–100 mg intramuscularly or orally, paraldehyde 8–15 ml orally or deep intramuscularly or chloral hydrate orally.

6. **Convulsions:** In such a case thiopental sodium 0.1 to 0.2 mg orally or intramuscularly, paraldehyde 8–15 ml orally or deep intramuscularly can be administered.

7. **Alkalosis:** Normal saline can be administered.

8. **Acidosis:** Sodium bicarbonate or sodium lactate is used.

9. **Acute hepatic insufficiency** may be seen in mushroom poisoning, yellow phosphorus, halothane, carbon tetrachloride, chlorpromazine or tetracycline, etc. Such a patient must be closely watched and further administration of toxic substance must be stopped.

10. **Acute renal insufficiency:** It may be seen as a result of shock, dehydration, electrolyte imbalance or nephrotoxic substances like heavy metals, carbon tetrachloride, ethylene glycol, kanamycin or neomycin. Condition requires proper monitoring of the renal output and replacement of the fluids and salt. Dialysis may be required in severe cases.

Administration of Antidotes

Antidotes are substances which counter act or neutralize the effects of poisons. Antidotes are of following types:

1. Mechanical antidotes
2. Chemical antidotes
3. Physiological antidotes

1. **Mechanical antidotes:** These antidotes neutralize poisons by mechanical action or by preventing their absorption:

   i. *Animal charcoal or activated charcoal:* It acts by adsorbing and retaining organic poisons or to some extent mineral poisons. It is administered in a dose of about 4 to 8 gm and is quite helpful in poisoning by atropine, morphine, strychnine, barbiturates and even in mercuric chloride.

   ii. *Demulcents:* These provide protective coating over the gastric mucosa and prevent absorption of poisons. Milk, starch, egg white, mineral oils, milk of magnesia or aluminum hydroxide act as demulcents.

   iii. *Bulky foods:* They also help by protecting the gastric mucosa like few bananas in case of ingestion of glass pieces.

2. **Chemical antidotes:** Chemical antidotes counter act the action of poisons by forming harmless or insoluble compounds or by oxidizing poisons by chemically reacting with them.

   i. Alkalis neutralize acids, however very weak solution is normally administered and carbonates are avoided as they form large amount of carbon dioxide gas which may cause rupture of the weak stomach.

ii. Acids to neutralize alkalis, in such cases harmless acids are normally used like vinegar, citric acid or lime juice.

iii. Common salt reacts with silver nitrate.

iv. Albumin precipitate mercuric chloride.

v. Dialyzed iron is used in arsenic poisoning.

vi. Potassium permanganate is used in 1:5000 strength for various alkaloids like present in opium or strychnine. It is also used in phosphorus, HCN and barbiturate poisoning. When it reacts with a poison it loses its pink colour hence the gastric lavage is continued till pink colour is there again in the stomach wash aspirate.

vii. Lugol's iodine, 15 drops in half glass of water to precipitate alkaloids.

viii. Tannic acid 4% can precipitate apomorphine, strychnine, cocaine, nicotine, salts of lead, copper, mercury or zinc.

ix. When exact nature of the poison is not known, following treatment can be administered:

Universal antidote is administered containing 2 parts of animal charcoal or burnt toast (to adsorb alkaloids), one part magnesium oxide (to neutralize acids) and one part tannic acid or strong tea (to precipitate alkaloids glycosides and certain metals). Tablespoonful is given in a glass of water and if required can be repeated again. It is advised not to use this, as its affectivity has not been properly established.

Coma cocktail: A combination of dextrose, flumazenil, naloxone and thiamine may be administered in emergency to comatosed patients when the nature of coma is not known. Some are not in favour of the combination and advocate specific treatment after proper diagnosis.

3. **Physiological antidotes:** These produce symptoms opposite to those produced by the poison or neutralizing their action and are mainly used when the poison has been absorbed into the circulation.

i. Atropine and physostigmine having opposite action on the nerve ending.

ii. Nalorphine or naloxone for morphine poisoning.

iii. Atropine for organophosphorus poisoning.

iv. Barbiturates and amphetamines.

v. Amyl nitrate in cyanide poisoning.

vi. *"Chelating agents"* to inactivate metals by combining with them and forming harmless compounds.

a. *Bal (british anti-lewisite) or dimercaprol:* This is a commonly used antidote for metal poisoning like arsenic, bismuth, mercury and copper.

As many of the metals have affinity for sulfhydryl (SH) radical of the respiratory enzymes of the cells. BAL has 2 unsaturated SH groups which combine with metals as there is substrate competition between enzyme radical and BAL, thereby preventing harmful effects of the metals.

Dose: 3 to 4 mg/Kg body weight is given as 2 ml of 10% BAL in 20% benzyl benzoate in arachis oil. It is given deep intramuscularly every 4 hourly for 2 days then twice daily for next 10 days or till recovery. It is contraindicated in liver damage. High doses may cause toxic symptoms like nausea; vomiting or tingling sensation for which 25 mg epinephrine sulphate should be given orally half an hour before the injection.

b. EDTA (ethylene diamine tetra acetic acid) or disodium versonate or calcium disodium edetate: This antidote is commonly used in lead and mercury poisoning, but can also be used in other metal poisons like copper, cobalt and iron.

Dose: 25 mg/Kg body weight is given in 250 to 500 ml of 5% glucose slowly over a period of 1 to 2 hours twice daily for 5 days and can be repeated after 2 to 3 days.

c. Penicillamine: It is hydrolyzed product of penicillin and has stable SH group.

Dose: 30 mg/kg body weight up to 2–4 gm/day orally in 4 divided doses for about 7 days. Blood count should be done regularly to watch for agranulocytosis and thrombocytopenia along with skin rashes and in some cases nephritic syndrome. It can also be given 1–3 gm intravenously in a very slow drip daily for 2 to 4 days.

d. *Desferoxamine:* It contains trivalent iron as chelating agent and hence useful in iron poisoning.

Dose: 8 to 12 gm daily orally in 100 ml of fluids or can be given in the dose of 1 gm intramuscularly and then 1/2 gm every 4 to 8 hourly.

Hastening Excretion of Absorbed Drugs:

1. **Renal route:** Poisons can be excreted by increasing urinary output.
   i. *Diuresis:* To increase urinary output large amounts of fluids or tea can be given orally. If required fluids like normal saline or 5% glucose, 500 ml/hour, can also be given by intravenous route.
   ii. *Forced diuresis:* This can be done by giving urea, mannitol infusion or chlorthiazide.

2. **Purgatives:** Unabsorbed poison still in the intestines can be eliminated by giving purgatives like 30 gm of sodium sulphate. Mag. sulphate is normally avoided in renal failure cases as it can cause depression. Purgatives should be avoided in corrosive poisoning or in severe diarrhea.

3. **Diaphoretics:** By increasing perspiration some poisons can be excreted faster. Diaphoresis can be achieved by application of hot water bottles or by giving 5 mg of subcutaneous pilocarpine or administration of salicylates.

4. **Dialysis:** May be required in some cases specially when there is renal shutdown.

a. Hemodialysis can be used especially in barbiturates, bromides, salicylates, methyl alcohol, amphetamines or alcohol poisoning.

b. *Peritoneal dialysis:* In case facilities for hemodialysis are not available peritoneal dialysis can be tried.

Legal and Other Aspects

1. **Preservation of evidence of poisoning:** In all cases of suspected poisoning or when requested by the investigative officer or absence of definitive cause of death, viscera is collected, preserved and handed over to the police. In routine cases following viscera is collected in clean containers:
   i. *Stomach and stomach contents:* Stomach is opened and the entire contents along with the stomach wall after it is examined is preserved in first bottle.
   ii. *Small intestines and contents:* Small intestine piece about 30 to 100 cm, along with contents are preserved in second bottle. Routinely these are preserved together in the first bottle along with stomach and its contents.
   iii. *Liver spleen and kidneys:* Piece of liver about 500 gm, half of spleen and half of each kidney are placed in third bottle.
   iv. *Blood:* Minimum of 30 ml of blood is collected from peripheral sites and placed in the 4th bottle.
   v. *Sample of preservative:* Preservative used is added in the 5th bottle.

Preservatives used: For preservation of viscera saturated solution of common salt (which is cheap and easily available) is preferred. Hand full of salt is added to the contents in each viscera bottle, which draws water from the viscera and make a saturated solution around it. Even though rectified spirit is the ideal preservative, still it is not used commonly as it is expensive and chances of pilferage are there. Spirit is also not used in alcohol, kerosene, ether, chloroform, phosphorus and related poisons. Blood sample is commonly preserved without any preservative, but in alcohol and cyanide poisoning potassium fluoride 10 mg and potassium oxalate 3 mg are used for each ml of blood. In carbon monoxide poisoning a layer of liquid paraffin is added over blood or the container is filled up to the brim. **Formalin should never be used as preservative for toxicological analysis.** In special cases total volume of urine sample is collected in a separate bottle. Urine is preserved by adding few crystals of thymol or phenyl mercuric nitrate. Hair sample from the head and pubic area are collected by plucking them from the roots. Skin sample preferably of 2 cm radius around the injection site should be incised and preserved. A 10 cm long bone piece from the shaft of the femur is preserved if required.

2. **Anticipating complications:** Treating doctor must be aware about the delayed complications and try to anticipate these complications and take appropriate action to combat them. In some cases the patient is discharged from the hospital after treating acute manifestations but may succumb to delayed complications, if not anticipated.

3. **Preventing further occurrence:** A patient, who has attempted suicide by consuming a poisonous substance, must undergo psychiatric evaluation, so that such a person is properly treated for depression and provided future guidance, before he is discharged. State is required to frame rules for the proper storage, labelling and availability of various poisons so as to prevent suicides.

36 | Corrosive Poisons

A corrosive is one that will destroy and damage other substances with which it comes into contact. It may attack a great variety of materials, including metals and various organic compounds, but in medical profession, doctors are mostly concerned with its effects on living tissues; as on contact it causes chemical burns. The word 'corrosive' is derived from the Latin verb *corrodere*, which means 'to gnaw'. Sometimes the word 'caustic' is used as a synonym but 'caustic' generally refers only to strong bases, particularly alkalis and do not include acids, oxidizers, or other nonalkaline corrosives.

CORROSIVE AGENTS

a. *Acids:*
   i. *Mineral acids:* These are sulfuric acid (car battery fluid), nitric acid (metal cleaners), hydrochloric acid (descalers) and hydrogen fluoride (rust removers).
   ii. *Organic acids:* These are formic acid, carbolic acids and acetic acid.
b. *Alkalis*
   i. Caustics or alkalis, such as hydroxide or carbonates of sodium, potassium, calcium and ammonia when anhydrous or in a concentrated solution.
   ii. Extremely strong bases (superbases) such as alkoxide, metal amides, (e.g. sodium amide) and organometallic bases such as butyllithium.

c. *Heavy metal salts:* Some of the heavy metal salts also have corrosive properties like calcium oxide, anhydrous zinc chloride, anhydrous aluminum chloride and mercuric chloride (corrosive sublimate).
d. Miscellaneous substances like formalin, elemental bromine, fluorine, chlorine and iodine, iodine tincture, concentrated hydrogen peroxide, etc.

Pathophysiology

Corrosive substances with a pH of less than 2 or greater than 12 are highly corrosive and can cause tissue necrosis. When tissues come in contact with acids, tissue proteins are transformed into acid proteins and hemoglobin is transformed into acid hematin, resulting in coagulation necrosis. This process leads to edema, erythema, mucosal sloughing, ulceration and necrosis of tissues. In case of alkalis, tissue proteins are transformed into proteinates and fats are converted into soaps, resulting in liquefactive necrosis.

Sulfuric acid at a high concentration is also a strong dehydrating agent, capable of dehydrating carbohydrates and liberating extra heat. This results in secondary thermal burns in addition to the chemical burns. Some corrosives, such as nitric acid and concentrated sulfuric acid, are strong oxidizing agents as well, which significantly contributes to the extra damage caused. Hydrofluoric acid does not necessarily cause noticeable damage upon contact, but produces toxicity after being absorbed painlessly.

When corrosives come in contact with the esophagus, it can produce perforation of the esophageal wall, mediastinitis and fatal outcome. The severity of the chemical burns that affect the entire gastrointestinal tract depends on several factors; nature of the corrosive substance; pH value; quantity; concentration and duration of exposure.

The pathologic classification of corrosive injuries of the upper gastrointestinal tract is similar to thermal skin burns and can be classified in similar manner.

First degree: It is characterized by superficial damage followed by onset of mucous edema and erythema. The affected mucous layer regenerates in a few days and usually does not manifest complications such as scars or stricture formation.

Second degree: It is characterized by penetration of corrosive substance through the submucosa into the muscular layer of the organ. Esophageal stenosis most frequently develops at the level of the aortic arch and tracheal bifurcation and the lower esophageal sphincter. Most gastric stenosis occurs in the pyloric antrum.

Third degree: This is characterized with perforation of the wall of the esophagus or stomach.

SULPHURIC ACID (H₂SO₄) (OIL OF VITRIOL OR BATTERY ACID)

Pure sulphuric acid is heavy, colourless, odorless, oily liquid. However commercially available sulphuric acid is brownish in colour due to impurities Anhydrous sulphuric acid reacts violently with water and organic material and generate heat. Concentrated sulphuric acid will oxidize, dehydrate, or sulfonate most organic compounds. It is capable of igniting finely divided combustible materials on contact. Sulphuric acid can corrode many metals.

Uses of Sulphuric Acid

1. Battery acid.
2. Preparation of some fertilizers and detergents.
3. Used in some toilet bowl and drain cleaners.
4. Used in industries for preparing indigo and chlorine.

Features of Sulphuric Acid Poisoning

a. Initial symptoms include severe dermal pain on contact.
b. Inhalation causes irritation of the eyes and nose with sore throat, cough, chest tightness, headache, tachycardia and confusion.
c. In case of ingestion there are burns in the mouth and throat with severe pain in the mouth and throat. Lips are swollen and excoriated.
d. Drooling mark with brown to black streak from angle of mouth and over chest.
e. Brown to black vomitus, with blood and shreds of mucosa. On addition of barium chloride solution to vomitus it gives white precipitates of barium sulphate.
f. Rapid development of low blood pressure.
g. Speech problems, voice may become husky due to inflammation of oropharynx and epiglottis.
h. Symptoms from breathing in or regurgitation of the poison may include bluish discoloration of skin, lips and fingernails along with breathing difficulty, chest tightness, choking and coughing.
i. May lead to blindness if eyes are affected.
j. Black swollen tongue.
k. *Chalky white* teeth.

Complications

a. Perforation of esophagus leading to mediastinitis or perforation of stomach.
b. Fibrosis and formation of strictures.
c. Secondary infections.
d. Renal impairment.

Fatal dose: In majority of cases it is 10 to 15 ml of concentrated sulphuric acid.

Autopsy Findings

Autopsy findings mainly depend on the amount and concentration of the sulphuric acid consumed.

1. **External findings**
   a. Brown to black corrosion streak from angle of mouth and over chest.
   b. Excoriation of lips and mucosa of the mouth.
   c. Chalky white teeth.

2. **Internal findings**
   a. Ulceration or perforation of esophagus which may result in mediastinitis.
   b. Inflammatory reaction may be seen in the larynx.
   c. Brown to black stomach wall and blotting paper appearance of stomach mucosa.
   d. There may be perforation of stomach leading to escape of acid into peritoneal cavity.
   e. The stomach may resemble a black spongy mass on postmortem.

Medicolegal Aspects

Mostly it is used for suicidal purposes. Accidental poisoning may take place when ingested by mistake. In some cases this acid is used to disfigure a person by throwing it on the face, which is known as vitriolage. It is rarely used to destroy evidence of homicide or body disposal like in the case of acid bath murderer.

Acid bath murderer

John George Haigh influenced an elderly widow to accompany him to a warehouse, where he shot her to remove some valuables from her body. Her body was then dumped in a steel tank filled with sulphuric acid. When the police emptied the tank they recovered part of left foot, some fragments of bones, gallstones and a set of dentures. Identification was established from these remnants. Haigh was charged with murder. He even confessed to similar disposal method adopted for some bodies earlier. He was found guilty and executed for the same.

Treatment

1. **Dermal exposure:**
   a. Remove patient from exposure.
   b. Remove all clothing and personal effects.
   c. Wash hair and all contaminated skin with copious amounts of water (preferably warm) and soap solution for at least 10–15 minutes. Decontaminate open wounds first and avoid contamination of unexposed skin. Pay special attention to skin folds, axillae, ears, fingernails, genital areas and feet.
   d. Cover affected area with a clean nonadherent dressing.

2. **Ocular exposure:**
   a. Immediately irrigate the affected eye thoroughly with water or normal saline for at least 10–15 minutes.
   b. Patients with corneal damage should be referred for urgent ophthalmological assessment.

3. **Inhalation:**
   a. Remove patient from exposure.
   b. Ensure a clear airway and adequate ventilation.
   c. Give oxygen to symptomatic patients.
   d. If the patient has clinical features of bronchospasm treat conventionally with nebulized bronchodilators and steroids.
   e. Endotracheal intubation, or rarely, tracheostomy may be required for life-threatening laryngeal edema.
   f. Apply other supportive measures as indicated by the patient's clinical condition.

4. **Ingestion**
   a. Maintain airway. In case of any indication of laryngeal burn with erythema and edema, which may lead to airway obstruction, such cases should be considered for early intubation or tracheostomy.
   b. Gastric lavage should not be attempted.
   c. Do not give neutralizing chemicals as heat produced during neutralization reactions may increase injury.

d. Monitor BP, pulse and oxygen saturation.

e. Treat hemorrhagic or hypovolemic shock by replacing lost fluids and blood intravenously to establish hemodynamic stability.

f. Apply other supportive measures as indicated by the patient's condition.

Vitriolage: Vitriolage or vitriol attack or acid throwing, is defined as the act of throwing acid or a similarly strong corrosive substance onto the body of another with the intention to disfigure, maim or torture that individual. Mostly the victims are females. The most common types of acid used in these attacks are sulfuric and nitric acid. Hydrochloric acid is also sometimes used. Vitriolage cases are seen all over the world but are more common in the southeast Asia.

Common reasons for this type of attacks are due to sexual rejections, rivalry, property disputes or gang wars between criminals.

Effects of acid attacks on the victim are extensive, as a majority of acid attacks are aimed at the face. The severity of the damage depends on the concentration of the acid and the time before the acid is thoroughly washed off with water or neutralized with a neutralizing agent. The acid can rapidly eat away skin, the layer of fat beneath the skin, and in some cases even the underlying bone. Eyelids may be completely destroyed and acid may cause blindness. The nose and ears get severely damaged; lips may be damaged exposing teeth. Acid vapors usually create respiratory problems.

The supreme court on July 16, 2013 has ruled that authorities must regulate the sale of acid. The buyers of such acids have to provide a photo identity card to any retailer when they make a purchase and the retailers must register the name and address of the buyer.

In 2013, section 326-A IPC was enacted by the Indian Parliament to ensure enhanced punishment for acid throwing.

Treatment

a. Remove all clothing and personal effects splashed with acid.

b. Wash contaminated skin and hair with copious amounts of water (preferably warm) and soap solution for at least 10–15 minutes. Decontaminate open wounds first and avoid contamination of unexposed skin. Pay special attention to eyes, skin folds, axillae, ears, fingernails, genital areas and feet.

c. Alleviate pain.

d. Cover affected area with a clean non-adherent dressing.

HYDROCHLORIC ACID (HCL) (MURIATIC ACID, HYDROGEN CHLORIDE SOLUTION OR SPIRITS OF SALT)

Hydrochloric acid is a nonflammable, transparent and colourless or light yellow liquid. It is a fuming liquid giving off hydrogen chloride gas at room temperature. Hydrogen chloride gas has a strong pungent odor. It is less destructive than sulphuric or nitric acids. It is a natural constituent of stomach.

Uses

a. Metal cleaner, i.e. pickling of steel to remove rust or iron oxide scales from iron or steel.

b. Toilet cleaner.

c. Flux for soldering.

d. In some industries like production of organic compounds such as vinyl chloride and dichloroethane for PVC and zinc chloride for the galvanizing industry and battery production, etc.

e. Leather processing.

f. Sometimes used to erase ink for forgery purposes.

Features of Hydrochloric Acid Poisoning

Similar features as seen in sulphuric acid poisoning are present.

1. When swallowed it causes burning of the mouth, throat and esophagus, vomiting,

diarrhea, collapse and possible death may result. Mucous membranes may be seen as grayish to brown or black in colour.

2. In eyes it can penetrate deeply causing irritation or severe burns depending on the concentration and duration of exposure. In severe cases, ulceration and permanent damage may occur.

3. When splashed on the skin it is capable of causing severe skin burns with deep ulceration. Corrosion will continue until removed. Severity depends on concentration and duration of exposure.

4. In case of inhalation irritation of the nose, throat and lungs would occur due to the corrosive nature of the product.

Usual Fatal Dose

15 to 20 ml when ingested.

Medicolegal Aspects

Mostly it is used for suicidal purposes. Accidental poisoning may take place when ingested by mistake. In some cases this acid is also used to disfigure a person by throwing on the face, which is known as vitriolage.

Treatment

Same treatment is employed as is done in case of sulphuric acid poisoning.

NITRIC ACID (HNO₃) (AQUA FORTIS)

Nitric acid is colourless, fuming liquid. Inhalation of fumes produces chocking sensation. It is strong oxidizing agent and produces picric acid when reacts with organic material staining them yellow (xanthoproteic reaction).

Uses of Nitric Acid

a. Fertilizers.
b. Substances used to clean metals (such as gun barrels).
c. Explosives.
d. Polymer industry, notably in the manufacture of polyurethanes and polyamides.

Features of Nitric Acid Poisoning

Symptoms from swallowing nitric acid may include:

a. Yellowish stains on the clothing.
b. Severe mouth throat and abdominal pain.
c. Lips tongue and mucous membrane of mouth is initially grayish but turns yellow.
d. Swelling in the throat leading to breathing problems.
e. Teeth are also stained yellowish.
f. Yellowish brown vomiting having altered blood. Abdomen is distended from the gases produced. However, perforation of stomach is less frequently seen.
g. Photophobia and excessive lachrymation from the fumes.
h. Oliguria or anuria may be present.

Inhalation of Fumes

a. Cough with bloodstained sputum.
b. Chocking sensation.
c. Tightness of chest, breathing difficulty or shortness of breath.
d. Dizziness and weakness.
e. Fall in blood pressure and rapid pulse.

Fatal Dose

About 10 to 15 ml.

Treatment

Treatment is undertaken in the similar manner in which sulphuric acid poisoning is treated.

Postmortem Findings

a. Stains are yellowish in colour.
b. Esophagus and stomach may be yellowish or brownish black due to formation of acid hematin.
c. Respiratory passage is more frequently involved.

Medicolegal Importance

Poisoning is mostly suicidal or accidental in nature, homicidal poisoning is rarely seen.

HYDROFLUORIC ACID (HF)

Hydrofluoric acid is a solution of hydrogen fluoride in water. It is a colourless liquid that is highly corrosive.

Uses

a. Oil refining
b. Cleaning agent
c. Rust remover
d. Glass etching.

Features of Poisoning

It is a contact poison initially produces painless burns which may delay the treatment but has potential for causing deep burns which are extremely painful. Hydrofluoric acid is a neutral lipid-soluble molecule penetrates tissue more rapidly than other mineral acids causing liquefaction necrosis. Once absorbed into blood through the skin; it reacts with blood calcium and may cause cardiac arrest. It can permanently damage corneas of the eyes and lungs leading to respiratory symptoms and death.

Treatment

Apart from the treatment instituted in any corrosive poisoning following additional steps may be required:

a. Initially decontaminate by irrigation with copious amounts of water.
b. Ice packs on the affected area or soaking the burnt area in icy solution of 25% magnesium sulphate.
c. If calcium gluconate gel or hexafluorine is available, apply liberally to the affected area.
d. Inject 10% calcium gluconate in and around the affected area.
e. Treat inhalation injuries with oxygen and 2.5% calcium gluconate nebulizer.
f. Control pain with opioid agents.

Postmortem findings

Postmortem findings are similar as seen in other corrosive acid poisoning except that in hydrofluoric acid tissue damage is more.

Medicolegal Significance

Majority of the cases are accidental in nature. Suicidal and homicidal cases are very rare.

CARBOLIC ACID (PHENOL)

Carbolic acid is one of the oldest antiseptic agents. It is colourless, needle shaped crystals which liquefy when exposed to air with characteristic smell. Commercial phenol is dark brownish liquid. Phenol acts both as locally corrosive agent and a general protoplasmic poison. Phenol derivatives are less toxic than pure phenol. Phenol is well absorbed by inhalation, dermal application, and ingestion.

Uses

a. Disinfectant
b. Plastic and bakelite industry
c. Preservation of sera and vaccines
d. Precursor to a large collection of drugs like aspirin
e. It is a component of industrial paint strippers
f. Preparation of cosmetics including sunscreens.

Fatal Dose

About 10 to 30 gm.

Features of Acute Poisoning

1. **Local manifestations:**
   a. Dermal exposure produces lesions which are initially painless white patches and later turn erythematous and finally brown.
   b. Nausea, vomiting, sweating, and diarrhea.
   c. Phenol produces mucosal burns and coagulum.
   d. They cause eye irritation and corneal damage.

2. **When ingested:**
   a. It causes extensive local corrosions, abdominal pain, nausea, vomiting, sweating, and diarrhea.

b. Severe gastrointestinal burns are uncommon and strictures are rare.

c. Inhalation produces respiratory tract irritation and pneumonia.

d. Systemic manifestations develop after few minutes to 30 minutes, both from ingestion or dermal application, and may produce nausea, vomiting, lethargy or coma, hypotension, tachycardia or bradycardia, arrhythmias, convulsions, acidosis, hemolysis and shock.

e. There may be renal damage. The patient excretes carbolic acid metabolites like *pyrocatechol* and *hydroquinone* in the urine. The urine turns smoky green after some time on exposure to air known as **"carboluria"**. Hydroquinone induced yellowish discolouration of the face, neck and photo exposed skin areas is known as "ochronosis".

Treatment

Phenol poisoning requires immediate medical evaluation and treatment. It is necessary to establish and maintain vital functions and establish vascular access.

a. If phenol is ingested, avoid emesis (it normally fails due to anesthetic effects of the phenol on the nerve endings), alcohol and oral mineral oil and dilution, because they may increase absorption.

b. Gastric lavage is usually not recommended but can be attempted with administration of olive oil or castor oil and activated charcoal by small bore nasogastric tube.

c. Treat shock by fluids and dopamine, arrhythmias with lidocaine and convulsions with diazepam.

d. Inhalation of 100% oxygen is recommended. Assisted ventilation might be necessary.

e. Metabolic acidosis should be managed by 1 to 2 mEq/kg of sodium bicarbonate.

f. Methemoglobinemia should be treated if greater than 30%, or in cases of respiratory distress, with methylene blue 1 to 2 mg/kg of 1% solution by slow intravenous infusion.

Postmortem Findings

1. **External findings:**

   a. Characteristic smell from mouth and skin lesions.

   b. Corroded areas are brownish in colour.

   c. Tongue is greyish white and swollen.

2. **Internal findings:**

   a. Stomach is hardened, greyish in colour and is leathery to feel (*leather bottle stomach*).

   b. Upper part of the duodenum and esophagus also show similar findings as seen in stomach. Portion of liver in contact with stomach may show white, hardened patches.

   c. Kidneys are inflamed and showing hemorrhagic spots.

   d. Other internal organs are congested.

Medicolegal Significance

Majority of cases are as a result of suicidal attempt, very rarely used for homicidal purposes. Accidental poisoning may occur from absorption from its application on the wounds or ulcerated surfaces.

OXALIC ACID (ACID OF SUGAR)

Oxalic acid is a colourless crystalline solid that forms a colourless solution in water. Oxalate is the most common component of kidney stones. Members of the spinach family, cabbage, broccoli and Brussels sprouts are high in oxalates.

Uses

a. Ink remover.

b. Cleaning or bleaching.

c. About 25% of produced oxalic acid is used as a mordant in dyeing processes.

d. It is used in rust removal agents.

Fatal Dose

Lethal oral dose is 15 to 30 gm.

Features of Poisoning

a. Symptoms and signs depend on the quantity and concentration of the oxalic acid consumed. In case a large dose is taken it may result in fulminating poisoning producing immediate death. It causes burns when comes in contact with skin, eyes or mucous membranes. Oxalic acid, if ingested, there is burning pain in the mouth and abdomen, tenderness, nausea, blood-stained vomiting, convulsions and shock.

b. Oxalic acid is extremely destructive to tissue of mucous membranes of the upper respiratory tract. In case it is inhaled, a burning sensation is felt in the respiratory tract, cough, laryngitis, shortness of breath, inflammation and edema of the larynx, inflammation and edema of the bronchi, pneumonitis and pulmonary edema may be seen.

c. Delayed toxicity of oxalic acid is mainly due to kidney failure caused by precipitation of calcium oxalate, the main component of kidney stones. Oxalic acid can also cause joint pain due to the formation of similar precipitates in the joints.

Treatment

a. Stomach wash is done with calcium lactate, calcium gluconate or lime water.

b. Calcium gluconate is given intravenously (10 ml of 10% solution).

c. Respiratory support.

d. Demulcents.

e. Other supportive measures.

Postmortem Features

a. There may be blister formation over the contact areas of the skin.

b. Corroded mucosa may appear whitish.

c. Cloudy swelling of the kidneys along with hyaline degeneration of the tubules.

d. Other visceral organs are congested.

Medicolegal Importance

Most of the poisoning cases are accidental in nature. It may be ingested in place of magnesium sulphate. Homicidal poisoning is very rare because of its bitter taste.

ALKALIS

Alkaline products include sodium or potassium hydroxide, Ammonium hydroxide and potassium permanganate. When pH is more than 12, the compound is likely to cause significant gastrointestinal ulceration. Corrosive potential varies with concentration of specific alkalis and liquid preparations are more likely to cause esophageal burns than powders. Alkaline agents penetrate local tissue rapidly and deeply, causing liquefactive necrosis. Unlike acidic products, very little pain may be evident upon initial contact with an alkaline product, which may encourage further contact and ultimately result in more extensive exposures.

Uses

1. Drain cleaners, oven cleaners, radiator cleaning agents.
2. Automatic dish washing liquids and powders.
3. Laundry detergents.
4. Alkaline batteries.
5. Portland cement.

Features of Toxicity

a. Clinical signs may not develop immediately, evidence of oral discomfort and inflammation generally develop within 2 to 4 hours, although the full extent of injury may not be evident until 12 hours after exposure.

b. Acute signs include hypersalivation, anorexia, oral inflammation or ulceration, drooling, dysphagia, refusing to eat and drink, vomiting which may be blood-stained in few cases, abdominal pain, melena and depression.

c. Significant hyperthermia (>104° F) may accompany oral inflammation.

d. Absence of mouth or pharyngeal ulcers does not preclude gastroesophageal lesions.

e. Pharyngeal and esophageal ulceration are more frequently seen. Gastric acid can neutralize alkali and the gastric volume and contents may prevent gastric injury from the exothermic neutralization reaction; however, large alkali volumes will still lead to gastric damage.

f. Inhalation of ammonia may result in coughing, dyspnea, and rhonchi.

g. Sequelae can include esophageal perforations and pleuritis or peritonitis from leakage. The most common complications are esophageal and gastric stenosis, which are found in greater percentage than in poisonings with acid substances.

Management

1. Activated charcoal should not be used.
2. If asymptomatic treat with fluid dilution: 10 ml/kg of water (maximum 250 ml).
3. If asymptomatic after 4 hours and able to eat and drink the patient can be safely discharged.
4. Treatment should include antibiotics, pain medication as needed, gastrointestinal protectants, (e.g. sucralfate), anti-inflammatory (corticosteroid use is controversial) and general supportive care. In cases with severe oral burns or esophageal burns, placement of a gastrostomy tube will facilitate nutritional support while allowing for mucosal healing. Esophageal lesions may take weeks to heal and there is risk of stricture formation, leading to impairment of esophageal function.

Postmortem Features

a. Features of corrosion and soapy feel on touching the affected area.
b. Esophageal corrosions along with inflammatory edema of the stomach wall.
c. Other visceral organs show congestion.

Medicolegal Importance

Mostly accidental poisoning is seen with alkalis when they are ingested by mistake. Ammonia poisoning may be encountered when nylon or wool is burnt in enclosed space releasing ammonia. Placing an open bottle of hydrochloric acid near the source may give white fumes of ammonium chloride.

37 | Metallic Poisons

Irritant poisons produce irritation to the gastrointestinal tract resulting in features of gastroenteritis. These are much milder in action than corrosives.

INORGANIC METALLIC IRRITANTS

Majority of the symptoms are as a result of causing irritation in the gastrointestinal tract but after absorption, to some extent, produces depression by acting on CNS. Most of the heavy metals are toxic when they form poisonous soluble compounds. Insoluble compounds as well as the metallic forms often exhibit negligible toxicity. Toxic metals like lead or mercury can bio-accumulate in the body resulting in chronic toxicity. Most commonly used metallic poisons for homicidal purposes are arsenic salts.

ARSENIC

Most of arsenic salts, arsine gas and organic arsenic compounds are toxic.

Uses

a. Calico printing
b. Dyes
c. Wall papers
d. Timber treatment against white ants
e. Rat killer
f. Sheep dips
g. Fly papers
h. Weed killer
i. Syphilis treatment under Indian system (Ayurveda).

Common Compounds of Arsenic

1. Arsenic trioxide or arsenious oxide or white arsenic or sankhya. It is white gritty, crystalline, heavy powder with a specific gravity of 3.669, odorless, colourless and insoluble in water. When added to water a thin layer is formed on the surface of water. One pinch of the salt weighs around 1 gm.
2. *Arsenites:* Copper arsenite (Sheel's green), copper acetoarsenite (Paris green) and potassium arsenite.
3. *Arsenates:* These are less toxic than arsenites. Some of such salts are sodium arsenate, potassium arsenate and calcium arsenate.
4. Arsenic acid is white crystalline solid.
5. *Arsenic sulphides:* These compounds are mostly seen in ores. Realgar is red arsenic disulphide and orpiment is yellow arsenic trisulphide.
6. Arsine gas (arsenic hydride) is a colourless gas having garlic odor. It is highly toxic having hemolytic action.
7. Other compounds of arsenic include trichlorides and tri-iodides.
8. Organic compounds of arsenic are: (a) cacodylic acid; (b) stovarsal; and (c) salvarsan.

Absorption

It is mainly absorbed from the GIT, but can also be absorbed from lungs. If applied to skin it can cause necrosis and sloughing. Rate of absorption depends upon the condition of the stomach. Narcotics delay absorption.

Distribution

It is initially stored in liver, in case a person survives for a day it is found in the muscles and subsequently in the nails and hair. Normal concentration in hair is 0.01 mg/kg to 0.5 mg/kg in case it exceeds 0.75 mg/kg then there is suspicion of poisoning.

Elimination

It is excreted in urine, feces and sweat but excretion is slow, hence there is cumulative effect.

Mode of Action

It has local action of irritation of the mucous membrane as well as remote action of CNS depression. Arsenic combines with sulfhydryl group of enzymes thus interfere with the cellular metabolism.

Features of Poisoning

Poisoning may be presented in three forms: (a) acute; (b) subacute; and (c) chronic form.

a. Acute Poisoning

Signs and symptoms are manifested in three forms.
1. Gastroenteritis form
2. Sudden collapse form
3. Neurotic form

1. **Gastroenteritis form:** Usually the symptoms start after about 30 minutes of ingestion. There is nausea, pain in throat and abdomen, eyes are congested, dysphagia, thirst, giddiness followed by vomiting which may be projectile. Vomiting is very severe and even after all the poison has been expelled it continues as small amounts of the absorbed poison is excreted back into the stomach. Purging occurs with pain and tenesmus. Initially the stools are dark in colour mixed with blood but later on they become watery. Oliguria is there due to dehydration and urine may contain RBC's and casts. Skin is dry; eyes are sunken; rapid feeble pulse from dehydration; convulsions; coma and death. As features resemble cholera, which can be differentiated in the manner mentioned in Table 37.1.

2. **Sudden collapse form:** This is seen in cases where large quantity of poison has been ingested. There are signs of collapse like cold and clammy skin, face is pale, eyes are sunken, pulse is feeble, dilated pupils and death occurs in a very short time. In such cases there may be very minimal signs of GIT irritation.

3. **Neurotic form:** In some cases of arsenic poisoning predominantly neurotic features are present. The patient may complain of giddiness, numbness, tingling sensation all over the body and tenderness of the

S.No	Feature	Arsenic poisoning	Cholera
		Table 37.1: Differences between Arsenic poisoning and Cholera	
1.	Onset	Abrupt	Takes 1–3 days
2.	Pain in throat	Before vomiting	Not present or after vomiting
3.	Vomiting	Before diarrhea	After diarrhea
4.	Vomit	Contains mucous and bile	watery
5.	Stools	Initially dark mixed with blood	Rice water
6.	Tenesmus	Marked	Absent
7.	Conjunctiva	Congested	Not congested
8.	Voice	Not affected	Rough and whistling
9.	Lab tests	Positive for arsenic	Vibrio cholera is detected
10.	Circumstantial evidence	Suggest poisoning	Usually in epidemic form

muscles. Gradually the patient becomes delirious and passes into coma and death.

Arsine gas poisoning: In arsine gas poisoning most of the features are as a result of hemolysis, hence there is burning sensation of the face, tightness of the chest, headache, giddiness, nausea, vomiting, pain abdomen, dark coloured urine as a result of hemoglobinuria, enlarged liver, jaundice, cyanosis, patient may collapse and die.

Organic arsenical compound poisoning: These compounds are less toxic than inorganic salts. Organic compounds are mostly administered through intravenous route and can give rise to anaphylactic reaction known as "Nitritoid crisis". The patient may present with giddiness, flushed face, nausea, pain in chest and joints and breathlessness. However in severe cases there is optic atrophy, severe stomatitis, diarrhea, dermatitis, jaundice and muscular cramps.

b. Subacute Poisoning

Subacute poisoning is seen in patient when he survives the initial acute poisoning or when small doses are given repeatedly.

Features of subacute poisoning: In the early stages the patient manifest only abdominal symptoms and signs like off and on pain abdomen, complaints of indigestion, foul smell from mouth, tenesmus and purging. Later on the patient complains of depression, there is blood mixed stools, signs of peripheral neuritis, cramps in muscles, paralysis and in some cases there is collapse and death. Patients recovering from subacute poisoning may show residual signs of paralysis.

Fatal dose: About 200 to 300 mg of arsenious oxide and 250 PPM of arsine gas are lethal.

Fatal period: Fatal period in acute poisoning is usually between 12 to 48 hours, whereas in subacute poisoning death may occur after several weeks.

Treatment

a. *Stomach wash:* It can be done with warm water or 1% sodium thiosulphate and should be repeated frequently so that particles sticking to the mucosal surface could be removed or neutralized.

b. *Chemical antidote:* Freshly prepared hydrated ferric oxide, which can be prepared by mixing 15 gm of magnesium oxide or sodium carbonate with 45 ml of ferric chloride solution. After filtration precipitates are given as tablespoonful dose at short interval of 2 to 3 hour. It reacts with arsenic and form harmless ferric arsenite.

c. *Demulcent:* Barley water, or milk with egg.

d. *Magnesium sulphate:* It is administered for reducing absorption.

e. *Antidotes:* British anti lewisite (BAL) is given 3 mg/kg body weight in 10% benzyl benzoate in arachis oil deep intramuscularly every 4 hours for 2 days then thrice daily for 10 days or till recovery. It acts by competition as there are two sulfhydryl bonds. Dimercapto succinic acid (DMSA) or 2, 3 dimercapto-1-propanesulfonic acid (DMPS) can also be administered.

f. Symptomatic treatment:
   i. Morphine for pain.
   ii. Bismuth kaolin for diarrhea.
   iii. Fluids for dehydration.
   iv. Blood transfusion.
   v. Massage for relieving cramps.
   vi. Oxygen administration.

g. Treatment of arsine gas poisoning:
   i. Remove patient to fresh air.
   ii. Oxygen inhalation.
   iii. Blood transfusion when hemolysis is present.
   iv. Hemodialysis in renal failure may be required.
   v. Alkaline drinks.

Postmortem Findings

a. **External findings:**
   i. Signs of dehydration like sunken eyes, wrinkled skin.
   ii. Jaundice especially in arsine poisoning.
   iii. Cyanosis.
   iv. Rigor mortis lasts longer than usual.

b. Internal findings:

i. Stomach contains white gritty powder.

ii. Stomach walls are inflamed red velvet covered with thick mucous with submucosal petechial hemorrhages.

iii. Small intestines show similar changes but of lesser degree.

iv. Heart may show subendocardial hemorrhages and fatty degeneration.

v. Kidneys show congestion, fatty degeneration and tubular necrosis.

vi. Other organs are congested.

c. Chronic Arsenic Poisoning

Chronic poisoning may result from: (a) ingestion of very small doses or drinking contaminated underground water with arsenic compounds; (b) working with compounds of arsenic; (c) consuming food articles having traces of arsenic; or (d) after an acute poisoning when the excretory functions are impaired.

Features of Chronic Poisoning

Features are seen in four stages:

1. **Stage one:** Most of the features are related to gastrointestinal or nutritional disturbances:

   a. Loss of appetite.

   b. Nausea.

   c. Salivation.

   d. Colic pain and constipation or diarrhea.

   e. Vomiting, vomitus may contain bile.

   f. Loss of weight.

   g. Gums are soft and red.

   h. White coated tongue.

2. **Stage two:**

   a. Initial stages produces milk and rose complexion, but later on there is cutaneous eruptions, rashes and hyperkeratosis.

   b. Bronchitis with hoarse voice.

   c. Congested eyes with photophobia.

   d. Intense running of nose later on there may be nasal septal perforations.

   e. Liver is enlarged.

f. Hair may fall off.

g. Nails become brittle and show transverse white bands known as "Mee's lines".

3. **Stage three:** After a month neurological disturbances are seen:

   a. Headache.

   b. Tingling sensation.

   c. Numbness of extremities.

   d. Hyperesthesia of skin.

   e. Cramps in muscles.

   f. Loss of knee and ankle jerks.

   g. Impotency.

4. **Stage four:**

   a. Peripheral neuritis.

   b. Weakness, ataxia.

   c. Paralysis like wrist drop or foot drop.

   d. Muscle cramps more severe at night.

   e. Bone marrow depression.

   f. Liver and kidney damage.

   g. Heart failure leading to death.

Treatment of Chronic Poisoning

After proper diagnosis following steps are taken:

a. Remove the source of poisoning.

b. Sodium thiosulphate 1 gm in 10 ml of distilled water is given intravenously every four hourly for first 24 hours.

c. BAL is administered deep intramuscularly every 6 hours for 2 days then once a day.

d. Vitamin B_1 for peripheral neuritis.

e. Strychnine in very small doses to increase muscular tone.

Postmortem Finding

Skin may show hyperkeratosis. "Mees" lines may be present in nails. Stomach and intestines may or may not show congestion. Liver is enlarged and show fatty degeneration. Kidneys may show signs of nephritis. Muscular atrophy may be observed in some cases.

Medicolegal Importance

1. Arsenic was commonly used as homicidal poison because it satisfied some of the criteria for ideal homicidal poison like

availability, cheap, small fatal dose, tasteless, odorless, can be mixed in food articles and signs and symptoms resemble cholera. Some of the disadvantages are; (a) it retards putrefaction; (b) it can be detected long after death; (c) it can be detected even in charred bodies; and (d) by analyzing the nail or hair one can know when the administration of arsenic took place, as arsenic starts depositing in hair after about 15 days of ingestion. Hair grows at 0.4 mm per day, whereas nails grow at 3 mm per month, this help in calculating the time of arsenic intake. However these days it is hardly used as homicidal poison as a result of restriction on sale and distribution imposed by the government. It is rarely used as suicidal poison. Accidental poisoning may occur.

2. *Arsenic tolerance:* Individuals who are in the habit of taking arsenic can develop tolerance. Such persons are known as "**Arsenophagist**" and can even tolerate fatal dose. However they suffer from chronic poisoning.

3. *Postmortem imbibition:* In some cases after exhumation doubts are raised regarding presence of arsenic in the organs; whether it is from imbibition from stomach contents or the earth around the body. Even though, the arsenic from soil is not imbibed by body organs as it is present in insoluble form. However, in all cases of exhumation samples of earth around the body are collected and preserved.

Serial Murderer Johann Otto Hoch

Hoch was a serial killer who in united states during 1892 to 1905 murdered many of his wives for financial gains. He used to move from one state to another in search of wealthy widows. He used to be friend them and after marriage took control over their wealth. New wife would become seriously ill from features of gastroenteritis and die. Authorities arrested him due to similarities in these deaths. During interrogations he confessed to have done many murders using arsenic. He was convicted and hanged in 1906.

MERCURY

Mercury is a liquid metal having bright silvery luster and is also known as "quick silver". It is volatile at room temperature and in vapour form it is poisonous.

Uses

a. Disinfectant.
b. Diuretic.
c. Dental amalgam.
d. Barometers.
e. Thermometers and blood pressure apparatus, at present there is government policy to discard mercury based thermometer and blood pressure apparatus.
f. Mercury vapours lamps.
g. Ceramics.
h. Fireworks.
i. Electroplating and electric industry.
j. Photography.
k. Paints, fingerprint powder.
l. Silvering of mirrors.
m. Embalming fluid.

Common Compounds of Mercury

In pure metallic form it is nonpoisonous, however vapours are toxic. Mercury in fine divided form when rubbed on the skin can be absorbed. Mercury forms two series of compounds (a) mercuric; and (b) mercurous. Mercuric compounds are soluble and are highly toxic whereas mercurous salts are less soluble and hence are less toxic.

a. *Mercuric chloride:* also known as corrosive sublimate or perchloride of mercury. It is white, heavy crystalline powder. It has nauseating metallic taste. It is used as antiseptic. It is highly toxic corrosive poison.

b. *Mercuric oxide:* It is brick red powder used in some ointments.

c. *Mercuric iodide:* It is scarlet red powder.

d. *Mercuric cyanide:* Similar to mercuric chloride it is highly toxic compound. It is seen in prismatic crystalline form having bitter metallic taste. When burnt it gives obnoxious fumes of mercury and form voluminous ash. Tablet of mercuric cyanide when burnt during Depawali time forms a snake like structure called "Pharaoh's serpent".

e. *Mercuric nitrate:* Crystalline substance used in painting over porcelain and also as veterinary medicine.

f. *Mercuric sulphide:* Deep red in colour used as vermilion, regarded as nonpoisonous but vapours are poisonous. It is used in tattooing.

g. *Mercuric sulphate:* White crystalline powder having corrosive properties.

h. *Mercuric methide:* Highly toxic liquid even vapour inhalation can cause death.

i. *Mercurous chloride:* (Calomel) Sold as Ras Kapoor. It was used in teething powder and caused pink disease in infants (acrodynia).

j. *Organic compounds:*
   i. Methyl and phenyl compounds are used as fungicide.
   ii. Mercury fulminate is used in the manufacture of detonators in firearms.
   iii. Novosurol and mersalyl are used as diuretics.
   iv. Mercurochrome is used as antiseptic.

Mode of action: Action of mercury is by causing depression of cellular enzymes by combining with Sulfhydryl group. It mainly affects nervous system and kidneys.

Features of Poisoning

Acute Poisoning

Mercuric chloride is the most toxic having corrosive properties. Hence majority of symptoms are seen in poisoning by corrosive sublimate. Symptoms usually start immediately or after 10 to 15 minutes.

Features of Acute Poisoning:
   i. There is acrid metallic taste.
   ii. Constriction in the throat and burning sensation during swallowing.
   iii. Pain in the epigastric region which increases on pressure.
   iv. Nausea followed by vomiting mixed with mucous and blood.
   v. Profuse purging with painful tenesmus.
   vi. Pulse is weak and irregular.
   vii. Tongue is white and shriveled.
   viii. Skin is cold and clammy.
   ix. Difficulty in breathing.
   x. Pronounced salivation.
   xi. Urine output increases for a short time then is depressed. Urine contains albumin and blood.
   xii. In some cases spasm of muscles, tremors, convulsions may be seen.
   xiii. After 1–3 days there is gingivitis and marked renal symptoms.
   xiv. Death is due to circulatory collapse or uremia.

Symptoms and signs are similar to arsenic poisoning but in mercury poisoning symptoms appear early, constriction of throat is more marked, vomitus and stool contain blood more frequently along with irritation to kidneys.

Fatal dose: About 200 to 300 mg of mercuric chloride.

Fatal period: Usually 3–5 days.

Treatment

a. Wash the stomach with warm water and preserve the first wash for chemical analysis. Give ½ liter of skimmed milk with 30 gm of glucose or 15 gm of sodium bicarbonate with 15 gm of egg white to form albuminates of mercury.

b. Activated charcoal orally.

c. Demulcents like barley water to protect stomach wall.

d. Sodium formaldehyde sulphoxylate 5 to 10% in 200 ml of water.

e. About 10 gm of sulphoxylate dissolved in 200 ml of distilled water can be slowly administered by intravenous route.

f. BAL is administered, 300 mg IM initially then 150 mg 2–3 times in next 12 hours.

g. Penicillamine in the dose of 250–300 mg 3 to 4 times a day.

h. High colonic wash with sulphoxylate; 1:1000 solution twice daily.

i. Fluids to combat shock.

j. Symptomatic treatment as required.

Postmortem Findings

a. Grayish white discolouration of mucosa of mouth lips esophagus and stomach.

b. Mucosa may show signs of corrosion.

c. Large intestinal mucosa is inflamed and ulcerated.

d. Kidneys show swelling with necrosis of tubules.

e. Liver and spleen are congested and may show cloudy swelling.

f. Heart shows fatty degeneration.

Chronic Poisoning

Chronic mercury poisoning (*erythrism or mercurialism*) may be as a result of any of the following:

1. Continuous accidental absorption by workers handling murcury salts.
2. Improper medical use.
3. A patient recovering from large intake.
4. Application of ointment containing mercury salt for long period of time.

Features of Chronic Poisoning

a. Initially in erythrism there is peculiar psychological disorder characterised by timidity, anxiety, lack of decision-making, lack of concentration and depression. This is followed by headache, fatigue, drowsiness or insomnia and in some cases there may be hallucinations.

b. Vasomotor disturbances include blushing and excessive sweating.

c. Gastrointestinal disturbances present as nausea, pain abdomen, diarrhea, salivation (ptyalism), gingivitis, foul smell from the mouth, painful salivary glands, brownish blue line over gums and loose teeth.

d. Tremors in erythrism are called *"Hatter's shake"*, *"Danbury shake"* or *"Mercurial tremors"*. There are course tremors effecting hands and progressing to arms, feet and legs. There may be difficulty in walking. These tremors can be demonstrated by drawing test, as they become more pronounced when any voluntary action is done.

e. Speech is slurred with hesitancy.

f. There are motor and sensory disturbances like ataxia, loss of postural sense and sensory loss.

g. *"Mercuria Lentis"* is a golden brown reflex from anterior capsule of the eye lens.

h. Kidneys due to tubular necrosis may show albumin and casts in urine. In later stages there is uremia.

i. Mild hypochromic anemia may be observed.

j. Pigmentation of the skin with small ulcerations known as powder holes.

Treatment

a. Stop exposure.

b. BAL can be administered.

c. Increased milk intake.

d. Gargles with potassium chlorate.

e. Purgatives if required.

Teratogenicity and Neurological Effects on Fetus and Young Children

There is strong evidence that exposure to mercury from eating fish contaminated with mercury during early pregnancy may have teratogenic effects on the fetus. The fetus may have mental retardation, cerebral atrophy, birth defects, and spasticity apart from other growth defects. During early childhood or developmental stages in children, exposure to mercury may lead to various neurological problems. Therefore, use of mercury has been banned in various countries.

LEAD

Lead is a heavy, steel grey metal. Lead in the pure metallic form is not poisonous, but when converted into salts by the actions of the enzymes and secretions in the GIT may cause toxicity.

Uses

a. Paint industry
b. Soldering
c. Plumbing and water pipes
d. Electric cable covering
e. Printing
f. Pigments.

Common Compounds of Lead

a. *Lead acetate:* It is also known as sugar of lead or salt of saturn. It is white, crystalline, having sweet astringent taste. It was used to sweeten wine in earlier times.
b. *Lead carbonate:* It is white crystalline powder used in paints. It can cause toxicity in small children who suck toys painted with this compound.
c. *Lead nitrate:* Crystalline salt used in calico printing.
d. *Lead chromate:* It is bright yellow in colour and used in pigment. It is also known as chrome yellow.
e. *Lead chloride:* White needle shaped crystals used as pigment.
f. *Lead iodide:* Bright yellow powder, which is odorless and tasteless.
g. *Lead sulphide:* Naturally found as cubic crystals but sold in powder form as Surma in place of antimony sulphide.
h. *Lead tetraoxide:* It is scarlet powder known as red lead or sindhur and used as pigment.
i. *Lead tetraethyl:* It is oily fluid, little volatile, lipid soluble, having sweetish odor and highly toxic. This was earlier added to petrol to prevent knocking. The mixture is known as ethyl petrol.

Absorption

Acute poisoning is rare as salts are slowly absorbed from the GIT. Fast absorption occurs in poisoning with lead tetraethyl by inhalation or by directly applying to skin surface. Mostly poisoning take place in industries when fine lead dust or fumes are inhaled.

Distribution

After absorption the highest quantities are seen in the liver and kidneys. Lead is deposited in bones as tertiary lead phosphate more near the epiphyseal end of the bone. This can be visualized as a dense line just behind the epiphyseal line or a ring of density around the ossification center, on X-ray examination. Factors which help in the deposition of lead in bones are high value of calcium and phosphate along with vitamin D. Once the lead is deposited in the bones it will not cause toxicity. Factors like acidosis, parathyroid hormones, iodides and bicarbonates help in the release of lead from bones. Before chelating agents were discovered, by giving suitable diet lead was deposited in bones and later on when conditions became suitable it was mobilized from bones for excretion.

Excretion of Lead

Lead is largely eliminated in feces and small quantities are excreted in urine, bile, saliva and milk. Lead portion which is present in plasma and not attached to RBC's is excreted out.

Features of Poisoning

Poisoning is seen in three forms (1) Acute; (2) Subacute; (3) Chronic.

1. Acute Poisoning

In acute poisoning following manifestations are seen:

a. Sweet metallic taste.
b. Burning and dryness in throat.
c. Salivation.
d. Nausea and vomiting, vomit is white with blood tinge.
e. Colicky pain relived on pressure.
f. Constipation, but rarely diarrhea with dark stools due to lead sulphide.
g. Weakness.
h. Scanty urine.
i. Insomnia, headache, vertigo and drowsiness.
j. Muscular cramps, convulsions, numbness and paralysis.
k. Death is mainly due to exhaustion.

Features of poisoning by lead tetraethyl:

a. Irritability, vertigo, nervousness and insomnia.
b. Headache.
c. Nausea and vomiting.
d. Tremors.
e. Muscular weakness.
f. Low blood pressure and bradycardia.
g. Hypothermia.
h. Delirium.
i. Convulsions and death.

Fatal dose: About 20 gm of lead acetate or 30 gm of Lead carbonate.

Fatal period: Death usually occurs in 2 to 3 days but fatal period may be prolonged.

2. Subacute Poisoning

Subacute poisoning is mainly seen from taking small doses of lead acetate and manifest following features:

a. Blue lead line on the gums.
b. Nausea, vomiting and pain abdomen.
c. Scanty urine, urine may be of red colour.
d. Numbness, vertigo, cramps and convulsions.
e. Flaccid paralysis of lower limbs.
f. Death is rare but may occur from coma.

Treatment:

a. Stomach wash is done with warm water then with 1% magnesium sulphate.
b. In case stomach wash is not possible emetics can be administered.
c. Cathartics like 30 gm of sodium or magnesium sulphate to remove lead from GIT.
d. Demulcents like milk, white of an egg or barley water.
e. Antidote: Calcium disodium versonate is given 25 to 35 mg/kg body weight. About 5 ml of 20% solution can be given intragastric or in 5% glucose solution by slow intravenous route, twice daily for 5 days and if required can be repeated after 2 days interval. This combines with lead and the nontoxic compound formed is excreted through urine. Penicillamine

can be given orally in the doses of 0.6 to 1.5 gm daily for 4 to 5 days. It can also be given intravenously in slow drip.

f. Calcium gluconate: About 2 gm in intravenous drip is given to relieve abdominal pain. 10 ml of 20% calcium chloride and 2 gm of calcium phosphate is given by mouth so as to deposit lead in the bones.
g. High dose of vitamin D, 100 mg of vitamin C and diet rich in calcium like milk is given for deposition of lead in bones.

Postmortem findings: In majority of cases features of acute gastroenteritis are present like mucosa of the stomach is inflamed and eroded at places. Lead line and evidence of tubular necrosis may be observed.

3. Chronic Poisoning

Chronic poisoning is seen in workers employed in industries using lead salts or from inhalation of lead dust:

a. Painters
b. Enamel workers
c. Electric light workers
d. Lead smelters
e. Plumbers
f. Glass blowers
g. Card players
h. Tinned food contaminated with lead.
i. In persons with prolonged use of hair dye or sindhur especially when the skin is abraded.

Prevention of poisoning can be achieved by proper ventilation in such industries, periodical medical checkup, personal cleanliness and diet rich in calcium like plenty of milk.

Features of Poisoning

Chief signs and symptoms of chronic poisoning are as follows:

a. *Colic and constipation (dry belly aches):* Pain is observed around umbilicus, which is relieved by pressure associated with constipation. There is metallic taste in the mouth, profuse sweating and vomiting may occur during colic.

b. *Lead line (burtonian line):* Blue line is seen over the gum margins near teeth when the oral hygiene is bad. Hydrogen sulphide generated from decomposition of food particles reacts with circulating lead in the gum margins to form lead sulphide.

c. *Anemia:* Moderate hypochromic anemia with reticulocytosis and punctuate basophilia is seen.

d. *Paralysis:* Typical paralysis of extensor group of muscles is seen like wrist drop or foot drop with wasting of involved muscles.

e. *Encephalopathy:* Mostly this is seen in infants. There is headache, loss of concentration and memory, insomnia, optic neuritis, convulsions, hallucinations delirium and coma.

f. *Cardiorenal manifestations:* Hypertension, arteriosclerotic changes, interstitial nephritis leading to albuminurea with copro-porphyrin-III and delta amino-leuvelinic acid secretion.

g. *Miscellaneous:* Other features include menstrual disturbances, abortions or miscarriage due to blastophoric effects seen in females and sterility in males as lead may reduce sperm count and produce changes in the sperm characteristics.

Diagnosis

Diagnosis of chronic poisoning mainly depends on following factors:

a. Details of occupation and related history.

b. Urine levels are more than 0.08 mg/liter in poisoning and blood levels are more than 0.8 mg/liter.

c. Estimation of urinary copro-porphyrin-III and delta amino-leuvelinic acid.

d. Glycosuria and amino acid in urine in children.

e. Increased X-ray densities like radio-opaque bands in metaphysis of long bones.

Treatment

a. Remove patient from the source of poisoning.

b. Vitamin K and iodine in medicinal doses.

c. Sodium bicarbonate about 20–30 gm/day in four divided doses to increase excretion.

d. Ammonium chloride capsule containing 500 mg every 4 hourly with plenty of water.

e. Low calcium diet for three weeks.

f. Intravenous calcium gluconate 15 ml or 10% calcium chloride to relieve abdominal pain.

g. Saline purgatives like sodium sulphate.

h. Calcium disodium versonate 25 to 35 mg/Kg body weight in slow drip.

Postmortem Features

a. Blue line over gums.

b. Paralytic muscles show fatty degeneration.

c. Intestines are thickened and contracted.

d. Tubular necrosis in kidneys.

e. Atheromatous changes in aorta.

f. Cerebral edema.

Medicolegal Significance

a. Acute poisoning is rarely seen but chronic poisoning is very common in specific industry workers.

b. Homicidal poisoning is very rare.

c. Red lead is used as abortifacient causing uterine contractions, degeneration of embryonic cells and chorionic epithelium.

d. Red lead is sometimes used as cattle poison mixed with arsenic.

e. Earlier syphilis was treated with lead salts leading to chronic poisoning.

f. Children may suffer from chronic poisoning if they ingest paint scrapings from toys.

g. Ladies using sindur over abraded skin may have chronic poisoning.

h. Mothers may pass on lead in the breast milk to the infants.

COPPER

Copper as a metal is nonpoisonous. It is one of the essential elements in the body required for metabolism.

Common Compounds

a. *Copper sulphate:* It is also known as blue vitriol (neela tutia). It is available in large blue crystals; soluble in water on heating it becomes white in colour. This salt is mainly used as colouring agent, fungicide, emetic, preservative for vegetables and also as astringent.

b. *Copper carbonate:* It is greenish in colour hence used as colouring agent.

c. *Copper subacetate:* It is bluish green crystalline compound.

Features of Poisoning

Poisoning is observed either in acute or chronic form.

Acute Poisoning

Acute poisoning is more commonly seen, mostly in suicidal attempts. Mostly the symptoms are observed after about half hour.

a. Astringent taste in mouth.

b. Salivation.

c. Headache.

d. Burning pain in epigastrium.

e. Nausea and vomiting.

f. Vomitus is bluish green in colour and can be differentiated from bile by adding ammonium hydroxide which reacts with copper salts giving deep blue colour.

g. Diarrhea with brown stool.

h. Oliguria, albuminuria and uremia.

i. Cramps in the legs, rarely paralysis of limbs.

j. Circulatory collapse if high doses are taken.

k. Death is due to shock due to vascular collapse, rarely from acute hemolysis or spasm of glottis causing asphyxia.

Fatal dose: About 30 gm of copper sulphate, however small doses taken on small intervals are more dangerous as large dose leads to emesis.

Fatal period: Usually in about 1 to 3 days.

Treatment

Normally emetics are not required.

a. *Stomach wash:* Initially with warm water to preserve the sample for chemical

analysis then with 1% potassium ferrocyanide which forms harmless cupric ferrocyanide. About 300 mg of potassium ferrocyanide can also be given by mouth if gastric lavage is not done.

b. Calcium EDTA 25 to 35 mg/Kg body weight can be given by mouth or intravenous route in slow drip.

c. BAL and penicillamine can also be used.

d. Symptomatic treatment like 10 to 15 mg of morphine for pain, diuretics for oliguria, intravenous fluids and corticosteroids for shock.

Postmortem Findings:

a. External findings:

i. Skin is yellowish due to jaundice.

ii. Greenish froth from mouth and nostrils.

iii. Lips and tip of tongue are blue tinged.

iv. Excoriation at the angles of mouth.

b. Internal findings:

i. Stomach and intestines are congested and excoriated.

ii. Stomach contents are bluish green.

iii. Colon may show large ulcerations.

iv. Rarely rectum may show perforations.

v. Liver is soft, fatty and yellowish stained.

vi. Kidneys show tubular degeneration especially of the proximal tubule.

vii. Bladder contains bloodstained urine.

Chronic Copper Poisoning

It is mostly seen in industries using copper salts. When food stored in copper utensils is consumed as acetic acid present in some food articles reacts with copper to form copper subacetate.

Features of Chronic Poisoning

Symptom complex known as *"Bronzed diabetes"*, *"Hemochromatosis"*, or *"Pigment cirrhosis"* is mentioned below:

i. Nausea and vomiting

ii. Headache and giddiness

iii. Dyspepsia

iv. Pain abdomen

v. Diarrhea

vi. Oliguria

vii. Anemia

viii. Green or purple line on gums

ix. Signs of peripheral neuritis

x. Jaundice

xi. Hair sweat and urine may become greenish.

Treatment

1. Remove the source of poisoning.
2. Keep the patient in fresh air.
3. Warm baths.
4. Antidote BAL may be used.
5. Symptomatic treatment.

Medicolegal Importance

1. Mainly due to colour and metallic taste it is not used for homicidal purposes.
2. Mostly it is used for suicidal purposes and rarely accidental poisoning is seen.
3. It is normal constituent of the body hence mere finding it in viscera is not indicative of poisoning. Normal intake is about 3 mg/day. The normal range for total copper in blood is 70 to 140 microgram per deciliter.
4. It is mainly eliminated through bile but also in saliva and mother's milk.

THALLIUM

Most of the thallium salts are easily soluble in water, tasteless and odorless compounds hence are used for homicidal purposes.

Uses

a. Hair removal creams.

b. Dye and glass industry.

c. Earlier used as medicine for ringworm, gout and venereal diseases.

d. Rat poison.

Features of Poisoning

a. Vomiting.

b. Diarrhea.

c. Lethargy, neuropathies, optic neuritis and features of psychosis.

d. Muscular weakness.

e. Hair loss is one of characteristic feature of thallium poisoning.

f. Mee's lines may be seen in nails.

g. Death is from respiratory failure.

Fatal dose: About 1 gm.

Treatment

a. Stomach wash

b. Activated charcoal

c. Prussian blue about 250 mg/kg body weight can be administered orally.

d. Chelating agents are usually not preferred.

Bovington Bug

An Englishman Graham Young had fascinations about various poisons from the younger age. He joined a factory producing high quality lenses using thallium in 1971. He used to serve tea to various workers in that factory. Suddenly many of his coworkers became sick showing nervous system manifestations known as "Bovington Bug". When two of his colleagues died he became a prime suspect because of his fascination with poisons. His diary revealed his involvement and was convicted and imprisoned for life.

38 | Nonmetallic Irritant Poisons

PHOSPHORUS

There are two common varieties of phosphorus, red and yellow phosphorus. Red phosphorus is relatively nontoxic but yellow phosphorus is highly toxic. In earlier days, yellow phosphorus was used in lucifer matchsticks before safety matches came into use (in safety matches, head has antimony sulphide and potassium chlorate, whereas, matchbox side has red phosphorus and powdered glass). Workers in factories manufacturing lucifer matchsticks used to suffer from phosphorus poisoning. Yellow phosphorus is translucent, waxy material having garlicky smell, which is stored under water as it ignites at room temperature. Aluminum or Zinc phosphide is commonly used as grain preservative giving off phosphine gas which is highly toxic.

Uses

a. Flares, tracer bullets, smoke screens.
b. Fireworks.
c. Rodenticides.
d. Red phosphorus is mainly used in safety matches and fertilizers.

Features of Poisoning

There are three types of poisoning seen with phosphorus, (a) fulminant; (b) acute; and (c) chronic poisoning.

1. **Fulminant poisoning:** It is commonly seen with heavy dose of phosphorus (more than 1 gm) leading to circulatory collapse and death in 12 to 36 hours.
2. **Acute poisoning:** Acute poisoning is manifested in two stages. Initial features include:
   a. Nausea, vomiting and diarrhea. Vomitus and stools are luminous in the dark.
   b. Garlicky odor from breath.
   c. Abdominal colicky pain.
   d. Intense thirst.

   These symptoms last for a day or two then they subside and patient is seen to improve. However these symptoms return with increased severity after few days.
   a. Apart from the above mentioned symptoms there is hepatomegaly with jaundice.
   b. Purpuric spots or even hematoma at places due to hypoprothrombinemia.
   c. Renal failure leading to oliguria.
   d. Convulsions, coma and death.

Treatment: In acute and fulminant cases following steps are taken. Demulcents, fatty foods or oils are not administered as they help in absorption.
   a. *Stomach wash:* It can be done with precautions by using 1:5000 potassium permanganate, 2% hydrogen peroxide or 0.2% copper sulphate.
   b. Sodium bicarbonate for acidosis.

c. Calcium gluconate, B complex, vitamin K and C should be administered.
d. Symptomatic and supportive measures.

Medicolegal importance: Yellow phosphorus was once used as a rat poison, which was sometimes consumed for suicidal purposes. Accidental poisoning especially in small children may take place from consuming rat poison or fire crackers. Homicidal poisoning is rare.

Ricketts murder case

Mr and Mrs Merrifield came to live with an old lady Mrs Ricketts with a promise to look after her. After some time Mrs Ricketts executed a will in the favour of Merrifields. One month after that a doctor was called to examine Mrs Ricketts but he found that there was nothing wrong with her. Later that night Mrs Ricketts became seriously sick and when the doctor was again called he found her to be dead. An autopsy was done and phosphorus was recovered from the viscera examined. Merrifield had administered the poison mixed with rum to mask the taste. Mrs Merrifield was convicted of murder and executed.

3. **Chronic phosphorus poisoning:** Chronic poisoning is seen in industrial workers by inhaling fumes of phosphorus. With advent of safety matches incidents of chronic poisoning are hardy observed.

   Features:
   a. Anorexia and giddiness.
   b. Toothache with loosening of teeth and necrosis of jaw with formation of sinuses known as *"Phossy Jaw"* or *"Lucifer's Jaw"*.
   c. Nausea and vomiting
   d. Joint pains
   e. Stomatitis and pain in epigastric area
   f. Liver damage with jaundice.

   Treatment:
   a. Prevent further absorption by removing the patient from source of poisoning.
   b. Dental care and treatment.

POISONING BY PHOSPHINE GAS

Aluminum phosphide is used as pesticide for stored grains very commonly. It is available as *quickphos, alphos, celphos, and fumigran,* etc. Each tablet of 3 gm on exposure to air and moisture liberates about 1 gm of phosphine gas. When such a tablet is ingested, the patient may manifest following features:
a. Garlicky smell from breath.
b. Nausea, vomiting and diarrhea.
c. Epigastric pain.
d. Headache and giddiness.
e. Hypotension, bradycardia, conduction or rhythm defects observed in ECG, myocarditis and heart failure.
f. Respiratory difficulty, crepitations and even respiratory failure.
g. Hepatomegaly with jaundice and renal failure.

The poisoning can be confirmed by placing a mask over the mouth and nostrils (soaked with silver nitrate in methanol and then dried), which turns black in case phosphine gas is present in breath.

Fatal dose: Fatal dose is 0.15 to 0.5 gm of aluminum phosphide.

Treatment of phosphine gas poisoning: Apart from the measures taken for acute phosphorus poisoning, magnesium sulphate is given 1 gm intravenously repeated after every 3–4 hours during the first 1–2 days then every 6 hours up to 5 days.

Postmortem Findings

a. Garlicky smell from the mouth and gastric contents
b. Gastric contents are luminous in dark
c. Stomach and intestines are congested
d. Enlarged liver with features of jaundice.
e. Kidneys and other organs are congested.

Medicolegal Importance

Suicidal poisoning with aluminum phosphide is especially seen with increased frequency in the agriculturists. Homicidal poisoning is rare.

IODINE

Iodine is a purple crystalline substance having characteristic smell and metallic taste. It gives off violet vapors at room temperature. Starch solution gives deep blue colour when added to iodine containing vomitus or stomach contents. Most of the poisoning cases are accidental in nature.

Uses

a. Medically used as antiseptic like Lugol's iodine, providone iodine and tincture of iodine.
b. Photography.
c. Industrial purposes.

Features of Poisoning

a. Nausea, vomiting and diarrhea.
b. Metallic taste.
c. Corrosion of skin and mucous membrane with brownish stains.
d. Renal failure.
e. Respiratory difficulty with pulmonary edema.

Fatal dose: About 3 to 4 gm.

Treatment

a. Administer milk or starch solution.
b. Sodium thiosulphate solution orally to convert iodine to iodide.
c. Symptomatic treatment.

Postmortem Findings

a. Brownish stains over skin or mucosa.
b. Corrosions and rarely perforation of GIT.
c. Congestion of visceral organs.

Chronic Poisoning

Chronic poisoning by iodine or iodism is seen in persons handling iodine frequently. Feature of chronic poisoning are as follows:

a. Urticaria.
b. Conjunctivitis and rhinorrhea.
c. Parotid swelling.
d. Anorexia and insomnia.

Treatment

Increase intake of common salt increases excretion through kidneys as chlorides are absorbed in comparison to iodides at the level of renal tubules.

MECHANICAL IRRITANT POISONS

Mechanical irritants are powder glass, diamond dust, pins, needles or sharp metallic pieces. A ball of hair may cause intestinal obstruction. Sharp ends or edges cause damage to the gastric or intestinal mucosa on ingestion. Sometimes it may lead to perforation of the intestines and resultant peritonitis and related complications.

Features

a. Pain abdomen.
b. Vomiting, vomitus may be bloodstained.
c. Sometimes features of perforation and resultant peritonitis may be seen.

Treatment

a. Mainly bulky food to protect the intestinal mucosa like bananas.
b. Symptomatic treatment.

Postmortem Features

a. Gastric and intestinal mucosa is inflamed and damaged.
b. Hemorrhage in the GIT
c. Perforation may be seen in few cases.

Medicolegal Importance

Ingestion is mostly accidental rarely it may be homicidal.

39 | Organic Irritant Poisons of Vegetable Origin

RICINUS COMMUNIS (Castor Plant or Arandi)

Castor plant grows all over India. The seeds are oval glossy brown and mottled. The seeds are of two varieties: (a) large variety and (b) small variety. Large variety seed oil is mainly used for lubricant purposes, however, small seed variety yields better quality of oil and is used for medicinal purposes. Castor seeds resemble croton seeds. The castor seeds are bright smooth reddish-brown with dark brown markings (Fig. 39.1), whereas the croton seeds are dull grayish brown in appearance. The active principal present in castor seeds is a water soluble toxalbumin known as *"ricin"*. The action of ricin resembles bacterial toxin causing agglutination of red blood cells with some amount of hemolysis.

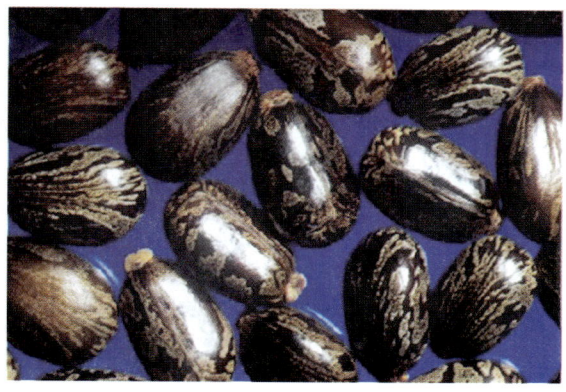

Fig. 39.1: Caster seeds

The residue (press cake) left after extraction of oil is highly toxic as ricin remains in the residue. Hence the residue should not be given to animals in the fodder. Even dust from the residue may lead to irritation in the eyes and nose along with allergic problems like dermatitis and asthma. Castor oil is pale yellow, viscid liquid and is nonpoisonous.

Uses

Castor oil is used as purgative, lubricant and in many other industries like soap, dye, polishes, nylon manufacturing, etc.

Features of Poisoning

Following signs and symptoms observed when crushed seeds are ingested:

a. Burning pain in throat.
b. Nausea, vomiting and colicky pain in abdomen.
c. Thirst and signs of dehydration.
d. Hemolysis and shock leading to vertigo, cold clammy skin and rapid feeble pulse.
e. Some cases may have oliguria and uremia.
f. Death usually results from shock.

Fatal dose: About 10 crushed seeds taken orally or 60 mg of ricin is lethal for an adult. However, through parentral route ricin is highly toxic and about 22 micrograms per kg of body weight is fatal.

Fatal period: Death usually takes place in about 2 days.

Treatment

a. Gastric lavage with warm water and potassium permanganate.
b. Activated charcoal can be administered.
c. Intravenous fluids for dehydration.
d. Sodium bicarbonate to alkalinize urine.
e. Symptomatic treatment.

Postmortem Findings

a. Fragments of the ingested seeds may be seen in the stomach.
b. Mucosa of the stomach and intestines is congested and inflamed. Ulcerations may be observed in some cases.
c. Hemorrhages are frequently seen in internal organs.

Medicolegal Importance

a. Accidental poisoning may be seen in children.
b. Powder may be put in the eyes to produce conjunctivitis.
c. Ricinoleate in castor oil is converted into ricinoleic acid in the intestines which is irritant hence it is used as purgative and also for causing illegal abortions.
d. Ricin when injected in pure form is highly toxic. However if small doses are injected subcutaneously antiricin may be formed in the body.
e. Rarely this has been used for homicidal purposes.

Umbrella Murder Case

A Bulgarian Mr. Markov, who defected to the west block, was waiting for a bus and felt that a by Stander's umbrella has poked him. That person apologized and moved away. After some time Markov had fever, vertigo and signs of shock. He subsequently died after three days. On autopsy examination a small pallet with holes was recovered from his thigh which contained ricin. The assassin was never captured who murdered Markov by firing a pellet containing ricin from a modified umbrella.

CROTON TIGLIUM (Jamal ghota)

Croton plant grows all over India. Seeds are very poisonous. They contain a toxalbumin "Crotin", which is similar to ricin in action but is less poisonous along with "Crotonoside" a glycoside. Seeds are oval, dull and grayish brown in colour (Fig. 39.2). The oil extracted from these seeds is brownish yellow in colour and of burning taste. It contains a powerful vesicating resin made chiefly of crotonoleic acid, tiglic acid and methyl crotonic acid along with some fatty acids.

Features of Poisoning

a. Hot burning taste in mouth extending to the epigastric region.
b. Salivation.
c. Vertigo.
d. Nausea and vomiting.
e. Pain abdomen, diarrhea with bloodstained stools.
f. Signs of dehydration.
g. Hemolysis may lead to jaundice, hemoglobinuria and anuria.
h. Features of shock like thready fast pulse and death from circulatory collapse.

Fatal dose: About 5 to 6 seeds or 1.5 ml of oil.

Fatal period: May occur early in 4 to 6 hours or delayed for 3 to 4 days.

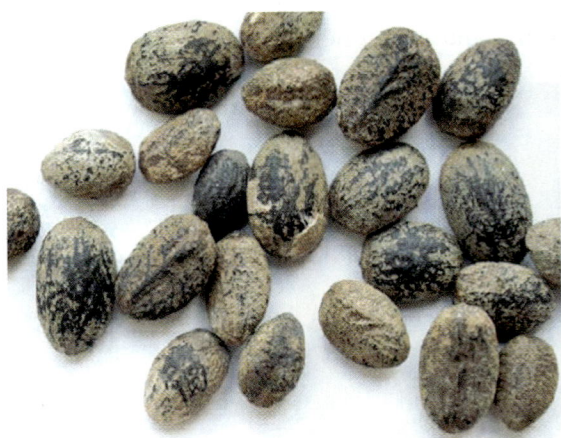

Fig. 39.2: Croton seeds

Treatment

a. Stomach wash.
b. Demulcent drinks.
c. Morphine for pain and stimulants if required.
d. Intravenous fluids to combat shock.

Postmortem Findings

a. Fragments of the seeds may be seen in the stomach.
b. Mucous membranes are congested and softened.
c. Mucosa may be eroded at places.
d. Kidneys may show cloudy swelling.
e. Other visceral organs are congested.

Medicolegal Importance

a. Earlier it was used as arrow poison.
b. Root of the plant or oil is used for illegal abortions.
c. Accidental poisoning is seen in some cases.
d. Rarely oil has been used for suicidal purposes.

ABRUS PRECATORIUS (Rati Seeds, Rosary Peas, Gunchi)

It is a climbing plant found all over India. Seeds are egg shaped scarlet in colour with a black spot at one end (Fig. 39.3). Few other varieties of dark red, black, yellow or white colour are also seen. Average weight of each seed is about 105 mg ($1^3/_4$ grains) and was used by gold smiths to weigh gold and silver.

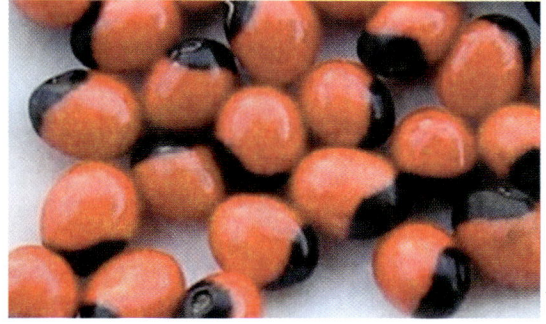

Fig. 39.3: Rati seeds

Seeds contain an active principal toxalbumin "Abrin" which is similar to ricin in action. In addition seeds contain poisonous proteins, fat splitting enzyme, abrussic acid, hemagglutinins and urease.

Abrin is tasteless, amorphous solid having pale gray colour. When taken orally it is inactivated to some extent by gastric juice and can also be deactivated by boiling. If installed in eyes it causes purulent conjunctivitis and even causes death from absorption through conjunctiva.

Features of Poisoning

When extract of the seeds is injected it results in following signs and symptoms, which resemble viper snake bite:

a. Inflammation, edema and necrosis of the site of injection.
b. Disinclination to take food.
c. Unable to move due to vertigo, giddiness and cardiac arrhythmia and convulsions.
d. Features of shock like cold clammy skin, irregular pulse and hemolysis.
e. Oliguria and uremia.
f. Death is due to cardiac paralysis.

Fatal dose: About 90 to 120 mg.
Fatal period: About 3 to 5 days.

Treatment

a. "Sui" if present should be extracted.
b. Inject Anti-Abrin serum if available.
c. Gastric lavage and emesis if ingested.
d. Mild hydrochloric acid and pepsin mixture by mouth.
e. Sodium bicarbonate 10 gm orally to alkalinize the urine.
f. Symptomatic treatment.

Postmortem Findings

a. Sui fragments may be seen at the site of injection.
b. Edema, inflammation and necrosis at the site of injection.
c. Petechial hemorrhages under the skin at the local site and also on pleura and peritoneum.
d. Other internal organs are congested.

Medicolegal Importance

a. Mostly for cattle killing "Sui" is used, which is made by mixing the decorticated seed extract with datura, opium, onion and spirit to form a paste. This is then rolled into spikes weighing from 90 to 120 mg and dried in sun. Two spikes are fixed on a wooden handle and thrust into the skin of an animal with intention of killing. Two spikes are used to mimic fang marks of a viper snake so as to avoid suspicion.

b. These spikes are sometimes used for homicidal purposes. A spike is kept between fingers before slapping the victim.

c. Orally the poison is not effective.

d. Sometimes this is also used as abortifacient.

e. It was used as an arrow poison.

SEMICARPUS ANACARDIUM (Marking nut)

Fruit of the Semicarpus anacardium is called Marking nut or Bhilawa (Fig. 39.4). Pulp of the fruit contains brownish acrid juice, which turns black when mixed with lime and exposed to air and is used for marking on the cloths. Juice contains semicarpol and bhilawanol.

Features of Poisoning

When taken in large dose it produces following signs and symptoms.

a. Blisters in the throat.

b. Severe gastrointestinal irritation, leading to nausea, vomiting and diarrhea.

c. Dyspnea, cyanosis and dilated pupils.

d. Hypotension and tachycardia.

e. Delirium, coma and death.

Fatal dose: About 5 to 10 gm.

Fatal period: About 12 to 24 hours.

Postmortem Findings

a. Blisters in the mouth

b. GIT congested and inflamed

c. Fatty degeneration of liver

d. Other visceral organs are congested.

Medicolegal Importance

a. Mainly used for producing false bruises.

b. Accidental poisoning occurs when used by quacks.

c. Homicidal poisoning is very rare.

d. Sometimes used for illegal abortions.

CALATROPIS GIGENTEA AND CALATROPIS PROCERA (Madar, Aak or Akdo)

Calatropis gigentea has purple flowers and grows all over India (Fig. 39.5), whereas procera has white flowers. Leaves and stalk when incised exude milky fluid. There are three active principals in the plant; calatoxin, calactin and uscharin.

Features of Poisoning

When applied to skin it causes redness and vesications, but on ingestion it causes following signs and symptoms:

a. Bitter taste

b. Pain in the throat

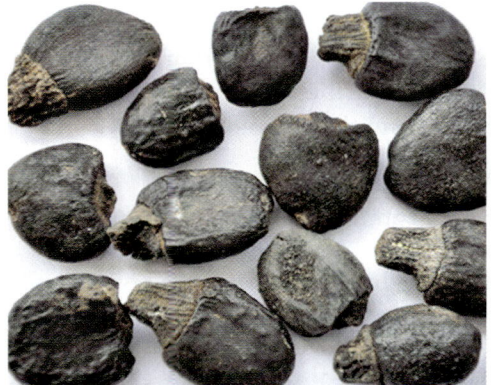

Fig. 39.4: Semicarpus anacardium

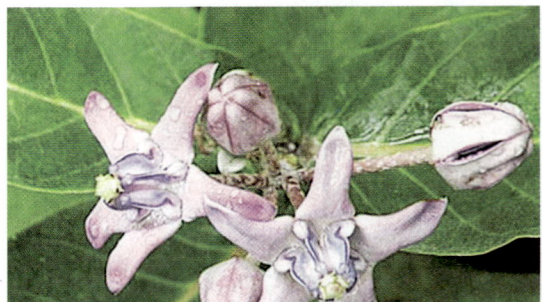

Fig. 39.5: Calatropis

Feature	Datura seed	Capsicum seed
	Tabe 39.1: Differentiating features between datura and capsicum seeds	
Size	Large and thick	Small and thin
Shape	Kidney shaped	Rounded
Colour	Dark or yellowish brown	Pale yellow
Margins	Double edge at convex boarder	Single boarder and sharp
Surface	Pitted with small depressions	smooth
Smell	Odorless	Pungent
Taste	Bitter	Pungent
Embryo	Curved outwards	Curved inwards

c. Epigastric pain
d. Salivation
e. Nausea, vomiting and diarrhea
f. Dilated pupils
g. Convulsions, collapse and death.

Fatal dose: Uncertain.

Fatal period: About 12 hours.

Treatment

a. Stomach wash.
b. Demulcents.
c. Symptomatic treatment.

Postmortem Findings

a. Froth at nostrils.
b. Stomatitis.
c. Inflammation of gastrointestinal tract.

Medicolegal Importance

a. Twig is used as abortifacient.
b. Juice is used as vesicant.
c. For cattle poisoning, juice of the plant is smeared on the cloth and inserted into the rectum of the animal.

CAPSICUM ANNUM (Lal Mirch)

Capsicum annum is commonly used household condiment. It contains capsaicin and capsicin having bitter or acrid taste. The seeds resemble datura seeds. Differentiating features are mentioned in Table 39.1.

Features of Poisoning

a. When applied to skin causes irritation and vesications.
b. When applied to eyes it causes burning and lacrymation.
c. In case of ingestion causes GIT irritation.

Treatment

a. No specific treatments, if applied to skin or eyes, wash with lots of water.
b. Use emollients.

Medicolegal Importance

a. Powder is used for confession of some guilt by introducing it into nostrils, eyes, vagina, rectum or rubbing it on the breasts.
b. So as to facilitate robbery, powder is thrown in the eyes.
c. Powder may be used for punishment.
d. Fumes from the burning chilies are highly irritating to the eyes and respiratory tract.
e. Powder is used by superstitious persons to drive away ghosts or spirits.
f. For self defence chili spray are used by women
g. It is proposed to use chili powder in hand grenades by security forces to control rioters.

40 | Organic Irritant Poisons of Animal Origin

SNAKES

There are more than 3000 species of snakes in the world out of which about 300 are poisonous. In India out of more than 200 species, about 52 are poisonous; however, six varieties of snakes are mainly responsible for envenomation in humans. Snakes have a long, thin scaly, legless bodies and unblinking, lidless eyes. Like all reptiles, snakes are cold blooded animals. Snakes use their tongue to smell. When a snake flicks its tongue it picks up chemical particles. Tongue carry these particles to special vomeronasal organ known as Jacobson's organ on the roof of the month.

Fatal snake bites have become a major public health concern in India. More than 81000 cases of snake bites with 11000 fatalities in India are reported every year. Those who survive the bite on the spot may subsequently die due to delay in getting proper treatment as they are unable to reach a hospital within the crucial golden hour or even some times from overdose of antivenom. In 2011 according to a report published in Times of India about 46000 deaths take place in India every year much more than the official figures.

Snakes belong to class reptilia, order squamata, suborder serpentes and super family ophidia. Ophidia includes all poisonous and nonpoisonous snakes. Poisonous snakes are divided into two groups or families.

1. **Colubridae:** These are egg laying snakes, have round pupils, head and neck is of same size, comparatively long tail, large scales on the head and have small grooved fangs. They have to close their jaws before they inject their venom. They are further sub-divided into two groups.
    i. *Elapidae:* These are land snakes and have round tail like king cobra, cobra, common krait, banded krait and coral snakes.
    ii. *Hydrophidae:* These are water snakes and have flattened tail with which they can swim in the water.
2. **Viperidae:** The word "viper" is derived from Latin word (*vivo* = "live" and *pario* = "give birth"). These are viviparous, have vertically split pupil, big triangular head, small tail and big canalized fangs. They can inject poison even when the bite is through some clothing. These snakes can inject venom as soon as the fangs enter the skin of a victim. They are found all over the world, except in Antarctica, Australia, New Zealand, Hawaii and some isolated islands.
    i. *Pitless vipers (Viperinae):* They do not have a pit between the eye and nostril. Following two varieties cause fatalities in South-East Asia.
        a. Russell's viper (*Daboia russelii*)
        b. Saw scaled viper (*Echis carinatus* or Phoorsa)

ii. Pitted vipers (Crotalinae): Pitted vipers are poisonous. Asian pit vipers are 2 to 5 feet long and are seen throughout Asia. Their bite cause severe tissue damage but rarely results in death.

Main poisonous snakes seen in India can be identified by noting the features unique to each variety.

a. **Cobra:** It is found throughout India. It is about 1.5 to 2 mtrs long with marked hood with a single or double spectacle mark. This mark is not visible in a dead snake. Snake can be identified from large 3rd supralabial shield touching the eye and nasal shield. There is a small shield between 4th and 5th infralabial shields, caudal scales are in double row and there is dark brown or white band after the hood (Fig. 40.1).

b. **King cobra**: Mostly seen in Himalayas, Assam, and forests of South India. They can grow up to 3 to 4 mtrs and the hood does not have the spectacle mark. Caudal scales are in a single row. There are less distinct white or yellow coloured bars on the back of the snake.

c. **Common krait:** Most common poisonous snake of India. They are shinning blue or steel black in colour with narrow white arches across the back. They are usually 1 to 1.5 mtrs long and can be identified from four shields on either side of the lower lip;

hexagonal scales on the back and the caudal scales are in a single row (Fig. 40.2).

d. **Banded krait:** They are from 1.5 to 2 mtrs long and are mainly seen in the northeast India. They can be identified from alternate black and yellow bands across the back (Fig. 40.3).

e. **Russell's viper** (Daboia russelii): They are light brown in colour and may grow up to 1.5 mtrs in length. They are identified from triangular head with a V shaped mark pointing forwards, tail is short, caudal scales are in two rows and the black-brown spots in the third row on the back has white edges (Fig. 40.4).

f. **Saw scaled viper** (Echis carinatus): They are small snakes of about half meter long mostly seen in Rajasthan and Maharashtra. They are brown or brownish grey in colour, There is a bird's footprint or arrow mark

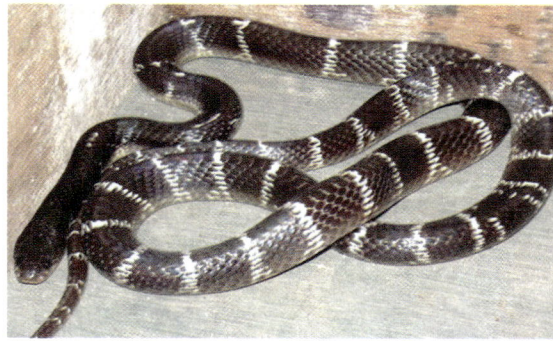

Fig. 40.2: Common krait

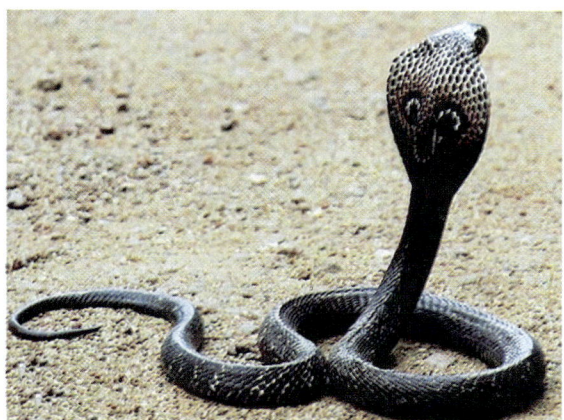

Fig. 40.1: Cobra

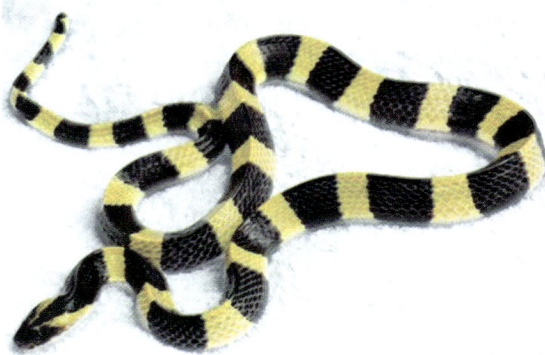

Fig. 40.3: Banded krait

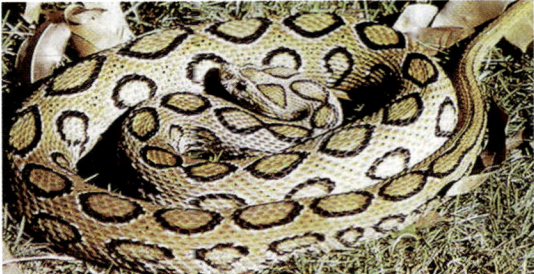

Fig. 40.4: Russell's viper

on the head, edges in the middle of scales are dented and the caudal scales are in a single row. Rough scales produce rustling sound when the snake moves (Fig. 40.5).

How to differentiate between poisonous and nonpoisonous snakes: Whenever a dead snake is brought along with the patient of snake bite, the treating doctor must examine the snake to find out whether the snake is poisonous or not. In case the bite is from a poisonous snake, then finding the variety of snake can help in administering proper treatment.

1. If Belly scales are wide so that they extend right across the width of the belly, the snake may be poisonous. Whereas in nonpoisonous snakes the belly scales are small. (Fig 40.6)
2. If the tail is compressed and flat it is sea snake and poisonous.
3. If the head scales are small with or without a pit it is viper and poisonous. Cobra, Krait and nonpoisonous snakes have large scales on the head.

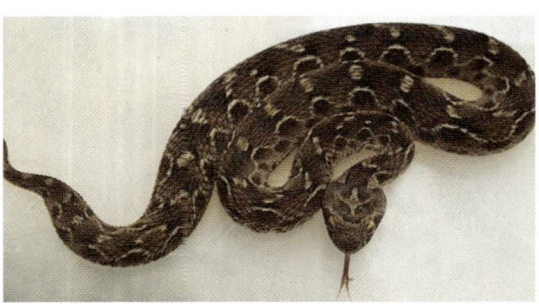

Fig. 40.5: Saw scaled viper

4. Cobra snake has large 3rd supralabial scale touching the eye and nasal scale and a small scale between 4th and 5th infralabial scales.
5. Triangular head and narrow neck is seen in viper snakes which are poisonous.
6. Hexagonal scales in the central row on the back are seen in Krait snakes which are poisonous. (Fig. 40.7)
7. Presence of fangs in poisonous snakes.
8. Compressed short tail is present in viper snakes.
9. Two fang marks are seen in the bite mark of a poisonous snake whereas multiple teeth marks are seen in an arc in non-poisonous snakes.
10. Poisonous snakes are mostly nocturnal in nature.

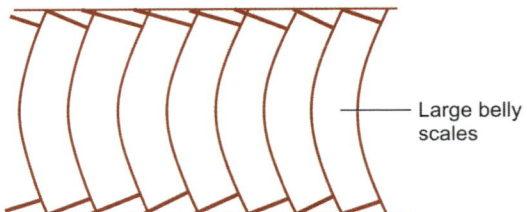

Poisonous or nonpoisonous snakes

— Large belly scales

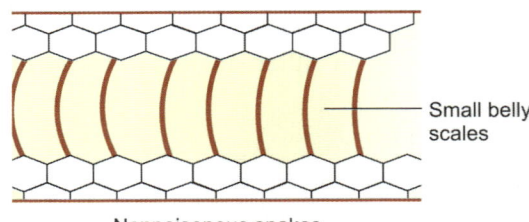

Nonpoisonous snakes

— Small belly scales

Fig. 40.6: Belly scales of snakes

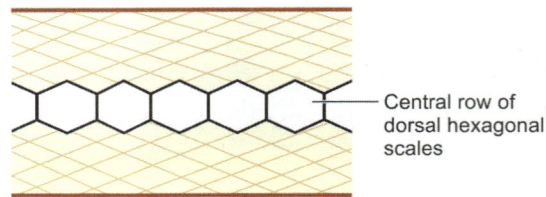

— Central row of dorsal hexagonal scales

Fig. 40.7: Back of Krait snake

Snake Venom

Snake venom is slightly yellowish in colour and is a complex mixture chiefly made up of proteins, many having enzymatic activity from 6000 to 30,000 molecular weight. Peptides present in the venom have specific receptor sites. Snake venom can be classified into three groups.

a. *Neurotoxic:* In this neurological findings are predominantly present, which is mainly seen in Elapidae snakes like Cobra and Krait.

b. *Hemotoxic:* In this predominantly hemolytic findings are present which is seen in Viperidae snakes like vipers.

c. *Myotoxic:* This type of venom causes muscular damage which is seen in Hydrophidae snakes or sea snakes.

Constituents of Snake Venom

i. Proteolytic enzymes like fibrinolysin and proteolysin act on the endothelium and muscles.

ii. Phosphatidases causing hemolysis and affect the heart.

iii. Thromboplastin along with phosphatidases is present in viper venom.

iv. Neurotoxins having curare like paralytic effects.

v. Cholinesterase's and neurotoxins are present predominantly in elapidae snake venom.

vi. Proteases.

vii. Erepsin.

viii. Hyaluronidases.

ix. Cardiotoxins.

x. Ribonucleases and desoxyribonucleases.

xi. Ophio-oxidases help in autolysis.

Features of Snake Bite (Ophitoxaemia)

Features mainly depend upon the type of snake and the amount of the venom injected. Following the immediate pain at the fang marks, which may increase in intensity at the site of the bite, local swelling and inflammation that gradually extends up the bitten limb and painful enlargement of the regional lymph nodes; however, bites by kraits, sea snakes may be virtually painless and may cause negligible local swelling.

a. *Elapidae snakes:* There is burning pain at the site, redness and some swelling. In Krait bite swelling and pain is minimal but abdominal pain and convulsions may be present. Early features include "heavy" eyelids, ptosis and abnormalities of taste and smell followed by other *neurological features* like drowsiness, paresthesia, external ophthalmoplegia, paralysis of facial muscles, difficulty in opening mouth and showing tongue and weakness of other muscles supplied by the cranial nerves, aphonia, difficulty in swallowing secretions, respiratory and generalized flaccid paralysis.

b. *Viperidae:* Local features are predominantly seen like pain, swelling, discolouration and ecchymosis. Then there are nausea, vomiting and *cardiovascular features* like dizziness, faintness, shock, hypotension, cardiac arrhythmias, pulmonary edema and cardiac arrest. Signs of collapse like cold clammy skin, thready pulse and dilated pupils are also observed. Patient may become unconscious in one to two hours. *Bleeding and clotting disorders* are manifested in the form of bleeding from recent wounds and spontaneous systemic bleeding from gums, epistaxis, bleeding into the tears, hemoptysis, hematemesis, rectal bleeding or Melena, hematuria, vaginal bleeding, bleeding into the skin and mucosa, subarachnoid hemorrhage and coma from cerebral hemorrhage. Later on sloughing and gangrene at the site may be observed.

c. *Hydrophidae:* There is little local reaction but after about half an hour stiffness and weakness of the muscles is seen. *Muscle damage* and *renal involvement* is manifested by lower back pain, hematuria, hemoglobinuria, myoglobinuria, oliguria or anuria, symptoms and signs of uremia.

Long-term complications (sequelae) of snake bite: At the site of the bite, loss of tissue may result from sloughing or surgical debridement of necrotic areas or due to amputation. In some cases chronic ulceration, infection, osteomyelitis or arthritis may be present, causing severe physical disability. Malignancy may be seen in rare cases in skin ulcers after a number of years.

Chronic renal failure occurs after bilateral cortical necrosis along with chronic hypopituitarism or diabetes insipidus after Russell's viper. Chronic neurological deficit is seen in the few patients who survive intracranial hemorrhages in Viperidae snake bite.

Factors determining the severity of the symptoms: It is reported that about 50% of Russell viper bites, 30% of cobra bites and 10% saw scaled viper bites do not cause envenomation. The severity of symptoms depends upon the following factors:

   i. *Type of snake:* As mentioned above features and severity depends on the variety of snake.

  ii. *Size of the snake:* Normally the larger snakes tend to inject more venom.

 iii. *Location of the bite:* Bite on the face, trunk and directly into a blood vessel is more dangerous. Bite in fatty tissues or extremities are less severe.

  iv. *Amount of the venom injected:* Amount of venom injected depends on the extent of anger or fear of the snake and conditions of the fangs weather broken or recently renewed.

   v. *Age and size of the victim:* Symptoms are more severe in children and persons suffering from debilitating diseases.

  vi. *Mode of bite:* Glancing bite is less serious than a direct bite. Moreover bite over clothing may give some protection in colubridae snakes as the poison flowing in the groove of the fang is absorbed by clothing.

 vii. First aid and medical treatment administered.

Fatal dose: Toxicity of dried venom of different types of snakes is as follows:
1. Cobra – 12 mg
2. Russell's viper 15 mg
3. Echis – 8 mg
4. Krait – 6 mg

Fatal Period: In Colubridae snakes it is 20 minutes to 6 hours and in Viperidae snakes it may be from 2 to 4 days.

Investigations/Laboratory tests

a. *Twenty minute whole blood clotting test (20 WBCT):* This is a very useful and informative bedside test. Place a few ml of freshly collected venous blood in a small glass vessel. Leave undisturbed for 20 minutes. If the blood is still un-clotted and runs out, the patient has hypofibrinogenemia. This is diagnostic of a viper bite and rules out an elapidae snake bite.

b. *Held breath count:* Patient is made to count while holding breath may indicate respiratory distress.

c. *Hemoglobin concentration:* There is a decrease in hematocrit values reflecting blood loss or, in the case of Russell's viper bite, intravascular hemolysis.

d. *Platelet count:* This may be decreased in victims of viper bites.

e. *White blood cell count:* An early neutrophils leukocytosis is present in systemic envenoming.

f. *Blood film:* Fragmented red cells are seen when there is hemolysis.

g. *Plasma/serum:* It may be pinkish or brownish if there is gross hemoglobinemia or myoglobinemia.

h. *Biochemical abnormalities:* In cases of Russell's viper or sea snake bites creatinine kinase will be elevated provided there is severe local damage or there is generalized muscle damage. Bilirubin is normally elevated following massive extravasation of blood. Creatinine, urea and blood urea nitrogen levels are raised in the renal failure due to Russell's viper, saw-scaled viper or sea snake bites.

i. *Arterial blood gases and pH:* Evidence of respiratory failure or metabolic acidosis may be seen in neurotoxic envenoming by examining pH and blood gases.

j. *Urine examination:* The urine should be tested for blood/hemoglobin/myoglobin. Red cell casts indicate glomerular bleeding. Massive proteinuria is an early sign of the generalized increase in capillary permeability in Russell's viper envenoming.

Treatment

a. Under the national snakebite management protocol, it is now recommended to adopt "Do it RIGHT" approach. Which include reassurance, immobilization as is done for a fractured limb, getting to hospital without delay and telling the symptoms to treating physician so as to facilitate treatment.

b. Most important aspect of treatment is reassurance to the victim as fright and consequent shock may result in fatalities in few cases. Anxiety from a snake bite or even suspected bite may lead to hyperventilation, paresthesia, even tetany, vasovagal reactions, agitation and a wide range of misleading symptoms.

c. First aid treatment includes immobilization of the limb as movement or muscular contraction increases absorption of venom into the bloodstream and lymphatics.

d. Bites by cobras, king cobras, kraits or sea snakes may lead, on rare occasions, to the rapid development of life-threatening respiratory paralysis. This paralysis might be delayed by slowing down the absorption of venom from the site of the bite. Pressure bandage the area by using crepe bandage or any long strips of cloth which is bound firmly around the entire bitten limb, starting distally around the fingers or toes and moving proximally, to include a rigid splint. The bandage is bound that much tight which can block the lymphatic flow but not the circulation of that limb. Pressure bandage should be avoided in viperidae snake bite, as it may lead to local necrosis.

e. Application of tourniquet or cauterization of the local site is not advised. Avoid any interference with the bite wound as this may increase absorption of the venom, introduce infection and increase local bleeding.

f. Arrange to shift the victim to nearby hospital or dispensary for medical treatment. While doing so, try to avoid movement of the affected limb.

g. On arrival, treating doctor must evaluate the patient. In case of respiratory failure, hypotension with shock or cardiac failure suitable resuscitative measures are provided.

h. Severity of envenoming can be made out by observing the signs and symptoms in the patient like spreading swelling, tender lymph nodes draining the area, signs of shock, neurological involvement like ptosis/ophthalmoplegia, bleeding from wounds with incoagulable blood shown by 20 WBCT, dark coloured urine along with nausea and vomiting. Only in such cases Antisnake venom should be administered.

i. *Administration of antisnake venom:* Monovalent antivenom neutralizes the venom of only one species of snake, whereas, polyvalent antivenom neutralizes the venoms of several different species of snakes. ASV is prepared at Haffkine institute Mumbai, central research institute kasauli, serum Institute Pune, King's Institute Chennai and Bengal Chemical and Pharmaceuticals Calcutta. The "polyvalent antisnake venom serum" neutralizes venoms of the four most important venomous snakes in India (Indian cobra, Indian krait, Russell's viper and saw-scaled viper). One ml of polyvalent ASV in India neutralizes 0.6 mg each of Cobra and Russell Viper venom and 0.45 mg each of Krait and saw scaled viper venom. **Antivenom treatment carries a risk of severe adverse reactions;** it should therefore be used only in patients in whom the benefits of antivenom treatment are considered to exceed the risks. Antisnake venom should not be administered under pressure from the relatives, when it is not required or in doses well in excess of the required amount. Skin and conjunctival "hypersensitivity tests" do not predict the large majority of early (anaphylactic) or late (serum sickness type) reactions. **Since these tests may delay treatment and can in themselves be sensitizing the patient, these tests are not recommended.**

j. *Polyvalent Antisnake venom (ASV)* is available as a lyophilized powder. It is reconstituted with 10 ml of distilled water and administered intravenously in a drip or slow injection The recommended initial dose of ASV is 8 to 10 vials administered over one hour which can be repeated after 1 to 2 hours in neurotoxic and after 6 hours in hemotoxic snake bites, if required. The maximum dose for neurotoxic snake bite is 20 vials whereas for hemotoxic snake bites it is 30 vials. It is most effective if given within 4 hours but its use is doubtful after 24 hours. In most of the cases the patients start showing improvement after 30 minutes to few hours.

k. The patient must be observed for initial one hour during administration of ASV for any adverse reaction. At first sign of adverse reaction intramuscularly adrenaline 0.5 mg is given (**must be available before starting ASV infusion**). Only when the patient stabilises the remaining dose of the ASV is administered. Antihistaminic and corticosteroids are also administered to prevent anaphylactic reaction of the ASV.

l. If a person has severe bleeding manifestations despite ASV administration, fresh frozen plasma and platelet concentrates can be given.

m. In viperidae snake bite ASV can be administered subcutaneously around the wound.

n. In cobra bite, patient with respiratory paralysis, neostigmine 0.5 mg preceded by atropine 0.6 mg is also administered. This can be repeated after half hour or more depending upon the response of the patient.

Neostigmine is effective in cobra venom which acts on the postsynaptic neurons. However clear respiratory passage must be maintained.

o. Heparin has no role in DIC caused by snake bite and may increase bleeding tendency.

p. Avoid NSAIDs for pain as it causes more bleeding, along with morphine which causes respiratory depression.

q. In terminal cases peritoneal dialysis can be performed.

r. Supportive treatment includes tetanus prophylaxis, antibiotics, surgical debridement of dead tissues, fasciotomy for intracompartment syndromes, endotracheal intubation and artificial ventilation if required.

Postmortem Findings

Two lacerated puncture mark, 1.2 to 2.5 cm deep in colubridae and viperidae snakes respectively with swelling, ecchymosis and cellulites around the wound.

In colubridae snakes features of respiratory depression like cyanosis, froth from mouth and nostrils and petechial hemorrhages are present. Nerve cells may show opacity and fragmentation of reticulum of the nuclei.

In viperidae snake bite there is marked swelling at the local site with blood oozing out. There are hemorrhages in various tissues. Kidneys are inflamed with interstitial nephritis. Intracerebral hemorrhages and necrosis of liver may be observed.

In the washing from the wound, cholinesterase is detected in colubridae and thromboplastin in viperidae snake bites.

Medicolegal Importance

Snake bites are most common accidental poisoning. Snakes have been used for homicidal purposes in rare cases. Cleopatra is reported to have committed suicide with a snake bite. Animal poisoning from snake venom is done with a banana, which a poisonous snake is made to bite, banana is then smeared on a cloth and inserted into the rectum of the animal.

SCORPION

Scorpions are a member of the Arachnida class and are closely related to spiders and mites. Scorpions have two pincers, 8 legs and an elongated body with a tail composed of segments. They range in length from about 2 to 20 cm. Some species are smaller and translucent. Last tail segment contains a hollow stinger or telson that transmits a toxin to the recipient of a sting. It communicates with venom gland by a connecting duct. Although about 2000 species exist but only about 25-40 species can deliver enough venom to cause serious or lethal damage to humans. Scorpion stings are painful and can be fatal, particularly in children.

Scorpions come in a variety of colours varying from tan to light brown to black. Dark coloured scorpions are more dangerous. Scorpions are found in highest numbers in arid or desert regions. However, they can be found occasionally in cold climates. Scorpions hunt at night and hide along rocks or trees during the days.

Scorpion venom: The cause of the scorpion's sting symptoms is clear and colourless venom that contains a mixture of proteins having neurotoxin, protein inhibitors, hemolysins, agglutinins and other substances.

Features of Scorpion Sting

In general, the sting usually causes discomfort that slowly decreases overtime. The discomfort, described below, usually ranges from moderate to severe.

i. A person who has been stung by a scorpion may feel a painful, tingling, burning or numbing sensation at the sting site. There is a red wheal with a sting hole in the middle. The area gradually becomes swollen and edematous.

ii. There is giddiness and severe headache.

iii. In severe cases, symptoms may include double vision or blurred vision, widespread numbness, salivation, thick-feeling tongue, difficulty in swallowing, muscle cramps and difficulty in breathing. In some cases it may result in death of the person especially in children.

Treatment

In most scorpion stings in adults, except in severe symptoms, treatment is simply supportive and can be done at home.

a. Wash the area with soap and water and remove all constricting jewelry like a ring on a finger that has got a sting, so that circulation is not hampered with swelling in that region.

b. Apply cool compresses, usually for 10 minutes at a time with a gap of 10 minutes, at the site of the sting.

c. Giving a cut and washing with dilute solution of potassium permanganate can be tried but it is not recommended these days.

d. Local anesthetic like 5% lidnocaine can be injected around the sting area to relieve pain.

e. Acetaminophen 1–2 tablets every 4 hours may be given to relieve pain.

f. Intravenous fluids are administered in shock. Calcium gluconate 10% can be added to relieve muscular cramps.

g. Antibiotics are not helpful unless the sting area become infected.

Medicolegal Importance

Contact with scorpions is usually accidental.

SPIDERS

Arachnidism is an injury resulting from the bite of a spider. Almost all spiders are venomous, but most of them are harmless and result in mild symptoms around the area of the bite and can be treated at home. Insect bites are usually misdiagnosed as spider bites and most presumed cases of spider bites are likely due to other conditions that mimic the symptoms of a spider bite.

Worldwide only two spider venoms have serious symptoms in humans; those of the widow spider and recluse spider. The wandering spider in Brazil and the funnel web in

Australia have lethal neurotoxic venom; however, death is rare from these spiders because of limited contact with humans.

Widow spider: This variety is found all over the world. Female is larger and mostly responsible for the bite. They may grow up to 5 cm (leg span). There is red hour glass mark on the back of the body. It is shiny black in colour. Venom is mainly neurotoxic.

Recluse spider: It is smaller than the widow spider and the leg span is up to 2–3 cm. There is a violin shaped mark on the back. It is mostly brown in colour. Venom is mainly necrotizing.

Venom: Spider venoms include various combinations and concentrations of necrotic agents, neurotoxins and serotonin.

Features of Spider Bite

Main characteristic symptom of spider bite is the pain at the site. Pain from nonvenomous, so-called "dry bites" typically lasts for 5 to 60 minutes while pain from venomous spider bites may last for longer than 24 hours. Other features include fever, nausea, vomiting, headache, abdominal pain, joint pain or stiffness, overall feelings of malaise, rash, and muscle cramps.

Widow spider injects neurotoxic venom which produces a condition known as *"latrodectism"*. Symptoms from a bite from the widow spiders may include pain which may be at the bite or involve the chest and abdomen, muscle cramps, vomiting along with activation of the sympathetic nervous system which leads to sweating, high blood pressure and gooseflesh.

Bites from the recluse spiders cause the condition *"loxoscelism"* in which local necrosis of the surrounding skin and widespread breakdown of red blood cells may occur. Headaches, vomiting and a mild fever may also occur.

Treatment

Most spider bites are managed with supportive care.

a. Wash the site of the spider bite well with soap and water.
b. Apply a cool compress or ice pack over the spider bite location.
c. Acetaminophen or ibuprofen for pain. Avoid aspirin in children. Morphine may be used if the pain is severe.
d. Antihistamines for itchiness.
e. Calcium gluconate intravenously for muscle cramps.
f. A tetanus booster shot may be necessary, depending upon the date of the patient's last immunization.
g. Antivenom exists (not available in India) for black widow spider venom, however, administration is associated with anaphylaxis in some cases.

Medicolegal Importance

Spider bites are mostly accidental in nature. This can occur from unintentional contact or trapping of the spider.

INSECT BITE

There are number of insects which can produce a bite in humans. Some of them are wasps, honey bees and ants. Stings and bites from insects are very common. They often result in redness and swelling in the bite area. Sometimes a sting or bite can cause a life-threatening allergic reaction or transmit pathogens to humans.

Most insects do not usually attack humans. Mostly bites and stings are defensive, when insects sting to protect their hives.

Venom: A sting or bite injects venom composed of toxic peptides, dopamine, histamine, neurotoxin, serotonin and other substances that may trigger an allergic reaction in the victim. The sting also causes redness and swelling at the site of the sting.

Mechanism of a sting: Bees, wasps, hornets and fire ants are members of the Hymenoptera family. Bees, wasps, and fire ants differ in how they inflict injury.

a. When a bee stings, it loses the entire barbed stinger as it gets firmly attached to the human skin. Eviscerated bee actually dies in the process.

b. A wasp can inflict multiple stings because it does not lose its injection apparatus after it stings.

c. Fire ants inject their venom by using their mandibles and rotating their bodies.

d. In contrast, bites from mosquitoes are not defensive; mosquitoes are looking to get blood for a meal. Mosquitoes cause mild allergic reactions but can inject pathogenic microorganisms like malaria, encephalitis, dengue, chikungunya and yellow fever.

e. Few other types of blood sucking insects or bugs are also responsible for spreading diseases in humans.

   i. Lice bites can transmit epidemic relapsing fever.

   ii. Sand fly bite may cause leishmaniasis.

   iii. Tsetse flies bite transmits protozoan trypanosomes.

   iv. Lice can spread epidemic typhus rickettsia.

   v. Ticks can transmit tick fever.

   vi. Bed bugs and mites cause localized itchiness and occasional swelling.

Features of Insect Bite

Mostly bites and stings from an insect result in pain, swelling, redness, and itching to the affected area, rarely blisters may be caused. Some cases the bite gets infected and may result in cellulitis. Anaphylactic reaction may be seen when the person is allergic to the bite. It may produce wheezing, shortness of breath, unconsciousness and even death in some cases. Multiple bee stings may cause kidney failure and death. Bites from a fire ant produce a pimple-like sore that is extremely itchy and painful.

Treatment

a. Look for stinger in honeybee bite and try to remove it by scrapping.

b. All insect bites should be treated with antihistamines.

c. Local antiseptic solutions may prevent infections.

d. Cold packs to reduce inflammation.

e. Anaphylactic reaction requires immediate administration of adrenaline in slow infusion and if required assisted ventilation with oxygen.

f. Corticosteroids can also be added in systemic manifestations.

CANTHARIDIN

Cantharidin is present in the powder of the Spanish fly, which may contain up to 5% of Cantharidin. It is highly irritant and is mainly responsible for its blistering properties. The crushed powder is of yellowish brown to brown-olive colour, disagreeable odor and bitter taste. It has been used as one of the world's oldest aphrodisiac. Cantharidin has been also used as nerve tonic, treatment of warts and abortifacient.

Features of poisoning: Powder of Spanish fly can be easily mixed with food and drinks and may go unnoticed. In some historical cases arsenic was also mixed with this for homicidal purposes. Accidental poisoning may result from overdose, as this is commonly used for aphrodisiac purposes.

Symptoms of cantharidin ingestion include burning of the mouth, nausea, hematemesis, dysphagia, bloody diarrhea, priapism in males and renal damage leading to gross hematuria and anuria. Convulsions may precede death.

Treatment

Mainly supportive and symptomatic treatment.

Arthur K Ford a Poisoner for Sex

Ford was infatuated by two female coworkers in a chemical factory during 1954. In order to gain their sexual attention he obtained cantharides. He mixed this poison in coconut candies and offered to three secretaries working in his office. All three ladies were hospitalized and two of them died. Ford confessed to his involvement and was sentenced to 5 years imprisonment.

SOMNIFEROUS GROUP

Various drugs included in the somniferous group include "*Opiates*" (natural or semi-synthetic preparations of alkaloids of poppy plant which bind to the opioid receptors) and "*Opioid*" (Any drug which binds to the opioid receptors in the CNS, hence includes Opiates and synthetic preparations acting on opioid receptors). These drugs primarily induce sleep hence included in the main group of "*Narcotic drugs*".

OPIUM

It is the dried juice of poppy plant (Papaver somniferum). The plant is mainly cultivated in China, India, Turkey, Russia and some other parts of the world. Unripe fruit while on the plant is given superficial incisions and the white juice which exudes out is collected after it dries (Fig. 41.1) Dry capsule contain very little quantity of opium, is used as a sedative drink known as Kasumbi. Poppy seeds (Khas khas) are harmless and are used as additives in food. Poppy seed oil is used for cooking and for lighting purposes.

Opium in fresh state is plastic but becomes hard and brittle after some time. It has characteristic odor. Crude opium contains about 25 alkaloids in combination with muconic, lactic and sulphuric acids. In crude opium morphine content varies from 7 to 14% but in "*standard opium*" the concentration of morphine is fixed at 10% (one such opium factory is located at Ghazipur UP).

Main alkaloids of opium are divided into two groups.

a. *Phenenthrine group:* Main alkaloids in this group are as follows:
   i. Morphine— About 10%
   ii. Codeine— About 0.5%
   iii. Thebaine— About 3% (convulsant)
b. *Isoquinoline group:*
   i. Papaverine— About 1%
   ii. Narcitine— About 6%

Morphine

This alkaloid has been named after "*Morpheus*" the god of dreams. It occurs as white powder

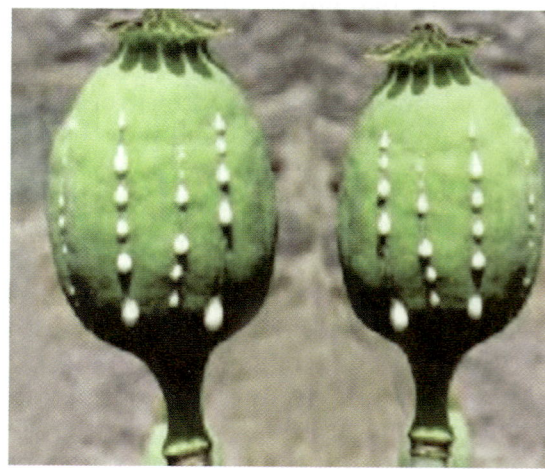

Fig. 41.1: Poppy capsules

or white crystals having bitter taste. Narcotic effect of opium is mainly due to morphine. Preparations for use are morphine hydrochloride and morphine sulphate, which are used in 8 to 20 mg doses.

Mode of Action

Morphine has depressant action on the cerebral cortex, respiratory center and cough reflex center in medulla, but stimulates vagus along with vomiting center and also stimulates spinal cord. Pain is relieved due to depression of cortex and some euphoric effects.

Semisynthetic Derivatives of Morphine

1. Heroin (diacetylmorphine)
2. Dionin
3. Oxymorphone
4. Dehydromorphine and hydromorphine.

Synthetic Derivatives

1. Fentanyl
2. Omnopan
3. Tramadol
4. Methadone
5. Pethidine or mepridine.

Codeine

It is chemically methyl morphine and found as colourless crystals. Codeine phosphate 10 to 60 mg is used in medical practice.

Codeine Poisoning

Poisoning resemble morphine poisoning but is less severe and convulsions are more common.

Thebaine Poisoning

This may result in strychnine like tonic convulsions.

Opium Poisoning

Manifestation of poisoning is mostly seen in acute or chronic form.

Acute Toxicity

Symptoms usually start after about half hour of ingestion but may depend upon route of administration. Symptoms are manifested in three stages:

a. *Stage of excitement or euphoria:* This stage is of very short duration and when higher dose is taken it may be absent. In children convulsions may be observed.
   i. There is sense of well-being
   ii. Restlessness and sometimes hallucinations.
   iii. Freedom from anxiety
   iv. Flushed face
   v. Tachycardia
b. *Stage of stupor:* This stage is characterised by CNS depression and may last from few minutes to few hours.
   i. Headache, nausea and vomiting
   ii. Drowsiness
   iii. Shallow breathing
   iv. Lethargy
   v. Uncontrollable desire to go to sleep
   vi. On examination there is constricted pupils and cyanosis of the lips.
c. *Stage of narcosis or coma:*
   i. The patient passes into deep coma.
   ii. Insensibility to pain.
   iii. Muscles are relaxed.
   iv. Reflexes are depressed or absent.
   v. Secretions are depressed except for perspiration.
   vi. Pupils are pin point constricted.
   vii. Cyanosis.
   viii. Pulse is slow and feeble.
   ix. Respiration is slow and deep.
   x. Smell of opium is present in breath.
   xi. If proper treatment is given, the patient may recover; otherwise death may occur from respiratory failure.
   xii. Some cases unusual symptoms may be observed like vomiting, diarrhea, convulsions, rise in body temperature due to convulsions and muscular rigidity.

Differential Diagnosis

Opium poisoning has to be differentiated from other conditions causing coma.

a. Cerebral stroke from hemorrhage, thrombosis or embolic phenomenon.
b. Head injury.
c. Uremic coma.
d. Diabetic coma.
e. Hepatic coma.
f. Postepileptic coma.
g. Acute alcoholic intoxication.
h. Acute barbiturate poisoning.
i. Carbolic acid poisoning.
j. Hysterical unconsciousness.

Cerebral Hemorrhage

a. This is mostly seen in people above 40 years of age.
b. Symptoms are abrupt with complete unconsciousness.
c. Convulsions are rare but muscular twitching is common.
d. Face is flushed and respiration is laboured.
e. Reflexes are commonly absent.
f. Cheyne-Stokes breathing.
g. When recovering hemiplegia is evident.

Thromboembolism

a. Most of the features are same as seen in cerebral hemorrhage.
b. Convulsions may be present at the onset.
c. Unconsciousness is rapid followed by hemiplegia.
d. Some cases may show murmurs suggestive of endocarditis.
e. Atherosclerotic changes in other vessels may be present.

Epilepsy

a. Insensibility follows convulsions.
b. All age groups may be involved.
c. Cyanosis and froth may be seen at nostrils and mouth.
d. Tongue may be bitten.
e. Pupils are dilated during convulsion phase.
f. Consciousness is gradually regained.

Uremia

a. Urine examination reveals abnormal constituents.

b. Cardiac enlargement is usually present.
c. Edema of the ankles and ascites may be present.
d. In some cases in place of convulsions, delirium may be seen.

Hysterical Coma

a. Person does not injure himself.
b. Convulsions are of mixed variety.
c. Foam may be seen at mouth.
d. Reflexes are normal.

Diabetic Coma

a. Could be due to hyperglycemia with blood sugar exceeding 200 mg% or from hypoglycemia when sugar levels fall below 70 mg%.
b. In hyperglycemia there is flushed skin, acetone small from the mouth, deep respirations and urine examination show high levels of sugar along with acetoacetic acid.
c. In hypoglycemia skin is usually white, no smell of acetone from breath, shallow respiration, profuse perspiration, tremors and confusion like drunkenness.

Head Injury

a. History of injury to head.
b. Conjunctiva show hemorrhage.
c. Bleeding from nose or ears.
d. CSF may escape from ear or nose.
e. Pupils are dilated (except in pontine hemorrhage).

Atropine Poisoning

a. Pupils are dilated and fixed.
b. Muttering or excited delirium.
c. Inarticulate speech and dysphagia.
d. Temperature is raised.

Barbiturate Poisoning

a. Initially there is nausea, vomiting, giddiness, headache, slurred speech and mental confusion.
b. Respiration is shallow.
c. Pupils are dilated in later stages.
d. Barbiturates can be detected in blood.

Alcoholic Intoxication

Features are similar to opium poisoning but characteristic smell of alcohol is detected.

Fatal dose: About 2 gm of opium and 200 mg of morphine.

Fatal period: Death usually takes place between 8 to 12 hours. Chances of recovery are more when the patient survives for more than 24 hours.

Treatment

In suspected opium overdose, check the respiration, skin colour for cyanosis, consciousness level and response to stimuli. In case he does not respond to stimulation immediate medical help is required. Following steps are taken to treat such a case:

i. Stomach wash: First wash is done with warm water then potassium permanganate 1:5000 solution is used. After completing stomach wash leave about 100 ml of the solution in the stomach to neutralize morphine secreted into the stomach. In case potassium permanganate solution is not available tannic acid or strong tea solution can be used. Stomach washes to be done even when morphine is given parenterally.

ii. In early stages keep him awake but do not try to make him walk.

iii. Emetics may fail due to cerebral depression.

iv. Artificial respiration and oxygen inhalation.

v. Purgatives like 30 gm of sodium sulphate with lot of water.

vi. Respiratory stimulants like amphetamines 30 mg intravenously or caffeine 0.5 gm or coramine 2 ml intravenously.

vii. Amiphinazole (Deptazole) 20–40 mg intravenously of intramuscularly.

viii. N-allyl-normorphine (lethidrone or nalorphine) is specific antidote to combat respiratory failure and is given 5 to 10 mg intravenously, which can be repeated after 15 to 30 minutes maximum up to 40 mg in 4 hours, till respiration becomes normal. It antagonizes respiratory depression, sedative and euphoric action of the morphine. Naloxone 0.01 to 0.02 mg/kg body weight can also be given. If nalorphine fails than lavallorphan can be given in 0.3 to 1.2 mg intravenously or subcutaneously every 15 minutes.

ix. For pethidine and methadone the treatment is the same.

Postmortem Findings

Postmortem findings are not characteristic; there are signs of asphyxia like cyanosis, froth at the mouth and nostrils, petechial hemorrhages. Stomach walls are congested and may contain opium lumps with characteristic smell. Lungs are congested and edematous. Other visceral organs are also congested.

Medicolegal Importance

a. Opium is very commonly used as suicidal poison.

b. It was used for killing infants.

c. Rarely used for homicidal purposes.

d. Opium can be detected in organs even after some time of death as it is not destroyed by putrefaction.

e. When potassium permanganate is used for gastric lavage, it is not detected in stomach contents.

Dr Death

Dr Harold Shipman a family physician was responsible for killing at least 215 individuals, mostly women. He used Opiates for his killings. His motive was to have power over others. He was convicted for 15 murders and sentenced for life. He committed suicide by hanging in the prison.

Opium Habit

a. Crude opium is commonly used.

b. Opium is sometimes smoked but in UP and West Bengal a person can be imprisoned for smoking opium.

c. Some places dried capsule of the opium fruit are taken in different form like concoction known is Kasumbi or used as Bhurji or Halwa.

d. Most commonly this is used for aphrodisiac purposes.

e. Addicts can take higher doses up to 10 gm in 24 hours.

Features of Opium Addiction

A person addicted to opium use may show anorexia, nausea, constipation, emaciation, signs of malnutrition, dry skin, pigmentation around mouth lids and cheek, impotence, melancholia or even features of mania. If the addict is deprived of drug he may stoop down to any level to obtain it.

Morphine addiction: Mostly seen in persons when the drug is used to relieve pain and gradually the person get addicted.

Heroin addiction: It is a highly addicting drug. (described under drug dependence).

Treatment

a. Hospitalise such cases.

b. Lecithin 10 gm 3 times a day

c. Glucose intravenously initially then orally.

d. Gradual reduction of drug and replacing it with methadone 100 mg tablet is used for treatment. 2 mg of heroin, 4 mg of morphine and 20 mg of pethidine can be substituted by 1 mg of methadone. These days **Buprenorphine** a semisynthetic preparation of thebain is used in 2 to 6 mg doses in place of methadone.

e. Other symptomatic treatment.

Inebriant poisons are characterised by producing initial excitement and followed by narcosis.

ALCOHOL

Alcohol is one of the important inebriant poisons. Alcohol in Arabic (Al-hok-l) means fine metallic powder. Term alcohol is mainly used for ethyl alcohol or ethanol. It is a transparent volatile liquid with characteristic smell and burning taste. The flovous and color of alcoholic beverages is mainly due to congeners produced during fermentation (higher alcohol and aldehydes). Alcohol is present in various concentrations in alcoholic beverages and laboratory reagents.

Laboratory Reagents

a. Absolute alcohol contains 99.95% of ethyl alcohol
b. Rectified spirit contains 90% of ethyl alcohol.
c. Methylated spirit contains 95% of ethyl alcohol with 5 % methyl alcohol and wood naphtha.

Alcoholic Beverages

1. **Distilled beverages:**
   a. Whisky, gin and brandy contain about 40% of ethyl alcohol.
   b. Vodka and rum contains about 50–60% of ethyl alcohol.

2. **Wines:**
   a. Wines contains 10 to 15% of ethyl alcohol.
   b. Port and sherry contains about 20% of ethyl alcohol.

3. **Fermented beverages:**
   a. Bear and ciders contain 4 to 12% of ethyl alcohol. Some larger bears may have slightly higher concentration.
   b. Champagne contains 10 to 15% of ethyl alcohol.

Depending upon the alcohol concentration beverages are sometimes grouped as mild moderate and hard drinks. In beverages the concentration of alcohol is mentioned as Proof (°) alcohol. The percentage of alcohol in a drink is divided by 0.571 which gives the Proof (°) of that drink e.g. 75° beverages will be having 43% alcohol (w/v).

Absorption

About 20% of alcohol is absorbed from stomach and the remaining 80% from the small intestines.

Factors which influence the rate of absorption:

a. *Empty stomach:* Alcohol if taken over an empty stomach is absorbed faster than when the stomach is full.
b. *Concentration of alcohol in the beverage:* Absorption is quick when the concentration of alcohol in the drink is between 10 to 20%. But in case the concentration is more

than 40% there is delay in absorption due to pyloric spasm and secretion of excessive mucous from the stomach wall as a result of irritation.

c. *Emptying time of stomach:* Fatty foods which delay stomach empting also slow down the absorption.

d. *Spirited liquors are absorbed faster than malted liquors.*

e. *Alcohol taken with large quantities of fluids:* Bears which have lower quantity of alcohol the absorption rate is slow.

f. *Height of a person:* It is observed that in tall persons the absorption is quick due to greater length of the small intestines providing more mucosal surface for absorption.

Distribution

Body tissues take up alcohol in proportion to the water content present. Hence blood and brain tissues have maximum affinity for alcohol, whereas bones and adipose tissues have lower levels of alcohol in them. Hence in ladies, as adipose tissues take up less alcohol, their blood alcohol levels are 20 to 25% more than in males of same weight and with the same quantity of alcohol intake.

Blood alcohol level builds up quickly and the peak levels are reached in half to one hour of ingestion. Plasma contains 20% more alcohol than in RBC's. For blood alcohol estimation, whole blood is utilized.

Metabolism

Most of the alcohol absorbed is oxidized in the body and remaining about 10% is excreted out in urine and breath. Very small quantity is excreted in saliva and sweat. On oxidation 1 gm of alcohol gives 7 calories of energy. About 10% of absorbed alcohol is incorporated in the body as fat, mostly in the form of neutral fats and cholesterol.

Oxidation of alcohol occurs mostly in the liver by the enzyme Alcohol Dehydrogenase (ADH) with coenzyme Nicotinamide Adenine Dinucleotide (NAD).

$$C_2H_5OH + NAD = CH_3CHO + NADH + H$$

Acetaldehyde a toxic substance thus formed is immediately oxidized into acetyl coenzyme A + acetate. Greater part of acetate enters Krebs's cycle and broken down to CO_2 and water, the remaining part is incorporated in the body as lipids. Oxidation of alcohol diminishes the breakdown of carbohydrates and lipids but does not affect the breakdown of proteins.

Presence of higher alcohols, glucose and fructose accelerate the oxidation of alcohol. Oxidation rate of alcohol is approximately 10 ml or 8 gm per hour (0.1 ml/kg/hr).

Excretion

About 10% of alcohol is excreted unchanged in urine, breath, saliva sweat and feces. Out of which majority is excreted out in urine.

Excretion of Alcohol in Urine

Concentration of alcohol is more in urine (1.3 times) than the blood alcohol level. Usually for routine purposes for calculating blood alcohol level from urinary alcohol levels a ratio of 2: 1 or half urinary level can also be used. The formula for calculating blood alcohol levels from urine alcohol level with about 1% error in calculations is as follows:

Concentration of alcohol in blood = 0.6582 × Concentration in urine – 0.608

Erroneous results may be obtained in following situations:

a. If urine is retained for some time, it will give higher values in comparison to the blood alcohol levels present at the time of testing.

b. If there is urine already present in the bladder before excretion of alcohol starts, the urine already present will dilute the alcohol and will give lower blood alcohol levels on calculations.

To avoid such false results two samples of the urine are collected; one before the start of examination of a drunken person and the second at the end of examination.

Excretion in Breath

It has been calculated that amount of alcohol present in 2100 ml of expired air is equal to the amount of alcohol present in 1 ml of blood. However, increase in the ambient temperature may increase the excretion. Various instruments are used for this purpose like *drunkometer, intoximeter, alcometer* and *breathanalyzer.*

Causes of erroneous results in breath analyses:
1. Due to higher concentration of alcohol remaining in mouth
2. Hyperventilation
3. Physical exercise
4. Emesis/regurgitation
5. If working in paint or solvent surrounding.

Excretion in Saliva

Small quantity (3% of blood level) of alcohol is excreted in saliva.

Calculation of Amount of Alcohol Consumed

Amount of alcohol consumed can be calculated from blood alcohol levels by "**Widmark's formula**".

$$A = PCr$$

A = Total amount of alcohol consumed in gm.
P = Weight of the body in kilograms.
C = Blood alcohol in mg/kg.
r = Constant for males 0.6 and for females 0.5.

Features of Alcohol Poisoning

These are manifested in two forms; acute intoxication and chronic alcoholism. Certain properties of alcohol must be kept in mind which may ascertain manifestations.
   i. Alcohol is CNS stimulant but causes selective depression of higher centers in cortex.
   ii. It does not increase mental or physical efficiency rather it impairs skill and thoughts.
   iii. It does not have true aphrodisiac properties. It enhances desire but affect performance.
   iv. It has hypnotic and diaphoretic properties.
   v. It creates a sensation of warmth by increased cutaneous circulation but increases heat loss.
   vi. In small doses it acts as appetizer.
   vii. Bear has diuretic action.

Acute Intoxication

Clinical picture depends upon following factors:
a. Amount of alcohol taken.
b. Rate of absorption.
c. Habituation or addiction.

Clinical signs and symptoms are seen in three phases:
   i. Phase of excitement or excitation.
   ii. Phase of incoordination or depression.
   iii. Phase of coma.

Phase of Excitement or Excitation

This stage is observed when the blood alcohol levels are between 50 and 150 mg percent.
a. Initially there is feeling of well-being with slight excitation.
b. Actions, speech and emotions are less restrained.
c. There is increased self-confidence. The patient is having flushed face with poor concentration and impaired judgment. He is talkative and may disclose certain secrets.
d. Rude behaviour.
e. Gradually there is loss of self-control.
f. O/E there is strong smell of alcohol in breath, pupils are slightly dilated but reacting to light and muscular incoordination in fine movements only. Alcohol gaze nystagmus may be observed.

Phase of Incoordination or Depression

This stage is observed when the blood levels of alcohol is 150 to 300 mg:
a. There is gradual depression of all brain centers.
b. During this stage sense of perception and skilled movements are affected.
c. Inherent desires and emotions take upper hand.
d. Reaction time is lengthened.

e. O/E there is slurred speech, person complaints of nausea and vomiting, face is flushed, pupils are dilated and temperature is subnormal. There is "positional lateral nystagmus" or "**alcohol gaze nystagmus**". Later on the person becomes stuperous but responding to stimuli. Gradually the person passes into the third stage of coma.

Phase of Coma

This stage is seen when the blood alcohol levels are more than 300 mg %:

a. Patient is insensitive.
b. Breathing is stertorous, indicating impending respiratory failure.
c. Pulse is rapid, temperature subnormal.
d. Pupils are slightly constricted but if a stimulus is given like pinching or slapping then the pupils dilate and slowly return to original position. This is known as "**McEwan's**" sign.
e. Mostly patient recovers unless a very large quantity is consumed in short duration.

If coma continues for more than 6 hours then the prognosis is bad but if it continue for more than 12 hours then chances of mortality increases from respiratory failure.

Based on blood alcohol levels, alcohol intoxication can also be divided into seven stages.

i.	10 to 50 mg%	Sober
ii.	50 to 100 mg%	Euphoric
iii.	100 to 150 mg%	Excitement
iv.	150 to 200 mg%	confusion
v.	200 to 300 mg%	Stupor
vi.	300 to 500 mg %	Coma
vii.	> 600 mg%	Death

Fatal dose: About 150 ml of absolute alcohol in a single dose is normally fatal; however, it may depend upon age, habit, duration and dilution.

Fatal period: Mostly deaths occur in 12 to 24 hours.

Alcohol tolerance: A person in habit of taking alcohol daily can consume alcohol in large quantities, however this is an acquired tolerance and may be lost if out of practice.

Acute Intoxication or Drunkenness

Special committee of British medical Association in 1927 defined drunkenness as " That the person concerned was much under the influence of alcohol as to have lost control of his mental and physical faculties to such an extent as to render him unable to execute safely the occupation in which he was engaged at that material time".

Hence, to prove acute intoxication it has to be established; (a) the person is under influence of alcohol; (b) there is loss of mental and physical faculties; (c) which is not safe for him or others; and (d) at that material time.

A person can be under the influence of alcohol but not drunk unless there is diminished skill or judgment required for that occupation.

Treatment

a. Stomach-wash with 5% sodium bicarbonate.
b. 30 ml of liquid paraffin to reduce absorption.
c. Person is kept warm by providing blankets or hot water bottles.
d. B-complex, B_6, 100 mg with fructose 300 gm intravenously in about half hour to increase metabolism of alcohol.
e. Fluids: 1000 ml of normal saline with 10% glucose and 10–15 units of insulin. 50 gm of sodium bicarbonate can also be added in the fluids.
f. Caffeine can be given in case coma deepens.
g. Artificial respiration and oxygen inhalation.
h. Mannitol or hypertonic glucose for cerebral edema.
i. For restlessness mephenesin can be given.
j. If required hemodialysis can be done in severe cases.

Postmortem Findings

These are nonspecific except for the smell of alcohol.

i. Rigor mortis is slightly delayed.

ii. Decomposition is also slightly delayed.

iii. Smell of alcohol on opening the body.

iv. Congestion of stomach.

v. Edema of brain along with congestion of meninges.

vi. Cloudy swelling of visceral organs.

HOW TO EXAMINE A CASE OF ALCOHOL INTOXICATION?

Clinical diagnosis is not an easy task; it depends upon combination of various symptoms and signs. Even though no single sign is diagnostic but smell of alcohol in breath taken together with other signs could help in concluding intoxication.

An individual can react differently to same amount of alcohol under different conditions and same amount of alcohol may show different effects on different persons.

An epileptic or who has received head injury some time back may show excessive reaction to same amount of alcohol. Hence all above factors are to be kept in mind while examining a person for alcoholic intoxication.

Before examining an intoxicated individual, it is desired that any injury or pathological condition which simulate alcoholic intoxication, as mentioned below, must be ruled out.

a. Head injury with intracranial hemorrhage.

b. Metabolic disorders:

i. Hypoglycemia.

ii. Hyperglycemic pre coma.

iii. Uremia.

iv. Hyperthyroidism.

c. Neurological conditions:

i. Intracranial tumors.

ii. Parkinsonism.

iii. Pre and postepileptic phase.

iv. Disseminated sclerosis.

d. Use of some drugs:

i. Antihistaminic.

ii. Morphine

iii. Atropine

e. Certain psychological conditions:

i. Hypomania

ii. GPI

f. High fever.

g. Carbon monoxide poisoning.

Medicolegal Report in a Case of Intoxication

Like any other medicolegal report there are three parts of alcoholic examination report.

Preliminary Information

This part include the basic information obtained from the patient or his relatives like name, age, address, time, date and place of examination, identification marks, consent for examination (section 53 CrPC an accused can be examined with reasonable force, without consent on the request of police officer). It also includes a short history of the relevant events, previous disease history along with quantity consumed and time of ingestion of alcohol.

Examination of an Alcoholic

1. **General behaviour and speech:**

a. Manner in which he is acting or behaving.

b. *State of clothing:* Whether cloths are soiled by vomitus or smelling of alcohol.

c. *Speech:* In alcoholic intoxication speech is thick, slurred or over precise. Earliest sign is slurring due to incoordination of tongue muscles. He can be tested with words like "British Constitution" but tongue twisting phases are avoided.

2. **Self-control:** An intoxicated person loses self-control easily.

3. **Memory and mental alertness:** He can be asked about recent events and solve simple arithmetic calculations.

4. **Writing:** He can be asked to copy few lines from a newspaper or any book and note the time taken, repetition or omission of words, ability to read his own handwriting. Under intoxication difficulty is seen with letter M, N and W. In case a

driving license is available, he can be asked to sign and signatures are compared. Handwriting sample can be taken.

5. **Pulse:** Pulse should be examined at the beginning and at the end of examination. Pulse is full and rapid during intoxication. Blood pressure is also slightly raised.

6. **Temperature:** Surface temperature is usually raised

7. **Skin:** Skin is examined to find whether it is flushed and moist or dry and pale.

8. **Mouth:** Note the smell of alcohol coming from mouth, state of tongue like dry, moist or furred. Presence of hiccups.

9. **Eyes:** Observe whether conjunctiva is congested or not. Pupils are examined as they are dilated in the second stage of intoxication and during this stage incoordination of extrinsic muscles are tested by lateral nystagmus or alcohol gaze nystagmus sign. Pupils are constricted during third stage when McEwan's sign is elicited for intrinsic muscles of eye.

10. **Hearing:** Hearing should be tested for any loss of acuity of hearing.

11. **Gait:** Patient is made to walk across the room and note: (a) manner of walking like staggering or reeling; (b) reaction time to turn and manner of turning; and (c) one leg stand test for balancing.

12. **Stance:** Note whether he can stand without swaying with open eyes.

13. **Reflexes:** Any delayed or sluggish reflexes are noted.

14. **Muscle incoordination:** Muscle incoordination is tested by any of the following tests:
    i. Finger nose test
    ii. Finger to finger test.
    iii. Picking a coin from the floor.

15. Heart, lungs and abdominal examination for detecting any abnormality.

16. **Collection of samples:** Blood and urine samples are collected. No spirit swab to be used. For blood 1/1000 mercuric chloride and 50 mg of sodium fluoride or 30 mg of potassium oxalate is added in 10 ml of blood as preservative in a glass stoppered bottle. Gaschromatography is more specific for medicolegal purpose.

Opinion

Opinion can be expressed in three ways:

i. *Not taken alcohol:* There is no smell of alcohol and the person does not show any feature of intoxication. However blood sample may be collected for analysis.

ii. *Taken alcohol but not under the influence of alcohol:* Presence of smell of alcohol, dilated pupils, normal reflexes and no muscular incoordination.

iii. *Taken alcohol and is under the influence of alcohol:* Smell of alcohol is present, conjunctiva congested, dilated pupils, muscle incoordination, alcohol gaze nystagmus, slurred speech, staggering gait and impaired conscious state.

Postmortem Findings

In suspected deaths from alcohol consumption, postmortem is very important to decide whether alcoholic intoxication is the cause of death or alcohol consumption is indirectly responsible for the death like involvement in an accident or violent behavior resulting in injuries and death.

In deaths due to alcohol there is invariably smell of alcohol emanating from the body or mouth. Signs of jaundice due hepatic damage or cyanosis from respiratory failure may be present. On opening the body stomach may smell of alcohol with signs of gastritis. Liver may show patchy or defuse cirrhosis. Pancreatitis, pneumonia or signs of aspiration may be present. Heart may show cardiomyopathies related to alcohol:

Postmortem Alcohol Estimation

Postmortem alcohol detection is of importance in diagnosing ingestion of alcohol or death from alcohol. However following important considerations must be kept in mind while estimating and interpreting alcohol in the viscera of the deceased:

a. Alcohol diffuses from stomach to the nearby structures which may show higher concentration of alcohol. Hence blood for alcohol estimation should not be drawn from nearby arteries or body cavities.

b. Blood alcohol level at the time of accident can be estimated from subdural hematoma which is not influenced by his survival period. Moreover it is suggestive of ante-mortem levels of alcohol.

c. Putrefaction also generates alcohol. Some studies have reported production of alcohol in body tissues with bacterial action seen in advanced putrefaction, up to 100 mg%, few authors have reported higher alcohol levels even up to 200 mg%.

d. Urine levels of alcohol in comparison to blood alcohol levels may be more helpful, as lower levels in urine indicate absorption phase (within 2 hours of intake). In case there is no alcohol in urine sample but is present in blood or viscera, is suggestive of postmortem production of alcohol.

CHRONIC ALCOHOL INTOXICATION OR ALCOHOLISM

An alcoholic is one whose habit of consuming alcohol on prolonged basis has produced substantial interference with a major area of life like health, socioeconomic status and interpersonal relationship.

Features of Alcoholism

It is characterised by:

i. Loss of appetite.
ii. Nausea, vomiting (indicative of gastritis).
iii. Diarrhea.
iv. Hepatic damage leading to jaundice.
v. Tremors of hand and tongue.
vi. Insomnia.
vii. Loss of memory.
viii. Impaired power of judgment.
ix. Hypoproteinemia.
x. Signs of peripheral neuritis.
xi. Dementia in some cases.

Cage Questionnaire

It is an easy to use questionnaire test for diagnosing problem drinking or alcoholism. These four questions are asked in a clinical setup:

a. *Cutting down alcohol intake:* The patient is asked whether he has ever considered cutting down his alcohol intake.

b. *Annoyance:* Does he feel annoyed when people criticized him for his drinking habit?

c. *Guilty feeling:* Does he patient have any guilty feeling about his alcohol intake?

d. *Eye opener drink:* Does he need a drink in the morning to steady him?

A total score of 2 or more is considered significant to identify alcohol drinking problem.

Alcohol Use Disorder Identification Test (AUDIT) is also a recommended test for diagnosing alcohol drinking problem.

Treatment

1. Individual or group psychotherapy.
2. Drug treatment
   a. *Emetics:* Emetine or apomorphine is used for creating aversion to alcohol.
   b. *Antabuse:* Disulphiram, 0.25 to 0.5 gm in a single daily dose is given. Adverse reaction are seen whenever alcohol is consumed by that individual.
   c. *Citrated calcium carbimide (temposil):* A 50 mg tablet is given daily. Temposil and antabuse does not cause any unpleasant effects on their own but when alcohol is consumed the patient suffers from head-ache, nausea, vomiting, vertigo, sweating and palpitations. These drugs prevent further metabolism of acetaldehyde resulting in above mentioned unpleasant features.
3. *Nutrition:* Person is provided with highly nutritive food.
4. *Socio-therapy:* So that he can be properly adjusted in his family and society, after he recovers.

Medicolegal Implications

1. Mostly persons under acute alcoholic intoxication are brought before a medical man for examination, when he has committed

some offence under any of the following categories:

a. Offences against intoxicating liquor laws.
b. Offences against highway laws.
c. Offences when alcohol is a contributing factor like sexual and aggressive offences.

2. Chronic alcoholism also becomes a medico-legal problem in conditions as alcoholic amnesia, delirium tremens, alcoholic hallucination, Korsakoff's psychosis and alcoholic intolerance.

   a. **Alcoholic amnesia:** It is quite common in alcoholism. During blackout periods behaviour of the individual is quite opposite to normal.

   b. **Delirium tremens:** This may be seen in chronic cases due to:
      i. Temporary excess.
      ii. Withdrawal of alcohol.
      iii. When some injury is sustained like fractures.
      iv. Acute infections occurring in alcoholics.

   The patient present as vigilant, fearful, sweating individual who is screaming for unknown horrors.

Clinical features:

a. Delirium or hallucinations.
b. Tremors.
c. Agitation.
d. Autonomous system stimulation like raised temperature, tachycardia and sweating.

Delirium tremens is considered as mental abnormality.

c. **Korsakoff's syndrome:** It is characterised by following manifestations:
   i. Loss of memory of recent events with confabulation.
   ii. Disorientation in time and place.
   iii. Polyneuritis.

Treatment of Above Conditions

a. Hospitalization.
b. Sodium pentothal intravenously.
c. Fluids with 15 units of insulin, vitamin B_1 and vitamin C.
d. Fructose to enhance breakdown of alcohol.
e. Sodium luminal 300 mg at bedtime.
f. Corticosteroids.

43 | Hypnotic and Sedatives

BARBITURATE POISONING

Barbiturates have depressant action on CNS but in higher doses depresses respiratory center in medulla and causes death by respiratory failure. Barbiturates also cause peripheral vasodilatation by decreasing sympathetic tone, leading to shock and diminished renal functions. They are seen as white powdery state with a faint bitter taste but without any odor. Long acting compounds are used to produce sedation and prevention of convulsions. Short acting barbiturates are used as hypnotics and the very short acting barbiturates are used for surgical anesthesia.

Classification

They are classified depending on their onset and duration of action:

a. *Long acting:* They have duration of action from 8 to 10 hours.
  i. Barbitone (discovered in 1903)
  ii. Phenobarbitone
  iii. Methyl phenobarbitone
  iv. Diallylbarbituric acid
  v. Mephibarbital
b. *Intermediate acting:* Their duration of action is from 4 to 8 hours:
  i. Amylbarbitone
  ii. Butobarbitone
  iii. Pentobarbitone and pentobarbitone sodium

iv. Probarbital
  v. Allobarbitone
c. *Short acting:* Having duration of action from 3 to 6 hours:
  i. Cyclobarbital
  ii. Hexabarbotone
  iii. Amobarbital
  iv. Sacrobarbital
d. *Ultra short acting barbiturates:*
  i. Pentothal sodium
  ii. Hexabarbitone sodium
  iii. Kemithal sodium.

Absorption, Distribution and Elimination

These drugs are rapidly absorbed from the GIT including rectum. Initially they concentrate for a short time in liver and then evenly distribute in the body fluids. They are partially inactivated in liver and excreted in urine.

Alkalization of urine increases the rate of excretion of barbiturates. It is given with caution in alcoholics and in persons with liver and kidney failure. Preferably it should not be given for at least 5 hours after anticoagulant drugs as barbiturates can cause tissue anoxia of extracellular type and also partially inhibit cytochrome enzyme system.

Features of Acute Poisoning

In therapeutic doses they produce quite normal sleep without any ill effects. Acute poisoning occurs when a large dose is taken at one time or small doses taken in short duration. Severe toxicity is caused when 15 to 20 times the hypnotic dose is taken which may prove fatal.

Features of acute poisoning mainly depend on following:

a. Type and amount of drug taken as short acting require small amount to produce unconsciousness.
b. Age of the person.
c. Route of administration.

Alcohol and barbiturates have synergistic action and sublethal dose in combination may prove fatal. Barbiturate overdose with other central nervous system depressants, such as opiates or benzodiazepines, is dangerous due to additive CNS and respiratory depressant effects.

Clinically acute barbiturate poisoning can be graded according to the severity of symptoms:

  a. Mild toxicity
  b. Moderate toxicity
  c. Severe toxicity

Mild Toxicity

a. This can be seen with slightly more than the therapeutic doses.
b. Patient is drowsy or sleepy and can be aroused by calling his name or shaking him.
c. Impaired judgment and disorientation.
d. Breathing, pulse and blood pressure are normal.
e. Drunken gait.
f. Speech is slurred.
g. Nystagmus may be present.
h. Incoordination in muscle movements.

Moderate Toxicity

a. This stage is observed when 5 to 10 times the therapeutic dose is consumed.
b. Patient is in deep sleep, can be aroused with difficulty but again goes to sleep.
c. Higher mental functions are depressed.

d. Breathing is slow.
e. There may be slight rise in blood pressure and pulse rate in some cases.
f. Depressed deep reflexes.
g. Corneal reflex is usually retained.

Severe Toxicity

a. This stage is seen when 15 to 20 times the therapeutic dose is taken.
b. Patient is in deep coma and cannot be aroused.
c. Higher mental functions cannot be assessed as patient is in deep coma.
d. Breathing is laboured, slow (3–4 per minute) and shallow.
e. Fast and thready pulse.
f. Low blood pressure and subnormal temperature.
g. Deep reflexes are depressed or absent, pupillary and corneal reflexes are lost.
h. Planters are extensors.
i. Patient may have pulmonary edema.
j. Cyanosis is usually present.
k. As narcosis deepens, cyanosis also increases with congestion of the face. Pupils are slightly dilated or normal in size. There may be spasm of muscles or tremors. Patient may develop bronchopneumonia as a consequence to deep coma. Anoxic blebs may be seen on pressure areas. Urine is suppressed or scanty and may contain sugar, albumin and hematoporphyrin. Jaundice may be seen in very severe cases.
l. Blood levels of barbiturates normally seen in comatosed patients:
  a. Short acting barbiturates it is normally > 2 to 3 mg%.
  b. Medium acting barbiturates it is normally > 4 to 6 mg%.
  c. Long acting barbiturates it is normally > 9 to 10 mg%.

Cause of Death

Deaths are mostly due to respiratory failure or ventricular fibrillation. Bronchopneumonia, anoxia from pulmonary edema may also contribute or result in death.

Diagnosis

1. Mainly from history and symptoms.
2. Estimation of barbiturates in blood and urine.
3. Characteristic pattern in ECG and arrhythmias.

Fatal Dose:

1. Barbitone   4–7 gm
2. Luminal   2–3 gm
3. Amytal, seconal, nembutal 1.5–2 gm

Fatal period: About 24 to 48 hours.

BARBITURATE AUTOMATISM

It is a state of mind in which a person who has taken a therapeutic dose, due to mental confusion does not remember that he has already taken the drug and goes on taking further doses and may die from overdose. However, some believe that this automatism is a myth and this hypothesis was propagated to safe guard the reputation of that person who has committed suicide.

Treatment

Management strategies generally fall into 3 major areas: supportive care, decontamination, and enhancement of elimination.

a. Ensure adequate airway, breathing, and circulation.
b. Aggressively initiate fluid therapy if the patient has a low blood pressure or appears to be in hypovolemic shock.
c. Gastric lavage with warm water and then with potassium permanganate, activated charcoal or tannic acid.
d. A single dose of 1 gm/kg activated charcoal may be given within an hour of overdose
e. Manganese sulphate for purgative action.
f. *Analeptics:* CNS stimulants have a very limited role; as under their influence, true clinical assessment becomes impossible. Also, they are associated with side effects like convulsions, cardiac arrhythmias vomiting and hyperpyrexia.

g. Alkalization of the urine with sodium bicarbonate along with forced diuresis. Since barbiturates are weak acids, enhanced renal elimination occurs through alkalization of the urine.
h. *Forced diuresis:* Normal saline and 5% glucose about 2500 to 3000 ml per day, to increase urinary output.
i. Artificial respiration with oxygen and 5% CO_2.
j. Patient should be kept warm.
k. Raise the foot end of the bed and remove mucous from the throat by aspiration.
l. Enema can be tried for bowel wash.
m. In cases of shock noradrenaline 2 mg in 5% glucose drip.
n. Dialysis preferably hemodialysis in long acting barbiturate poisoning. If facilities are not available peritoneal dialysis can be tried.
o. Exchange transfusion.
p. Antibiotic to prevent pneumonia.

Postmortem Findings

1. Externally main findings are those of asphyxia like cyanosis, petechial hemorrhages, anoxic bulla especially on the pressure areas.
2. Internal findings include:
   a. White particles may be seen in the stomach with congestion of the stomach wall.
   b. Lungs are congested and edematous.
   c. In some cases pneumonic consolidation may be present.
   d. Petechial hemorrhages over lung and heart surface.
   e. Kidneys show degenerative changes of the tubules.
   f. Brain is edematous with softening of globus pallidus and small hemorrhages in the white matter.

Chronic Barbiturate Poisoning

It normally occurs due to long time consumption of barbiturates. Mostly it is seen in persons having easy access to barbiturates like nurses and doctors or sometimes in patients prescribed with barbiturates who continue to take them even after the requirement is over.

Features of Chronic Poisoning

a. Slurred speech
b. Nystagmus
c. Vertigo
d. Ataxia
e. Hypotonia
f. Tremors
g. Diplopia
h. Diminished reflexes
i. Poor memory
j. Suicidal tendency
k. Acute toxic psychosis manifested as confusion, hallucination and disorientation.

Treatment

1. Hospitalize the case of chronic barbiturate poisoning for evaluation.
2. Stabilize him by giving short acting barbiturates, e.g. sodium seconal 200 to 300 mg every six hours. After a week reduce the dose by 100 mg daily till the dose becomes half of the original daily dose. Continue the same for 4 days and again start reducing the dose by 100 mg daily till it is one-fourth of the original dose. Continue the same for 4 days and then again reduce the dose by 100 mg daily till the drug is completely withdrawn.
3. Supportive measures including psychotherapy.
4. Rehabilitation is required to prevent relapses.

Delirium is normally referred to altered consciousness, disorientation, and hallucination. Some of the following plants have anticholinergic alkaloids, which are responsible for deliriant action on ingestion:

a. Datura (thorn apple)
b. Atropa belladonna
c. Cannabis

DATURA (Thorn Apple)

Datura grows wildly all over India. All parts of the plant are poisonous; especially the fruits and seeds have higher concentration of alkaloids. Fruits are spherical having spines also known as thorn apple (Fig. 44.1) and contain about 450 to 500 yellowish brown kidney shaped seeds. Weight of 100 seeds is equal to 1 gm. Alkaloids present in datura are hyoscine (scopolamine), hyoscyamine and traces of atropine.

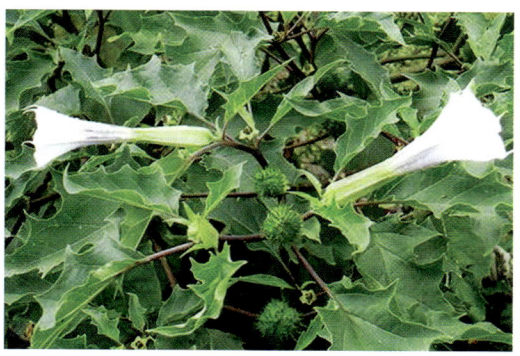

Fig. 44.1: Datura plant

Common species found in India are datura fastuosa, datura atox and datura metel. There are two varieties of the datura fastuosa:

a. Datura alba having white flowers
b. Datura niger having deep purple flowers.

Mechanism of Action

Alkaloids present in datura block the acetylcholine receptors and produces sympathomimetic or parasympatholytic action.

Main action is on CNS. Active ingredients initially cause stimulation of the higher centers and motor system with excitement and followed by depression, delirium and paralysis of the vital centers of medulla. Inhibitory fibers of vagus becomes paralyzed. Respiratory system is stimulated followed by depression. Heart rate is increased.

Features of Poisoning

Contact with datura causes dermatitis. In case seeds are taken, signs and symptoms appear in about half hour but in case decoction of seeds is taken they appear in few minutes. Signs and symptoms are described by a phrase *"Hot as a hare, blind as a bat, dry as a bone, red as a beat and mad as a wet hen"*.

Most of the features start with letter "d"; however some authors categorize them under 9 Ds as marked below:

a. There is bitter taste, dryness of mouth and throat[1] and thirst.

b. Dysarthria[2] and dysphagia[3].

c. Burning pain in stomach along with vomiting.

d. Voice become hoarse and difficulty in talking.

e. Face is flushed, dilatation of cutaneous vessels[4].

f. Pupils are dilated; conjunctiva is congested and patient complaints of diplopia[5].

g. Patient is confused; there is giddiness and staggering/drunken gate[6].

h. Skin is dry and hot[7].

i. Pulse is fast (120–140/minute) full and bounding but later on becomes thready and weak.

j. Respiratory rate is also increased.

k. Body temperature is raised.

l. Muscle tone and reflexes are increased.

m. There may be muscular spasm.

n. Patient is restless, talkative, excited, noisy and may run away from bed. Delirium[8] is there and patient is seen to pull imaginary threads from fingertips or may thread imaginary needle.

o. Hallucinations of sight or hearing may be present.

p. Gradually as the level of intoxication increases, the excitement phase passes off and patient becomes drowsy[9] and gradually sinks into deep coma.

q. Death if it occurs, take place from respiratory paralysis.

Fatal dose: 80 to 100 seeds or about one gram of crushed seeds.

Fatal period: About 24 hours.

Treatment

After assessing the patient the treatment is done on following lines:

i. *Emetics:* Apomorphine does not act, as there is depression of vomiting center.

ii. *Stomach wash:* Normally done with potassium permanganate solution or 5% tannic acid.

iii. *Purgative:* Sorbitol or sodium sulphate by mouth.

iv. *Enema:* Can help in removing the seeds from large intestine.

v. *Physostigmine:* It is administered in 1–2 mg slow intravenously or intramuscularly every 1 to 2 hours and is more effective than pilocarpine, as it crosses blood–brain barrier.

vi. *Prostigmine:* About 0.5 to 1 mg is given subcutaneously.

vii. *Pilocarpine nitrate:* It can be administered in 6 to 15 mg doses subcutaneously repeated every 2 hours but does not counter the CNS effects of datura.

viii. Short acting barbiturates or chloral hydrate for delirium.

ix. Artificial respiration along with oxygen.

x. Morphine is contraindicated.

Postmortem Features

a. *External features:* There may be signs of asphyxia like cyanosis and rarely froth at mouth and nostrils.

b. *Internal features:* Seeds may be detected in stomach and should be differentiated from capsicum seeds by examining the embryo. Seeds normally resist putrefaction and may be seen in decomposed bodies. Stomach is congested, subendocardial petechial hemorrhages and other visceral organs may be congested.

Medicolegal Importance

a. Datura seeds are mainly used as stupefying agent to facilitate robbery, rape or kidnapping. It is normally given as "Prasad" or mixed with foodstuff or tea or coffee.

b. Not used for suicidal purposes; however, accidental poisoning may take place especially in small children.

c. Poisoning may result when used as abortifacient.

d. Seeds have been used for aphrodisiac purposes.

e. Sometimes the seeds are smoked with tobacco or ganja.

f. Rarely used as love filter.

g. Sometimes it is mixed with alcohol to enhance its effects (Kick).

Dr Crippen the mild Mannered Murderer

Dr Crippen was a small statured man having affair with his secretary. One day his wife Cora disappeared and the secretary moved into Dr Crippens house which aroused suspicion. He was interrogated by the Scotland Yard. During interrogations he initially informed the police that his wife has gone to America and died. Later on he said that his wife has gone with another man. When he left for Canada with disguised secretary, his house was searched and remains of his wife were discovered. Hyoscine was found in the tissues, may be the first case of use of this alkaloid as homicidal poison. Dr Crippen was apprehended while disembarking at Canada port. He was tried, found guilty and was hanged on 23rd November 1910. His statue is on display in Madam Tussaud's Museum.

ATROPA BELLADONNA

It is a small shrub having spiny leaves, purple flowers and berries. It is also known by different names like deadly nightshade, devil's herb, love apple and witches berry. Belladonna literally means beautiful lady as it was used to dilate the pupils to enhance beauty. Main active alkaloids present are hyoscine, hyoscyamine and traces of atropine. All parts of the plant are poisonous. Although the root is having the highest concentration of the alkaloids but most of the accidental cases are from eating nice looking berries (Fig. 44.2).

Features of Poisoning

Features are similar to datura poisoning. Features of poisoning are slow to develop but last for few days. There is dryness of the mouth, difficulty in speaking and eating, blurred vision, tachycardia, drowsiness, confusion, disorientation, hallucinations, delirium convulsions, coma and death.

Fatal dose: Uncertain

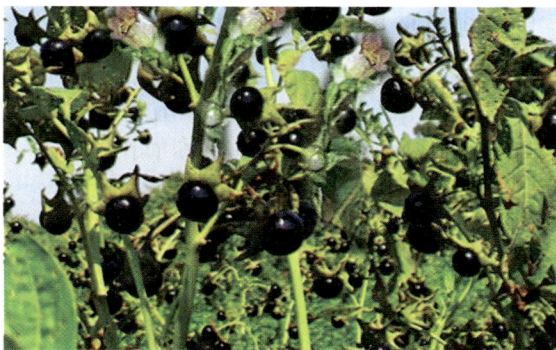

Fig. 44.2: Atropa belladona

Postmortem Findings

Signs of asphyxia and congested internal organs are present.

Treatment

It is also done on the similar lines as done in datura poisoning.

Medicolegal Importance

Mostly poisoning is accidental in nature, suicides and homicides are rare. Poisoning may occur from the eyedrops in case they are swallowed.

CANNABIS (Indian Hemp)

Cannabis is a flowering plant which grows wildly in central Asia and Indian subcontinent (Fig. 44.3). There are three main varieties of

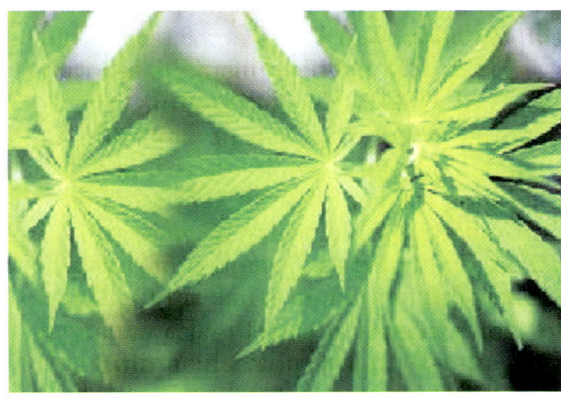

Fig. 44.3: Cannabis leaves

the plant known as Cannabis sativa, Cannabis Indica and Cannabis ruderalis. Sativa plant is a taller variety growing up to 4 to 6 mtrs and primarily used as source of fiber and is seen in many tropical and humid parts of the world. Cannabis indica is of medium height seen in Indian subcontinent whereas Cannabis ruderalis is a small variety. The term hemp is used for soft fibers obtained from plant stem.

This plant has separate sexes with staminate in male plant and pistillate in female plants. Cannabis plant produces many cannabinoids out of which two are present in significant quantities which are Δ-tetrahydrocannabinol (THC) and cannabidiol. Main active psycho-active component is Δ-tetrahydrocannabinol. Cannabidiol has mild stimulant action and may control features of anxiety present on consumption of THC.

Cannabis was used as analgesic, anti-convulsant, and for the treatment of anorexia and even asthma. It has been banned all over the world. However, THC is being tried these days for treating nausea and vomiting following chemotherapy in terminally ill cases of malignancy.

Cannabis use has been mentioned in earlier Hindu scriptures and referred as *"Food for Gods"*. Consumption of cannabis as a ritual is routinely observed during Holi festival in India.

Preparations of Cannabis

a. *Bhang:* Preparation made from dried leaves and taken orally mixed with milk.
b. *Majun:* Sweet preparation made from the leaves.
c. *Ganja:* Made from flowering tops of the female plant.
d. *Marijuana:* Dried flower buds mainly used for smoking, contain 1–2% of THC.
e. *Hashish (Charas):* Resin obtained from flowering top of female plant and contains about 10 to 20% THC. Usually found in the form of brown or black cake of resinous material.

f. *Hashish oil:* Various extracts, colourless to brown or black from cannabis plant are collectively known as Hashish oil mostly smoked with tobacco.
g. *Sinsemilla:* It a preparation of flowering tops without seeds.

Most of the times cannabis is smoked mixed with tobacco in a cigarette. Cannabis is frequently mixed with other drugs of abuse.

Features of Intoxication

When smoked, symptoms appear within few minutes and last from 30 minutes to one hour but on ingestion it may take half an hour to appear but may last from 12 to 24 hours.

1. With mild to moderate dose, following features are seen:
   a. Excitement
   b. Euphoria
   c. Talkativeness
   d. Disorientation
   e. Incoordination
   f. Giddiness
   g. Ataxia
   h. Tachycardia
   i. Congested eyes, blurred vision and constricted pupils
   j. Increased appetite and thirst
   k. The person may laugh uncontrollably.
2. Higher doses may also lead to confusion, delusions and hallucinations.

Gradually person passes into deep sleep and recovers fully on waking up.

Fatal dose: Bhang; it is 10 gm/kg body weight, charas; it is 2 gm and ganja; about 8 gm is fatal. However death from use of cannabis is extremely rare.

Fatal period: About 12 hours.

Treatment

a. Gastric lavage with warm water or emesis.
b. Activated charcoal.
c. Haloperidol for psychotic manifestations. Diazepam is given to control aggression.
d. Psychotherapy.

Postmortem Findings

Nonspecific except in some cases signs of asphyxia may be present.

Chronic Intoxication

Prolonged use may lead to tolerance, the person becomes lethargic, disoriented, confused, frustrated and sometime commits homicide or suicide. The term used for such behaviour is "**Running Amok**", when a person goes berserk, behave uncontrollably and disruptively. Such an individual may kill a person with real or imaginary enmity then killing any other person in his way. He may surrender to the law enforcing agency or commit suicide. A person suffering from this condition is not considered mentally normal and is not punished for his crimes.

Cannabis withdrawal symptoms are mild and normally a person may manifest anorexia, irritability and insomnia and are not life-threatening.

45 | Hallucinogens

These are drugs which produce alteration of sensory perception, mood and thought patterns in normal or small doses and include LSD, phencyclidine, cannabis, peyote and certain mushrooms. These drugs are primarily consumed for their psychedelic effects. There are few other drugs which also produce hallucinations in high doses but are not grouped under hallucinogenic drugs.

LYSERGIC ACID DIETHYLAMIDE (LSD)

Lysergic acid diethylamide (LSD) is one of the most potent psychedelic drugs. It is almost 3000 times potent than mescaline. This drug was first synthesized by Albert Hofmann in 1938 from ergotamine. In pure form it is colourless, odorless and tasteless. A small oral dose of 20 to 30 micrograms is capable of producing psychedelic effects. Other names of LSD are *"acid"* and *"blotters"*.

Route of Administration

In majority of cases it is either taken orally or sublingually. It is absorbed on sugar cube, blotting paper or gelatin for oral use. In liquid form it can be administered parenterally. Even when it is injected the onset is not quick as seen in other drugs of abuse. The effect of the drug may last from 6 to 12 hours depending on the dose consumed, tolerance level and body weight.

Features of Acute Intoxication

a. Somatic manifestations include nausea, dilated pupils, hypertension, tachycardia, flushing, sweating, loss of appetite, drowsiness, paresthesia, pyrexia, piloerection, tremors and ataxia.

However a large dose may lead to respiratory arrest, cardiac arrhythmias or intracranial hemorrhage. Rarely patient may be comatosed.

b. Psychedelic effects include sensory experience after about half an hour of ingestion. There are visual hallucinations, (animated objects or moving geometrical patterns of colours) and auditory hallucinations. A person may have enhanced spiritual experience or *"out of the body"* experience.

c. Adverse effects may include panic attacks of extreme anxiety known as "bad trip" or suffer from "Flash backs" where he experience recurrence of the LSD's subjective experiences long after the drug has been discontinued. *"Hallucinogen persisting perception disorder"* (HPPD) may be seen in some cases where the visual perception are persistent and leads to constant distress. There are few reported cases of psychosis after prolonged use.

Tolerance

LSD tolerance may be seen with prolonged use. Cross tolerance has been observed between various psychedelic drugs like LSD, mescaline and psilocybin.

Diagnosis

Diagnosis is primarily made from the available history and physical examination along with laboratory analysis by radioimmunoassay techniques, high performance liquid chromatography or gas chromatography.

Treatment

a. Reassure the patient in stress free environment.
b. Gastric lavage or emesis is not required as it is rapidly absorbed. It may be done within 30 minutes in case a massive dose is taken.
c. In agitated patients benzodiazepines or haloperidol can be administered.
d. Respiratory support and endotracheal intubation may be required in case large dose is ingested.
e. Other complications like tachycardia or hyperthermia should be symptomatically treated.
f. Psychotherapy.

Postmortem Features

Postmortem findings are nonspecific.

Medicolegal Importance

LSD was very commonly used as recreational drug during sixties and early seventies in western countries. Homicides are rare; however suicidal deaths or accidental deaths have been encountered in LSD addicts. LSD use is rarely seen in India.

PHENCYCLIDINE (PCP)

Phencyclidine was originally developed for use as anesthetic agent in 1950 but the use was discontinued in 1965 because of post-anesthetic delirium and extreme agitation. It is a white crystalline powder or clear yellow liquid. During late seventies it became a popular street drug sold under various names like *angel dust, peace pill, super kool, crystal joint, rocket fuel, super grass, tic tac and wack,* etc.

It is normally snorted, smoked as a joint, sprinkled over a cigarette, ingested or taken intravenously. It mainly acts on CNS causing both stimulation and depression. It has sympathomimetic, anticholinergic and cholinergic actions along with action on nicotinic and opioid receptors. It also has effect on the action of dopamine.

Features of Poisoning

Signs and symptoms start appearing within few minutes and may last up to several hours. Fluctuating symptoms are observed, as PCP is fat soluble and release from fat stores is erratic.

a. Somatic manifestations include nystagmus especially rotator type, miosis, hypertension, tachycardia, violent actions and ataxia.

When a high dose is taken there is catatonia, seizures, dystonia, myocardial infarction and coma without respiratory failure. Death is mostly from hypertensive crisis, renal failure or rhabdomyolysis.

b. Psychedelic effects include euphoria, agitation, amnesia, disorientation, distorted sensory perception and bizarre or violent behaviour.

Diagnosis is primarily made from the available history and physical examination along with laboratory analysis by radioimmunoassay techniques.

Fatal dose: About 20 mg or above may result in coma and death.

Treatment

a. Evaluate and stabilize the patient's airway, breathing, and circulation (ABCs).
b. Physical restrain if agitated or having seizures, administer benzodiazepines.
c. Place patient in dark quite room.
d. Hydrate the patient to increase urinary output.

e. Activated charcoal under proper supervision is helpful especially when a large dose in ingested.
f. Haloperidol, if prominent psychotic symptoms are present.
g. Symptomatic treatment for hypertension and hyperthermia.

Postmortem Features

These are nonspecific.

Medicolegal Importance

It is rarely used in India as drug of abuse. A structurally related anesthetic drug *Ketamine* is used as date rape drug.

46 | Cardiac Poisons

Cardiac poisons include various plants having cardiac glycosides or alkaloids having main action on the heart along with other actions. Digitalis was prescribed for the treatment of heart failure during the last few decades of eighteenth century. There are number of plants having cardiotoxicity; important cardiac poisons are mentioned below:

i. Digitalis
ii. Aconite
iii. Nicotine
iv. Quinine

DIGITALIS

It is flowering shrub with tubular flowers which are white, pink or yellow in colour from the family scrophulariaceae. There are about twenty species out of which most common is digitalis purpurea, also known as foxglove as the flower fits over a finger (Fig. 46.1). This plant is native to central Asia, southwestern Europe, Australia and some parts of Africa. The entire plant is toxic including roots and seeds.

Active principles are glycosides like digoxin, digitoxin and gitoxin. Digitalis glycosides were used to increase the cardiac contractibility and improve the function of the failing heart. It is also used these days as antiarrhythmic agent. Digitalis works by inhibiting sodium-potassium ATPase. This leads to an increase in calcium concentration in cellular cytoplasm, which improves cardiac contractility.

Features of Poisoning

a. There is nausea, vomiting, salivation, headache and diarrhea initially.
b. Dilated pupils, blurred vision or yellow vision (Xanthopsia) and blue halos around the source of light.
c. Loss of appetite.
d. Abnormal heart rate and cardiac arrhythmias.
e. Weakness, wild hallucinations, tremors, seizures, collapse and death.

Diagnosis is made from the available history and laboratory analysis by radio-immunoassay techniques.

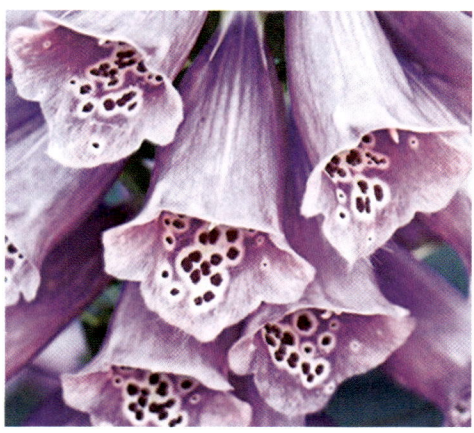

Fig. 46.1: Digitalis flowers

Treatment

a. Evaluate and stabilize the patient's airway, breathing, and circulation (ABCs). Especially close monitoring of cardiac functions.
b. Active charcoal can be used for decontamination, preferably within one hour of ingestion.
c. For ventricular fibrillation lidocaine is more commonly used.

Fatal dose: About 2 gm of digitalis, 4 mg of digitoxin and 15 mg of digoxin.

Postmortem Features

They are nonspecific.

Medicolegal Importance

Mostly the poisoning is accidental in nature like drinking water from a vase having digitalis plant. Homicides are rare.

ACONITE

Aconite is a plant having blue or white flowers with prominent upper hood hence given the name *"Monk's hood"*. This plant is also known by many other names like *wolf's bane, mouse bane, Devil's helmet, mithazahar, bish, queen of all poisons or blue rocket,* etc. There are more than 250 species of plants belonging to the family Ranunculaceae. Some of these species like Aconitum ferox, Aconitum luridum and Aconitum balfourii are found in the Himalayan region of India. It is used as arrow poison in Ladakh, Nepal and some other parts of the world.

All parts of the plant are toxic, but root is the most toxic part of the plant having resemblance to horse-radish root. Dry roots are dark brown, conical, shriveled having longitudinal folds or wrinkles and bitter sweet to taste (Fig. 46.2).

Aconite root has been traditionally used in chinese, ayurvedic, homeopathic, greek and roman medicines for neurological and cardiac problems.

Main alkaloids present in aconite plant are aconitine, mesaconitine, hypaconitine, jesaconitine, pseudaconitine and many others. Pure aconitine is seen as rhombic white crystals.

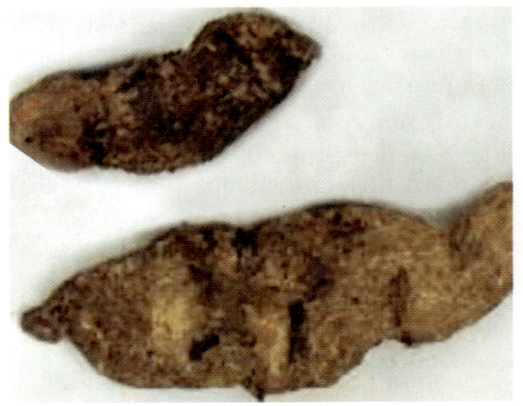

Fig. 46.2: Aconite root

Mechanism of Action

Aconite alkaloids have cardiotoxic and neurotoxic properties. These alkaloids affect the voltage sensitive sodium channels of the cell membranes. Through hypothalamus these alkaloids also produce hypotension and bradycardia. They also release acetylcholine resulting in strong contractions of ileum. However they do not affect higher centers of the brain controlling consciousness.

Features of Poisoning

Symptoms appear early after the ingestion of aconite root:

a. Initial features are nausea, vomiting and salivation.
b. These are followed by neurological features like tingling sensation and numbness of mouth, face and throat, giddiness, vertigo, headache and restlessness. In case large dose is ingested the tingling sensation may spread to limbs.
c. There is burning sensation in the abdomen.
d. Cardiovascular features include hypotension, sinus bradycardia and ventricular arrhythmias.
e. Hypothermia and difficulty in breathing may be encountered.
f. Muscular weakness, twitching of muscles or muscular spasms.
g. Impaired vision with alternate contraction and dilatation of pupils **(Hippus sign)**.

h. The main causes of death are ventricular arrhythmias, systole or paralysis of the respiratory centre.

Fatal dose: About 1 to 2 gm of root or 2 to 5 mg of pure aconitine.

Fatal period: Death normally occurs in 2 to 6 hours. It may be immediate if a large dose is taken.

Treatment

a. Evaluate and stabilize the patient's airway, breathing, and circulation (ABCs). Especially close monitoring of cardiac functions.
b. Active charcoal can be used for decontamination, preferably within one hour of ingestion.
c. Rest of the treatment is mainly supportive. Atropine is used for bradycardia induced hypotension. Lignocaine for ventricular arrhythmia or cardiopulmonary bypass if symptoms are refractory to drugs.

Postmortem Features

Features are nonspecific.

Medicolegal Importance

a. The poison is not easily detected on chemical analysis hence may be used for homicidal purposes.
b. However deaths are mostly accidental in nature. The root can be differentiated from horse-radish by the pink colour which develops after the cut surface of the aconite root is exposed to air for some time.
c. Poisoning may also result while collecting flowers without wearing gloves. Tingling sensation is felt in hands which extends to arm followed by cardiac manifestations.

Dr George Henry Lamson

Dr Lamson was in need of funds to finance his morphine addiction. He tempered some raisins in the cake slice with alkaloids of aconite, which he offered to his handicapped bother-in-law. Who after suffering from stomach ailments, died. While Dr Lamson was trying to sell the inside story to a new paper, he was apprehended and on conviction for the murder was hanged.

QUININE

Quinine is obtained from the bark of cinchona plant from the family Rubiaceae. Cinchona plant bark is also known as *red bark, Jesuit's bark, China bark, fever tree bark*, etc. Cinchona bark contains alkaloids like quinine, quinidine, cinchonine, and cinchonidine. These alkaloids are readily absorbed from the lungs or GIT.

Quinine is seen as needle shaped, odorless but intensely bitter, crystalline substance in pure form and mainly used for the treatment of the malaria. It has also been used for cramps, internal hemorrhoids and varicose veins.

Quinine was taken for antimalarial action in the colonial India in the form of *"Tonic Water"* mixed with alcohol, especially Gin. Even these days tonic water contains small quantities of quinine.

Features of Poisoning

A person may suffer from **Cinchonism** on ingestion of these alkaloids in an overdose or in repeated doses. It stimulates and then causes depression of the CNS:

a. Initially there is pain in abdomen and vomiting.
b. Visual disturbances, blindness and ringing in the ears.
c. Giddiness, confusion, muscular weakness and severe headache.
d. Convulsions and hypotension.
e. In very high doses there may be oliguria and hematuria.
f. Respiratory depression leading to cyanosis and death.

Fatal dose: A single 2 to 8 gm oral dose may be fatal.

Fatal period: About 6 hours.

Treatment

a. Evaluate and stabilize the patient's airway, breathing, and circulation (ABCs). Especially close monitoring of cardiac functions.
b. Gastric lavage or activated charcoal.
c. Urine acidification if required.
d. Supportive treatment.

Postmortem Findings

Features are nonspecific.

Medicolegal Significance

Deaths are from accidental poisoning. Rarely suicides or homicides are attempted with quinine.

NICOTINE

Nicotine is an alkaloid present in the Nicotiana Tabacum and related plants from the family Solanaceae. It is a stimulant drug having parasympathomimetic action. It is made in the roots of the plant and gets accumulated mainly in the leaves which contain about 1 to 8% of nicotine. All parts of the plant are toxic except ripe seeds.

Nicotine in small doses acts as stimulant as well as relaxing agent. It is highly addictive as it leads to euphoria. Nicotine is associated with cardiovascular diseases, potential birth defects and poisoning. Prolonged cigarette smoking and tobacco chewing has been associated with lung and mouth cancers.

Nicotine is seen as oily substance with burning taste and peculiar odor.

Features of Poisoning

a. Initially there are neurological symptoms like dizziness, headache, confusion, anxiety, insomnia and weakness. These are followed by seizures, panic attacks and tingling sensation.

b. Cardiovascular symptoms include palpitations and increased blood pressure.
c. Patient may complain of chest pain.
d. There is reduced appetite, nausea, vomiting and abdominal pain.
e. There may be blurred vision, tinnitus and cold sweats.
f. Respiratory failure or cardiovascular complications may cause death.

Fatal dose: About 50 to 100 mg of nicotine can be fatal.

Fatal period: About 10 to 30 minutes.

Treatment

a. Evaluate and stabilize the patient's airway, breathing, and circulation (ABCs).
b. Gastric lavage with potassium permanganate or administer activated charcoal.
c. Benzodiazepines for convulsions or seizures.
d. Control hypotension.
e. Symptomatic treatment.

Postmortem Findings

They are nonspecific. In some cases traces of tobacco leaves may be seen in stomach. Signs of asphyxia like cyanosis may be observed.

Medicolegal Importance

Poisoning is mostly accidental; homicidal or suicidal cases are rare. Some cases of poisoning are seen in tobacco cultivators when handling leaves may result in poisoning known as *"Green tobacco sickness"*.

STRYCHNOS NUX VOMICA (KUCHILA)

Plant commonly grows in jungles of Tamil Nadu, Malabar and Coramandal coast. Seeds of the plant are poisonous. They are flat, circular discs of about 2.5 cm in diameter and half centimeter in thickness at the periphery. They are slightly concave on one side and convex on the other side. Seeds are ash grey in colour and have a satin like appearance due to silky hair present on the surface. Internally they are horny, tough and translucent, they are bitter in taste but having no odor (Fig. 47.1).

There are two main alkaloids present in the seeds *strychnine* and *brucine* along with small quantities of glycoside *Lagonin*. Other parts of the plant only contain brucine. Brucine has similar properties as strychnine but less potent, about 1/20 strength of strychnine.

Strychnos tieute (Upas tree) is used for making poisonous arrows.

Strychnine

In pure form it is colourless, odorless, rhombic crystals having intense bitter taste. It is used 2 to 8 mg in medicinal doses. It is very stable and is not destroyed in decomposition hence can be detected in putrefied dead bodies for quite some time.

Uses

a. Nerve tonic.
b. Respiratory stimulant.
c. Rodenticides.
d. Ingredient of vermicide.
e. Killing dogs.

Brucine

It is colourless, prismatic crystals with bitter taste and resembles strychnine in chemical and physiological action.

Salts of strychnine and brucine are soluble in water but get precipitated in alkaline mixture.

Absorption

They are readily absorbed from GIT, mainly from the small intestines. It can also be administered parenterally. Uncrushed seeds are not poisonous. Greater part of the absorbed salt

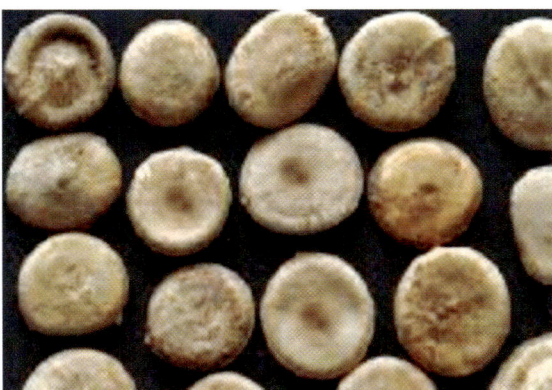

Fig. 47.1: Strychnos nux vomica seeds

is destroyed in liver and some part is excreted unchanged in urine. In about 3 hours 25% of the absorbed alkaloids are excreted hence longer the patient survives better are his chances of recovery. In body it is mainly found in liver and kidneys.

Features of Poisoning

Signs and symptoms start in 15 to 45 minutes after ingestion of crushed seeds:

i. Person gets intense bitter taste on swallowing, which can be detected in 1:100000 dilutions.

ii. There is chocking sensation in the throat.

iii. Within short time there is stiffness of the muscles starting from the neck muscles then jaw muscles and then the limbs are involved.

iv. Twitching of muscles followed by generalized contractions caused by acting as antagonist of glycine, preventing inhibitory effects of glycine on the postsynaptic neuron in the spinal cord.

v. Initially convulsions are clonic but then are tonic as the interval becomes shorter and paroxysm longer. Convulsions are painful. Features are drawn into a grin known as *Risus Sardonicus*. Body is arched known as opisthotonus, but sometimes emprosthotonus (forward bending) or rarely pleurosthotonus (sidewise bending). Any sensory stimulus or movement, noise even light can initiate convulsions.

vi. During paroxysm the face becomes cyanosed with froth at the mouth.

vii. There is anxious apprehensive look of impending death.

viii. Mind is clear till death.

ix. There is sweating, but vomiting is rarely seen.

x. Contraction of the respiratory muscles causes a sensation of suffocation which ends in asphyxia. Death is from asphyxia or from exhaustion.

Fatal dose: About 30 to 120 mg for an adult. One seed of Nux Vomica contains about 20 mg of strychnine.

Fatal period: About 1–2 hours.

Treatment

1. Convulsions are controlled first even before removing poison.
2. Patient is kept in dark room free from any noise or other disturbances.
3. Inhalation anesthesia is effective when given in between attacks, as person is not able to inhale during convulsions.
4. Short acting barbiturates like pentobarbital sodium 0.3 to 0.6 gm intravenously can be administered.
5. Stomach-wash with warm water followed by potassium permanganate solution.
6. Activated charcoal to adsorb the poison.
7. Mephansin 30 mg/kg body weight in slow drip to control fits.
8. Chloral hydrate and bromides at frequent intervals.
9. Symptomatic treatment depending upon the requirements.

Postmortem Features

Postmortem features are not very characteristic:

1. Rigor mortis appear early.
2. Signs of asphyxia like cyanosis, froth at mouth and nostrils and petechial hemorrhages.

Biological test to detect poisoning can be done on the frogs by injecting into lymph sac can produce convulsions (not advocated there days).

Medicolegal Importance

1. Mostly poisoning is accidental in nature.
2. Suicides are very rarely observed.
3. Few cases of homicidal poisoning have also been reported.
4. It is mostly used for killing cattle especially dogs.

Table 47.1: Differentiating features of strychnine and tetanus

Feature	Strychnine	Tetanus
Onset	Sudden	Gradual
History	H/O intake of bitter substance	H/O injury
Convulsions	All muscles are affected simultaneously	All muscles are not affected at a time. (Tonic)
Lower jaw	Do not start from lower jaw	Start from lower jaw
Muscles between attacks	Muscles are relaxed	Muscles are rigid.
Fatal period	1–2 hours	Rarely in 24 hours
Chemical analysis	Strychnine is detected	No chemical found

5. It has also been used as aphrodisiac; some person can consume up to 1 gm on prolonged use.
6. Used as arrow poison.
7. Poisoning has to be differentiated from tetanus. Differentiating features are mentioned in Table 47.1.

The Lambeth poisoner

Dr Thomas Cream used to offer capsules containing strychnine to prostitutes under the pretext to improve their complexion. He was caught when he offered to disclose the identity of poisoner for thousands of pounds. He was placed on trial, found guilty and was hanged.

48 | Peripheral Neurotoxic Poisons

CURARE

Curare is an arrow poison used by native South American people. It is obtained from the bark of Strychnos curare and strychnos toxifera. The paste prepared by the natives is dark, viscid having bitter taste. Bark and leaves of these plants are boiled for two days filtered and boiled again till a thick paste is available. This paste is used as arrow poison or in poisonous darts used from blow guns. Main active alkaloids present are D-tubocurarine, Curarine and Poto-curarine.

Curare act by reversibly inhibiting nicotinic acetylcholine receptors at neuromuscular junction. In small doses it causes muscular weakness, but when sufficient dose is administered it causes paralysis of muscles and result in asphyxial death from respiratory paralysis. In case artificial respiration is provided to a patient he recovers without any side effects, hence it is used as muscle relaxant in anesthesia or convulsant conditions like strychnine poisoning or tetanus. Moreover, it does not affect cardiac muscles.

Features of Poisoning

As this poison is not effective when taken orally, hence, the route of administration is intramuscular or intravenous.

There is paralysis of the skeletal muscles leading to respiratory paralysis. There may be associated headache, blurred vision and dilated pupils. The person remains conscious but is not able to speak or make gestures till he loses consciousness.

Treatment

1. Artificial respiration is the main stay of the treatment. When facilities are not available even continuous mouth to mouth respiration may save the life.
2. Muscular paralysis can be reversed by administering cholinesterase inhibitors like physostigmine, but the patient must be closely observed.
3. Absorption from the injected limb can be reduced by bandage as done in snake bite.

Fatal dose: It is about 60 mg of curare.

Postmortem Features

Asphyxial features are present like cyanosis, petechial hemorrhages, and congestion of internal visceral organs. By close examination injection prick mark may also be detected.

Medicolegal Importance

It is used as arrow poison and as a muscle relaxant in anesthesia. Homicidal and suicidal poisoning is very rare.

49 | Asphyxiants

Asphyxiants are primarily irrespirable gases or gases responsible for producing "Anoxic anoxia" (carbon dioxide), "Anemic anoxia" (carbon monoxide) or "Histotoxic anoxia" (anesthetic gases like chloroform) resulting in improper oxygenation of the body tissues. Hydrogen sulphide gas may result in anoxia due to formation of methemoglobin along with paralysis of respiratory center.

CARBON MONOXIDE

Carbon monoxide (CO) is a colourless and nonirritant gas which is lighter than air; however impurities give it a garlicky odor.

Sources

Wherever there is incomplete combustion of any carbonaceous material, carbon monoxide gas is produced like in charcoal fires, refineries, furnaces, brick kilns, gas refrigerator and house on fire. This is present in the exhaust gases of motor vehicles and also in small quantities in the tobacco smoke.

Mode of Action

Carbon monoxide displaces oxygen from the combination with hemoglobin and form a relatively stable compound known as carboxyhemoglobin. The relative affinity to combine with hemoglobin of carbon monoxide is 300 times more than oxygen. Therefore, oxygen carrying capacity of the blood is reduced leading to "Anemic Anoxia". Carbon monoxide poisoning will result after few minutes of exposure to 0.4% concentration in air, whereas 0.2% concentration in air can cause death in about 4 hours. Safe limit of carbon monoxide is 0.01%.

In a closed garage, if a 20 horse power motor is on, the carbon monoxide present in the exhaust can kill a person in few minutes. Exhaust gases leaking inside the car may result in poisoning to the occupants and can be cause of an accident. A person smoking 20 cigarettes a day may have about 6% carboxyhemoglobin in his blood.

Features of Poisoning

Features of carbon monoxide poisoning are simply because of lack of oxygen and resultant subanoxia.

Signs and symptoms depend upon following factors:

a. Time and duration of exposure.

b. Concentration of carbon monoxide in the air.

c. Physical activity of the person which increases intake.

Blood concentration of carbon monoxide and resultant features:

i. 0 to 10%: There are no appreciable symptoms.

ii. 10 to 20%: Breathlessness on moderate exertion and headache in some cases.

iii. 20 to 30% : Headache, nausea, giddiness, muscular weakness, ringing in the ears, irritability, fatigue and disturbed judgment.

iv. 30 to 40%: Fainting attacks, rapid breathing dimness of vision, vomiting low blood pressure and rapid pulse.

v. 40 to 60%: Weakness, incoordination, mental confusion, intermittent convulsions and patient may collapse.

vi. 60 to 70%: Unconsciousness and respiratory failure leading to death.

vii. 80% or more: Certain death.

Saturation required to cause death varies with age, health of the person (anemia or cardiovascular diseases) or when barbiturates are taken, lower concentration is required.

An elevated COHb level of 2% for non-smokers and >9% COHb level for smokers strongly support diagnose of CO poisoning.

Common Differential Diagnosis of CO Poisoning

a. Acute respiratory distress syndrome
b. Diabetic ketoacidosis
c. Altitude sickness
d. Meningitis
e. Migraine and other headache
f. Chronic fatigue syndrome
g. Depression
h. Flu
i. Opioid or alcohol poisoning.

Treatment

a. Remove the patient to fresh air immediately if the patient is conscious usually no treatment is needed as half of the inhaled gas is eliminated in about half hour.
b. When the condition of the patient is bad, give artificial respiration with 5% carbon dioxide as stimulant.
c. Hypodermic injection of 0.5 ml of adrenaline.

d. Coramine which can be repeated if required.
e. Keep the patient hot by giving hot water bottles.
f. Exchange transfusion in severe cases.
g. To reduce cerebral edema mannitol or 50% glucose can be administered intravenously.
h. Hyperbaric oxygen at 2 to 2.5 times atmospheric pressure if available *is the treatment of choice.*
i. Antibiotics to prevent lung infections.

Postmortem Findings

a. Cherry red postmortem staining.
b. Fine froth at mouth and nostrils.
c. Anoxic blebs may be seen over pressure points.
d. Internal organs are also of cherry red in colour and congested.
e. Bronchopneumonia in some cases when they survive for some time.
f. Pericardial hemorrhages.
g. Brain is edematous and may show bilateral symmetrical necrosis of lenticular nuclei, punctate hemorrhages in white matter and infarction of globus pallidus and Ammon's horns.

Diagnostic test: Spectroscopic examination is characteristic of carboxyhemoglobin. There are two bands between D and E lines as seen in diluted blood having oxyhemoglobin but when ammonium sulphide is added there is no change in CO poisoning, whereas a single broadband is seen in reduced hemoglobin.

Medicolegal Importance

a. Accidental poisoning is very commonly seen especially of elderly persons in closed rooms with coal fires in winter months or from exhaust gases in a closed garage or in coal mines.
b. Suicide is rare and homicides are uncommon.

CARBON DIOXIDE

This is a colourless, odorless gas resulting from combustion or fermentation process. It is a normal constituent of the air we respire. At low concentrations, gaseous carbon dioxide appears to have little toxicological effect. Main mode of action of carbon dioxide is as an asphyxiant, although it also exerts toxic effects at cellular level. As it is heavier than normal air, it tends to settle in the lower confines of an ill ventilated room. Moreover, presence of carbon dioxide in manholes, cellars or deep holes, makes it dangerous for workers.

Dry ice (carbonic acid gas) is solid form of the carbon dioxide. Handling dry ice without proper precautions may result in dry ice burns or dry ice frostbite. In case it is warmed rapidly, large amount of carbon dioxide is generated, which can be dangerous, particularly within a confined area.

Features of Poisoning

Hypercapnia is the term used to express excess carbon dioxide in the blood. Permissible exposure limit or threshold limit for CO_2 is equivalent to 0.5% by volume of air for an 8 hour work day. A 30 minutes exposure to 5% concentration produces intoxication, and concentrations greater than 10% produce unconsciousness.

Early features of hypercapnia include flushed skin, headache, bounding pulse, tachycardia, dyspnea, muscle twitching and raised blood pressure. In severe cases there is disorientation, hyperventilation, convulsions, pulmonary edema, coma and death.

Fatal dose: Concentrations greater than 10% produce unconsciousness; concentration more than 25% may result in fatal consequences and concentration exceeding 50% may be fatal immediately.

Treatment

The management of carbon dioxide poisoning requires immediate removal of the patient to fresh air, administration of oxygen and appropriate supportive care. In severe cases, assisted ventilation may be required.

Dry ice burns require thawing of the tissue and suitable analgesia. Healing may be delayed and surgical intervention may be required in severe cases.

Postmortem Features

Features of anoxia are prominently present like cyanosis, dilated pupils, petechial hemorrhages, and froth from mouth and nostrils. Internal organs are congested and cyanosed.

Medicolegal Importance

Death from carbon dioxide is mostly accidental in nature. Person involved in cleaning of sewer well or ship holds may get accidental poisoning. In rare anesthetic mishaps carbon dioxide may be supplied in place of oxygen gas.

HYDROGEN SULPHIDE

Hydrogen sulphide (H_2S) is a colourless, flammable gas with highly lipid solubility that has strong odor of rotten eggs. However, continuous exposure to low concentrations of hydrogen sulphide result in olfactory paralysis and loss of the ability to smell or detect the gas. It is produced from the decay of sulphur containing organic material and commonly encountered in sewers, liquid manure pits, ships' holds, sulphur springs or as result of volcanic eruptions. It is also produced due to putrefaction of dead bodies. Hydrogen sulphide is often encountered as a by product of the petroleum, viscose rayon, rubber, and mining industries.

It has local irritant effects along with arrest of cellular respiration. Hydrogen sulphide forms a complex bond causing inhibition of mitochondrial cytochrome oxidase thereby arresting aerobic metabolism. High concentrations have the potential to cause sudden death due to hydrogen sulphide's action on the respiratory center.

Features of Poisoning

Low-level exposures to hydrogen sulphide usually produce local irritation to eye and mucous membrane along with headaches, asthenia, and bronchitis.

High-level exposures of hydrogen sulphide result in more neurologic and pulmonary symptoms like cough, dyspnea, vertigo, confusion, nausea, vomiting, loss of consciousness and in some cases hemoptysis.

Very high concentrations lead to myocardial infarction, sudden loss of consciousness, seizures and cardiopulmonary arrest.

Treatment

a. Initial treatment of hydrogen sulphide exposure requires immediate removal of the patient from the contaminated area to fresh-air.
b. Intubation may be necessary for ventilatory support.
c. Ventilation with 100% oxygen and possible use of positive pressure ventilation may lead to recovery in majority of the cases.
d. Based on the similarities in cyanide and hydrogen sulphide toxicity, induced methemoglobinemia may be used in hydrogen sulphide toxicity. Methemoglobin concentrations should be closely monitored and kept below 30%. Symptomatic treatment includes the use of bronchodilators for patients with bronchospasm.

Postmortem Features

External features are predominantly that of asphyxia like cyanosis and petechial hemorrhages. Postmortem staining is bluish green in colour. On opening the body, characteristic smell of hydrogen sulphide is detected. Early decomposition of the body is also observed.

Medicolegal Importance

Death in majority of cases is accidental in nature in persons working in deep sewers, liquid manure pits or ships' holds. However, mixing of household chemicals like bath sulphur mixed with toilet bowl cleaner to create hydrogen sulphide is increasingly used as means of committing suicide.

HYDROCYANIC ACID

Hydrocyanic acid (HCN) or cyanogen is widely distributed in nature. Many fruits and leaves such as cherry, bitter almonds, apricot, plums, peaches and bamboo shoots contain a glycoside known as "Amygdaline", which in presence of water and enzyme emulsin readily gets hydrolyzed into hydrocyanic acid, glucose and benzaldehyde. Consumption of such food articles may result in chronic exposure. Bad effects of such toxicity can be minimized by vitamin B_{12} (hydroxycobalamin) intake.

Hydrocyanic acid is chiefly used to fumigate houses, ships and railways. It can be obtained by distilling KCN or potassium ferrocyanide with dilute sulphuric acid. In pure form it is colourless, highly volatile, boils at 26°C, solidifies below 14°C and has bitter almond smell.

Mechanism of Action

Cyanide results in histotoxic hypoxia, because the cells are unable to utilize oxygen, primarily through the inhibition of cytochrome oxidase enzyme.

Absorption and Excretion

Cyanide gas is rapidly absorbed from the respiratory system. Cyanide salts are also readily absorbed from stomach. HCN can also be absorbed from abraded skin. Absorption from the stomach is delayed when taken on full stomach or with alcohol. When KCN or NaCN is ingested, hydrochloric acid present in the stomach reacts with it and liberate HCN.

After absorption, HCN detoxification takes place by the mitochondrial enzyme rhodanese. Small amount is eliminated unchanged in breath and rest is excreted through urine.

Features of Poisoning

Death is most rapid and in some cases there may not be any manifestations. Symptoms usually occur at once or after about a minute during which the person may perform some voluntary acts. If a large dose is taken there is immediate collapse with muscular twitching, convulsions, unconsciousness, froth from mouth, eyes are fixed and glistening, pupils are dilated, rapid feeble pulse, patient is gasping and death occurs from heart and respiratory failure.

In case small but lethal dose is taken there is bitter burning taste, constriction or numbness of the throat, salivation, nausea, headache, confusion, giddiness, loss of muscular power, face is congested, froth at mouth, eyes are glossy and prominent, pupils are dilated rapid feeble pulse, laboured breathing, convulsions, insensibility and death from respiratory failure.

In poisoning by sodium or potassium cyanides the appearance of symptoms may be slightly delayed up to 15 to 20 minutes and there is corrosive effects seen in throat and stomach.

Fatal dose: About 50 to 60 mg of HCN; 200 to 300 mg of NaCN or KCN. Concentration of 1/500 in air of cyanide gas can cause immediate death.

Fatal period: Few minutes when HCN is taken but may be up to to half an hour in NaCN or KCN.

Treatment

Immediate treatment is started when there is suspicion of cyanide poisoning even without waiting for laboratory confirmation. Principle of treatment is to activate cytochrome oxidase enzyme, this is achieved by converting hemoglobin into methemoglobin which combines with cyanide and form harmless nontoxic cyanomethemoglobin thus cytochrome oxidase enzyme is spared.

a. Break 0.2 ml ampule of amyl nitrite in a handkerchief and hold over the nose of the patient for half a minute and repeated after every 2 minutes or till sodium nitrite is given.

b. Hydroxycobalamin, 10 ml of 40% solution intravenously, which is considered as the drug of choice, combines with cyanide to form cyanocobalamin, which is cleared from the kidneys.

c. 300 mg of sodium nitrite in 10 ml of distilled water is given slowly intravenously is considered as second line of treatment as it can cause life-threatening toxicity.

d. This is followed by sodium thiosulphate about 12.5 gm in 50 ml of water given in a slow infusion. This help in converting cyanide to thiocyanates which is easily excreted.

e. Half dose of nitrite and thiosulphate is given after one hour if recovery is not achieved with earlier treatment.

f. Stomach wash is given after nitrite treatment with 3% hydrogen peroxide or 10% sodium thiosulphate or 0.2% potassium permanganate. Leave 200 ml in the stomach after stomach wash.

g. Low blood pressure can be treated with nor adrenaline drip.

h. Blood transfusion and oxygen inhalation is also required in some cases.

i. Other methods of forming methemoglobin are mentioned below:
   i. Methylene blue 1% solution of 50 ml is infused.
   ii. 4-dimethylaminophenol (4-DMAP) can be used intravenously which produces methemoglobin.
   iii. PAPP (Para-amino propiophenone) can also be administered.
   iv. A mixture of ferrous and ferric sulphate with potassium carbonate which forms Persian blue.

j. Dicobalt edentate or dicobalt-EDTA can chelates cyanide as cobalt cyanide, which is then excreted.

k. Symptomatic treatment as per requirements of the patient is provided.

l. Patients should be re-evaluated 7–10 days after discharge from the hospital. Delayed onset of Parkinson-like syndrome or neuropsychiatric sequelae may be noted on follow-up.

Postmortem Features

a. Rigor mortis appear early but lasts longer.
b. Eyes are prominent, bright and glistening.

c. Froth at nostrils and mouth.
d. Postmortem staining is brick red in colour.
e. There is bitter almond smell from the stomach. Some individuals are unable to smell hydrogen cyanide and it is thought that ability to smell is genetically controlled by a recessive gene.
f. Congestion of organs.
g. Edema of lungs.
h. Mucosa of stomach is congested.
i. NaCN and KCN may cause corrosion of the mouth and stomach wall.
j. In case a person survives for some time then necrosis of the lenticular nuclei may be seen.

Medicolegal Importance

a. Commonly used for suicidal purposes as death is fast.
b. Accidental poisoning may be seen.
c. Decomposition destroys cyanide.

50 | Insecticides and Weed Killers

These are classified either based on their toxicity or on the basis of chemical nature of various compounds.

CLASSIFICATION BASED ON THE TOXICITY

i. *Virtually harmless:* Copper oxide, oxychlorides a fungicide and lime sulphur washes used as fungicide in orchards.

ii. *Comparatively harmless:* Sodium chlorate used as mass herbicide along railway tracks and 20% sulphuric acid used as weed killer.

iii. Mild to moderate toxic: Include chlorinated hydrocarbons used as insecticides.

   a. *Chlorobenzene derivatives:* DDT (dichloro diphenyl trichloroethane) and TDE.

   b. *Benzene hexachloride compounds:* Lindane.

   c. *Polycyclic chlorinated compounds:* Aldrin and endrin.

iv. Highly toxic:

   a. *Arsenic compounds:* Sodium arsenite and Paris green.

   b. *Nicotine compounds:* Used in horticulture.

   c. *HCN and thiocyanates:* Used as disinfectant.

   d. Dinitrophenols.

   e. *Organophosphorus compounds:* Parathion, melathion, diazinon, etc.

CLASSIFICATION BASED ON CHEMICAL STRUCTURE OF COMPOUNDS

1. *Organophosphorus compounds:* Parathion, melathion, diazinon, etc.
2. *Chlorinated hydrocarbons:* DDT, TDE, lindane, etc.
3. *Carbamates:* They are also cholinesterase inhibitors but action is readily reversible like baygon, sevin, metacil, etc.
4. Dinitrophenols.
5. *Miscellaneous group:*
   a. Arsenical compounds
   b. Compounds of natural origin like nicotine
   c. HCN, thiocyanates.

ORGANOPHOSPHORUS COMPOUNDS

These are derivatives of phosphoric acid. Organophosphorus compounds are readily available as they are used extensively in agriculture. Depending upon chemical structure these compounds can be divided into two groups.

1. **Alkyl phosphates:**
   i. HETP (Hexaethyltetraphosphate)
   ii. TEPP (Tetraethylpyrophosphate)
   iii. OMPA (Octamethylpyrophosphate)
   iv. Dimefox
   v. Isopestox
   vi. Melathion
   vii. Systox
   viii. Dipetrex

2. Aryl phosphates:
  i. Paraoxon
  ii. Parathion
  iii. Methyl parathion
  iv. Diazinon (Tick-20)
  v. Chlorothion

Absorption

These compounds can be easily absorbed from skin, GIT and respiratory tract.

Mode of Action

Action of organophosphorus compounds is due to their inhibitory action on cholinesterase enzyme at myoneural junction and ganglionic synapses. Their action can be divided into main two groups apart from other actions.

a. *Muscarinic effects:* Parasympathetic post-ganglionic cholinergic fibers are affected resulting in nausea, vomiting anorexia, abdominal cramps, sweating, salivation, increased bronchial secretions, bronchial spasm, pupillary constriction and blurred vision.

b. *Nicotinic effects* These are due to stimulation of preganglionic sympathetic fibers followed by paralysis resulting in twitching, fasciculation, arrhythmias, tachycardia followed later on by weakness, relaxation of sphincters and paralysis.

c. *Effects on CNS.* These include giddiness, restlessness, headache, tremors, ataxia, insomnia, disorientation and coma leading to death.

d. *Chromodacryorrhea (red tears):* Patient may shed red tinged tears due to accumulation of porphyrin in the lachrymal glands.

Features of Poisoning

Symptoms and signs of organophosphorus poisoning start within half hour or maximum up to 2 to 8 hours of ingestion.

a. In the early phase there is headache, nausea, giddiness, defective vision, miosis and profuse frothing.

b. During the late stages there is vomiting, sweating, twitching, tremors, incoordination, muscular weakness, abdominal cramps, diarrhea, incontinence, delirium, pulmonary edema and coma leading to death.

Fatal dose: TEPP is most toxic and 100 mg orally or 50 mg parenterally can cause death. Parathion can result in death with 175 mg orally or 80 mg intravenously and 1 gm of melathion or diazinon orally can be fatal.

Prophylactic Measures

So as to prevent poisoning while using these compounds in agriculture, following precautions are recommended:

  i. Protective clothing including overall, hood for head and gloves while spraying insecticides.
  ii. Thorough washing of hands after spraying.
  iii. Working should be limited to 2 hours a day.
  iv. Any person suffering from cold and bronchitis should not spray.
  v. Use of proper instructions like standing on the side wind is blowing, while spraying.
  vi. No eating or drinking while spraying.

Diagnosis

The diagnosis is based on history, signs and symptoms. Symptoms are normally seen when cholinesterase level falls by 20%. It can also be diagnosed by administering atropine. When 2 mg of atropine is administered intravenously signs of atropinisation appear in a normal person which are not seen in organophosphorus poisoning. This method is also used to differentiate this poisoning from morphine poisoning.

Diagnosis in living can be confirmed from RBC cholinesterase levels which is reduced to below 40% in severe toxicity.

Treatment

a. Ensure adequate airway, breathing, and circulation (ABCs).

b. *Decontamination:* Remove clothing when contaminated and wash skin with soap and water or mild alkaline solution.

c. Stomach wash, when poison is ingested, with warm water followed by potassium permanganate solution.

d. *Antidote:* Atropine is administered from 2 to 4 mg intravenously or intramuscularly and repeated after 10 to 30 minutes interval depending upon severity of the poisoning, till symptoms are markedly reduced or features of atropinisation appear like dry mouth, flushed skin and dilated pupils.

e. *Specific reactivator oximes:* Specific reactivator oximes are administered along with atropine to reactivate cholinesterase enzyme.

   i. P_2AM (Pyridine-2-aldoxime methiodide) is given in a dose of 50 mg/Kg body weight in slow infusion. Usually 1 gm is administered and is repeated after 3 to 4 hours.
   ii. DAM (Dactylmonoxide) is given slowly in the dose of 2 gm intravenously.
   iii. P_2S (Pyridine 2 aldoxime methane sulphonate), 1 gm is administered slowly.
   iv. Protopam chloride, 1 gm is given slowly in 250 ml of saline.

f. *Supportive treatment:*

   i. Oxygen inhalation and artificial respiration.
   ii. Correct dehydration and electrolyte imbalance.
   iii. Antibiotics for prevention of infection.
   iv. Exchange transfusion if required.

(Avoid morphine, aminophylline along with mouth to mouth respiration).

Postmortem Findings

These are nonspecific suggesting asphyxial death like pulmonary edema, froth from mouth, petechial hemorrhages and kerosene like smell from the stomach contents.

Medicolegal Importance

As these compounds are very commonly used in agriculture hence accidental poisoning is commonly encountered. Moreover these compounds are readily available, quick in action and cheap, therefore, frequently used for suicidal purposes. Homicidal poisoning is possible but is rarely seen.

CARBAMATES

Carbamates, just like organophosphorus compounds act by inhibiting cholinesterase. However, their action is readily reversible, hence the toxicity not as severe as seen in organophosphorus poisoning. These are organic compound derived from carbamic acid.

Various compounds of carbamates are divided into methyl carbamates, ethyl carbamates and polyurethane groups. Some of the commonly used insecticides from this group are baygon, sevin and metacil.

Features of Poisoning

Signs and symptoms are similar to those seen in organophosphorus compounds poisoning except these are not very severe.

Treatment

Treatment is also done on the same lines as is done for organophosphorus poisoning. Apart from decontamination, treatment is primarily done by administration of anticholinergic atropine and supportive therapy. Role of reactivator oximes is controversial because of the potential toxicity caused by combination of oximes with carbamates. However, these days use of oximes is advocated in carbamates poisoning as benefits of using oximes outweigh the low level of this potential risk.

CHLORINATED HYDROCARBONS

DDT and endrin are the compounds commonly used as insecticide. These are soluble in kerosene oil hence in this form they can be readily absorbed from skin, GIT or respiratory tract.

Features of Poisoning

In acute poisoning there is apprehension, salivation, nausea, vomiting, abdominal pain, frothing from the mouth, vertigo, tremors, incoordination, ataxia, blurred vision, mental confusion convulsions, coma and death from respiratory failure.

Fatal dose: For DDT fatal dose is about 30 gm and as endrin is 3 time potent than DDT hence fatal dose is about 6 to 10 gm.

Fatal period: It is half hour to several hours. Mostly death takes place in first two days.

Mode of Action

It is mainly neurotoxic. After absorption it is stored in body fat and other visceral organs.

Treatment

1. Stomach wash and emesis.
2. Symptomatic treatment like artificial respiration for respiratory depression, barbiturates for convulsions, calcium gluconate intravenously, large doses of carbohydrate and B complex.

Postmortem Findings

Externally there is froth at mouth and nostrils, congested conjunctiva, smell of kerosene and nails show cyanosis.

Internal examination show all organs are congested, there are petechial hemorrhages, pulmonary edema and trachea have blood-stained froth.

PARAQUAT

Paraquat (dipyridylium) is primarily used as herbicidal or weeds killer.

Features of Poisoning

a. Burning in the throat, vomiting.
b. Difficulty in breathing due to respiratory depression.
c. Nasal bleeding.
d. Stomach pain.
e. Shock.
f. Jaundice.
g. Renal failure.

Treatment

There is no specific treatment for this poisoning; hence the treatment is mainly supportive in nature.

a. Wash the area of the skin with soap and water.
b. Activated charcoal immediately when poison is ingested.
c. Symptomatic treatment includes respiratory support and oxygen administration.

51 | Common Household Poisons

There are innumerous items in a house which if ingested may produce ill effects or even prove fatal especially in case of children or pets. Some of the common household products can be grouped as mentioned below:

a. Drugs like pain medicines, vitamins, iron pills, antihistamines, sedatives, antidepressants, etc.

b. Hydrocarbons like kerosene, paint removers, petroleum products, etc.

c. Drain cleaners like alkalis and acids.

d. Pesticides like organophosphorus compounds, carbamates, etc.

e. Cosmetics.

f. Deodorants.

PARACETAMOL

Paracetamol is an antipyretic and pain reliever drug which is very frequently used these days. After taken orally, paracetamol is absorbed from the stomach and small intestine. Peak plasma concentration is achieved in about one hour, but this may be early if taken in liquid form.

It is inactivated by the liver by conjugation leading to two metabolites; glucuronide and paracetamol sulphate, which are then excreted through urine. When taken in overdose a toxic metabolite, N-acetyl-p-benzoquinone imine (NAPQI) is produced which is inactivated by glutathione. When glutathione stores are depleted to less than approximately 30%, necrosis of the liver and renal tubules is caused by NAPQI.

Risk factors: Alcohol-related or other liver disease, malnutrition, fasting, rifampicin and phenobarbital increase the risk of liver damage from paracetamol.

Features of Poisoning

Features of paracetamol toxicity are seen in three stages. Within few hours of high dose nonspecific symptoms are present like nausea, vomiting and sweating which may be seen in the first 24 hours. Massive overdose may lead to metabolic acidosis and coma.

Second stage of toxicity is seen between 24 to 72 hours, mainly consisting of increasing liver damage. There is pain in the right hypochondria. Liver function tests are deranged. There is rise in the hepatic transaminases, bilirubin and prolonged coagulation times. Acute renal failure may be seen in some cases of toxicity.

The third stage which is seen during 3rd to 5th day is as a result of massive hepatic necrosis. This may be manifested in the form of coagulation defects, hypoglycemia, jaundice, cerebral edema and hepatic encephalopathy terminating into coma and death. There are features of renal damage or multiorgan failure. If the patient survives this stage then there is gradual recovery in few weeks. Severity of liver and renal damage depends upon the dose taken and the treatment given.

Toxic dose: A single dose above 10 gm or 200 mg/kg of bodyweight, have a reasonable likelihood of causing hepatic toxicity. Fatal results are normally seen with higher doses of 10 to 25 gm depending upon the susceptibility of the person.

Diagnosis of Poisoning

Detection of paracetamol levels in blood, both in living as well as in dead, is diagnostic of paracetamol poisoning. Any level above 30 mg/liter is indicative of overdose. Plasma level of the drug can be estimated by gas or liquid chromatography.

Treatment

a. Hospitalise the patient with history of overdose as the liver and renal failure may manifest after few days.

b. Gastric decontamination is required to be done as early as possible. Paracetamol is normally absorbed in about two hours; hence gastric lavage is done within this period. In case some preparations which causes delayed release of the drug or other drugs leading to delayed empting time of the stomach, the stomach wash can be attempted after two hours.

c. Activated charcoal can adsorb paracetamol and can be administered, but is of no use after 8 hours of ingestion of paracetamol.

d. Acetyl cysteine should be administered immediately either orally or intravenously. Initial dose of 140 mg/kg body weight is given followed by half that dose every four hours maximum for 2 to 3 days. Activated charcoal may also adsorb acetylcysteine hence they are not given together. Preferred route is intravenous; 300 mg/kg body weight is administered slowly in dextrose solution over 20 hours and can be repeated. Acetylcysteine or N- Acetylcysteine (NAC) is helpful in increasing the synthesis of glutathione.

e. Methionine, 2.5 gm is administered orally and is repeated every 4 hours till a full dose of 10 gm is administered. Methionine acts by increasing the synthesis of glutathione.

f. Supportive measures like vitamin K and fresh plasma for bleeding tendency, electrolytes and for cerebral edema hypertonic glucose may be administered.

g. In severe cases blood transfusion is helpful.

h. Liver transplant is the only option in severe hepatic damage.

Postmortem Features

On external examination there are features of liver damage in the form of jaundice. Petechial hemorrhages or skin rashes may also be seen.

On internal examination congestion of the GIT, signs of centrilobular hepatic damage, acute tubular necrosis and cerebral edema are present.

Medicolegal Significance

In many instances suicides are committed by consuming overdose of paracetamol. In long term use of paracetamol may result in hepatic toxicity more so in cases were some predisposing factor is present.

SALICYLIC ACID

Aspirin (acetylsalicylic acid) is the most common salicylic acid compound associated with salicylic acid poisoning. Methyl salicylate (oil of wintergreen) is another therapeutic preparation for local application causing toxicity, but it is an infrequent cause of death. Sodium salicylates and bismuth subsalicylate are some of the other therapeutic preparations.

Elimination of aspirin at therapeutic concentrations is predominantly by hepatic route with only 10–20% eliminated unchanged in the urine. In an overdose situation urinary excretion of free salicylates becomes even more significant, accounting for 60–85% of total elimination if urine is made alkaline.

Uses

a. Antipyretic

b. Analgesic

c. Keratolytic

d. Antirheumatic

Fatal dose: Serious toxic reaction is seen when 300 to 500 mg per kg body weight of aspirin is consumed and potentially lethal toxic reaction is expected with consumption of more than 500 mg/Kg body weight.

Normal fatal dose of aspirin is 15 to 20 gm and methyl salicylates it is 10 to 20 ml in a single dose.

Features of Poisoning

1. **Gastrointestinal:** Nausea, vomiting, epigastric pain usually occur early following an acute ingestion. Hematemesis may be seen in few cases. Gastric perforation following massive aspirin overdose may be seen in rare cases.

2. **Metabolic abnormalities:**
   a. Significant hyperpyrexia requiring cooling.
   b. Acid-base disturbances (respiratory alkalosis, metabolic acidosis)
   c. Dehydration (orthostatic pressure changes are observed)
   d. Electrolyte imbalance (increased potassium excretion as well as systemic acidosis in salicylate overdose leads to hypokalemia.)

3. **Central nervous system:**
   a. In mild toxicity there is lethargy and tinnitus, in moderate cases patient may complain of irritability, disorientation and vertigo and in serious cases hallucinations, seizures, and coma may be present. Presence of seizures indicates a serious prognosis.
   b. Key clinical manifestations of chronic salicylate intoxication, especially in cases involving elderly patients are confusion, bizarre behaviour, stupor, movement disorders and cerebral edema.

4. **Respiratory:** There is pulmonary edema, tachypnea and respiratory alkalosis.

5. **Cardiovascular:** Patient may show features of shock.

Treatment of Poisoning

1. **Emergency and supportive measures:** Maintain airway and assist ventilation if necessary. Administer oxygen and establish intravenous access.

2. **Prevention of absorption:**
   a. Gastric lavage is the preferred route of stomach evacuation. Patients may require gastric lavage with warm water and sodium bicarbonate if possible. Gastric lavage can be performed up to several hours postingestion, especially when tablets are ingested.
   b. Following gastric lavage, administer activated charcoal. Ideally, a 10:1 ratio of activated charcoal to ingested aspirin is administered to bind all the salicylate and prevent absorption.

3. **Fluid and electrolytes:** Fluid and electrolyte deficits may be significant due to vomiting and hyperventilation. Optimal hydration is of great importance in the treatment. Although aggressive fluid therapy is advised, treating doctor must use caution because excessive fluid administration may contribute to pulmonary edema. Potassium replacement is necessary.

4. **Temperature control:**
   a. Begin external cooling with cold sponging and fanning.
   b. Iced gastric or colonic lavage or even ice-water immersion may lower core temperature.
   c. Cooling may help in the control of seizures and agitation.

5. **Enhanced elimination:**
   a. Urinary alkalization is required to enhance urinary excretion of salicylate. 100 mEq of sodium bicarbonate to 1 liter of normal saline, and infuse intravenously at 200 ml/hour (3–4 ml/kg hour).

If the patient is dehydrated, start with a bolus of 10–20 ml/kg.

Unless renal failure is present, add potassium, 30–40 mEq, to each liter of intravenous fluids (potassium depletion inhibits alkalization).

b. Hemodialysis is the most effective way of removing salicylate from the body.

Postmortem Features

a. Stomach and intestines may show hemorrhagic patches.
b. Heart may show subpericardial and endocardial hemorrhages.
c. Pulmonary edema.
d. Kidneys are congested along with other visceral organs.

Medicolegal Importance

Accidental poisoning is common in small children. Some cases of suicidal attempts with aspirin have also been reported, as it is freely available. Homicidal cases are extremely rare.

HYDROCARBONS

Hydrocarbons are those substances that are formed with combination of only hydrogen and carbon atoms. Most of the petroleum product like petrol and kerosene are included in this group.

KEROSENE (Lamp oil, Coal oil)

Kerosene oil is used as a fuel for lamps, as well as for heating and cooking. Kerosene is poorly absorbed by the gastrointestinal tract but there is often aspiration into the respiratory tract especially if the patient vomits, which is commonly seen in small children. This causes pneumonitis which may be so severe as to cause pulmonary edema and hypoxemia.

Features of Poisoning

Swallowing kerosene may cause damage to the linings of the mouth, throat, esophagus, stomach, and intestines resulting in abdominal pain, vomiting, diarrhea and mucosal burns.

If kerosene gets into the lungs, serious and possibly permanent lung damage may result.

Symptoms of aspiration are seen within few hours but may be delayed for a day after ingestion and the patient manifests breathlessness or difficulty in breathing and high fever apart from other features like cough, tachycardia, cyanosis, pulmonary crepitations and rhonchi. However a chest X-ray often shows pulmonary consolidation or collapse, especially on the lower lobes of right lung.

There is blurred vision or loss of vision when eyes are involved. Skin may show irritation and burns. Central nervous system complications are variable but may include lethargy and in few cases especially in children there is convulsions and coma followed by death. Bone marrow toxicity, hemolysis, atrial fibrillation, ventricular fibrillation, hepatic and renal failure are some of the rare complications.

Treatment

a. First priority is to remove the patient from the source of the poisoning and ensure that the airway is patent.
b. Remove contaminated clothing and thoroughly wash the skin with soap and water. If the chemical is in the eyes, flush with lots of water for at least 15 minutes.
c. Give oxygen if indicated. Intubation and mechanical ventilation may be needed in a patient with severe hypoxia, respiratory distress or depressed consciousness.
d. Avoid gastric lavage because of the risk of inhalation and hence pneumonitis. If very large amounts of kerosene have been ingested less than an hour earlier then lavage may be considered provided airway is protected by means of a cuffed endotracheal tube. Use of activated charcoal is not recommended as charcoal poorly adsorbs petroleum products and may cause distension of abdomen resulting in vomiting.
e. Use of antibiotics and corticosteroids is recommended but has a very limited role.

How well a person recovers, depend on the amount of poison swallowed and how fast treatment was given. Damage can continue to occur for several weeks after the poison was swallowed. Death may occur as long as a month later.

Fatal dose: Normal fatal dose in an adult is about 15 ml.

Postmortem Features

Externally finding of asphyxia like cyanosis, froth from mouth and petechial hemorrhages may be seen. Smell of kerosene may be detected from clothing.

Internal features include inflammation and congestion of the gastrointestinal tract. Characteristic smell from stomach contents is detected. Signs of pulmonary edema and consolidation are seen. Prolonged use may cause damage to liver and kidneys along with bone marrow depression.

Medicolegal Importance

Most of the deaths from kerosene poisoning are due to accidental consumption when kerosene is consumed by mistake for water, from an unmarked bottle. Kerosene has also been associated with bride burning or self-immolation. In cases body is charred, presence of soot in trachea is helpful in deciding whether the death was antemortem or not.

52 | Drugs of Abuse and Date Rape Drugs

During the last few decades the problem of drug abuse has almost reached epidemic proportions. It is difficult to obtain actual data on drug abuse.

REASONS FOR NONMEDICAL USE OF DRUGS

i. Over the counter availability of certain drugs.
ii. Self-medication.
iii. Some are curious to know about the effects of certain addicting drugs.
iv. Sometimes drugs are used to treat a condition for which it is not relevant or in excess doses.

However a physician is primarily concerned with those drugs which are habit forming because apart from behaviour problems they may cause psychotic reaction (from a bad trip) leading to their involvement in a crime.

Earlier there were various terminologies used to describe conditions due to use of these drugs apart from drug abuse.

a. **Drug addiction:** It is a state of periodic or chronic intoxication produced by repeated consumption of a drug. Characteristic of drug addiction include following features:
   i. Overpowering desire to continue taking that drug and obtain it by any means.
   ii. Tendency to increase the dose (due to tolerance).

iii. Psychic and physical dependence.
iv. Detrimental effects on the individual and society.

Mostly the term of drug addiction is used when there is physical dependence, but in case of cocaine use even though there is no physical dependence this term is used.

b. **Drug habituation:** This is a condition where the repeated consumption of drug leads to psychological or emotional dependence on that drug. According to the WHO, habituation is defined as "becoming accustomed to any behaviour or condition, including psychoactive substance use" and includes four features:
   i. A desire (but not a compulsion) to continue taking the drug for the sense of improved well-being.
   ii. Little or no tendency to increase the dose.
   iii. Some degree of psychic dependence on the effect of the drug, but absence of physical dependence and hence of an abstinence syndrome.
   iv. Detrimental effects, if any, primarily on the individual.

c. **Drug dependence:** In 1964 WHO expert committee on addiction producing drugs recommended that the term drug dependence should replace drug addiction and drug habituation terms. It is defined as "A state, psychic or sometimes physical resulting from interaction between a living organism and a drug, characterised by behavioural and other responses including a compulsion to take that drug on a continuous or periodical basis in order to avoid the discomfort of absence. Tolerance may or may not be present".

Most person use drugs of dependence with certain discrimination and in such cases little harm usually results. However, indiscriminate use of these drugs may produce mental, physical and moral deterioration of the individual and in some cases may lead to sexual perversions or crimes.

DRUGS USED FOR DRUG DEPENDENCE

Drugs to which dependence develop act on the central nervous system, some are depressant whereas others are stimulant:

i. Opiates and their semi-synthetic or synthetic analogues like heroin or pethidine.
ii. Barbiturates and other sedatives like diazepam or methaqualone.
iii. Alcohol
iv. Coca leaves and cocaine.
v. Amphetamine and related stimulants
vi. Cannabis and other hallucinogenic drugs like LSD.

Inspite of restriction in their use by Indian government as well as other countries, there is increase in drug dependence cases. Apart from alcohol, other drug majority of people get addicted, is heroin.

Reasons for drug dependence: In various studies it has been found that major reasons for use of drugs of dependence are:

a. Pleasure
b. Curiosity
c. Group pressure (stressing that it is the thing to do).

Risk factors: Predisposing or risk factors responsible for drug dependence are as following:

i. Broken homes.
ii. Unhappy family relations.

iii. Depression with regular use of depressant drugs.
iv. Excessive use of alcohol or depressant drugs by parents.
v. Poor academic achievements.
vi. Lack of ambition for future.
vii. Drug use amongst friends.
viii. Regular cigarette use.
ix. Not a believer in religion.

HEROIN DEPENDENCE

Heroin is used in many parts of the world as drug of dependence. Preferred route of administration varies from place to place.

a. Some smoke or take it in a snuff. **Chasing the dragon** is a form of heroin smoking, originating in or near Hong Kong in the 1950s, and refers to the intake of heroin by inhaling the vapours which result when the drug is heated-typically on tin-foil above a flame. Chasing the dragon has now been reliably reported from many parts of the world.

b. Inexperienced inject it subcutaneously known as "**skin popping**". Small nodules are present over the accessible areas of the body where subcutaneous injections have been given over a period of time.

c. More experienced take it intravenously known as "**main liners**". Veins used by addicts range from those in the arms, on the back of hand, legs or even under the tongue. Place where addicts take heroin is known as "**shooting gallery**". Majority of drug addicts injecting in the arm; select an area where overlying skin show a tattoo mark. Common practice is to burn some cotton taken from the shoe and put a small spoon having heroin and water over it, so that it boils. This solution is then taken into a syringe and injected. As there are impurities in the solution injected and syringe is not sterilized, these addicts may suffer from complications like hepatitis, endocarditis, tetanus, meningitis, HIV, Pulmonary abscess, renal failure, etc.

"Drug trafficking" or drug smuggling across the international borders is a very common practice. With multi-trillion dollar global market for illicit narcotics, drug traffickers have a clear incentive to get their products down the supply chain to their customers, despite the legal and moral objections to their activities. Drug lords employ very ingenious methods like hiding drugs in various appliances such as wheel-chairs, walking sticks or carriers are employed where they carry the drug in side their body in the form of implants like breast implant or plastic wrapped drug packets hidden in any of the body cavities. They are known as "**Body Packers**" and carry the drugs wrapped in plastic balloons or condoms which are either ingested or put in any of the body cavities like rectum or vagina. Death may occur in case the packet ruptures. Body scanners present on the airports can detect such carriers; earlier X-ray or CT scans were the diagnostic modalities.

Withdrawal symptoms: They appear after drug has been stopped after prolonged use. They may appear as early as 6–8 hours or delayed for 24 to 48 hours depending upon the drug consumed.

a. *Initial stage of 1–12 hours:* There is improvement in mental and neurological picture.

b. *Early symptoms or first stage seen in 12–30 hours:* There is chilliness, restlessness or uneasiness, yawing, rhinorrhea, agitation, insomnia, nausea, vomiting, abdominal cramps, orthostatic hypotension and twitching of muscles.

c. *Second stage seen in 30–48 hours:* Respiration becomes laboured, goose skin (cold turkey), lacrymation, tremors, "yen sleep" (a trance-like state), involuntary leg movements (kicking the habit or restless leg syndrome), tachycardia and anorexia may be observed.

d. *Third stage seen during 48–96 hours:* There is gradual improvement in the symptoms and the person may go to sleep.

e. *Fourth stage seen during 5–6 day:* On awakening the symptoms become severe along with assuming fetal position, tachycardia, fever, diarrhea, cramps and hallucinations with slight disorientation along with frightful dreams are present. Gradually they subside and may take about 10 days before they disappear.

f. *Later stage seen after 10th day:* Most of the symptoms disappear except for visual hallucinations which may persist in few cases for 3 to 4 months.

Treatment

a. Hospitalize the person.
b. Drug treatment depending upon the drug of dependence.
c. Psychotherapy:
   i. Individual psychotherapy.
   ii. Group therapy.
d. Rehabilitation.

Recidivism

Majority of drug addicts try to get back to their addiction unless they are properly rehabilitated after psychotherapy.

Cause of Death

1. Overdose (hot shot).
2. Complications.

Postmortem Findings

There are characteristic external and internal findings observed depending upon the drug used and route of administration. Mostly the body is malnourished or emaciated showing poor body hygiene. There may be skin popping or injection prick marks with hardened veins. Internal examination mostly shows multiple pus pockets especially under the diaphragm, in the liver or lungs.

AMPHETAMINES

Amphetamines are a type of central nervous system stimulant and are known as *"ice"*, *"speed"*, *"glass"*, *"crank"* or *"crystal"*. They provide a sense of increased wakefulness, energy, attention, concentration, sociability, self-confidence, improved mood, and decreased appetite. Commonly used preparations include benzedrine, dexedrine (dexamphetamine) and ritalin (methylphenidate). Amphetamines are used to treat attention deficit hyperactivity disorder, narcolepsy and obesity. They are also used as mood elevators. Amphetamines cause the release of neurotransmitters or catecholamines, in particular dopamine. Pathways producing pleasure feelings are acted upon by dopamine; which is responsible for the addiction. Tolerance is very common and contributes toward addiction.

Features of Intoxication

a. Initially in acute intoxication there is euphoria, increased self-confidence, increased respiratory rate, tachycardia, raised blood pressure, dilated pupils, depressed appetite, fatigue, hyperpyrexia, tremors, insomnia and over talkative.
b. When a large dose is taken there is manic like presentation and person may even go into cardiovascular shock.
c. Chronic users apart from craving for the drug, show lower social inhibitions leading to aggressive behaviour and altered sexual behaviour. There may be abdominal pain, blurred vision, skin disorders and seizers. He suffers from delusions, hallucinations especially tactile or auditory in nature. There are features of malnutrition and chest pain. In some cases coma leads to death.

Withdrawal Symptoms

These include fatigue, unpleasant dreams, suicidal tendency, depression, anxiety, short term memory loss and difficulty in staying awake.

Treatment

Acute intoxication without life-threatening signs is treated symptomatically with sedatives (diazepam) and cold sponging or antipyretics. Patient is kept in a dark room or soothing environments. When drug is in-gested, gastric lavage is done. Urine is made alkaline to facilitate excretion. Diuretics are administered to manage pulmonary edema.

Complications may require procedures to establish airway management or fluid resuscitation or to initiate vigorous cooling measures including ice bath. Agitation or persistent seizers may require benzodiazepines. Cardiac arrhythmias may require defibrillation and antiarrhythmic drugs. Cardiogenic pulmonary edema can be managed with nitroglycerin and diuretics.

Medicolegal Importance

Aggressive behavior may lead to criminal acts or sexual assaults by the intoxicated person. Overdose or complications may cause death.

As majority of the drug ingested is excreted unchanged in the urine of an addict, hence urine of addicts, known as "**Liquid Gold**", is sold in the market as an economical substitute for other addicts.

COCAINE

Cocaine is one of the most potent stimulant acting on the central nervous system. This is extracted from the leaves of the coca plant erythroxylum coca (Fig. 52.1). This plant is native of South America, where it was used for relieving fatigue by either chewing or making a concoction like tea. It is known by different names like *"Snow"*, *"Coke"* or *"Cadillac"*.

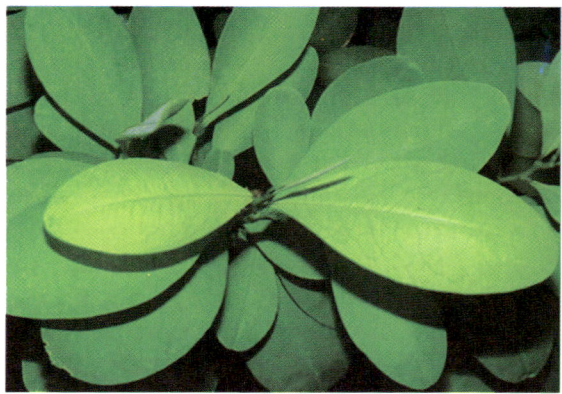

Fig. 52.1: Coca plant

Pure cocaine is colourless, crystalline substance with bitter taste. Inspite of this drug being on the banned list in most of the countries, it remains as one of the common drugs of abuse. It was one of the constituent of "Coca-Cola" earlier. Mixture of cocaine with alcohol is *"liquid lady"* and combination with heroin is *"speed ball"* or *"crank"*.

Cocaine is administered by various routes like snorting, smoking, chewing, ingesting or intravenously. Cocaine is well absorbed from the lungs on inhalation and from the mucosal surfaces of nose or gastrointestinal tract. Vasoconstrictive properties of cocaine delay the rate of absorption from mucosal surface prolonging the effects. It is mainly used for giving pleasant feeling or as an aphrodisiac.

Features of Intoxication

In the initial phase cocaine acts as CNS stimulant leading to increased alertness, increased motor activity, over confidence, increased sexuality and euphoria. Cocaine is responsible for increasing the levels of neurotransmitters dopamine and serotonin in the pleasure giving centers of the brain.

a. A patient may have bitter taste in the mouth.
b. Dryness of the mouth.
c. Restlessness.
d. Flushed face.
e. Dilated pupils.
f. Hyperpyrexia.
g. Tachycardia and increased respiratory rate.
h. High dose may result in anxiety, teeth grinding, muscle incoordination, twitching leading to convulsions.
i. There may be hallucinations, delusions in some cases resulting in violent behaviour.

The stage of stimulation is followed by stage of depression with suicidal tendencies. Respiratory and cardiac failure along with increased blood pressure, leading to cerebral hemorrhage or stroke, may results in fatal consequences. Cocaine use during pregnancy may lead to premature labour.

Fatal dose: About 1 gm taken orally is usually fatal. Small doses may cause death when smoked or snorted.

Treatment

a. Incase cocaine is ingested, gastric lavage with potassium permanganate or tannic acid may be done. Activated charcoal also adsorbs this alkaloid. When it is taken as snort, the nasal cavity should be washed with normal saline.
b. Diazepam is helpful in reducing heart rate and blood pressure.
c. Only alpha-blockers are to be used; use of beta-blockers are not recommended.
d. Hyperpyrexia seen in cocaine intoxication must be controlled immediately. Peripheral vasoconstriction reduces heat loss from the body and may cause muscle cell destruction and myoglobinuria leading to renal failure. Paracetamol and application of ice or wet blanket can help in controlling hyperpyrexia.
e. Symptomatic treatment as required may be provided.

Chronic Poisoning: (Cocainism or Cocainophagia)

Individual addicted to cocaine show weight loss from anorexia, dilated pupils, insomnia, running nose, nasal bleeding, weakness, tremors, tactile or visual hallucinations (Feeling of sand particles under the skin or ants crawling on the skin are known as **Magnan's symptoms**) impotency, sexual perversions, loss of inhibitions, moral degradation and insanity. Teeth and tongue of cocaine eater are black stained. In cases where cocaine is taken as snort, damages the nasal septum like ulceration or perforations, due to vasoconstrictor property. Other complications due to use of infected syringe may be hepatitis, AIDs, abscesses and endocarditis. Bronchitis may be associated with smoking habit.

Chronic addiction is thought to be more common with a particular variant of a gene in addicts. Such addicts normally move in a group and continue using cocaine inspite of financial or legal problems.

Withdrawal Symptoms

Withdrawal symptoms are as a result of psychological dependence on the drug include unpleasant dreams, nausea, insomnia, agitation or depression, aggressive behaviour and increased appetite.

Treatment

a. Effective abstinence from cocaine use by gradually withdrawing the drug which may be achieved by offering incentives.
b. Methylphenidate, amantadine or lithium can be used to treat cocaine addiction.
c. Cognitive behavioural therapy to address the reasons for the addiction.
d. Rehabilitation of the addict in the society.

Postmortem Features

Postmortem findings depend upon the route of administration. When it is taken as a snort *"nasal ulcerations"* or perforations may be seen; if leaves are eaten there is *"black staining of the teeth"* and in case injected then telltale injection prick marks are seen over arms or neck. On internal examination congestion of visceral organs and features of various complications like hepatitis, AIDs, abscesses and endocarditis may be observed.

Medicolegal Importance

a. Most of deaths are accidental overdose in nature. Homicides and suicides are rare.
b. Addiction is seen in upper social circles of the society due to the high cost of the drug.
c. It is commonly used as aphrodisiac. Some persons rub it on the glance penis to increase the duration of sexual act. Prostitutes may apply this in vagina to give sense of local constriction and with absorption may give sexual stimulation to the male partner.
d. Like heroin, it is also commonly transported by "body packers".

DATE RAPE DRUGS (PREDATOR DRUGS)

These are drugs when administered; incapacitate that individual to an extent that *"Drug Facilitated Sexual Assaults"* (DFSA) or rape could be perpetrated, even when woman is not a willing partner. Majority of such cases alcohol is consumed by the victim either voluntarily or administered surreptitiously. Other commonly used date rape drugs are rohypnol, chloral hydrate, ketamine, gamma-hydroxybutyrate (GHB), cannabis, cocaine, sedatives or barbiturates. They are sometimes referred as *"party drugs "or "recreational drugs"*.

"Drink spiking" is the term used when any of the above mentioned drugs are mixed surreptitiously in the drinks offered for committing any robbery, assault or DFSA. Such drugs are detected in the blood or urine of the victim if tested within two days of administration, however, GHB may not be detected in the samples if it is taken after 12 hours of consumption.

Alcohol is the most common date rape drug as most of the cases especially in western countries where it is taken voluntarily by the victim. Alcohol is known to have effects related to sexual and aggressive behaviour. It reduces the ability to resist advances made by the assailant.

Benzodiazepine tranquilizers are also frequently used as date rape drug. Flunitrazepam (Rohypnol) is commonly used for this purpose and is also known as *"Roofies"*, *"Rope"*, *"forget pill"* or *"Roaches"*. It leads to confusion, disassociation, sleepiness, dizziness, incoordination or difficulty in moving their limbs, amnesia and even unconsciousness. After the effect of the drug is over victim may not be able to remember about any event while she was under its influence. The drug can be detected in the urine up to 72 hours of consumption.

GHB (Gamma-hydroxy-butyrate) is odorless but tastes salty and act as CNS depressant. When ingested it produces euphoria, loss of inhibitions and promote sexual urges. It is available in the market as *"Liquid-E"* or *"Liquid-X"*. Gradually it is being favoured as date rape drug because it is easily available, cheap and not easily detectable after 12 hours of use.

Chloral hydrate is also used as DFSA and is known as *"Knockout drops"* or *"Mickey finn"*.

So as to avoid being a victim of such drugs women attending any party or a date are advised not to drink from a punch bowl; not to leave their drink unattended and avoid any drink which was not opened in their presence.

53 | Chemical, Biological, Radiological and Nuclear Warfare Agents

Chemical, biological, radiological and nuclear warfare agents (CBRN) are materials that can be used to produce great harm in battle field and can pose great threats in the hands of terrorists. Army mostly use these agents in weaponized form so that they can be delivered using conventional bombs or enhanced blast weapons known as dirty bombs. Nonweaponized materials are most likely used by terrorists by contaminating food or water sources.

WAR GASES (Chemical Warfare Agents, CWA's)

In chemical warfare the term "gas" is applied to any chemical substance, whether solid, liquid, or vapour (including toxic smokes), which is used for its poisonous, irritant, or blistering effects. They are mainly used at the time of war and sometimes to control unruly mob.

Germans in April, 1915, on the Western Front used chlorine gas initially, followed by phosgene gas which was countered by allied forces wearing special face mask or box respirator. Germans then used arsenicals (lewisite) and mustard gas having a very faint smell and causing no immediate irritation proved to be highly successful during First World War.

These war gases are described as "persistent" or "nonpersistent". Nonpersistent gases are those which, when released into the air, disperse quickly. Persistent gases are mostly observed in the form of liquids which evaporate slowly, therefore, remain dangerous for long-time.

The effective use of gas may be markedly influenced by wind speed, temperature and moisture. Therefore clear nights, low wind velocity, moderate temperature and absence of rain are most favourable conditions to use these gases. During wars they are used in the artillery shells with which the enemy lines are bombarded or dropped from the war planes.

Primary object of using these gases is to cause mortality or to disable enemy troops. They are also used to contaminate food and army supplies so that it becomes dangerous to handle them or reduce mobility of the enemy troops. Lachrymators or tear gases are normally used for dispersing unruly mobs.

Classification of War Gases

War gases have been classified depending upon their physical or physiological properties. During First World War a broad classification of these chemicals were made into *"Lethal"* and *"Harassing"* types. Later on they were classified into *"Persistent"* and *"nonpersistent"* gases. However, from medical point of view these are classified depending on their mode of action.

1. **Vesicants or blistering gases:** This group includes **mustard gas** (dichlordiethyl sulphide) and **lewisite** (dichlorarsine).

These substances whether in the liquid, solid or vapour state will damage any part of the body with which they come in contact. They are fired in artillery shells. Effects of the vapour are acute conjunctivitis, inflammation of the mucous membranes lining the respiratory tract, nausea, vomiting, abdominal pain and burning of the skin varying from erythema to vesications. Liquid coming in contact with skin causes severe vesications.

Death may occur after the inhalation of mustard gas, it is due to aseptic bronchitis along with bronchopneumonia. Very extensive vesications may result in fatalities from secondary shock.

Treatment primarily includes decontamination by washing with soap and water and weak sodium bicarbonate solution for eyes and administration of BAL for lewisite

2. **Asphyxiant:** These gases, which include *Chlorine, Chloropicrin (PS), Phosgene (CG)* and *Di-phosgene*, are essentially lung irritants exerting their main action on the respiratory passages and deeper tissues of the lungs. They are used primarily as lethal agents, and, in the absence of an efficient respirator, their action usually results in the production of a pulmonary edema which may be fatal.

Treatment includes decontamination and removal of the patient to fresh air and respiratory support.

3. **Paralysants:** This group includes gases such as hydrocyanic acid and hydrogen sulphide. These highly toxic gases were found to be not much effective in war situations. In high concentration, both these gases can produce death rapidly through paralysis of the respiratory centre. Treatment includes decontamination and removal of the patient to fresh air. Amyl nitrite by inhalation and sodium nitrite in slow intravenous injection can be administered.

4. **Arseniuretted hydrogen:** This gas exerts its poisonous action only after absorption through the lungs into the body. It causes destruction of the red corpuscles in the blood, hemoglobinuria, jaundice and anemia associated with damage to the kidneys and liver.

5. **Nerve agents:** These are esters of phosphoric acid and similar in action to organophosphorous compounds as they also inhibit acetylcholine esterase. Symptoms and signs are thus similar to organophosphorous compounds. Treatment is also done on the similar lines using atropine and oximes in combination.

6. **Lachrymators:** These are also known as *"teargases"* and include *ethyliodo-acetate (KSK), bromo-benzyl-cyanide (BBC),* and *chloro-aceto-phenone (CAP).* Even low concentrations of the gases given off by these compounds will immediately irritate the eyes, causing profuse lachrymation and intense spasm of the eyelids. Symptoms, however, disappear after some time on leaving the contaminated area. In very high concentrations they may act as lung irritants and may require decontamination and respiratory support.

7. **Nasal irritants:** These are organic arsenical compounds such as *diphenyl-amine-chloroarsine (DM)* and *diphenyl-cyanoarsine (DC).* These solid arsenicals, when suitably dispersed, produce clouds of minute particles which, if inhaled even in exceedingly low concentration, will produce symptoms of acute physical distress. These symptoms are intense pain in the nose and chest, with lachrymation, salivation and even vomiting. The symptoms, however, although alarming at the time, usually subside within an hour after removal from the affected area.

8. **Miscellaneous group:**
   a. *Screening smokes:* Various chemicals are used in warfare to produce smoke for screening movements of troops. Substances as *phosphorus, chlorosulphonic acid, titanium tetrachloride,* and a number of the *chlorinated-hydrocarbon series* are utilized for this object. These smokes are nontoxic

in the open field, but serious effects may follow the bursting of such projectiles in confined space. Yellow phosphorus is primarily used for incendiary purposes in military. However, burning of large quantities of yellow phosphorus generates phosphorus oxide (P_4O_{10}) in dangerous proportions which may lead to increase in the number of cancers and birth defects.

b. *Carbon monoxide:* Whenever combustion occurs in the absence of an adequate supply of oxygen carbon monoxide is generated. Typical instances occur in confined spaces following the burst of a highly explosive shell. This causes interference with the respiratory functions of the blood. *Ordinary respirators give no protection.*

c. *Methyl isocyanate:* This may lead to acute irritation to the eyes, blurring of vision, chest pain and respiratory distress. Sodium thiosulphate can be used as antidote.

d. *Fire fumes:* In case of a big fire at the time of wars, there is risk of inhalation of carbon monoxide and possibly nitrous fumes. Moreover, such an atmosphere may be seriously deficient in oxygen.

BIOLOGICAL WARFARE AGENTS (BW)

Numerous bacterial, viral agents and toxins can pose public health risk in the event of a bioterrorist or biological warfare attack and can cause large number of causalities and may pose many difficulties in containing the attack. There are many instances when smallpox or plague has been used on enemy troops.

Biological agents are easy to acquire, synthesize, transport and use. Dissemination of BW agents may occur by various methods, including aerosol sprays, food or water contamination. The use of an explosive device to deliver and disseminate biological agents is not very effective, since such agents tend to be inactivated by the heat of the blast.

Detection of biological agents involves either finding the agent in the environment or medical diagnosis of the agent's effect on human or animal victims. Early detection of a biological agent in the environment allows for early specific treatment and time during which prophylaxis would be effective. Most aerosolized biological agents do not penetrate unbroken skin.

Multilayered HEPA masks can filter 99.9% of 1 to 5 μm particles, but face-seal leaks may reduce the efficacy by as much as 10–20%. Thorough showering with soap and water removes 99.99% of organisms left on the victim's skin after disrobing. Latex gloves and universal precautions provide sufficient protection when treating.

Various biological warfare agents: Following are some of the important biological agents.

a. *Bacterial agents:*
   i. Anthrax
   ii. Plague (Pneumonic)
   iii. Brucellosis
   iv. Tularemia
   v. Melioidosis
   vi. Cholera
   vii. Q fever
   viii. Rocky mountain spotted fever.

b. *Viruses:*
   i. Smallpox
   ii. Venezuelan equine encephalitis
   iii. Yellow fever
   iv. Japanese B encephalitis
   v. Marburg hemorrhagic fever.

c. *Toxins:*
   i. Botulism
   ii. Staphylococcal enterotoxin-B
   iii. Ricin
   iv. T-2 mycotoxin.

Bacterial Agents

1. **Anthrax:** Anthrax is caused by *Bacillus anthracis*, which is a large, aerobic, gram-positive, spore-forming, nonmotile bacillus. Humans become infected by contact with infected animals or contaminated animal products.

As a biological warfare agent spores are released in aerosol form. Initial manifestations on inhalation are nonspecific and include headache, malaise, fatigue, myalgia, and fever. This is followed by the sudden onset of increasing respiratory distress with dyspnea, cyanosis and increased chest pain. Edema of the chest and neck may be present. The onset of respiratory distress is followed by the rapid onset of shock and death within 24–36 hours.

Penicillin historically has been the preferred therapy for the treatment of anthrax. Penicillin, amoxicillin, doxycycline and ciprofloxacin are used to treat anthrax infections.

2. **Plague:** Plague is caused by *Yersinia pestis*, a gram-negative cocco-bacillus. Plague has been the cause of three great human pandemics in the 6th, 14th, and 20th centuries.

Plague is characterized by the abrupt onset of high fevers, painful lymphadenopathy, and bacteremia. Septicemic plague sometimes can ensue from untreated bubonic plague. Main features of pneumonic plague are severe malaise, headache, vomiting, chills, cough, abdominal pain, chest pain, high fever, bloodstained sputum, septic shock and meningitis.

Streptomycin has been the treatment of choice for bubonic, septicemic, and pneumonic plague. chloramphenicol, gentamicin, doxycycline, ciprofloxacin and ofloxacin may be used as alternatives.

Pakur murder case:

While Mr Amarendra was waiting for a train on Hawrah station, he felt an injection prick. He suffered from high fever, toxaemia and lymph node swelling and died after about 9 days. Blood culture revealed plague bacilli. After police investigations it was submitted to the court that his brother Mr Benoyendra had procured Plague bacilli from Hoffkine institute through his contacts, which was injected by a hired assassin in Mr Amarendra. Mr Benoyendra was convicted and sentenced to death, which was commuted to life imprisonment later on.

3. **Cholera:** Cholera is an acute and potentially severe gastrointestinal disease caused by the bacteria *Vibrio cholerae*. To be effective as a biological weapon water supplies have to be contaminated for this agent to be effective.

The symptoms start suddenly with intestinal cramps, vomiting, feeling ill and painless (rice-water) diarrhea. Headache often accompany the diarrhea, especially early in the illness. The rapid loss of body fluids often leads to more severe illness and even death.

Treatment includes replacement of fluids and electrolytes. Antibiotics such as tetracycline or doxycycline are normally used to treat. The antibiotics ciprofloxacin or erythromycin also may be used.

4. **Tularemia:** Tularemia is caused by the gram-negative, intracellular bacterium *Francisella tularensis*. The disease is characterized by localized skin or mucous membrane ulceration, regional lymphadenopathy, and occasionally pneumonia. Symptoms consist of fever, chills, headache, cough and myalgia. Patients may also complain of chest pain, vomiting, arthralgia, sore throat, abdominal pain, diarrhea, dyspnea, back pain, or neck stiffness.

Streptomycin is the drug of choice for tularemia. Gentamicin is also effective.

5. **Brucellosis:** Brucellosis is a zoonotic infection caused by an organism of the genus Brucella. This may be useful as a BW agent as it can be easily transmitted by aerosol. Symptoms are observed after few days of getting infected. There is fever, chills, weakness, joint and back pain.

Doxycycline along with the addition of streptomycin is effective in the treatment of most forms of brucellosis.

6. **Q fever:** Human infection with *coxiella burnetii* is usually the result of inhalation of infected aerosols. Most common signs and symptoms are diaphoresis, malaise, myalgia, fatigue, and anorexia.

Doxycycline is the drug of choice. Erythromycin, azithromycin and trimethoprim/Sulfamethoxazole are also effective.

Viral Agents

1. **Smallpox:** Variola, the causative agent of smallpox and represents a significant threat as a BW agent. Variola is highly infectious and is associated with a high mortality rate. After the incubation period of 10 to 14 days, symptoms begin acutely with high fever, headache, rigors, malaise, myalgia, vomiting, and abdominal and back pain. After 2–3 days, an exanthema develops on the face, hands, and forearms and extends gradually to the trunk and lower extremities. Death occurs in the second week and is attributed to toxemia.

   Treatment of smallpox is mainly supportive. The antiviral agent cidofovir is effective.

2. **Viral encephalitis:** The viral encephalitis includes Venezuelan equine encephalitis (VEE) virus, Western equine encephalitis (WEE) virus, and Eastern equine encephalitis (EEE) virus. Patients with VEE develop sudden fever, chills, headache, malaise, myalgia, sore throat, and photophobia. CNS manifestations range from mild confusion and lethargy to seizures, paralysis, and coma.

   No specific treatment is available for the viral encephalitis.

Biological Toxins

1. **Staphylococcal enterotoxin B:** Staphylococcal enterotoxin B (SEB) is one of the best-studied and, therefore, best-understood toxins. Staphylococcal enterotoxin is one of the most common causes of food poisoning. Following ingestion of contaminated foodstuffs, nausea, vomiting, and diarrhea are normally present.

2. **Ricin:** Ricin a plant alkaloid derived from the seeds of the castor plant is one of the most toxic and easily produced of the plant toxins. The worldwide availability of castor seeds and the ease with which toxin can be produced give it significant potential as a biological weapon. Ricin is approximately 1000-fold less toxic than botulinum toxin.

3. **Botulinum toxin:** *Clostridium botulinum* is anaerobic, spore-forming, gram-positive bacillus, which produces botulinum toxins. Depending on the subtype botulinum toxins are 10000–100000 times more toxic than chemical nerve agents. Even less than 0.01 mg can cause death. In most of the cases death takes place in one to two days.

   Initial signs and symptoms include blurred vision, mydriasis, ptosis, dysphagia, and dysarthria, dysphonia, and muscle weakness. Anticholinergic signs and symptoms, such as dry mouth, urinary retention, paralytic ileus, and constipation are present.

   After 24 to 48 hours, neuromuscular manifestations progress to symmetric descending paralysis and respiratory failure.

   Apart from decontamination, polyvalent botulinum antitoxin vial can be administered slowly in saline solution. If available, botulinum immune globulin, 50 ml can be given intravenously.

RADIOLOGICAL AND NUCLEAR WEAPONS

Radiological weapons of mass destruction have been suggested as a possible weapon of terrorism used to create panic and casualties in densely populated areas.

Radiological weapons are widely considered to be militarily useless for a states-sponsored army and are initially not hoped to be used by any military forces. Firstly, the use of such a weapon is of no use to an occupying force, as the target area becomes uninhabitable (due to the fallout caused by radioactive poisoning of the involved environment).

Furthermore, area-denial weapons are generally of limited use to an attacking army, as it slows the rate of advance.

A dirty bomb is a radiological weapon dispersed with conventional explosives.

A **nuclear weapon** is an explosive device that derives its destructive force from nuclear reaction, either fission (fission bomb) or a combination of fission and fusion (thermo-nuclear weapon). Both reactions release vast quantities of energy from relatively small amounts of matter. Nuclear weapons have been used twice in nuclear warfare, both times by the United States against Japan near the end of World War II. The first fission (atomic) bomb test released the same amount of energy as approximately 20000 tons of TNT.

The heart of a nuclear explosion reaches a temperature of several million degrees centigrade. Over a wide area the resulting heat flash literally vaporizes all human tissue. People inside buildings or otherwise shielded will be indirectly killed by the blast and heat effects as buildings collapse and all inflammable materials burst into flames. The immediate death rate will be over 90%. Various individual fires will combine to produce a fire storm as all the oxygen is consumed. Outside the area of total destruction there will be a gradually increasing percentage of immediate survivors. However most of these will suffer from fatal burns, will be blinded, bleeding from glass splinters and will have suffered massive internal injuries. Many will be trapped in collapsed and burning buildings.

Survivors will be affected within a matter of days by radioactive fallout. The effects of exposure to high levels of radioactive fallout include hair loss, bleeding from the mouth and gums, internal bleeding and hemorrhagic diarrhea, gangrenous ulcers, vomiting, fever, delirium and terminal coma. There is no effective treatment and death follows in a matter of days.

Radiation-induced cancers will affect many, often over twenty years later. Certain cancers such as thyroid cancer in children are particularly associated with exposure to radiation.

The children of those exposed to radiation are statistically more likely to be born with abnormalities and suffer from leukemia.

Chemical, biological, radiological and nuclear defense (CBRN defense or CBRND) is protective measures taken in situations in which chemical, biological, radiological or nuclear warfare (including terrorism) hazards may be present. CBRN defense consists of CBRN passive protection, contamination avoidance and CBRN mitigation. Dealing with a CBRN event always starts at the local level. Along with the detection and analysis of causative agent, zoning, triage, decontamination, and treatment should be initiated promptly.

Scene management is very important in such an eventuality. Scene of incident must be approached with caution. All responders must take appropriate measures to protect themselves before entering the contaminated area by using Personal Protective Equipment (PPE). Different types of PPE may be used depending on the hazard present. Such protective equipment refers to the respiratory equipment, garments, and barrier materials used to protect rescuers and medical personnel from exposure to biological, chemical, and radioactive hazards. Team of assessors must determine type of incident; estimate the number of casualties and carry-out primary triage.

Try to setup treatment facilities in the cold zone in the nearby area. After receiving emergency care, a casualty must go through the decontamination station before receiving more definitive care in a designated definitive care center.

The Indian Army is presently equipped with CBRND mobile units developed by the defense research and development organization.

54 | Food Poisoning

Food poisoning is an acute gastroenteritis caused by ingestion of food or drinks contaminated by bacteria, bacterial toxins or any poisonous substance of organic or chemical in nature. Mostly there is history of consumption of some food article by a large number of persons manifesting same features. Food articles mainly associated with food poisoning are meat and poultry products.

TYPES OF FOOD POISONING

Food poisoning can be classified depending on the type of contamination present in food.
1. *Bacterial:* They can be of two types:
   i. Infective type due to
      a. Living bacteria which multiply in the GIT and secrete toxins like *Vibrio cholera or E. coli.*
      b. Bacteria invade intestinal mucosa like *Salmonella* or *Shigella* and result in toxicity.
      c. Bacteria cause toxicity by entering bloodstream like *Salmonella typhi.*
   ii. Toxic type due to presence of preformed bacterial exotoxins in the ingested food like staphylococcal food poisoning or botulism.
2. Nonbacterial food poisoning is due to contamination with poisonous fungus, viruses, plants or chemicals.
3. Miscellaneous food poisoning may result in few cases from consumption of following types of food substances:
   i. Food consumed is itself poisonous like some poisonous fishes, mushrooms or toxic honey.
   ii. Food allergies or idiosyncrasies due to hypersensitivity to some foods items like egg, milk or chocolates.

INFECTIVE BACTERIAL FOOD POISONING

Mostly bacterial food poisoning is encountered with *salmonella, shigella,* and campylobacter species, worldwide. Food articles can be contaminated at any stage during food production, food processing, distribution or handling while the food is consumed.

However, most of times the person himself is responsible for contamination of the food articles resulting in food poisoning when food is prepared without washing hands, using unclean utensils, consumed food was not properly refrigerated, raw food not washed properly before use, undercooked food or using untreated water.

Following are some of the bacteria responsible for infective bacterial food poisoning.

Salmonella Food Poisoning

Common *Salmonella* species associated with human outbreaks are *S. typhimurium* and *S. enteritidis.* A person may get infected by consuming prepared farm food like milk, milk products, meat or eggs. Food may get infected through food handlers, infected animals or sometimes by rats which contaminate the food by their urine or feces. There are two main clinical manifestations as mentioned below:

a. *Gastroenteritis:* It takes about 12 to 24 hours for the symptoms to appear as organisms multiply in the intestines to cause illness after consumption of the contaminated food. There is nausea, vomiting, diarrhea, headache, abdominal pain and fever.

b. *Enteric fever:* There is gradual onset of fever with abdominal tenderness. Diarrhea and fever are the main symptoms.

Shigella may cause gastroenteritis by consuming contaminated water or from swimming pool. Incubation period for manifestation of symptoms is between 12 to 48 hours.

Campylobactor is also responsible for bacterial food poisoning from consuming infected meat or poultry products. This is more prevalent during summer months. There is acute diarrhea along with nausea, vomiting, abdominal pain and fever. In severe cases blood and mucous may be present in the stools.

Yersinia is mainly found in the pork and other pork based food articles.

Toxic Bacterial Food Poisoning

Toxic bacterial food poisoning from the preformed toxin present in the food. There is bacterial growth in the food substance due to contamination and improper storage or food kept at a temperature which favours bacterial growth. These bacteria produce enterotoxin resulting in food poisoning on consumption of such food substances. Mostly dairy products and meat preparations are responsible for such outbreaks of food poisoning. Symptoms of such food poisoning appear early, i.e. within an hour or in some cases it may take few hours as preformed toxin are present in the ingested food. However, duration of symptoms is short and mostly the patient recovers early.

Staphylococcal food poisoning is seen from *Staphylococcus aureus,* which is mostly transmitted through milk, milk products, meat, eggs or salads. They multiply in the food and produce thermostable enterotoxin which directly acts on the intestines. Some strains may result in toxic shock syndrome or causes toxic food poisoning.

Vibrio cholera produces enterotoxin leading to excessive secretion of water and electrolytes resulting in diarrhea.

Treatment of Bacterial Food Poisoning

a. Oral rehydration fluid is given initially, if not successful intravenous fluids can be administered.

b. Administration of lactobacillus can be helpful in reducing diarrhea in children.

c. Antibiotics depending upon the infection can be administered. Chroramphenicol, ampicillin or sulphamethoxazole and trimethoprim combination is used in salmonella infection. Tetracycline or ampicillin is used to treat *shigella* food poisoning.

Postmortem Appearance

Congestion of the mucosa of the stomach and intestines and other visceral organs is present. Sometimes ulceration of the intestinal mucosa may be seen.

MUSHROOMS POISONING

Severe poisoning cases are sometimes encountered after consumption of mushrooms. Mushrooms are flesh fungi and lack chlorophyll. Most of the mushrooms are edible and safe to consume. There are thousands of species of mushrooms, but about 15 to 20 species of mushrooms are lethal if ingested.

Common poisonous mushrooms species causing human fatalities are *Amanita phalloides* (death cap) and *Amanita muscaria. Amanita phalloides* contains Cyclopeptides, alpha and beta amanitins, phallotoxins and virotoxins, whereas, *Amanita muscaria* contains alkaloid muscarine.

Features of Poisoning

In mushroom poisoning when the clinical manifestations appear as early as < 3 hrs, effects are mostly not very severe and may not result in fatalities but when the clinical signs appear after 6 hour of ingestion the poisoning is severe and life-threatening. Clinical features depend upon the species consumed, amount ingested, preparation method and individual's susceptibility to the toxins present in the mushrooms.

a. Initial symptoms are constriction of throat, nausea, vomiting, sweating, headache, diplopia, constricted pupils, twitching and convulsions leading to coma.
b. Late symptoms are seen around 24 hours include damage to the liver.
c. Delayed features seen mostly after a day of ingestion mainly in the form of nephrotoxicity.

Treatment

When the mushroom poisoning has been identified, main thrust of treatment is on supportive measures by administering fluids and correcting electrolyte imbalance. Activated charcoal may be administered with an hour of ingestion to decontaminate GIT.

a. In cases of amatoxin (cyclopeptides) poisoning: (i) intravenous benzyl penicillin to reduce uptake of amatoxin by hepatocytes; (ii) cimetidine to reduce conversion of alpha amanitin into hepatotoxic metabolites; and (iii) N-acetyl cysteine for antioxidant activity.
b. In cases of muscarine poisoning, if patient is having excessive bronchial secretions, atropine sulphate can be administered intravenously.
c. Hemodialysis may be helpful. In severe hepatic damage, liver transplant may be considered.

Postmortem Features

Congestion of the stomach and intestine along with fatty degeneration of liver and kidneys is common. Congestion of the brain and other internal organs may be seen.

Medicolegal Aspects

Mushroom poisoning mainly results from wrong identification of the variety of the mushroom or accidental consumption by children. Rarely it may be due to consumption of mushrooms for euphoric effects. About 95% of the poisoning cases are due to accidental consumption.

Multiple Choice Questions

LEGAL PROCEDURE

1. Before proceeding to conduct inquest, police officer must inform:
a. Incharge of the police station
b. Area/executive magistrate
c. Session judge
d. Concerned doctor

2. Age of consent for age determination is:
a. 12 years
b. 16 years
c. 18 years
d. 21 years

3. Police cannot conduct inquest in a case of:
a. Unnatural death
b. Suspected death
c. Dowry death
d. Accidental death

4. Magistrate is not required to hold inquest in:
a. Exhumation
b. Dowry deaths
c. Death in jail
d. Homicidal deaths

5. Leading questions are not allowed in:
a. Examination in chief
b. Cross examination
c. Questions by judge
d. Hostile witness

6. Person telling a lie under oath is:
a. Hostile witness
b. Charged with perjury
c. Professional liar
d. Professional misconduct

7. Person telling a lie under oath is punished under:
a. Section 190 IPC
b. Section 191 IPC
c. Section 192 IPC
d. Section 193 IPC

8. Presiding officer of the court which can award death sentence is:
a. First class magistrate
b. Chief judicial magistrate
c. Assistant session judge
d. Session judge

9. Conduct money is given to:
a. Witness in civil case
b. Witness in criminal court
c. Doctors for conducting autopsy
d. Any witness for good conduct

10. Time limit for cross examination is:
a. Fixed by presiding judge
b. Time available during that day
c. Equal to examination in chief
d. No limit

11. Volunteering of a statement can be made by:
a. Common witness
b. Expert witness
c. Hostile witness
d. Defence lawyer

12. **Open verdict in coroner's inquest is:**
    a. Verdict declared to accused
    b. Verdict declared in open court
    c. Case kept pending
    d. Case referred to higher court

13. **Dying declaration can be recorded by:**
    a. Magistrate
    b. Doctor
    c. Police officer
    d. Anyone of the above

14. **A judge can ask questions during:**
    a. Examination in chief
    b. Cross examination
    c. Re-examination
    d. Any time during the trial

15. **An accused can be examined by a doctor without consent under section:**
    a. 44 IPC
    b. 53 IPC
    c. 53 CrPC
    d. 44 CrPC

IDENTIFICATION

16. **Nuclear sexing is negative in:**
    a. Turner's syndrome
    b. Klinefelter's syndrome
    c. Down's syndrome
    d. Female pseudohermaphroditism

17. **Incidence of Turner's syndrome is:**
    a. 1 : 500
    b. 1 : 1000
    c. 1 : 1500
    d. 1 : 2500

18. **Person with XO genotype will have following except:**
    a. Broad chest
    b. Tall stature
    c. Amenorrhea
    d. Webbed neck

19. **Most common cardiac anomaly in Turner's syndrome is:**
    a. Coarctation of aorta
    b. Bicuspid aortic valve
    c. Aortic stenosis
    d. Aortic bifurcation

20. **Congenital adrenal hyperplasia is responsible for:**
    a. Female pseudohermaphroditism
    b. Male pseudohermaphroditism
    c. True hermaphroditism
    d. Gonadal dysgenesis

21. **Most reliable criterion of Gustafson's method is:**
    a. Secondary dentine deposition
    b. Root transparency
    c. Attrition
    d. Cementum opposition

22. **Most common pattern fingerprint is:**
    a. Whorls
    b. Loops
    c. Composite
    d. Arches

23. **Basi-occipital and basi-sphenoid bones fuse at the age of:**
    a. 10–12 years
    b. 15–16 years
    c. 18–20 years
    d. 24–26 years

24. **Locard's system is study of:**
    a. Pores of sweat glands
    b. Pores of sebaceous glands
    c. Palmar ridges
    d. Ridges and sweat glands

25. **Ridges on the fingertips are detected up to the depth of:**
    a. 0.2 mm
    b. 0.4 mm
    c. 0.6 mm
    d. 0.8 mm

26. **First fingerprint bureau was established in:**
    a. London
    b. Paris
    c. New York
    d. Calcutta

27. **After removal of Tattoo marks, their presence can be inferred from presence of pigment in:**
    a. Deep dermis
    b. Subcutaneous tissue
    c. Regional lymph nodes
    d. Underlying muscles

28. Cephalic index is used to estimate:
    a. age
    b. Race
    c. Sex
    d. Stature
29. Karyotype of Turner's syndrome is:
    a. 45XO
    b. 46XY
    c. 47XXY
    d. 46XX
30. Anterior fontanel normally closes by:
    a. At birth
    b. At birth to 6 months
    c. At 1½ to 2 years
    d. At 5 years
31. Posterior fontanel normally closes by:
    a. At birth
    b. At birth to 6 months
    c. At 1½ to 2 years
    d. At 5 years
32. First carpal bone to show ossification centre is:
    a. Capitate
    b. Triquetral
    c. Lunate
    d. Scaphoid
33. At what age a person under guardian appointed by court attains majority:
    a. 16 years
    b. 18 years
    c. 21 years
    d. 25 years
34. Which site is important to access age of 18 years in a female:
    a. Wrist
    b. Elbow
    c. Ankle
    d. Clavicle
35. Age for full criminal responsibility is:
    a. 7 years
    b. 10 years
    c. 18 years
    d. 21 years

36. Age of a scar when it is white glistening and tough is:
    a. 1–2 weeks
    b. 2–4 weeks
    c. 1–2 months
    d. > 6 months
37. Shovel shaped incisor tooth is present in:
    a. Negroes
    b. Red Indians
    c. Europeans
    d. Chinese
38. First primary incisor to erupt is:
    a. Lower central incisor
    b. Lower lateral incisor
    c. Upper medial incisor
    d. Upper lateral incisor
39. Stack method of dental age determination is done in:
    a. Fetus
    b. Infant
    c. Adult
    d. Elderly
40. Primary dentition is complete by:
    a. 2 years
    b. 2.5 years
    c. 3 years
    d. 6 years
41. Number of permanent teeth at 8 years:
    a. 6
    b. 8
    c. 12
    d. 16
42. Human bone most helpful in sex determination is:
    a. Skull
    b. Femur
    c. Pelvis
    d. Mandible
43. Sex from long bones can be determined up to:
    a. 75%
    b. 80%
    c. 85%
    d. 90%

44. Chilotic line is helpful in determination of:
    a. Age
    b. Sex
    c. Stature
    d. Race
45. Pearson's formula is used to find out:
    a. Age
    b. Sex
    c. Race
    d. Stature
46. Comparative thickness of cortex from medulla of human hair is:
    a. Half
    b. Equal
    c. Double
    d. Thrice or more
47. Fetal shadow can be detected on X-ray of the mother after:
    a. 8 weeks
    b. 12 weeks
    c. 16 weeks
    d. 20 weeks
48. Length of the fetus at 5th month is:
    a. 20 cm
    b. 25 cm
    c. 30 cm
    d. 35 cm
49. Minimum age of a child which can be punished under railways act is:
    a. 5 years
    b. 7 years
    c. 10 years
    d. 12 years
50. Greater sciatic notch in females is:
    a. Smaller
    b. Narrower
    c. Deeper
    d. Wider
51. Normal weight of skeleton in comparison to his weight, of an adult person is:
    a. 5%
    b. 15%
    c. 25%
    d. 50%

52. Preauricular sulcus is seen in:
    a. Pelvis
    b. Skull
    c. Femur
    d. Scapula
53. Human skeleton is made of:
    a. 450 bones
    b. 806 bones
    c. 206 bones
    d. 600 bones
54. Age at which four carpals are ossified:
    a. 2 years
    b. 3 years
    c. 4 years
    d. 5 years
55. Daily growth of facial hair is:
    a. 0.1 mm
    b. 0.2 mm
    c. 0.4 mm
    d. 0.6 mm

THANATOLOGY

56. Suspended animation may be seen in following conditions except:
    a. Drowning
    b. Hypothermia
    c. Hyperthermia
    d. Electrocution
57. Postmortem caloricity after death means:
    a. Livor mortis
    b. Recording of temperature
    c. Increase in body temperature
    d. Fall of body temperature
58. Algor mortis is:
    a. Cadaveric spasm
    b. Cadaveric rigidity
    c. Cooling of body
    d. Hypostasis
59. For transplantation cornea can be removed from dead up to:
    a. 6–8 hrs
    b. 12–14 hrs
    c. 18–20 hrs
    d. 24–26 hrs

60. Intraocular tension becomes nil after death in:
    a. 1 hour
    b. 2 hours
    c. 3 hours
    d. 4 hours

61. After stoppage of circulation muscles can live up to:
    a. 10 mts
    b. 30 mts
    c. 3 hrs
    d. 6 hrs

62. Postmortem caloricity can be seen in poisoning from:
    a. Arsenic
    b. Opium
    c. Cyanide
    d. Strychnine

63. Fixation of hypostasis is seen by:
    a. 1 hour
    b. 3 hours
    c. 6 hours
    d. 12 hours

64. Patchy hypostasis can be seen by:
    a. Immediately after death
    b. Half to one hour after death
    c. 2–4 hours
    d. 6–8 hours

65. Postmortem lividity is well developed within:
    a. 2 hrs
    b. 4 hrs
    c. 6 hrs
    d. 8 hrs

66. Fall of temperature after death can help in calculating time since death up to:
    a. 6–8 hours
    b. 12–18 hours
    c. 24–36 hours
    d. 36–48 hours

67. Inner core temperature does not appreciably fall till what time after death:
    a. 15–30 mts
    b. 30–60 mts
    c. 60–90 mts
    d. 90–120 mts

68. Inner core temperature is taken from:
    a. Rectum
    b. Axilla
    c. Mouth
    d. Groin

69. Muscular rigidity seen immediately after death is:
    a. Rigor mortis
    b. Cadaveric rigidity
    c. Cadaveric spasm
    d. Algor mortis

70. First structure to show rigor mortis in body is:
    a. Eyelids
    b. Heart
    c. Intestines
    d. Lip muscles

71. Rigor mortis starts when ATP level in muscle is reduced below:
    a. 50%
    b. 35%
    c. 15%
    d. 5%

72. Which occurs immediately after death:
    a. Pugilistic attitude
    b. Cadaveric spasm
    c. Cold stiffening
    d. Gas stiffening

73. Cadaveric spasm commonly seen in:
    a. Legs
    b. Hands
    c. Neck muscles
    d. Involuntary muscles

74. Cutis anserina of rigor mortis due to stiffness of:
    a. Erector pilorum
    b. Biceps
    c. Cremaster
    d. Diaphragm

75. Rigor mortis may be seen in fetus after:
    a. 2 month
    b. 5 months
    c. 7 months
    d. 9 months

76. Heat stiffening occurs when body exposed to temperature:
    a. 40°–45°C
    b. 45°–50°C
    c. 55°–60°C
    d. 65°–75°C

77. Rate of putrefaction in air in comparison to buried body is:
    a. Half
    b. Same
    c. Four times
    d. Eight times

78. First external sign of putrefaction is seen over:
    a. Around umbilicus
    b. Rt. iliac fossa
    c. Lt. Hypochondrium
    d. Rt. Hypochondrium

79. Combustible gas of autolysis is:
    a. Nitrogen dioxide
    b. Hydrogen sulphide
    c. Methane
    d. Carbon dioxide

80. First internal organ to putrefy is:
    a. Heart
    b. Brain
    c. Larynx/trachea
    d. Kidney

81. Maggots appear in natural orifices of dead in summer in about:
    a. 2–4 hrs
    b. 6–8 hrs
    c. 8–12 hrs
    d. 12–24 hrs

82. After death blood level of following decrease:
    a. Chloride
    b. Potassium
    c. Magnesium
    d. Creatinine

83. Odor of mummified body is:
    a. Pungent
    b. Putrid
    c. Offensive
    d. Odorless

84. Bacteria helpful in formation of adipocere:
    a. *B. proteus*
    b. *E. coli*
    c. *Staphylococcus*
    d. *Cl welchii*

85. Bacterial enzyme helpful in adipocere formation is:
    a. Lecithinase
    b. Phospholipase
    c. Streptokinase
    d. Hyaluronidase

86. Greenish colour of putrefaction is due to:
    a. Reduced hemoglobin
    b. Carboxyhemoglobin
    c. Methemoglobin
    d. Sulphmethemoglobin

87. Organ which putrefy late is:
    a. Heart
    b. Kidney
    c. Ovaries
    d. Prostate

88. For embalming chemicals are injected into:
    a. Femoral artery
    b. Abdominal cavity
    c. Chest cavity
    d. Skull cavity

89. Microscopic changes are not observed after myocardial infarction before:
    a. 2 hours
    b. 4 hours
    c. 8 hours
    d. 16 hours

90. In maceration all are correct except:
    a. Sweetish disagreeable smell
    b. Happens in sterile conditions
    c. Fetus is flaccid
    d. Greenish discolouration of the skin

91. Preservative used for preserving viscera for chemical analysis:
    a. Normal saline
    b. 10% formalin
    c. Saturated salt solution
    d. Methylated spirit

92. Reliable time since death estimation from vitreous humour is done from:
    a. Sodium levels
    b. Urea levels
    c. Potassium levels
    d. Glucose levels

93. Tache noire refers to:
    a. Postmortem staining
    b. Flaccidity of eyeball
    c. Wrinkled dark patch on sclera
    d. Maggot growth

94. Exhumation is:
    a. Preservation of body
    b. Cremation of a body
    c. Removing body from grave
    d. Sponification of the body

95. Exhumation in India can be done up to:
    a. 10 years
    b. 20 years
    c. 30 years
    d. No limit

96. For virology study tissue should be preserved in:
    a. Sodium chloride
    b. Rectified spirit
    c. Absolute alcohol
    d. Glycerine

97. Presence of less than 7 amino acids indicate bone are at least:
    a. 1–2 years old
    b. 5–10 years old
    c. 20–50 years old
    d. >100 years old

98. Under section 108 IEA a person is presumed dead if not seen or heard for:
    a. 3 years
    b. 5 years
    c. 7 years
    d. 10 years

INJURIES

99. Injury is illegal harm caused to a person in:
    a. Body
    b. Mind
    c. Reputation
    d. All of above

100. A brush burn is a form of:
     a. Electric burn
     b. Filigree burn
     c. Grazed abrasion
     d. Chemical burn

101. Most common type of abrasion seen in traffic accidents is:
     a. Scratch abrasion
     b. Graze abrasion
     c. Pressure abrasion
     d. Imprint abrasion

102. Pus can be seen in a wound after:
     a. 6–12 hours
     b. 12–18 hours
     c. 18–24 hours
     d. 36–48 hours

103. Proper scab is formed over an abrasion in about:
     a. 4–6 hours
     b. 6–12 hours
     c. 12–24 hours
     d. 3 to 5 days

104. Green colour in abruise is due to:
     a. Reduced hemoglobin
     b. Hemosiderin
     c. Hematoidin
     d. Bilirubin

105. Contusion may not show typical colour changes if present on:
     a. Forehead
     b. Genitalia
     c. Conjunctiva
     d. Axilla

106. Colour changes in a bruise start from:
     a. Centre of the bruise
     b. Periphery of the bruise
     c. Area towards centre of the body
     d. Uniformly all over the bruise

107. Rail track bruise is caused due to:
     a. Fall on the railway track
     b. Railway accident
     c. Hit with a whip
     d. Hit with an iron rod

108. Tissue tags bridging across the wound is seen in:
   a. Incised wound
   b. Incised looking wounds
   c. Stab wounds
   d. Chop wounds

109. Bevelling refers to:
   a. Flap wound
   b. Overhang margins
   c. Undermined margin
   d. Irregular margins

110. Incised looking wounds may be seen over:
   a. Hand
   b. Neck
   c. Chest
   d. Scalp

111. Characteristics of incised wounds include following except:
   a. Clean margins
   b. Tailing may be present
   c. Bleeding is more
   d. Length of the blade is usually equal to the length of the wound

112. Hesitational cuts are present in:
   a. Homicides
   b. Suicides
   c. Accidents
   d. Fall from height

113. Depth of a stab wound is normally:
   a. Equal to length of blade
   b. Less than length of blade
   c. More than length of blade
   d. Not related to length of blade

114. Lines of langer in a stab wound will determine:
   a. Direction of the wound
   b. Gaping
   c. Depth of the wound
   d. Bevelling

115. Constituent of black gunpowder present in a cartridge is:
   a. Lead styphnate
   b. Mercury fulminate
   c. Barium nitrate
   d. Potassium nitrate

116. Smokeless gunpowder may contain following except:
   a. Nitrobenzene
   b. Nitrocellulose
   c. Nitroglycerine
   d. Nitroguanidine

117. Amount of gases produced from 1 gm of smokeless power is:
   a. 3000–4000 cc
   b. 5000–7000 cc
   c. 12000–13000 cc
   d. 15000–16000 cc

118. What is wobbling of a bullet:
   a. Tail of the bullet move around the flight path
   b. Entire bullet move around the flight path
   c. Bullet rotate during the flight
   d. Bullet explode on hitting the target

119. Puppe's rule is related to:
   a. Sequence of colours in bruise
   b. Related to age estimation
   c. Sequence of bullets entering skull
   d. Related to sex determination

120. Wounding power of the bullet depend more on:
   a. Mass
   b. Weight
   c. Size
   d. Velocity

121. Tattooing in a gunshot injury is due to:
   a. Wads
   b. Smoke
   c. Powder particles
   d. Pellets

122. Primary markings on the bullet are also known as:
   a. Class characteristics
   b. Individual characteristics
   c. Manufacturing defects
   d. Marks produced during removal of bullet

123. Paradox gun is:
   a. Shotgun with rifling at the muzzle end
   b. Clockwise rifling grooves
   c. Anticlockwise rifling grooves
   d. Narrowing at the muzzle end

124. **Large central hole with peripheral holes in a shotgun are seen at:**
    a. 0.5 mtr
    b. 0.5 to 1 mtr
    c. 2 to 3 mtr
    d. 4 to 5 mtr

125. **Cruciate splitting of firearm entrance wound is seen in:**
    a. Contact wounds
    b. Near contact wounds
    c. Near range wounds
    d. Distant range

126. **Singeing of hair in shotgun may be seen up to a distance of:**
    a. 15 cm
    b. 30 cm
    c. 45 cm
    d. 60 cm

127. **Gunshot residue is detected from hand by:**
    a. Benzedine test
    b. Takayama test
    c. Phenolphthalein test
    d. Diphenylamine test

128. **Spread of pellets in cm is roughly equal to:**
    a. Same distance of fire in meters
    b. Half the distance of fire in meters
    c. 2½ times the distance of fire in meters
    d. 5 times the distance of fire in meters

129. **Near range of a gun is up to:**
    a. Range of flame
    b. Range of smoke
    c. Range of powder particles
    d. Complete spread of pellets

MEDICOLEGAL IMPORTANCE OF INJURIES

130. **Grievous injuries include following except:**
    a. Emasculation
    b. Fracture of a bone
    c. Dislocation of a tooth
    d. Admission in a hospital for 20 days

131. **Injury has been defined under section:**
    a. 319 IPC
    b. 320 IPC
    c. 44 IPC
    d. 351 IPC

132. **Fabricated wounds are mostly:**
    a. Abrasions
    b. Incised wounds
    c. Contusions
    d. Lacerations

133. **Sections related to grievous hurt include following except:**
    a. 320 IPC
    b. 326 IPC
    c. 331 IPC
    d. 319 IPC

134. **On postmortem finding a fist size clot indicate blood loss of:**
    a. 100–200 ml
    b. 200–300 ml
    c. 300–400 ml
    d. 400–500 ml

135. **Secondary hemorrhage is normally seen:**
    a. 8 hours after surgery
    b. 1 day after surgery
    c. 3–5 days after surgery
    d. 7–14 days after surgery

136. **Most common variety of pulmonary embolism is:**
    a. Amniotic
    b. Thrombus
    c. Air
    d. Fat

137. **Patient of long bone fracture with breathlessness, likely diagnosis is:**
    a. Pneumonia
    b. Fat embolism
    c. Air embolism
    d. Thromboembolism

138. **Enzyme which increases after one hour of injury is:**
    a. Aminopeptidase
    b. Alkaline phosphatase
    c. Acid phosphatase
    d. Esterase

139. **Socket of a knocked out tooth is filled by soft tissues by:**
    a. One day
    b. 1–2 weeks
    c. 6–8 weeks
    d. 8–12 weeks

140. **Cause of death from crush syndrome is:**
    a. Local infection
    b. Fat embolism
    c. Acute renal failure
    d. Damage to heart

REGIONAL INJURIES

141. **Minimum air which can result in fatal pulmonary embolism:**
    a. 50 ml
    b. 100 ml
    c. 200 ml
    d. 500 ml

142. **Atheromatous changes are most commonly seen in which coronary artery:**
    a. Anterior descending
    b. Left circumflex
    c. Right coronary trunk
    d. Left coronary trunk

143. **Diastatic fracture of the skull is:**
    a. Fracture up to medullary cavity
    b. Spiral fracture
    c. Fracture through skull suture line
    d. Depressed fracture of skull

144. **Facture of the roof of the orbit may occur due to:**
    a. Blow on the jaw
    b. Blow on the forehead
    c. Fall on the back
    d. Blow on the parietal region

145. **Feature of anterior cranial fossa fracture:**
    a. Black eye
    b. CSF otorrhea
    c. Pupillary dilatation
    d. Battle sign

146. **Battle sign indicates:**
    a. Orbital fracture
    b. Basilar fracture
    c. Fracture of cribriform plate
    d. Facture of nasal bones

147. **A person with a head injury can tell about the circumstances during:**
    a. Lucid interval
    b. Concussion
    c. Retrograde amnesia
    d. Automatism

148. **In contrecoup impact lesion is present:**
    a. At site of impact
    b. At a site opposite to impact
    c. At a site lateral to impact
    d. Anywhere in the body

149. **Extradural hemorrhage mainly occurs from rupture of:**
    a. Superior sagittal sinus
    b. Middle meningeal artery
    c. Dural sinus
    d. Rupture of aneurism

150. **Commonest traumatic intracranial hemorrhage is:**
    a. Extradural
    b. Subdural
    c. Subarachnoid
    d. Intracerebral

151. **Rupture of berry aneurysm commonly produces:**
    a. Extradural hemorrhage
    b. Subarachnoid hemorrhage
    c. Intracerebral hemorrhage
    d. Subdural bleed

152. **Whiplash is most frequently seen in:**
    a. Hyperflexion of neck
    b. Hyperextension of neck
    c. Lateral flexion of neck
    d. Judicial hanging

153. **Main damage in whiplash injury is present between:**
    a. C1–C2
    b. C2–C3
    c. C3–C4
    d. C4–C5

154. **"Undertaker's fracture" due to backward falling of head occurs at:**
    a. L5–S1
    b. T12–L1
    c. C6–C7
    d. C1–C2

155. **In a blunt abdominal trauma commonest injury is:**
    a. Rupture of stomach
    b. Laceration of liver
    c. Laceration of spleen
    d. Laceration of kidney

156. **Ring fracture of the base of skull is caused by following except:**
    a. Landing on feet in a fall
    b. Landing on buttocks in a fall
    c. Blow on the chin
    d. Blow on the side of the face

157. **Signature fracture on the skull is caused by:**
    a. Blow with a stick
    b. Blow with a hammer
    c. Glancing blow from a sword
    d. Gunshot injury

158. **Commonest intracranial hemorrhage in a boxer is:**
    a. Extradural and intraventricular
    b. Subdural and pontine
    c. Subarachnoid and intracerebral
    d. Intracerebral only

159. **Cephal hematoma is:**
    a. Hemorrhage between skull and pericranium
    b. Subdural hemorrhage
    c. Subarachnoid hemorrhage
    d. Intracerebral hemorrhage

160. **Retrograde amnesia is associated with:**
    a. Concussion
    b. Compression
    c. Coup and contrecoup injuries
    d. Rupture of aneurism

161. **Visible capsule in subdural hemorrhage is formed by:**
    a. 1 week
    b. 3 weeks
    c. 5 weeks
    d. 10 weeks

162. **Diffuse axonal injury is diagnosed by damage at:**
    a. Junction of white and grey matter
    b. White matter

    c. Basal ganglion
    d. Internal capsule

163. **Cardiac temponade can result from:**
    a. 50–100 ml of blood
    b. 100–150 ml of blood
    c. 200–300 ml of blood
    d. 400–500 ml of blood

THERMAL INJURIES

164. **Hypothermia is when body temperature falls below:**
    a. 35°C
    b. 30°C
    c. 25°C
    d. 20°C

165. **Heatstroke is when the body temperature goes above:**
    a. 37°C
    b. 39°C
    c. 41°C
    d. 43°C

166. **Sweating is absent in case of:**
    a. Heat exhaustion
    b. Heat syncope
    c. Heatstroke
    d. Heat cramps

167. **Frostbite occurs when there is continuous exposure to temperature between:**
    a. 5 to 10°C
    b. 2 to 4°C
    c. –2.5° and below
    d. –10°C and below

168. **Which part of the body frostbite is very common:**
    a. Lips
    b. Nose
    c. Cheeks
    d. Hand

169. **Burn type relatively painless:**
    a. Epidermal burns
    b. Dermoepidermal burns
    c. Deep burns
    d. None

170. **Blister formation is included in which type of burns:**
    a. First degree
    b. Second degree superficial
    c. Second degree deep
    d. Third degree superficial

171. **Under rule of 9, perineum burns constitute:**
    a. 1%
    b. 5%
    c. 9%
    d. 18%

172. **Most common cause of death in burns:**
    a. Primary shock
    b. Secondary shock
    c. Toxemic shock
    d. Septicemic shock

173. **Percentage of carboxyhemoglobin in blood indicative of antimortem death is more than:**
    a. 2%
    b. 5%
    c. 10%
    d. 15%

174. **Heat hematoma is located in:**
    a. Scalp
    b. Extradural space
    c. Subdural space
    d. Subarachnoid space

175. **Minimum temp to produce burn is:**
    a. 40°C
    b. 44°C
    c. 50°C
    d. 60°C

176. **Curling ulcer in burn cases is seen in about:**
    a. 1–2 days
    b. 3–5 days
    c. 7–10 days
    d. 12–14 days

177. **Hemoglobinuria occurs when burnt skin surface exceeds:**
    a. 20%
    b. 30%
    c. 50%
    d. 70%

178. **Scalding is caused when liquid in contact has temperature above:**
    a. 44°C
    b. 50°C
    c. 60°C
    d. 80°C

179. **Which finding is not seen in heatstroke:**
    a. Hyperpyrexia
    b. Contracted pupils
    c. Sweating
    d. Rapid pulse

180. **Pugilistic attitude is due to:**
    a. Protein digestion
    b. Protein coagulation
    c. Carbohydrate coagulation
    d. Low ATP levels

181. **Pugilistic attitude is helpful in deciding whether burns are:**
    a. Antemortem
    b. Postmortem
    c. Due to defending himself
    d. Cannot differentiate between antemortem and postmortem burns

182. **Most important aspect of management of burns in initial 24 hours is:**
    a. Fluid administration
    b. Cleaning of wounds
    c. Antibiotics
    d. Application of antiseptics

183. **In burns parkland formula is to calculate administration of:**
    a. Ringer lactate
    b. Dextrose
    c. Albumin
    d. Antibiotics

184. **Crocodile skin is seen in:**
    a. Electric entrance burn
    b. Drowning
    c. Mummification
    d. High voltage flash burn

185. **Bone pearls are seen in:**
    a. Burns
    b. Burnt bones
    c. Lightening
    d. High voltage arc injuries

186. The most resistant body tissue to electrical injury is:
    a. Dry skin
    b. Muscles
    c. Bones
    d. Blood and body fluid

187. Filigree burns are as a result of:
    a. Electric flash burns
    b. Lightening
    c. Radiation burns
    d. Chemical burns

188. Characteristics of antemortem burns include following except:
    a. Red line of demarcation
    b. Elevated levels of CO in blood
    c. Soot particles in trachea
    d. Pugilistic attitude

ASPHYXIA

189. Anoxic anoxia produced by all except:
    a. High altitude
    b. Narcotic poisoning
    c. Cyanide poisoning
    d. Traumatic asphyxia

190. Reliable sign of hanging is:
    a. Congested face
    b. Protruded tongue
    c. Hard parchment like ligature mark
    d. Dribbling of saliva

191. Ligature mark of hanging is:
    a. Transversely placed
    b. Placed below thyroid cartilage
    c. Completely around neck
    d. Hard, pale and parchment like

192. Fracture of cervical vertebrae in judicial hanging is present between:
    a. Base of skull and C1
    b. C1-C2
    c. C2-C3
    d. C5-C6

193. Adduction fracture of hyoid bone is present in:
    a. Hanging
    b. Ligature strangulation
    c. Manual strangulation
    d. Bansdola strangulation

194. Le facies sympathique is seen in:
    a. Strangulation
    b. Hanging
    c. Traumatic asphyxia
    d. Smothering

195. Atypical hanging means:
    a. Body is completely suspended
    b. Some part of the body is touching the ground
    c. Knot is present on the back of head
    d. Knot is present on the right mastoid region

196. A type of homicidal strangulation is:
    a. Lynching
    b. Smothering
    c. Burking
    d. Garrotting

197. Transverse tear of intima in the carotid artery is present in:
    a. Complete hanging
    b. Partial hanging
    c. Judicial hanging
    d. Smothering

198. Weight acting on the ligature which can block trachea is:
    a. 2 kg
    b. 5 kg
    c. 10 kg
    d. 15 kg

199. Death in café-coronary is due to:
    a. Coronary insufficiency
    b. Myocardial infarction
    c. Laryngeal spasm
    d. Heart failure

200. Accidental deaths are commonly seen in:
    a. Lynching
    b. Garrotting
    c. Smothering
    d. Traumatic asphyxia

201. Garrotting is a type of:
    a. Hanging
    b. Suffocation
    c. Strangulation
    d. Drowning

202. **Tardieu spots in hanging are commonly seen at the following sites except:**
    a. Scalp
    b. Eyebrow
    c. Chest wall
    d. Face

203. **Tardieu's spot are also seen in:**
    a. Septicemia
    b. Endocarditis
    c. Meningococcemia
    d. All of the above

204. **Hyperkalemia is seen in:**
    a. Dry drowning
    b. Fresh water drowning
    c. Sea water drowning
    d. Immersion syndrome

205. **Cause of death in hydrocution is:**
    a. Asphyxia
    b. Cardiac arrest
    c. Pulmonary edema
    d. Electrolyte imbalance

206. **Death in dry drowning is:**
    a. Laryngeal spasm
    b. Vagal inhibition
    c. Hyperkalemia
    d. Exhaustion

207. **Hyperventilation deaths are:**
    a. Accidental
    b. Suicidal
    c. Homicidal
    d. None of the above

208. **Most important feature of antemortem drowning is:**
    a. Cutis anserina
    b. Washer woman's hand and feet
    c. Weeds held firmly in hands
    d. Wet clothing

209. **Skin of hands and feet is bleached in drowning after:**
    a. 2–4 hours
    b. 6–10 hours
    c. 12–24 hours
    d. 28–36 hours

210. **Burking deaths were produced by:**
    a. Choking and strangulation
    b. Gagging and smothering
    c. Gagging and traumatic asphyxia
    d. Smothering and traumatic asphyxia

211. **Emphysema equosum is seen in:**
    a. Fresh water drowning
    b. Secondary drowning
    c. Dry drowning
    d. Immersion syndrome

212. **Important external sign of drowning seen on postmortem is:**
    a. Goose skin
    b. Washerwoman's hands
    c. Peeling of the skin
    d. Fine froth at the mouth and nostrils

213. **Peltauff's hemorrhages are seen in:**
    a. Lungs
    b. Heart
    c. Kidney
    d. Brain

IMPOTENCY, STERILITY AND PREGNANCY

214. **Quad is a person who is:**
    a. Impotent
    b. Potent
    c. Surgery made him potent
    d. Impotent for a particular lady

215. **Satyriasis in a male is:**
    a. Sexual perversion
    b. Dislike for sex
    c. Increased desire for sex
    d. Impotency

216. **Precocious puberty may result from:**
    a. Adrenal tumour
    b. Thyroid dysfunction
    c. Pituitary tumour
    d. Testicular tumour

217. **Test to differentiate psychological and organic cause of impotency in males:**
    a. Drug induced penile erection
    b. Nocturnal penile tumescence
    c. Serum testosterone levels
    d. Squeeze method

218. Commonest cause of impotence in male is:
    a. Adrenal dysfunction
    b. Testicular failure
    c. Mal developed penis
    d. Psychogenic

219. Frigidity is:
    a. Absence of desire for sexual act in a female
    b. Absence of desire for sexual act in a male
    c. Premature ejaculation
    d. Inability to conceive in a female

220. **Sterility in female may result from chronic poisoning with:**
    a. Arsenic
    b. Antimony
    c. Lead
    d. Aluminium

221. **PH of seminal fluid is:**
    a. 6
    b. 7
    c. 7.4
    d. 8.2

222. **Highest levels of HCG in pregnancy are seen after last menstrual period at:**
    a. 30 days
    b. 60 days
    c. 90 days
    d. 120 days

223. Fecundation-ab-extra means:
    a. Twin pregnancy
    b. Birth of a child after death of father
    c. Insemination without penetration
    d. Pregnancy in rape

224. **Fetal heart sounds can be heard earliest on ultrasound:**
    a. 4 weeks of pregnancy
    b. 6 weeks of pregnancy
    c. 8 weeks of pregnancy
    d. 12 weeks of pregnancy

225. **Superfetation means:**
    a. Two ova fertilized with one act of coitus
    b. Two ova of same cycle fertilized with two acts of coitus
    c. Fertilization of second ovum in a pregnant woman
    d. Uniovular twin pregnancy

226. **Fraternal twins are:**
    a. Dizygotic twins
    b. Uniovular twins
    c. Twins are always males
    d. Twins are always females

227. **Softening of cervix from below up-wards is known as:**
    a. Goodell's sign
    b. Hegar's sign
    c. Chadwick's sign
    d. Palmer's sign

228. **Uterus is felt just after delivery at the level of:**
    a. Just below umbilicus
    b. At the level of umbilicus
    c. Between umbilicus and pubic symphysis
    d. Just above pubic symphysis

229. **Uterus become a pelvic organ after delivery in:**
    a. 1 week
    b. 2 weeks
    c. 3 weeks
    d. 4 weeks

RAPE

230. **In a sexual assault on a small child:**
    a. Hymen ruptures as it is thin
    b. Hymen may not rupture because it is deeply located
    c. Hymen may not rupture because it is thick
    d. Hymen may rupture because it is situated superficially

231. **Statutory rape means:**
    a. Rape of a married woman
    b. Rape in police station
    c. Rape of a girls who is <18 years
    d. Rape under judicial custody

232. **Punishment for disclosing name of a rape victim is under:**
    a. Section 375 IPC
    b. Section 376 IPC
    c. Section 354 IPC
    d. Section 228-A IPC

233. **Hymen rupture in sexual act is normally located at:**
    a. 3 o'clock
    b. 5 o'clock
    c. 9 o'clock
    d. 11 o'clock

234. **Transvestism means:**
    a. Wearing cloths of opposite sex to attract attention
    b. Wearing cloths of opposite sex to be associated with opposite sex
    c. Wearing cloths of opposite sex for sexual gratification
    d. Wearing cloths of opposite sex for curiosity sake

235. **Most suitable test for seminal stain in aspermic person in:**
    a. Florence test
    b. Barberio test
    c. Takayama test
    d. Acid phosphatase test

236. **Vaginal cells can be detected in a smear by:**
    a. Precipitin test
    b. Barberio test
    c. Takayama reagent
    d. Lugol's iodine

237. **Sexual act not punishable under Indian law is:**
    a. Incest
    b. Rape
    c. Adultery
    d. Pederasty

238. **Motile sperm can be normally detected in vaginal aspirate after coitus up to:**
    a. 6 hours
    b. 9 hours
    c. 12 hours
    d. 18 hours

239. **Lesbianism is also known as:**
    a. Tribadism
    b. Nymphomania
    c. Satyriasis
    d. Masochism

240. **Active partner in lesbianism is known as:**
    a. Bugger
    b. Catamite
    c. Dyke
    d. Femme

241. **Catamite is:**
    a. Active agent in sodomy
    b. Passive agent in sodomy
    c. Small child acting as passive agent in sodomy
    d. Female acting as passive agent in sodomy

242. **Presence of smegma on the glace of accused indicates:**
    a. Sexual act done recently
    b. Sexual act not done in last 24 hours
    c. Sexual act not done in last 48 hours
    d. Sexual act not done in last one week

DELIVERY

243. **Premature expulsion of products of conception before full term is legally:**
    a. Stillbirth
    b. Abortion
    c. Miscarriage
    d. Premature birth

244. **Natural abortions are most common during:**
    a. First trimester
    b. Second trimester
    c. Third trimester
    d. Any time during pregnancy

245. **Most common cause of first trimester abortions is:**
    a. Chromosomal abnormalities
    b. Endocrine disturbance
    c. Anatomical abnormality of uterus
    d. Infections

246. **Medical termination under MTP act by a single doctor can be done up to:**
    a. 8 weeks
    b. 10 weeks
    c. 12 weeks
    d. 20 weeks

INFANTICIDE

247. Infanticide is unlawful destruction of a child under the age of:
a. 15 days
b. One month
c. Six months
d. One year

248. In stillbirth age of fetus should be above:
a. 180 days
b. 196 days
c. 210 days
d. 220 days

249. Spalding sign indicates:
a. Viable child
b. Stillbirth
c. Live birth
d. Dead birth

250. Condition when hydrostatic test is not required except:
a. Dead born
b. Nonviable child
c. Monster child
d. Stillbirth

251. Weight of the lungs in a live birth increase after respiration by:
a. 15 gm
b. 25 gm
c. 35 gm
d. 50 gm

252. Aseptic autolysis is known as:
a. Maceration
b. Mummification
c. Adipocere
d. Decomposition

253. Live birth as per Indian law is:
a. Living child is completely born
b. Any part of a living child comes out
c. Child cries after being completely born
d. Child respires after completely born

254. Specific gravity of unrespired lung is:
a. 0.80
b. 0.85
c. 0.90
d. 0.95

255. Ductus venosus is completely closed after birth by:
a. 1st day
b. 2nd day
c. 5th day
d. 10th day

256. In a child level of fetal hemoglobin at 3rd month is:
a. 16%
b. 8%
c. 4%
d. 2%

257. Lanugo hair appear in a fetus at:
a. 2nd month
b. 3rd month
c. 4th month
d. 5th month

258. Testes are completely descended by:
a. End of 7th month
b. End of 8th month
c. End of 9th month
d. At birth

259. Radiological signs of fetal death includes all except:
a. Overlapping of skull bones
b. Hyperextension of spine
c. Collapse of spinal column
d. Gas in aorta

260. Presence of gas in heart and great vessels in a dead born child is known as:
a. Spalding sign
b. Chadwick's sign
c. Ploucquet's test
d. Robert's sign

261. On postmortem presence of ossification centre to confirm viability of the child is seen in:
a. Talus
b. Calcaneum
c. Lower end of femur
d. Medial end of clavicle

262. In precipitate labour umbilical cord is usually be torn:
a. Near fetal end
b. Near placental end
c. In the middle
d. Not torn

263. **Birth length of a child is double at:**
    a. 1 year
    b. 2 years
    c. 3 years
    d. 4 years
264. **Umbilical cord separates from the child on:**
    a. 3rd day
    b. 6th day
    c. 10th day
    d. 14th day
265. **Birth weight of a child becomes triple at:**
    a. 6 months
    b. 1 year
    c. 2 years
    d. 4 years
266. **Casualty medical officer may diagnose battered baby syndrome by:**
    a. Finding injuries of different durations
    b. Presence of serious injuries
    c. Presence of multiple injuries
    d. Presence of few injuries
267. **Cafey's syndrome is also known by:**
    a. Cot death
    b. Battered baby syndrome
    c. SIDS
    d. Death from choking
268. **Common injury seen in shaken-baby syndrome is:**
    a. Intracranial hemorrhage
    b. Cervical vertebrae damage
    c. Lung laceration
    d. Laceration of liver
269. **Concealment of birth is punishable under:**
    a. Section 312 IPC
    b. Section 315 IPC
    c. Section 317 IPC
    d. Section 318 IPC
270. **Length of 7 months old fetus is:**
    a. 25 cm
    b. 30 cm
    c. 35 cm
    d. 40 cm

TORTURE

271. **Falanga used for torture is:**
    a. Using a roller over thighs
    b. Beating over feet with a stick
    c. Slapping over both ears
    d. Beating over buttocks
272. **Term telephono is used for:**
    a. Made to hear loud voice
    b. Slapping over both ears
    c. Pulling both ears
    d. Cutting of both external ears

MEDICAL JURISPRUDENCE

273. **Professional death sentence is awarded to a doctor by:**
    a. Session court
    b. Indian medical council
    c. Indian medical association
    d. State medical council
274. **Doctors are prohibited to participate in torture under:**
    a. Geneva declaration
    b. Oslo declaration
    c. Tokyo declaration
    d. Helsinki declaration
275. **Moral principles guiding medical profession are known as:**
    a. Medical ethics
    b. Medical etiquettes
    c. Medical norms
    d. Professional courtesy
276. **Medical qualifications awarded by other countries are registered by MCI act under:**
    a. First schedule
    b. Second schedule
    c. Part I of third schedule
    d. Part II of third schedule
277. **Medical etiquettes are related to:**
    a. Medical ethics
    b. Courtesy observed between doctors
    c. Professional misconduct
    d. Moral principles followed by doctors
278. **Examining a patient without consent amounts to:**
    a. Assault
    b. Medical negligence
    c. Indecent assault
    d. Unethical act

279. **Contributory negligence is:**
   a. Negligence only by the doctor
   b. Negligence only by the patient
   c. Negligence by the paramedical staff
   d. Negligence by the patient along with doctor

280. **Doctor can examine a person in emergency without consent under:**
   a. Section 87 IPC
   b. Section 90 IPC
   c. Section 89 IPC
   d. Section 92 IPC

281. **Declaration of helsinki is about:**
   a. Human experimentation
   b. Organ transplant
   c. Torture
   d. Oath for doctors

282. **Burden to prove defence lies with doctor in cases of:**
   a. Res judicata
   b. Mens rea
   c. Res ipsa loquitor
   d. Vicarious responsibility

283. **Onus to prove civil negligence case against a doctor lies with:**
   a. Doctor
   b. Patient
   c. Judge
   d. Police

284. **Doctrine of common knowledge is same as:**
   a. Calculated risk doctrine
   b. Novus acta interveniens
   c. Res ipsa loquitor
   d. Vicarious responsibility

285. **Contributory negligence is used as defence in:**
   a. Civil negligence
   b. Criminal negligence
   c. Departmental inquiry
   d. Professional misconduct

FORENSIC PSYCHIATRY

286. **Mental health act deals with persons known as:**
   a. Lunatic
   b. Mad
   c. Insane
   d. Mentally ill

287. **A delusion is a disorder of:**
   a. Thought
   b. Orientation
   c. Perception
   d. Reasoning

288. **Hallucination is:**
   a. False interpretation of a stimulus
   b. False sense perception without stimulus
   c. False belief
   d. Irresistible desire

289. **Obsession is appearance of irresistible:**
   a. Thought
   b. Impulse
   c. Emotion
   d. All of above

290. **Pyromania is a type of:**
   a. Impulse
   b. Delusion
   c. Illusion
   d. Obsession

291. **IQ of a moron as per Indian law is between:**
   a. Below 20
   b. 20 to 50
   c. 50 to 75
   d. Above 75

292. **Maximum duration up to which a mentally ill person can be kept under medical observation is:**
   a. 10 days
   b. 20 days
   c. 30 days
   d. 50 days

293. **Testamentary capacity of a person means:**
   a. Capacity to give evidence in court
   b. Capacity to make a valid will
   c. Capacity to file a case in the court
   d. Capacity to self-attest a document

294. **Legal section applied for criminal responsibility of a mentally ill person is:**
   a. 44 IPC
   b. 84 IPC
   c. 324 IPC
   d. 204 IPC

295. **McNaughten's rule is also known as:**
    a. Irresistible impulse rule
    b. Inability to adhere to right
    c. Loss of capacity to obey law
    d. Right or wrong test

296. **A person may be held responsible under:**
    a. Delirium tremens
    b. Somnambulism
    c. Postepileptic phase
    d. Hypnosis

GENERAL TOXICOLOGY

297. **Vaccine and sera are included in drugs and cosmetic rule 1945 under:**
    a. Schedule C
    b. Schedule E
    c. Schedule F
    d. Schedule H

298. **For gastric lavage length of stomach tube introduced is:**
    a. 30 cm
    b. 40 cm
    c. 50 cm
    d. 60 cm

299. **Method used to avoid aspiration during gastric lavage in a comatose patient is:**
    a. Putting the head of the patient at a lower level than his feet
    b. Putting the patient in the left lateral position
    c. Introduction of a cuffed endotracheal tube before lavage
    d. Continuous suction of the fluid from the trachea

300. **Gastric lavage can normally be done in the poisoning by:**
    a. Kerosene
    b. Phenols
    c. Sulphuric acid
    d. Strychnine

301. **Wall scrapings can be administered as an antidote in:**
    a. Hydrochloric acid
    b. Carbolic acid
    c. Salicylic acid
    d. Oxalic acid

302. **Animal affected by poisoning in similar manner to humans is:**
    a. Cat
    b. Dog
    c. Guinea pig
    d. Frog

303. **NDPS act repeal:**
    a. Poison act 1919
    b. Dangerous drug act 1930
    c. Drugs and cosmetic act 1940
    d. Drugs control act 1950

304. **Strength of potassium permanganate used for gastric lavage is:**
    a. 1:50
    b. 1:500
    c. 1:1000
    d. 1:5000

CORROSIVES

305. **Antidote used in mineral acid poisoning is:**
    a. Sodium carbonate
    b. Potassium bicarbonate
    c. Potassium hydroxide
    d. Magnesium oxide

306. **Chalky white teeth are seen in poisoning by:**
    a. Carbolic acid
    b. Oxalic acid
    c. Nitric acid
    d. Sulphuric acid

307. **Yellowish discolouration of skin is seen in:**
    a. Sulphuric acid
    b. Hydrochloric acid
    c. Nitric acid
    d. Hydrofluoric acid

308. **Substance used for removing stains is:**
    a. Carbolic acid
    b. Oxalic acid
    c. Acetic acid
    d. Acetyl salicylic acid

309. **Hypocalcemia is normally present in poisoning by:**
    a. Carbolic acid
    b. Salicylic acid
    c. Oxalic acid
    d. Hydrogen sulphide

310. **Leather bottle stomach is seen in poisoning by:**
    a. Carbolic acid
    b. Oxalic acid
    c. Salicylic acid
    d. Copper sulphate

311. **Ochronosis may be seen in poisoning by:**
    a. Phenols
    b. Oxalic acid
    c. Boric acid
    d. Nitric acid

312. **Urine becomes greenish after some time in poisoning by:**
    a. Carbolic acid
    b. Oxalic acid
    c. Copper sulphate
    d. Sheel's green

313. **Damage to esophagus is more in poisoning by:**
    a. Hydrochloric acid
    b. Nitric acid
    c. Sulphuric acid
    d. Sodium hydroxide

IRRITANTS

314. **Which of the following poisons retards putrefaction:**
    a. Abrin
    b. Ricin
    c. Arsenic
    d. Phosphorus

315. **One pinch (1 gm) of sankhiya can kill:**
    a. 1 person
    b. 2 persons
    c. 5 persons
    d. 10 persons

316. **Rain drop pigmentation in skin is caused in chronic poisoning by:**
    a. Arsenic
    b. Copper
    c. Lead
    d. Mercury

317. **Antidote used while doing gastric lavage in acute arsenic poisoning is:**
    a. Potassium permanganate
    b. Potassium ferrocyanide
    c. Ferrous sulphate
    d. Hydrated ferric oxide

318. **Vermilion used by Hindu ladies is:**
    a. Mercurous chloride
    b. Lead tetraoxide
    c. Copper arsenite
    d. Lead sulphide

319. **Route of administration of BAL is:**
    a. Oral
    b. Subcutaneous
    c. Intramuscular
    d. Intravenous

320. **Mee's lines are seen in:**
    a. Gums
    b. Nails
    c. Cornea
    d. Abdomen

321. **Milk rose complexion followed by hyperpigmentation is seen in chronic poisoning by:**
    a. Lead
    b. Antimony
    c. Arsenic
    d. Copper

322. **Hatter's shake is seen in the chronic poisoning by:**
    a. Mercury
    b. Antimony
    c. Arsenic
    d. Copper

323. **Mercurial lentis reflex on slit lamp examination is demonstrable from:**
    a. Anterior lens capsule
    b. Posterior lens capsule
    c. Anterior corneal surface
    d. Posterior corneal surface

324. **Ulcerative gingivitis is present in poisoning by salts of:**
    a. Arsenic
    b. Lead

c. Copper

d. Mercury

325. **Chemical antidote used in acute mercury poisoning is:**
   a. Ferric chloride
   b. Potassium ferrocyanide
   c. Sodium formaldehyde sulphoxylate
   d. Magnesium sulphate

326. **Symptom most frequently present in chronic lead poisoning is:**
   a. Lead line over gums
   b. Lead palsy
   c. Encephalopathy
   d. Dry belly aches

327. **Blue line in the gingival margin in case of lead poisoning is due to deposition of:**
   a. Lead chromate
   b. Lead sulphide
   c. Lead subacetate
   d. Lead iodide

328. **Burtonian line is seen in the chronic poisoning with:**
   a. Arsenic
   b. Mercury
   c. Lead
   d. Copper

329. **Punctate basophilic stripling is seen in chronic poisoning by:**
   a. Arsenic
   b. Mercury
   c. Lead
   d. Iron

330. **Metal fume fever is commonly seen the chronic poisoning by:**
   a. Arsenic
   b. Lead
   c. Iron
   d. Zinc

331. **In chronic lead poisoning, raised levels are present:**
   a. Porphobilinogen
   b. Bilirubin
   c. Urobilinogen
   d. Delta-amino levulinic acid

332. **Pharaoh's serpent is produced by burning a tablet of:**
   a. Mercury cyanide
   b. Mercuric chloride
   c. Mercuric oxide
   d. Mercuric sulphide

333. **Garlic like smell is detected in poisoning by:**
   a. Cyanide
   b. Carbolic acid
   c. Yellow phosphorus
   d. Organophosphorus

334. **Antidote used in phosphorus poisoning:**
   a. Demercaprol
   b. Potassium ferrocyanide
   c. Penicillamine
   d. Copper sulphate

335. **Poisoning during Diwali celebrations may be due to:**
   a. Phosphorus
   b. Lead
   c. Arsenic
   d. Copper

336. **One of the substances present on the side of safety matchbox is:**
   a. Potassium chlorate
   b. Antimony sulphide
   c. Lead styphnate
   d. Red phosphorus

337. **Yellow fatty liver is seen in poisoning by:**
   a. Datura
   b. Abrus precatorius
   c. Yellow phosphorus
   d. Opium

338. **Artificial bruise is produced by application of:**
   a. Ricinus communis
   b. Abrus precatorius
   c. Croton tiglium
   d. Semicarpus anacardium

339. **Active ingredient present in nux vomica is:**
   a. Atropine
   b. Abrin
   c. Ricin
   d. Strychnine

340. Dry mouth and dilated pupils are present in poisoning by:
    a. Morphine
    b. Organophosphorus
    c. Barbiturates
    d. Datura

341. Active principle present in a "sui" resembling viper snake bite is:
    a. Abrin
    b. Crotin
    c. Ricin
    d. Bhilawanol

342. Most common snake of India is:
    a. Cobra
    b. Krait
    c. Russell's viper
    d. Saw scaled viper

343. Vertically slit pupils are seen in:
    a. Cobra
    b. Krait
    c. Viper
    d. Sea snakes

344. Single central line of hexagonal scales on the back is seen in:
    a. Cobra
    b. Krait
    c. Viper
    d. Sea snakes

345. Third supralabial shied touching eye and nasal shield is seen in:
    a. Cobra
    b. Krait
    c. Viper
    d. Sea snake

346. Polyvalent antisnake venom is prepared against:
    a. Cobra, king cobra and krait
    b. Cobra, common krait, russell's viper and saw scaled virus
    c. Cobra, banded krait, russell's viper and saw scaled virus
    d. King cobra, common krait, russell's viper and saw scaled virus

347. Priapism is seen in poisoning with:
    a. Abrus precatorius
    b. Viper snake
    c. Spider bite
    d. Cantharides

348. Drug used to treat muscarinic effects of cobra bite is:
    a. Naloxone
    b. Nalorphine
    c. Neostigmine
    d. EDTA

SOMNIFEROUS AND INEBRIENTS

349. Concentration of morphine in standard opium is:
    a. 5%
    b. 7%
    c. 10%
    d. 13%

350. Fatal dose of opium is:
    a. 0.2 gm
    b. 0.4 gm
    c. 1 gm
    d. 2 gm

351. Alkaloid of opium showing convulsant action is:
    a. Morphine
    b. Papaverine
    c. Narcoline
    d. Thebaine

352. Pin point pupils are seen in:
    a. Opium poisoning
    b. Datura poisoning
    c. Alcohol poisoning
    d. Charas poisoning

353. Antidote preferred in opium poisoning is:
    a. Naloxone
    b. Nalorphine
    c. Lavallorphan
    d. Atropine

354. Highly addicting drug is:
    a. Bhang
    b. Charas
    c. Amphetamine
    d. Heroin

355. Amount of ethyl alcohol present in methylated alcohol is:
    a. 50%
    b. 80%
    c. 90%
    d. 95%

356. Amount of alcohol metabolized in the body per hour is:
    a. 5 ml
    b. 10 ml
    c. 15 ml
    d. 20 ml

357. Most frequently used addicting drug in the world is:
    a. Alcohol
    b. Heroin
    c. Charas
    d. Amphetamine

358. McEvans sign is diagnostic of:
    a. First stage of alcohol intoxication
    b. Second stage of alcohol intoxication
    c. Third stage of alcohol intoxication
    d. Not used in alcohol intoxication

359. Alcohol gaze nystagmus becomes detectable when alcohol level is above:
    a. 20 mg%
    b. 40 mg%
    c. 100 mg%
    d. 150 mg%

360. Metabolite of methyl alcohol responsible for optic atrophy is:
    a. Acetaldehyde
    b. Acetone
    c. Formaldehyde
    d. Direct effect of methyl alcohol

361. As per motor vehicles act alcohol levels in blood is punishable if above:
    a. 10 mg%
    b. 30 mg%
    c. 50 mg%
    d. 100 mg%

362. Pressure affecting the nerve in saturday night palsy is:
    a. Ulnar nerve
    b. Radial nerve
    c. Median nerve
    d. Trigeminal nerve

363. Widmark's formula is used to calculate:
    a. Alcohol levels in blood form quantity of alcohol consumed
    b. Alcohol consumed from blood alcohol level

    c. Blood alcohol from breath level
    d. Blood alcohol from urine alcohol

364. Alcohol levels in a female in comparison to a male of same weight on consumption of same amount of alcohol is:
    a. 10% more
    b. 25% more
    c. Same
    d. 10% less

365. Criminal responsibility of alcohol intoxicated person is under:
    a. Section 82 IPC
    b. Section 83 IPC
    c. Section 84 IPC
    d. Section 85 IPC

366. Delirium tremens is seen in:
    a. Acute alcohol intoxication
    b. Chronic alcoholic
    c. Opium addiction
    d. Charas addiction

367. Wirnicke-Korsakoff syndrome is due the deficiency of:
    a. Vitamin A
    b. Vitamin B_1
    c. Vitamin B_6
    d. Vitamin B_{12}

368. Chemical used to estimate alcohol in breath is:
    a. Potassium dichromate
    b. Potassium chloride
    c. Potassium ferrocyanide
    d. Diphenylamine

369. Disulfiram is used in chronic addiction by:
    a. Heroin
    b. Morphine
    c. Charas
    d. Alcohol

370. Treatment of methyl alcohol is done with:
    a. Calcium gluconate
    b. Ethyl alcohol
    c. Amphetamine
    d. Phenothiazine

371. Knock out drops used for robbery or rape purposes is:
    a. Datura
    b. Amphetamine
    c. Chloral hydrate
    d. Ketamine

DELIRIENTS

372. Muttering delirium is present in the poisoning by:
    a. Datura
    b. Cocaine
    c. Charas
    d. Chloral hydrate

373. Hot as hare, blind as bat, dry as bone, red as beet and mad as wet hen is seen in poisoning by:
    a. Cocaine
    b. Atropa belladonna
    c. Ricinus communis
    d. Abrus precatorius

374. Antidote preferred in datura poisoning is:
    a. Physostigmine
    b. Pilocarpine
    c. Neostigmine
    d. Pethidine

375. Ganja is preparation of cannabis made using:
    a. Dried leaves
    b. Dried flowering tops of female plant
    c. Sweat preparation with leaves
    d. Resin collected from tops of female plant

376. Most potent preparation of cannabis is:
    a. Bhang
    b. Majun
    c. Hashish
    d. Charas

377. Run amok is a condition seen in chronic poisoning by:
    a. Cannabis
    b. Opium
    c. Datura
    d. Cocaine

378. Magnan's symptoms are present in chronic poisoning by:
    a. Cannabis
    b. Opium
    c. Datura
    d. Cocaine

379. Black discolouration of teeth is seen in chronic poisoning by:
    a. Sulphuric acid
    b. Cocaine
    c. Copper
    d. Iron

380. Tears may be red tinged in poisoning by:
    a. Heroin
    b. Datura
    c. Organophosphorus
    d. Cocaine

381. Smell of bitter almond is present in:
    a. Phosphorus
    b. Oxalic acid
    c. Carbolic acid
    d. Prussic acid

382. Amygdaline is converted by the action of emulsion into:
    a. Tetrahydrocannabinol
    b. Hydrocyanic acid
    c. Cannabidiol
    d. BOAA

383. Route of administration of amyl nitrate in cyanide poisoning is:
    a. Subcutaneous
    b. Intramuscular
    c. Intravenous
    d. Inhalation

384. Hippus sign is present in the poisoning by:
    a. Aconite
    b. Heroin
    c. Cocaine
    d. Charas

385. Mechanism of action of cyanide in the body is:
    a. Inhibiting SH containing enzymes.
    b. Formation of cyanmethemoglobin
    c. Reducing oxygen carrying capacity of blood
    d. Inhibiting cytochrome oxidase

386. Hemodialysis is not useful in poisoning with:
    a. Alcohol
    b. Barbiturates
    c. Kerosene
    d. Acetyl salicylic acid

387. Nonpoisonous salt of cyanide is:
    a. Potassium cyanide
    b. Sodium cyanide
    c. Hydrocyanic acid
    d. Potassium ferrocyanide

388. Usual fatal period in poisoning by potassium cyanide is:
    a. Immediate
    b. 2 to 10 minutes
    c. 10–20 minutes
    d. About 30 minutes

389. Speedball is combination of:
    a. Heroin and cannabis
    b. Heroin and quinine
    c. Brown sugar and cocaine
    d. Brown sugar and strychnine

390. Heroin is also known as following except:
    a. Smack
    b. Junk
    c. Dope
    d. Speed

391. Amphetamine is also known as:
    a. Junk
    b. Crystal
    c. Dope
    d. Smack

392. Cocaine is also known by followings except:
    a. Snow
    b. Coke
    c. Cadillac
    d. Glass

393. Predator drugs include following except:
    a. Alcohol
    b. Chloral hydrate
    c. Ketamine
    d. Carbamates

394. Poisonous effects of sewer gas is mainly from:
    a. Carbon dioxide
    b. Hydrogen sulphide
    c. Methane
    d. Ammonia

395. Affinity of carbon monoxide to combine with hemoglobin in comparison to oxygen is:
    a. Equal
    b. 10 times
    c. 100 times
    d. 200 times

396. Shooting gallery term in addiction is used for:
    a. Place for storing heroin
    b. Place used for smoking heroin
    c. Place used for injecting heroin
    d. Place used for making heroin

397. Term chasing the dragon is used in addiction for:
    a. Place for storing heroin
    b. Place used for smoking heroin
    c. Place used for making heroin
    d. Place used for injecting heroin

398. Blistering gas is:
    a. Lewisite
    b. Phosgene
    c. Hydrogen sulphide
    d. Chloroacetophenone

399. Main route of excretion of methyl alcohol is:
    a. Urine
    b. Breath
    c. Sweat
    d. Feces

400. Ethanol intoxication is mainly diagnosed by:
    a. Euphoria and sense of well-being
    b. Muscular incoordination
    c. Increased confidence
    d. Effects on judgment

ANSWERS TO MCQs

1. (b)	2. (a)	3. (c)	4. (d)	5. (a)	6. (b)	7. (d)	8. (d)	9. (a)
10. (d)	11. (b)	12. (c)	13. (d)	14. (d)	15. (c)	16. (a)	17. (d)	18. (b)
19. (b)	20. (a)	21. (b)	22. (b)	23. (c)	24. (a)	25. (c)	26. (d)	27. (c)
28. (b)	29. (a)	30. (c)	31. (b)	32. (a)	33. (c)	34. (a)	35. (c)	36. (d)
37. (d)	38. (a)	39. (b)	40. (b)	41. (b)	42. (c)	43. (b)	44. (b)	45. (d)
46. (d)	47. (c)	48. (b)	49. (b)	50. (d)	51. (b)	52. (a)	53. (c)	54. (c)
55. (c)	56. (c)	57. (c)	58 (c)	59. (a)	60. (b)	61. (b)	62. (d)	63. (c)
64. (b)	65. (b)	66. (b)	67 (b)	68. (a)	69. (c)	70. (b)	71. (c)	72. (b)
73. (b)	74. (a)	75. (c)	76 (d)	77. (d)	78. (b)	79. (b)	80. (c)	81. (d)
82. (a)	83. (d)	84. (d)	85 (a)	86. (d)	87. (d)	88. (a)	89. (c)	90. (d)
91. (c)	92. (c)	93. (c)	94 (c)	95. (d)	96. (d)	97. (d)	98. (c)	99. (d)
100. (c)	101. (b)	102. (d)	103. (c)	104. (c)	105. (c)	106. (b)	107. (c)	108. (b)
109. (c)	110. (d)	111. (d)	112. (b)	113. (d)	114. (b)	115. (d)	116. (a)	117. (c)
118. (b)	119. (c)	120. (d)	121. (c)	122. (a)	123. (a)	124. (c)	125. (a)	126. (b)
127. (d)	128. (c)	129. (c)	130. (d)	131. (c)	132. (b)	133. (d)	134. (d)	135. (d)
136. (b)	137. (b)	138. (d)	139. (b)	140. (c)	141. (b)	142. (a)	143. (c)	144. (c)
145. (a)	146. (b)	147. (a)	148. (b)	149. (b)	150. (b)	151. (b)	152. (b)	153. (d)
154. (c)	155. (b)	156. (d)	157. (b)	158. (b)	159. (a)	160. (a)	161. (b)	162. (a)
163. (d)	164. (a)	165. (c)	166. (c)	167. (c)	168. (b)	169. (c)	170. (b)	171. (a)
172. (b)	173. (c)	174. (b)	175. (b)	176. (c)	177. (b)	178. (c)	179. (c)	180. (b)
181. (d)	182. (a)	183. (a)	184. (d)	185. (d)	186. (c)	187. (b)	188. (d)	189. (c)
190. (d)	191. (d)	192. (c)	193. (c)	194. (b)	195. (d)	196. (d)	197. (c)	198. (d)
199. (c)	200. (d)	201. (c)	202. (c)	203. (d)	204. (b)	205. (b)	206. (a)	207. (a)
208. (c)	209. (c)	210. (d)	211. (a)	212. (d)	213. (a)	214. (d)	215. (c)	216. (a)
217. (b)	218. (d)	219. (a)	220. (c)	221. (c)	222. (b)	223. (c)	224. (b)	225. (c)
226. (a)	227. (a)	228. (a)	229. (b)	230. (b)	231. (c)	232. (d)	233. (b)	234. (c)
235. (d)	236. (d)	237. (a)	238. (a)	239. (a)	240. (c)	241. (c)	242. (b)	243. (b)
244. (a)	245. (a)	246. (c)	247. (d)	248. (b)	249. (d)	250. (d)	251. (c)	252. (a)
253. (b)	254. (d)	255. (c)	256. (b)	257. (d)	258. (c)	259. (b)	260. (d)	261. (a)
262. (a)	263. (d)	264. (b)	265. (b)	266. (a)	267. (b)	268. (a)	269. (d)	270. (c)
271. (b)	272. (b)	273. (d)	274. (c)	275. (a)	276. (b)	277. (b)	278. (a)	279. (d)
280. (d)	281. (a)	282. (c)	283. (b)	284. (c)	285. (a)	286. (d)	287. (a)	288. (b)
289. (d)	290. (a)	291. (c)	292. (c)	293. (b)	294. (b)	295. (d)	296. (d)	297. (c)
298. (c)	299. (c)	300. (b)	301. (d)	302. (a)	303. (b)	304. (d)	305. (d)	306. (d)
307. (c)	308. (b)	309. (c)	310. (a)	311. (a)	312. (a)	313. (d)	314. (c)	315. (c)
316. (a)	317. (d)	318. (b)	319. (c)	320. (b)	321. (c)	322. (a)	323. (a)	324. (d)
325. (c)	326. (d)	327. (b)	328. (c)	329. (c)	330. (d)	331. (d)	332. (a)	333. (c)
334. (d)	335. (a)	336. (d)	337. (c)	338. (d)	339. (d)	340. (d)	341. (a)	342. (b)
343. (c)	344. (b)	345. (a)	346. (b)	347. (d)	348. (c)	349. (c)	350. (d)	351. (d)
352. (a)	353. (a)	354. (d)	355. (d)	356. (b)	357. (a)	358. (c)	359. (b)	360. (c)
361. (b)	362. (b)	363. (b)	364. (b)	365. (d)	366. (b)	367. (b)	368. (a)	369. (d)
370. (b)	371. (c)	372. (a)	373. (b)	374. (a)	375. (b)	376. (d)	377. (a)	378. (d)
379. (b)	380. (c)	381. (d)	382. (b)	383. (d)	384. (a)	385. (d)	386. (c)	387. (d)
388. (d)	389. (c)	390. (d)	391. (b)	392. (d)	393. (d)	394. (b)	395. (d)	396. (c)
397. (b)	398. (a)	399. (b)	400. (b)					

Index